DATE DUE

PRINTED IN U.S.A.

Sexually Transmitted Infections

Diagnosis, Management, and Treatment

Edited by

Jonathan M. Zenilman, MD
Professor of Medicine
Johns Hopkins University School of Medicine

Chief
Infectious Disease Division
Johns Hopkins Bayview Medical Center
Baltimore, Maryland

Mohsen Shahmanesh, MD, FRCP
Honorary Consultant in Genitourinary Medicine and HIV
Whittall Street Clinic
Birmingham, United Kingdom

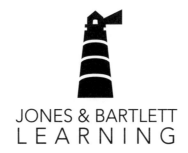

JONES & BARTLETT
LEARNING

World Headquarters

Jones & Bartlett Learning
40 Tall Pine Drive
Sudbury, MA 01776
978-443-5000
info@jblearning.com
www.jblearning.com

Jones & Bartlett Learning Canada
6339 Ormindale Way
Mississauga, Ontario L5V 1J2
Canada

Jones & Bartlett Learning International
Barb House, Barb Mews
London W6 7PA
United Kingdom

Jones & Bartlett Learning books and products are available through most bookstores and online booksellers. To contact Jones & Bartlett Learning directly, call 800-832-0034, fax 978-443-8000, or visit our website, www.jblearning.com.

Substantial discounts on bulk quantities of Jones & Bartlett Learning publications are available to corporations, professional associations, and other qualified organizations. For details and specific discount information, contact the special sales department at Jones & Bartlett Learning via the above contact information or send an email to specialsales@jblearning.com.

Production Credits

Publisher: Michael Brown
Editorial Assistant: Teresa Reilly
Associate Production Editor: Kate Stein
Senior Marketing Manager: Sophie Fleck
Manufacturing and Inventory Control
   Supervisor: Amy Bacus

Composition: Arlene Apone
Art: diacriTech
Cover Design: Kristin E. Parker
Cover and Interior Image: © Sebastian Kaulitzki/Dreamstime.com
Printing and Binding: Courier Westford
Cover Printing: Courier Westford

Library of Congress Cataloging-in-Publication Data

Zenilman, Jonathan M.
  Sexually transmitted infections : diagnosis, management, and treatment / Jonathan M. Zenilman and Mohsen Shahmanesh.
    p. ; cm.
  Includes bibliographical references and index.
  ISBN-13: 978-0-7637-8675-5 (hardcover)
  ISBN-10: 0-7637-8675-6 (hardcover)
  1. Sexually transmitted diseases. I. Shahmanesh, Mohsen. II. Title.
  [DNLM: 1. Sexually Transmitted Diseases. WC 140]
  RA644.V4Z46 2012
  616.95'1--dc22

                 2011000574

6048

Printed in the United States of America
15 14 13 12 11   10 9 8 7 6 5 4 3 2 1

Dedication

To Carol and Jaleh

Contents

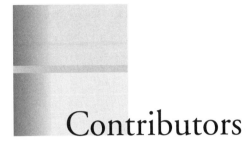

Contributors

Jean R. Anderson, MD
Department of Obstetrics and Gynecology
Johns Hopkins University School of Medicine
Baltimore, Maryland

Andrew F. Angelino, MD, DFAPA
Associate Professor
Department of Psychiatry and Behavioral Sciences
Johns Hopkins University School of Medicine
Baltimore, Maryland

Michael Augenbraun, MD, FACP
Professor of Medicine
SUNY-Downstate College of Medicine
Brooklyn, New York

Susan Blank, MD, MPH
Assistant Commissioner
Bureau of STD Control
New York City Department of Health and
    Mental Hygiene
New York, New York

Christine A. Bowman, MA, BMBCh, FRCP
Consultant Physician
Department of Genitourinary Medicine
Sheffield Teaching Hospitals NHS Foundation Trust
Royal Hallamshire Hospital
South Yorkshire, United Kingdom

M. Gary Brook, MD, FRCP
Consultant Physician
Central Middlesex Hospital
London, United Kingdom

Louise Brown, BSc, RGN
Service Improvement Lead
Whittall Street GU Medicine Clinic
Birmingham, United Kingdom

Gale R. Burstein, MD, MPH
Associate Professor
Department of Pediatrics
University at Buffalo
Division of Adolescent Medicine
Women and Children's Hospital of Buffalo
Buffalo, New York

Roy Chan, FRCP, Dip Ven, FAMS
Director National Skin Centre
Head STI Control Programme
Singapore

Verapol Chandeying, MD
Associate Professor
Faculty of Medicine
Prince of Songkla University
Hat Yai, Thailand

Janette Clarke, MBChB, FRCP
Consultant Physician
Department of Genitourinary Medicine
Leeds General Infirmary
Leeds, United Kingdom

Elizabeth Claydon, MBChB, FRCP
Consultant in Genitourinary Medicine and HIV
North Devon District Hospital
Barnstaple, United Kingdom

Richard A. Crosby, PhD
DDI Endowed Professor and Chair
Department of Health Behavior
College of Public Health
University of Kentucky
Lexington, Kentucky

Michael Dan, MD
Head, Infectious Diseases Unit and the Clinic
    for Genitourinary Infections
E. Wolfson Hospital, Holon
Associate Professor of Medicine
Tel Aviv University School of Medicine
Israel

Deblina Datta, MD
Division of Sexually Transmitted Diseases
Centers for Disease Control and Prevention
Atlanta, Georgia

Eileen F. Dunne, MD
Division of Sexually Transmitted Diseases
Centers for Disease Control and Prevention
Atlanta, Georgia

Sarah Edwards, MBBS, MA
Consultant Physician
Department of Genitourinary Medicine
West Suffolk Hospital
Suffolk, United Kingdom

Charles Ebel
Director
Proposal Operations
Research Computing Division RTI International
Research Triangle Park, North Carolina

Emily J. Erbelding, MD, MPH
Associate Professor of Medicine
Division of Infectious Diseases
Johns Hopkins University School of Medicine
Baltimore, Maryland

Harneet Ranu Eriksson, MBBS, MRCP, MSc Clin Derm
National Skin Center
Singapore

Kevin A. Fenton, MD, PhD, FFPH
Director
National Center for HIV/AIDS, Viral Hepatitis, STD,
    and TB Prevention
Centers for Disease Control and Prevention
Atlanta, Georgia

Patrick French, MBChB, FRCP
Consultant Physician
Camden Primary Care Trust
Mortimer Market Centre
London, United Kingdom

Allison Friedman, MS
Health Communication Specialist
Centers for Disease Control and Prevention
Atlanta, Georgia

Samuel R. Friedman, PhD
National Development and Research Institutes, Inc.
New York, New York

Joel C. Gaydos, MD, MPH
Science Advisor
Armed Forces Health Surveillance Center
U.S. Department of Defense
Silver Spring, Maryland

Charlotte A. Gaydos, MD
Professor of Medicine
Johns Hopkins University School of Medicine
Baltimore, Maryland

Penny Goold, MBBS, MRCP
Consultant Physician in GU Medicine and HIV
Whittall Street Genitourinary Medicine Clinic
Birmingham, United Kingdom

Holly Hagan, PhD
Center for Drug Use and HIV Research
NYU School of Nursing
New York, New York

Hans-Jochen Hagedorn, MD
Medizinale Untersuchungsstelle
    im Regierungsbezirk
Bad Salzuflen, Germany

Klaus-Peter Hunfeld, MD, MPH
Institute of Laboratory Medicine
North West Medical Centre
Medical Faculty
Academic Teaching Hospital
Goethe-University Frankfurt
Frankfurt, Germany

Nikki N. Jordan
Epidemiologist
U.S. Army Public Health Command (Provisional)
    Disease Epidemiology Program
Aberdeen Proving Ground, Maryland

Benny Jose Kottiri, PhD
Health Science Administrator
Bureau for Global Public Health, USAID
Washington, DC

Jean M. Keller, PA
Department of Obstetrics and Gynecology
Johns Hopkins University School of Medicine
Baltimore, Maryland

Doshi Hemendra Kumar
Dermatovenerologist
Klinik Kulit Dan Kelamin Shriji
Selangor, Malaysia

Ahmed S. Latif, MBChB, FCP, FRCP, MD, FAFPHM
Medical Director, Sunrise Health Service
    Aboriginal Corporation
Katherine, NT, Australia
Formerly Dean of Medicine
University of Zimbabwe
Harare, Zimbabwe

Lamont Law, MB, Dip GU Med
Associate Specialist in Genitourinary Medicine
Prostatitis Clinic
Churchill Hospital
Oxford, United Kingdom

Hillary Liss, MD
Clinical Assistant Professor
Department of Medicine
University of Washington
Seattle, Washington

Graz Luzzi, DM, FRCP
Consultant in Genitourinary Medicine
Wycombe Hospital
High Wycombe, United Kingdom

Lauri Markowitz, MD
Division of Sexually Transmitted Diseases
Centers for Disease Control and Prevention
Atlanta, Georgia

Jeanne M. Marrazzo, MD, MPH
Associate Professor
University of Washington
Seattle, Washington

Raymond Maw, MB, FRCP
Consultant Physician
Department of Genitourinary Medicine
Royal Victoria Hospital
Belfast, Northern Ireland

Kelly T. McKee Jr., MD, MPH
Vice President
Public Health and Government Services
Quintiles Transnational Corp.
Durham, North Carolina

Beth Meyerson, MDiv, PhD
President/CEO
Policy Resource Group, LLC
Indianapolis, Indiana

Sharon Moses, MBChB, MSc, MRCOG, MFSRH, Dip GUM
Consultant Reproductive and Sexual Health
BRASH, Contraception and Sexual Health Services
Birmingham, United Kingdom

David Mutimer, MBBS, MD
Reader in Hepatology and Consultant Hepatologist
Liver Unit
Queen Elizabeth Hospital
Birmingham, United Kingdom

Robyn Neblett, MD, MPH
Medical Director, Druid STD Clinic
Baltimore City Department of Health
Baltimore, Maryland

Farah M. Parvez, MD, MPH
Director
Office of Correctional Public Health
NYC Department of Health and Mental Hygiene
New York, New York

Raj Patel, FRCP
Senior Lecturer
University of Southampton
Southampton, United Kingdom

David C. Perlman, MD
Beth Israel Medical Center
New York, New York

Keith Radcliffe, MS, FRCP
Consultant Physician
Whittall Street Clinic
Birmingham, United Kingdom

Gary Remafedi, MD, MPH
Director
Youth and AIDS Projects
Associate Professor of Pediatrics
University of Minnesota
Minneapolis, Minnesota

Karen Elizabeth Rogstad, MBBS, FRCP
Consultant
Department of Genitourinary Medicine
Royal Hallamshire Hospital
Sheffield Teaching Hospitals NHS Foundation Trust
Sheffield, United Kingdom

Anne Rompalo, MD, ScM
Professor of Medicine
Johns Hopkins University School of Medicine
Baltimore, Maryland

Jonathan D. C. Ross, MD, FRCP
Professor of Sexual Health and HIV
Whittall Street Clinic
Birmingham, United Kingdom

Darren Russell, MBBS, FRACGP, DipVen, FAChSHM
Clinical Associate Professor
University of Melbourne
Director
Cairns Sexual Health Service
Queensland, Australia

Nadim Salomon, MD
Beth Israel Medical Center
New York, New York

Mona Saraiya, MD
Division of Sexually Transmitted Diseases
Centers for Disease Control and Prevention
Atlanta, Georgia

Jane R. Schwebke, MD
STD Program
University of Alabama at Birmingham
Birmingham, Alabama

C. Wayne Sells, MD, MPH
Director, Division of Adolescent Health
Associate Professor of Pediatrics
Department of Pediatrics
Oregon Health and Science University
Portland, Oregon

Taraneh Shafii, MD, MPH
Director of Teen Health Services
Harborview Medical Center
Assistant Professor
Division of Adolescent Medicine
Department of Pediatrics
University of Washington
Seattle, Washington

Maryam Shahmanesh, MA, PhD, MRCP
Clinical Lecturer
Centre for Sexual Health and HIV Research
University College London
London, United Kingdom

C. Sonnex, MD, FRCP
Consultant
Department of GU Medicine
Addenbrooke's Hospital
Cambridge, United Kingdom

Hiok-Hee Tan, FRCP, FAMS
Senior Consultant Dermatologist
National Skin Centre, Singapore
Head
DSC Clinic
Honorary Secretary
Chapter of Dermatologists
College of Physicians
Philadelphia, Pennsylvania

Alan L. F. Tang, FRCP, Dip GUM, DFFP
Consultant Physician
The Florey Unit
Royal Berkshire NHS Foundation Trust
Reading, United Kingdom

T. Thirumoorthy, MD
Associate Professor
Duke-NUS Graduate Medical School
Senior Consultant Dermatologist
Singapore General Hospital
Singapore

Steven K. Tobler
U.S. Army Public Health Command (provisional)
Aberdeen Proving Grounds, Maryland

Glenn J. Treisman, MD, PhD
Professor
Department of Psychiatry and Behavioral Sciences
Johns Hopkins University School of Medicine
Baltimore, Maryland

Terri Warren, CRNP, ANP
Westover Heights Clinic
Portland, Oregon

Jan Welch, MD, MBE, BSc, FRCP, FFFLM
Consultant Physician
King's College Hospital
London, United Kingdom

Harold C. Wiesenfeld, MDCM
Department of Obstetrics, Gynecology and
    Reproductive Sciences
Magee-Womens Hospital
Pittsburgh, Pennsylvania

Janet D. Wilson, MBChB, FRCP
Consultant Physician
Department of Genitourinary Medicine
Leeds General Infirmary
Leeds, United Kingdom

Mark H. Yudin, MD, MSc, FRCSC
Department of Obstetrics and Gynecology
University of Toronto
Toronto, Canada

About the Editors

JONATHAN M. ZENILMAN, MD

Dr. Jonathan Zenilman is Professor of Medicine and Chief of the Infectious Diseases Division at Johns Hopkins Bayview Medical Center. His career in sexually transmitted infections (STIs) started at the Centers for Disease Control and Prevention, where he was responsible for developing the national gonococcal isolate surveillance system. His STI-related activities have included being the director of clinical services at the Baltimore City Health Department and a translational research program in the epidemiology of gonococcal resistance, behavioral interventions, and HIV/STI interactions. He is a former president of the American STD Association.

MOHSEN SHAHMANESH, MD, FRCP

Dr. Mohsen Shahmanesh was born in Teheran, Iran. He completed his medical training in the United Kingdom and specialized in endocrinology with his MD thesis on the pituitary-hypothalamic control of gonadotrophin secretion.

Between 1975 and 1981, he was associate professor of medicine and endocrinology at Shiraz University, Iran. Returning to England in 1983, he retrained in genitourinary medicine at St. Thomas' Hospital, and in 1988 became consultant in GU medicine and HIV at Birmingham General Hospital and the University of Birmingham, United Kingdom. Among a number of senior posts in the speciality, he pursued his deep interest in teaching by becoming chairman of the specialist advisory committee for GU Medicine at the Royal College of Physicians of London. Between 1996 and 2002, he edited the journal *Sexually Transmitted Infections* (changing its name from *Genitourinary Medicine*). He was a member of the Department of Health's expert advisory group on AIDS. In 2008 he was awarded life fellowship by the British Association of Sexual Health and HIV. He retired from clinical medicine in January 2010. His research interests include nongonococcal urethritis; the neurological complications of HIV; and the effects of currently used antiviral treatment regimens for HIV on glucose, cortisol and lipid metabolism, and adipocyte gene expression.

1

Introduction

Jonathan M. Zenilman and Mohsen Shahmanesh

Sexually transmitted infections (STIs) are some of the most commonly encountered infectious diseases and affect up to 25–30% of adolescents and young adults. STIs are treated in a variety of clinical settings, including outpatient clinics, adolescent clinics, family planning clinics, hospitals, and public traditional health clinics. They are also seen by a large variety of practitioners, including subspecialists, such as infectious disease specialists, primary care physicians, nurse practitioners, and paraprofessionals, again in a large variety of clinical settings.

Although the World Health Organization (WHO), the U.S. Centers for Disease Control and Prevention (CDC), the U.K. National Health Service, and other countries and organizations issue guidelines, clinical guidance for sexually transmitted infections management and treatment is often difficult to access outside of either very brief guidelines and decision-tree documents or large comprehensive textbooks. Those of us who work in clinical and public health settings need a resource that provides comprehensive discussion of diagnosis, management, and epidemiology, albeit in an accessible format for the busy clinician.

The coeditors of this book were the editor-in-chief and the associate editor of *Sexually Transmitted Infections* between 1996 and 2007 and interacted with STI specialists and practitioners around the world. Our desire is to provide an accessible volume that provides up-to-date clinical information on the epidemiology, management, and strategies for sexually transmitted infection intervention and control.

This book contains several unique parts. In addition to the traditional epidemiology, diagnosis, and management chapters, we also provide chapters on managing STIs in a variety of settings and populations. These include such populations as homosexual men and women, military populations, correctional settings, and adolescent populations; these populations are at extremely high risk for STIs and have their own unique social aspects. From the standpoint of intervention, we also were interested in developing strategies to provide the practitioner with up-to-date information on HIV counseling and testing, but recognizing more recent trends, we provide specific counseling messages for practitioners who deal with herpes and HPV infections, which are increasingly seen as the primary reason for visits, especially in developed countries.

We have recruited authors from around the world, primarily from the United Kingdom and the United States, as well as experts from Africa, Asia, and the Middle East, to provide their unique insights on sexually transmitted infections. We recognize that STI is a global problem and a global issue and hope that this book will provide information and insights into improving the care of sexually transmitted infections and other reproductive tract infections.

2

The Sexual History

Verapol Chandeying

WHY TAKE A SEXUAL HISTORY?

Although sexual health issues are some of the most common problems encountered in clinical practice, stigma is still encountered at both the patient and the provider level. The clinical and cultural contexts may also affect patients' openness in sharing their sexual history with providers. Often, patients will substantially edit their sexual history. Therefore, providers need to be able to ask the important and pertinent questions and to establish a nonjudgmental environment where patients can feel comfortable sharing responses to highly sensitive questions.

Training providers to obtain a sexual history and experience are two major factors that will affect obtaining accurate information. A challenge is that sexual health services are delivered in a variety of clinical settings, which may require focusing on a separate menu of clinical problems and services. These include (Chandeying 2005):

1. Primary care settings

2. Family planning counseling and clinical services: focusing on contraception and sexually transmitted infections (STI) prevention

3. Maternal and child health: education and service for prenatal care, safe, delivery, and postnatal care, especially breast-feeding and infant and women's health care

4. Abortion services and postabortion contraception and STI prevention

5. Adolescent reproductive health: information, education, counseling, and services, providing transition and education into developing a sexual identity

6. Couple reproductive health: counseling, information, education, treatment of sexual dysfunction, counseling for couples with dichotomous STI status (e.g., herpes)

7. Clinics for STIs and human immunodeficiency virus (HIV) and acquired immunodeficiency syndrome (AIDS): prevention, reduction, and care

8. Older adults information, education, and care

The sexual history provides important information on specific STI risk and on developing patient- and couple-centered counseling for addressing specific problems.

BARRIERS TO TAKING A SEXUAL HISTORY

In primary care, sexual health issues often are managed in a reactive mode—in response to a symptom or diagnosis of STI, and sexual health issues are not discussed until a problem arises. However, studies in multiple cultural settings have demonstrated that the patient expects the physicians and nurses to have some knowledge of sexual health, and there is enormous patient-based desire for practitioners to open the conversation. A major barrier is that the practitioner may be embarrassed, especially if the practitioner has known the patient for some time. Practitioners often voice concern about embarrassing the patient or asking sensitive questions that may sound judgemental from the patient's perspective. However, in contrast, patients are often eager to share their sexual history details as long as confidentiality is assured and patients are certain that sexual health questions are routine and part of a general clinical evaluation (Presswell and Barton 2000).

Unless the presenting complaint is a primary STI symptom, such as genital ulcer or urethral/vaginal discharge, patients generally will not share sexual concerns unless their clinician prompts them. Health professionals are often reluctant to address sexual health issues for the following four reasons: (1) embarrassment in asking about sexuality, (2) inadequate training in asking questions and modulating their own nonverbal responses, (3) belief that sexual history is not relevant to the chief complaint, and (4) time constraints.

■ SEXUAL HISTORY: CREATING A POSITIVE ATMOSPHERE AND CONFIDENTIALITY

The sexual history should be seen as a specific application of medical history taking. Setting the environment and tone is critical. Introduce yourself in a professional manner, and ensure that the interview takes place in a quiet and private room. At the outset, discuss confidentiality guidelines with the patient, including alleviating fears about notifying partners or parents (if patients are adolescents). The patient should be informed that the interview will be complete and that you will be asking sensitive questions related to their body and sexuality using culturally appropriate language. If a trainee or student is present in the room, ask the patient permission for him or her to remain and indicate that they are all bound by the same confidentiality rules. However, at the patient's request, the trainee or student observer may have to leave.

Often, patients may wish to have friends, partners, or family members present because they do not know that the clinician plans to ask sexual and other personal questions. If a patient expresses interest in having someone else present, indicate that your policy is not to discuss personal or sexual issues in the presence of anyone but the patient. If necessary, include the other person in the opening discussion of general health issues, but, at some point, ask the accompanying person to leave the room.

Good Opening Statements

The physicians may start sexual history with an opening statement that puts the subject in context and makes it normative. For example, the practitioners might say,

"Sexual health is important to everyone's overall health and might also help me in making a diagnosis in your case. It is therefore a normal part of the routine that we always follow. Of course, all of your answers will be totally confidential."

Screening Sexual History

Various example questions related to screening sexual history are as follows:

Are you currently sexually active? If no, when was the last time you were sexually active?

If yes,

Was this person of the opposite sex to yourself?

Have you had sex with someone of the same sex as yourself?

Do you have any discomfort during sexual activity?

Do you have any questions or concerns about your sexual functioning? About your partner's sexual functioning?

Questions to determine sites of exposure (ask questions directly):

When you have sex, what types of activity do you have?

For heterosexual men: Do you place your penis in your partner's vagina, anus, or throat? Do you place your mouth on your partner's vagina or anus?

For homosexual men: Do you place your penis in your partner's anus or throat? Does your partner insert his penis into your throat or rectum?

For heterosexual women: Does your partner place his penis into your throat, rectum, or vagina? Does your partner place his mouth on your vagina or anus?

For homosexual women: Do you place your mouth on your partner's vagina or anus? Does your partner place her mouth on your vagina or anus?

■ SPECIFIC ELEMENT OF SEXUAL HISTORY

Where the patient presents with a specific sexual problem, such as a possible STI, a possible sexual dysfunction, or questions about sexual functioning, specific sexual history should be taken appropriately to his or her problem and concern. Those include STI/HIV/AIDS, menstrual, obstetric, perimenopausal, sexual relationship, sexual behavior, and sexual intercourse history.

The specific sexual history can be obtained in depth as it relates to the specific problems of the patients, such as organic cause of sexual dysfunction, desire disorder, arousal and erectile disorder, lubrication and penetration disorder, and orgasmic disorder history.

A general medical history is a critical part of the sexual history and should include a full review of other medical problems faced by the patient, as well as a complete list of current medications. For example, a large number of medications and diseases such as diabetes may interfere with sexual function and may not be elucidated unless specifically asked.

Drug allergy should be specifically assessed, as presence of a drug allergy, especially to beta-lactams, may affect therapeutic choices. When inquiring about drug allergy, the clinician should be careful to note that often patients confuse toxic reactions or drug side effects with allergy. For example, a history of mild gastrointestinal upset after taking azithromycin is not a drug allergy or a contraindication to taking the drug again.

Because there may be myriad underlying etiologies, and because of the sensitivity of the subject matter, at the end of the interview, two concluding, open-ended questions are suggested:

What do you attribute your problem to?

Is there anything that I have not asked but you would like to add?

STI/HIV History

The STI history is by definition an assessment of a patient's risk factors and provides an excellent opportunity for preventive counseling and prompts further clinical action, such as testing or treatment. Never assume that older patients are not sexually active or not at risk. In particular, older adults embarking on new relationships following separation, divorce, or death of a long-term partner may be at particular risk and may not be forthcoming unless specifically asked. Never assume that older patients can negotiate condom use better than other patients. How does a woman negotiate the issue of condom use? The risk assessment and sexual behavior questions, aimed at identifying the patient's risk for an STI, are modified from Cachay and coworkers (2004) and include:

Earlier age at first sexual activity

Exposure to an STI

History of past STI and treatment

Last sexual intercourse

Number of recent sex partners

Unprotected sexual risk behaviors with someone with STI

Improper or inconsistent condom use

Use of drugs/alcohol during sex

History of blood or blood products transfusion

IV drug use

Sexual practices (vaginal, oral, and anal sex)

Recent sexual activities

Multiple partners

New partner

Casual partners

Various Example Questions Related to Risk Assessment

What are you doing in your life that you think might be putting you at risk for STI/HIV?

How many sexual partners have you had in the past year?

Does your sexual behavior change as a result of travel outside your home area, that is, vacation/business trips?

Have you had sex abroad?

What do you know about the sexual practices of your partner(s)?

Have you ever exchanged drugs or money for sex?

What is you experience with drug use?

What is your experience with shooting up drugs?

How do drugs or alcohol influence your STI or HIV risk behaviors?

Condom Use

When you have sex, how often do you use a condom—all of the time, some of the time, or none of the time?

When or with whom do you have sex without a condom?

What would be the difference between when you would use condoms versus when you might not?

When was the last time you had unprotected sex?

Examples of Questions to Ask Patients with High-Risk Behaviors to Elicit Information About HIV Status

Have you had sex with someone who you know or suspect has HIV? If yes, when was the last time?

Do you have any concerns regarding HIV testing?

Have you been tested for HIV? If yes, when and at which facility?

When were you last tested for HIV, and what was the result? If not, what are the reasons you haven't been tested for HIV?

Do you have any concerns regarding STI testing?

Have you been tested for STI? If so, where were you last tested for STI and what were the results? If not, what are the reasons you haven't been tested for STI?

Do you have any concerns regarding STI testing?

During risk assessment, it is worth assessing experience with condom use, as appropriate.

What do the symptoms of STI/HIV/AIDS look like? Many people are unaware that they may be infected with an STI. Some STIs do not present obvious symptoms in either men or women. Emphasize to the patient that an STI diagnosis cannot be made based on symptoms and visible signs. Symptoms of STI can vary from person to person and can resemble the symptoms of many other illnesses. The questions in Table 2-1 may be asked and followed by probing questions. Probing questions should always follow the classic medical-history-taking model of asking the length of time of symptoms, quality, quantity, and exacerbating and mediating factors.

The clinical symptoms of acute HIV infection closely resemble other viral infections. Patients with acute HIV infection may present to either their primary care providers, emergency care providers, or an STI care provider, depending on the specific symptoms. Symptoms associated with acute HIV may be nonspecific and include fevers, rash, the presence of oral aphthous ulcers and oral lesions, lymphadenopathy, and gastrointestinal complaints, such as nausea, vomiting, diarrhea, and abdominal pain. Patients in whom acute HIV is suspected should be referred for immediate evaluation and testing for HIV, including measurement of viral RNA. Standard HIV serological tests will give false-negative negative within the "seroconversion window" of acute HIV, and because HIV transmission is extremely high during this period, patients should be advised not to have sexual activity until the test results are available and proper counseling can be provided.

TABLE 2-1   Clinical STI-Related Symptom Questions

Have you had a sore or blister on your genital area, your anus, or your mouth?
Have you had any warts or other "bumps" in your genital area (or other areas of exposure?)
Have you had any rash?
Do you have a sore throat?
Have you had any recent fevers or chills?
Have you had any swollen glands?
Have you had discomfort or pain when urinating?

Men

Have you had a discharge from your penis?
Have you had any swelling in your testicles?
Are you circumcised? (If not, has your foreskin been swollen?)

Women

Have you had a vaginal discharge? If yes—is it different than your "normal" discharge?
Have you had any abdominal pain?
Do you have pain on intercourse or with penetration?

■ MENSTRUAL, OBSTETRICAL, AND PERIMENOPAUSAL HISTORY

A menstrual history should be obtained if possible, even among women who are postmenopausal. In older women and in women who have stopped menstruating, perimenopausal symptoms that affect sexual activity, such as vaginal dryness and loss of libido, should be directly and nonjudgmentally questioned. In perimenopausal women who are sexually active, contraception should be discussed because they may not realize their potential for getting pregnant. Protection from unintended pregnancy is important until women are truly menopausal.

An obstetrical history should be obtained, such as prenatal, intrapartum, postpartum, and neonatal problems. Injuries from forceps and vacuum extraction can result in chronic pelvic pain, dyspareunia, and urinary and fecal incontinence. The suggested questions include:

Menarche, interval, duration, regularity (when)

Last menstrual period

Bleeding, pain, or discomfort associated with menses or sexual intercourse

Premenstrual tension

Contraception

Parity

Pregnancy-related problems

Menopausal/perimenopausal symptoms (older women)

■ SEXUAL RELATIONSHIP, BEHAVIOR, AND INTERCOURSE HISTORY

This applies to the patient who has a problem or concern, related to his or her sexual functioning or sexual dysfunction or his or her partner's sexual functioning. Ensure there is privacy and the patient is comfortable. Be both verbally and nonverbally nonjudgmental and avoid labeling the patient's behavior and sexual orientation. However, never make assumptions about the patient's sexuality or sexual practices based on how they dress, speak, or act. If possible, allow frequent opportunities for the patient to raise questions and concerns.

The terminology used by the healthcare worker to phrase inquiries must be understood by and acceptable to the patient. Similarly, information supplied by the patient must be specific rather than ambiguous. Begin with the least-threatening questions, and leave crude questions for later or at the end. Never invite a negative answer, and never assume that people know what words mean. The example sentences should use open-ended questions where possible as follows:

Tell me about your sexual partner.

How did you meet your current partner?

What happened physically in the early stages of the relationship?

What happened when you first had intercourse with your partner?

Do you have any sexual concerns?

How often do you have sexual intercourse?

Do you have one or more than one partner? If so, male or female?

How is the relationship going?

Is there anything you would change about your sexual activity?

Tell me about your current sexual intercourse pattern.

Does your partner touch your genitals?

Do you have any problems with lubrication?

Do you have pain with sexual activity?

Does your partner have pain with sexual activity?

How long and how often have you or your partner had painful sexual intercourse?

Do you have orgasms?

Are you sexually satisfied?

How often do you have complete sexual satisfaction when making love?

Have you ever touched yourself?

When was the last time you masturbated?

Organic Cause and Risk Factors of Sexual Dysfunction History

The causes of sexual dysfunction can generally be classified as either organic or psychological. Psychological causes include performance anxiety, stress, depression, and marital conflict. The possible organic causes and risk factors of male and female sexual dysfunction, summarized from various studies, are listed in Table 2-2. All chronic illnesses, medical and surgical, can be a factor for sexual dysfunction, both the disease and its psychological aspects. Thus, cancer patients may be affected by sexual dysfunction throughout the entire course of the disease. Sexual health among this group is largely under-evaluated and undertreated.

TABLE 2-2   Possible Organic Causes and Risk Factors of Male and Female Sexual Dysfunction

Organic Causes/Risk Factors	Remarks
Arthritis: osteoarthritis, rheumatoid	Sexual dysfunction due to pain and disability, affects both male and female
Cancer	A variety of cancers are commonly associated with treatment-related sexual dysfunction, especially genitourinary and rectal cancer
Chronic alcoholism	Suppresses central nervous system and causes sensory inactivity in male, while it may cause vaginal dryness and ovarian dysfunction in female
Chronic obstructive pulmonary disease	Shortness of breath inhibits all physical activity
Chronic pelvic pain syndrome	Psychological and organic cause
Chronic prostatitis	Pain and psychological
Diabetes mellitus: microvascular complications, polyneuropathy	Affects male because of microvascular complication and polyneuropathy, but female study is limited
Endocrine disorders of sex steroid hormones (female)	Various endogenous hormones impairment includes estrogen, testosterone, progesterone, and prolactin
Endocrine disorders of sex steroid hormones (male)	Leads to hypogonadism
Endocrinopathy	Addison's disease (chronic adrenocortical insufficiency, sexual dysfunction due to weakness, fatigability, and other medical ills) Cushing's syndrome (hypercortisolism, sexual dysfunction owing to multiple illnesses)
Epilepsy	Disorder and antiepileptic drugs disturb production of sex hormones
Exercise-induced amenorrhea	Affects female due to hypothalamic dysfunction with low gonadotropin-releasing hormone
Gynecological conditions	Endometriosis, pelvic floor relaxation, uterine prolapse, uterine fibroids, episiotomy scar, senile vaginal atrophy, vulvovestibulitis, vaginismus, clitoral adhesion, and bartholinitis may cause various degrees of sexual dysfunction
Hypertension	Affects both male and female
Lower urinary tract infection	Strongly linked with sexual dysfunction, both male and female
Myocardial infarction	Fear of bringing on another attack may produce sexual dysfunction
Multiple sclerosis	Disability-related sexual dysfunction
Parkinson's disease	Decreased agility and flexibility associated with autonomic nervous system
Peyronie's disease	Affects male only, owing to build up of scar tissue in the penis
Prolonged heavy smoking	More erectile disorders than nonsmoker in male, but in female needs more study
Renal disease	Uremia associated with autonomic neuropathy
Spinal injury	Depends on degree of the injury and its location
Stroke	Psychological and social factors
Vaginal infection	Sexual pain syndrome–related sexual dysfunction

Desire Disorder

Currently, the most common sexual dysfunction in women is hypoactive, or low, sexual desire, which is one of the most troubling sexual problems, affecting up to one-third of women. Several female reproductive-life experiences may uniquely affect sexual desire. These events include menstrual cycles, hormonal contraceptives, postpartum states and lactation, oophorectomy and hysterectomy, and perimenopausal and postmenopausal states. While the prevalence in male is 15%, both are associated with a wide variety of medical and psychologic causes. Questions to ask about desire disorder, adapted from Ross and Channon-Little (1991), are as follows:

How often do you have sexual intercourse?

How long have you had the loss of desire?

How is this problem affecting you? Are you concerned about or bothered by it?

How is your loss of desire affecting your relationship?

Is it always a problem? Is it a problem only at certain times or in certain situations?

Has the problem changed over time? If so, how?

Does anything appear to improve your libido or make it worse?

Does your partner have any sexual difficulties?

Do you have any idea about what may be causing your loss of desire? Does your partner?

Have you seen anyone else about this problem? If so, what was suggested? What steps were taken?

Is there anything in your current situation that makes sex unpleasant or difficult?

Arousal and Erectile Disorder

Sexual arousal disorders, including erectile dysfunction in men and female sexual arousal disorder in women, are found in 10% to 20% of men and women and are strongly age-related in men. Questions to ask about arousal disorder, adapted from Ross and Channon-Little (1991), are as follows:

How often do you have sexual intercourse?

How do you and your partner initiate intercourse?

Do you and your partner usually welcome the idea?

What happens during foreplay?

How do you feel when your partner inserts his penis?

Do you touch yourself?

Have you had any unpleasant experiences with sex?

Is there anything in your current situation that makes sex unpleasant or difficult?

Lubricant and Penetration Disorder

Painful vaginal penetration during intercourse is a common primary symptom. Questions to ask about lubricant and penetration disorder, adapted from Ross and Channon-Little (1991), are as follows:

How often do you have sexual intercourse?

Do you and your partner start with foreplay? How long? Long enough?

Do you begin to lubricate during foreplay?

Do you have painful penetration?

Is penetration successful?

Is your penis able to remain stiff for insertion? Loses stiffness?

How do you feel when you or your partner starts pelvic movement?

How does you partner feel about your response?

Orgasmic Disorder

Orgasmic disorder is parallel in both male and female; it includes early orgasm, delayed orgasm, impaired orgasm, and absence of orgasm. Questions to ask about orgasmic disorder, adapted from Ross and Channon-Little (1991), are as follows:

Tell me what happened the first time you had sexual intercourse.

Did you have any unpleasant experiences with sex?

How did you feel about it at the time?

What were your physical responses?

Tell me about experiences after that.

How often do you have sexual intercourse?

What features are you interested in?

Do you have any problems with lubrication?

Do you touch yourself?

How long do you and your partner use for foreplay? Does it satisfy you?

After you admit the penetration, about how long does it take before you achieve orgasm?

After you insert your penis, about how long does it take before you ejaculate?

How do you feel during pelvic movement? Active or passive role?

How do you feel after sexual intercourse?

Drug-Induced Sexual Dysfunction

Sexual desire disorders are sexual dysfunctions characterized by alteration in sexual desire: (1) hypoactive sexual desire disorder is a sexual dysfunction consisting of persistently or recurrently low level or absence of sexual fantasies and desire for sexual activity; (2) sexual aversion disorder is feelings of repulsion for and active avoidance of genital sexual contact with a partner, causing substantial distress or interpersonal difficulty. Sexual arousal disorders are characterized by alterations in sexual arousal: (1) female sexual arousal disorder is a sexual dysfunction involving failure by a female either to attain or maintain lubrication and swelling during sexual activity, after adequate stimulation; (2) male erectile disorder is a sexual dysfunction involving failure by a male to attain or maintain an adequate erection until completion of sexual relations.

The influence of drugs on neurogenic, hormonal, and vascular mechanisms may result in diminished libido, impotence, ejaculatory and orgasmic difficulties, inhibited vaginal lubrication, menstrual irregularities, and gynecomastia in men or painful breast enlargement in women. Parasympatholytic agents, which interfere with cholinergic transmission, may affect erectile potency, while adrenergic-inhibiting agents may interfere with ejaculatory control. Central nervous system depressants or sedating drugs, drugs producing hyperprolactinemia, and antiandrogenic drugs also may affect the normal sexual response. Drugs such as antihypertensive and antipsychotic agents may induce sexual dysfunction that can result in patient noncompliance. Usually, drug-induced side effects are reversible with discontinuation of the offending agent (Aldridge 1982).

Possible drug-induced sexual dysfunctions are described in Tables 2-3, 2-4, and 2-5 and are not meant to be complete but rather to serve as a guide.

The final part of history taking is for the practitioner to decide what is to be done next. A management plan should then be discussed and agreed to with the patient. At this point, they should decide whether the patient's partner should be invited for a joint meeting if he or she has not been present. In this way, the patient will feel that a partnership exists with the doctor, and treatment is much more likely to succeed. Many practitioners are

TABLE 2-3   Possible Drug-Induced Desire Disorder

Medications That Cause Desire Disorder
Antipsychotics
Barbiturates
Benzodiazepines
Beta blockers
Bupropion
Cardiovascular and antihypertensive medications
Clonidine
Danazol
Digoxin
Fluoxetine
Fluvoxamine
GnRh agonists
Histamine H2-receptor blockers and promotility agents
Hormonal preparations
Indomethacin
Ketoconazole
Lipid-lowering medications
Lithium
Moclobemide
Nefazodone
Oral contraceptives
Phenytoin sodium
Psychoactive medications
Selective serotonin reuptake inhibitors
Sertraline
Spironolactone
Tricyclic antidepressants

fully qualified to diagnose and treat certain commonly encountered sexual health problems for which there are well-established treatment protocols. In other cases, referral to a specialist may be indicated. When referring a patient, couch the recommendation in terms that will reassure patients that the problem they face is not unusual and that a referral to a therapist or other specialist is common practice.

TABLE 2-4   Possible Drug-Induced
Arousal Disorder

Medications That Cause Arousal Disorder
Anticholinergics
Antihistamines
Antihypertensives
Benzodiazepines
Bupropion
Fluoxetine
Fluvoxamine
Moclobemide
Monoamine oxidase inhibitors
Nefazodone
Psychoactive medications
Selective serotonin reuptake inhibitors
Sertraline
Tamsulosin
Tricyclic antidepressants

TABLE 2-5   Possible Drug-Induced
Orgasmic Disorder

Medications That Cause Orgasmic Disorder
Amphetamines and related anorexic drugs
Antipsychotics
Benzodiazepines
Bupropion
Fluoxetine
Fluvoxamine
Methyldopa
Moclopromide
Narcotics
Nefazodone
Selective serotonin reuptake inhibitors
Sertraline
Trazadone
Tricyclic antidepressants*
*Also associated with painful orgasm.

■ KEY POINTS

- The sexual history is critical to directing investigations and developing a diagnostic plan.

- A complete sexual history includes a general medical history background, current medications, assessment of type of sexual activity and risks, and specific symptoms.

- Ensuring confidentiality and developing a comfortable, nonjudgmental environment are key elements in obtaining a valid history.

- Questions about sexual exposures and types should be direct.

- Questions about sexual symptoms should be general and then include symptoms specific to each organ system.

- Patients expect clinicians to ask detailed questions related to their sexual history.

REFERENCES

Aldridge SA. Drug-induced sexual dysfunction. *Clin Pharm.* 1982;1:141–147.

Bull SS, Rietmeijer C, Fortenberry JD, et al. Practice patterns for the elicitation of sexual history, education, and counseling among providers of STD services: results from the gonorrhea community action project (GCAP). *Sex Transm Dis.* 1999;26:584–589.

Cachay E, Mar-Tang M, Mathews WC. Screening for potentially transmitting sexual risk behaviors, urethral sexually transmitted infection, and sildenafil use among males entering care for HIV infection. *AIDS Patient Care STDs.* 2004;18:349–354.

Chandeying V. Sexual health promotion in Thailand. *Sex Health.* 2005;2(3):129–134.

Mackay HT. Gynecology. In: Tierney LM, McPhee SJ, Papdakis MA, eds. *Current Medical Diagnosis and Treatment.* 4th ed. New York: Lange Medical Books/McGraw-Hill; 2005:704–738.

Merrill JM, Laux LF, Thornby JI. Why doctors have difficulty with sex histories. *South Med J.* 1990;83:613–617.

Pan American Health Organization and World Health Organization. Promotion of sexual health: recommendations for action. In: Proceeding at a regional consultation of the Pan American Health Organization and World Health Organization, in collaboration with the World

Association for sexology; May 19–22, 2000; Antigua, Guatemala.

Phillips NA. Female sexual dysfunction: evaluation and treatment. *Am Fam Physician*. 2000;62:127–136, 141–142.

Presswell N, Barton D. Taking a sexual history. *Aust Fam Physician*. 2000;29:535–539.

Rosen RC. Prevalence and risk factors of sexual dysfunction in men and women. *Curr Psychiatry Rep*. 2000;2:189–195.

Ross WR, Channon-Little LD. In: Ross WR, Channon-Little LD, eds. *Discussing Sexuality: A Guide for Health Practitioners*. Artarmon, Australia: MacLennan & Petty; 1991.

3

Examination of the Male Patient

Keith Radcliffe

During a consultation for a possible sexually transmitted infection (STI) in a man, the first question concerning the physical examination that the clinician must consider is: "Do I need to carry out an examination in this case?"

In answering this question, the main point to consider is whether the patient has any symptoms. If he has, then a physical examination is mandatory, but frequently, he does not and is attending because of concern about the possibility of having acquired an STI following sexual contact with one or more partners. Depending on the nature of this contact, the concerns might be more or less real; anxiety over objectively low-risk activity is not an infrequent reason for seeking a consultation and the patient may be a candidate for noninvasive screening tests.

▇ WHEN TO CARRY OUT A PHYSICAL EXAMINATION

In general, the physical examination may be safely omitted in a male patient who is without symptoms provided that the clinician is in a position to carry out full and reliable testing for all relevant important pathogens in a timely manner. This is because it is important to obtain a microbiologically confirmed diagnosis whenever possible before prescribing treatment or initiating partner notification, but also because the examination of large numbers of otherwise healthy men is likely to be unproductive in most cases. Even when there are findings, these will most often be nonspecific and hence will need to be confirmed or excluded by the results of laboratory investigations, so that in either case the performance of the examination will have no effect on the care of the person.

Recent advances in diagnostic tests have also contributed to making the routine examination of asymptomatic men less relevant. Traditionally, testing for STI in the heterosexual man would require taking a urethral swab to test for gonorrhea and chlamydia. In this case, it made sense for the clinician to carry out a genital examination at the same time as taking the swab, but with the arrival of the ability to test reliably for these infections using a urine sample, this argument no longer applies. The patient can be instructed to produce a urine sample privately, sparing him the inconvenience of a genital examination and saving time for the clinician. Similarly, in asymptomatic men who have sex with other men (MSM), then self-taken pharyngeal and rectal swabs have been shown to be a satisfactory method of testing for STI at those anatomical sites.

In some cases, it might be indicated to carry out a physical examination even in the absence of symptoms if the clinician believes that the patient is at high risk of STI. This is likely to be because they are in a high-risk group such as MSM, are clients of commercial sex workers (CSW), or because they give a history of unprotected sex with multiple partners. It is not possible to be dogmatic on this point, and the clinician must exercise a judgment based on their knowledge of the probability of disease in their own individual practice and the resources that are available.

▇ WHAT TO EXAMINE

Any part of the body and any organ system may be involved in a patient with an STI, especially where the infection has disseminated beyond the genital area, for example, in secondary syphilis.

However, the parts of the body most likely to be involved are those directly employed in sexual activity, that is, the genitalia (see Figure 3-1), followed by the adjacent perianal and suprapubic areas. In MSM, then, the perianal area and rectum, and the mouth and oropharynx, are also frequently affected especially where there is a history of recent receptive oral, anal, or oro-anal sex.

It is these areas therefore that should be the focus of the physical examination, while remembering to extend it to other parts of the body depending on any symptoms or risk factors (sexual or other, e.g., injecting drug use) that have been elicited during the consultation. The healthcare worker also needs to consider their knowledge of the epidemiology of STI both locally and generally. Thus, for example, if syphilis is known to be prevalent among MSM at that time and place, and if the patient gives a history of high-risk sexual behavior, then even in the absence of symptoms it would be appropriate to extend the examination beyond the anogenital region to actively seek evidence of secondary syphilis, that is, to inspect the skin and mucous membranes (especially to look in the mouth) and to palpate for generalized lymphadenopathy.

■ CHAPERONE

Before embarking on a genital examination, the clinician must consider whether to have a chaperone present. It is a mistake to believe that this is only an issue that arises when a male healthcare worker conducts an intimate examination of a female patient: it is relevant whatever the genders of the clinician and the patient. A chaperone can serve several purposes: helping to reassure the patient and to prevent inappropriate behavior by the examining healthcare worker; protecting the latter against malicious allegations of unprofessional behavior; and providing practical assistance to the clinician doing the examination. Some men, particularly teenagers, find the presence of a female nurse as a chaperone embarrassing. In deciding on a chaperone, the clinician must remember the legal and other regulatory imperatives applicable in their country and region of practice, but a good baseline position is probably to always offer a chaperone, but in most cases not to insist on one if the patient objects. Surveys show that only a small proportion of male patients (less than 1 in 20) will accept. The offer, and whether it is accepted or refused, should be documented in the case notes.

FIGURE 3-1   Side View of the Male Reproductive Organs

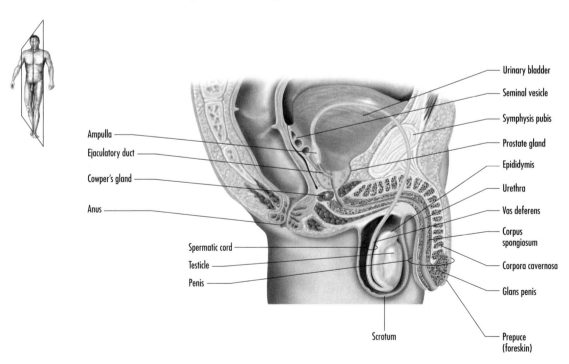

Ampulla

Ejaculatory duct

Cowper's gland

Anus

Spermatic cord

Testicle

Penis

Scrotum

Urinary bladder

Seminal vesicle

Symphysis pubis

Prostate gland

Epididymis

Urethra

Vas deferens

Corpus spongiosum

Corpora cavernosa

Glans penis

Prepuce (foreskin)

A related question is whether anyone else will be present during the examination. Usually this means a trainee who will be taught by observing, and possibly by carrying out, an examination or other practical procedures. The trainee could be a medical student, a nursing student, or a qualified healthcare worker who is trained in the field. The principle must be that the patient's permission is always sought in advance and that this request is not made in front of the trainee, as many patients will be uncomfortable refusing in front of the person and may therefore feel that they are under some duress.

■ THE EXAMINATION

There is no single best way of carrying out the physical examination: over time, each individual clinician will develop his or her own method. It is helpful to establish a personal sequence of steps that is logical and then to follow it as a routine. This will lead to the most efficient use of time and will make it less likely that any step will be omitted even when working under pressure of time.

It is natural that the patient will feel nervous and embarrassed about undergoing a genital examination. The clinician should attempt to put the patient at ease by explaining what is happening, using straightforward language and avoiding medical terminology. A confident and professional manner also helps.

Show respect for the dignity and privacy of the patient. The examination should be carried out in a room behind closed doors, with adequate soundproofing. A cubicle separated from a public area with only a drawn curtain is inadequate, as any necessary conversation occurring during the examination may be overheard, or the patient will certainly fear that it might be. The examination room should be properly equipped for the purpose. It should be warm and well lit, with a flexible light source that can be directed at all areas to be examined. There should be a comfortable, adjustable examination couch. All necessary equipment should be prepared in advance and be laid out, ready for use such as swabs, culture media, proctoscope, and so forth.

The patient should be told what clothing to remove and then left in privacy to undress. As a minimum, the patient should be exposed from the waist down to the knees. It might be necessary to ask the patient to undress completely if the examination needs to be extended beyond the anogenital area if evidence is sought of systemic disease due to HIV infection or syphilis or the clinician needs to look for evidence of a dermatological condition, such as psoriasis or eczema, involving the genitalia.

General Examination

An abbreviated general examination is performed prior to evaluating the anogenital area. While taking the history, the astute examiner will be able to assess the patient's overall health and risk-taking profile. Observation of the skin on the extremities or trunk will provide important clues to the diagnosis of secondary syphilis, dermatoses, and systemic manifestations of diseases such as HIV, herpes and disseminated gonococcal infection. Particular attention should be paid to the extensor surfaces, trunk and palms and soles. Assessment of cervical, axillary and femoral lymphadenopathy can also be rapidly performed. Many young men often do not routinely seek primary health care.

Groin, Penis, and Urethra

The genital examination is most easily performed with the patient lying. The first step is to carefully inspect the genitalia looking for abnormalities such as enlarged inguinal lymph nodes, ulcers, warts, rashes, and visible urethral discharge. Remember to extend the inspection to the perigenital area, including the pubic hair for signs of pubic lice (eggs), and to the suprapubic area and inner thighs where skin lesions from molluscum contagiosum or scabies may be seen.

Then palpate the genitalia, starting by feeling for enlarged inguinal lymph nodes before proceeding to the penis. If nodes are palpable, assess number, size, and tenderness. Remember that enlarged lymph nodes might be due to malignancy as well as to infection, and if they are due to infection, they might not be sexually transmitted (e.g., tuberculosis, tularemia, plague).

Palpate the body of the penis for areas of induration that might be due to Peyronie's disease, tumors, or a foreign body. If a male patient is uncircumcised, gently retract the prepuce or ask the patient to do so, both to exclude a phimosis and to inspect the glans penis, urethral meatus, and inner surface of the prepuce for lesions. There may be a visible abnormality of the meatus, such as a hypospadias or, less commonly, an epispadias. The metal opening should be carefully examined for the presence of meatal or intraurethral condylomata.

If there is a urethral discharge, note whether it is profuse or slight in amount and whether its consistency is purulent, mucoid, or mucopurulent. If no discharge is visible, determine whether discharge is elicited by "milking," or "stripping," the urethra. This is done by holding the glans penis between the index finger and thumb of one hand in the 12 o'clock and 6 o'clock positions, and using the fingers of the other hand to exert gentle pressure on the underside of the shaft of the penis, moving them from the base of the penis toward the glans to see whether this produces a discharge visible at the meatus. This is the appropriate time to take a urethral swab for microscopy (if available) and microbiological tests, if required.

Specimen Collection

The most widely used tests for gonocorrhea and chlamydia are nucleic acid amplification assays, which can use either urethral swabs or first void urine samples. Gram stains can be performed on discharge, by adsorbing expressed discharge onto a glass microscope slide and delivering to the laboratory for staining and analysis. Urethral swabs are performed if there is no expressed discharge present, or if a culture is being performed. Urethral swabs are performed with narrow swabs, typically calcium alginate wire swabs. The swab is passed 1-2 centimeters into the urethra and then rapidly withdrawn. If a culture is performed, the swab is then immediately rolled across the surface of the culture media.

If genital ulcers are found during the examination, they should be gently blotted with a moist sterile gauze. If cultures for HSV are performed, a sterile swab should be pressed into the ulcer, to ensure that the surface cells and exudates are adsorbed onto the swab. For darkfield examination for syphilis, a clean glass slide is pressed against the base of the ulcer. As soon as it is removed, a drop of sterile saline may be added to keep it moist and it is covered immediately with a glass cover slip.

Scrotum

Next, palpate the scrotal contents, using both hands to palpate each side in turn. Feel the testis, noting whether it is present or absent (cryptorchidism), and if so, whether it is of normal size and tender. If a lump is felt in the testis, then investigate to exclude a malignancy (the testis is the commonest site of a malignancy in the younger male). A swelling in the scrotum may be a hydrocele; attempt to transilluminate it using a small light.

If the testis is unusually small, this may be due to atrophy, which can be congenital or result from prior infection (e.g., mumps), surgery (e.g., for maldescent of the testis), or torsion. Small firm testes are also a feature of Kleinfelter's syndrome, which affects 0.2% of men and is due to the presence of an additional X chromosome (i.e., XXY) and is associated with infertility. A swollen and painful testis is most likely due to epididymo-orchitis (see Chapter 21), but could also result from torsion of the testis. Torsion most commonly occurs in the adolescent male (younger than 18 years of age) and is a surgical emergency since delay of a few hours can lead to avoidable loss of the testicle. Finally, palpate the spermatic cord up to where it exits the scrotal sac. A swelling here is most likely due to a varicocoele with a distinctive "bag of worms" character but can also be due to a hydrocele or inguinal hernia. The genital examination can be concluded once swabs have been obtained for microbiological tests.

Perianal Area

Examination of the perianal area and rectum is indicated in the MSM who has reported recent receptive anal or oro-anal sex and in all men who report symptoms relating to the anus (pain or lump), rectum (rectal discharge or bleeding, pain on defecation), or prostate (poor urinary stream, nocturia, terminal dribbling of urine at the end of micturition, perineal pain, hematuria) (see Chapter 27).

The patient should be asked to move into the left lateral position and to draw his knees up toward his body. The clinician should then separate the buttocks and inspect the perianal area and natal cleft. Lesions in this area can indicate STI (e.g., condylomata acuminata due to human papillomavirus infection, condylomata lata due to secondary syphilis, ulceration due to herpes simplex virus) or other pathology (e.g., external hemorrhoids, anal fissures, or fistulas). In the absence of symptoms, this part of the examination can be completed by obtaining samples for microbiological tests by inserting a swab blindly through the anus. If the patient has reported rectal symptoms, then proctoscopy should be performed using a well-lubricated instrument. This allows the rectum to be visualized and swabs can be taken through the proctoscope.

Finally, if there is a history of prostatic symptoms, then a digital rectal examination should be carried out using the lubricated index finger of the examiner's gloved hand. The size and consistency of the prostate gland should be assessed and any tenderness noted. A normal prostate has a diameter of approximately 4 centimeters, a rubbery consistency, and both lobes and the dividing median sulcus are palpable. Unusual tenderness suggests infection, and an enlarged prostate might be due to benign prostatic hyperplasia, malignancy, calculi, or infection (see Chapter 27). It might be possible to palpate the seminal vesicles lateral to the prostate and extend superiorly.

Rarely, these are enlarged due to a pathological process (e.g., malignancy, tuberculosis). A rectal mass might be felt. Sometimes, painful perianal conditions (e.g., herpes simplex virus infection, thrombosed external hemorrhoids) will prevent digital or proctoscopic examination, and these may need to be deferred to a subsequent visit. Once the examination has been completed, the clinician should tell the patient what the next stage in the consultation will be and then leave them to dress in privacy.

■ KEY POINTS

- A physical examination is usually unnecessary in a male patient who has no symptoms, unless the patient is judged by the clinician to be at particularly high risk of STI.

- Undergoing a genital examination is embarrassing. Minimize this for the patient by a good bedside manner, by explaining what will be done in advance and reinforcing this during the examination, and by respecting the patient's privacy and dignity at all times.

- Consider in advance whether to have a chaperone present. In general, a chaperone should be offered but not insisted upon if the patient refuses the offer.

- Remember to extend the genital examination to other areas, depending on the sexual history and symptoms. In particular, carry out on a general physical examination if disseminated disease is possible: examine for lymphadenopathy and inspect the skin and mucous membranes (especially the mouth) if syphilis or HIV is suspected.

REFERENCES

Alexander S, Ison C, Parry J, et al. Self-taken pharyngeal and rectal swabs are appropriate for the detection of *Chlamydia trachomatis* and *Neisseria gonorrhoeae* in asymptomatic men who have sex with men. *Sex Transm Infect.* 2008;84:488–492.

Bignell CJ. Chaperones for genital examination. *BMJ.* 1999; 319:137–138.

Cohen CE, McLean KA, Barton SE. Chaperoning in GUM clinics. *Sex Transm Infect.* 2004;80:250.

Cohen C, McLean K, Barton S. Chaperones protect both parties. *BMJ.* 2005;330:846–847.

Gaydos CA, Ferrero DV, Papp J. Laboratory aspects of screening men for *Chlamydia trachomatis* in the new millennium. *Sex Transm Dis.* 2008;35(11):S45–S50.

General Medical Council. Maintaining boundaries. http://www.gmc-uk.org/guidance/current/library/maintaining_boundaries.asp. Accessed September 2009.

Krieger JN, Graney DO. Clinical anatomy and physical examination of the male genital tract. In: Holmes KK, Sparling PF, Stamm WE, et al, eds. *Sexually Transmitted Diseases.* 4th ed. New York: McGraw-Hill; 2008.

Van der Pol B, Ferrero DV, Buck-Barrington L, et al. Multicenter evaluation of the BDProbeTec ET system for detection of *Chlamydia trachomatis* and *Neisseria gonorrhoeae* in urine specimens, female endocervical swabs, and male urethral swabs. *J Clin Microbiol.* 2001;39: 1008–1016.

Van der Pol B, Quinn TC, Gaydos CA, et al. Multicenter evaluation of the AMPLICOR and automated COBAS AMPLICOR CT/NG tests for detection of *Chlamydia trachomatis. J Clin Microbiol.* 2000;38:(3):1005–1112.

4

Examination of the Female Patient

Jean M. Keller, Jean R. Anderson, and Elizabeth Claydon

■ OVERVIEW

Examination of the female urinary and reproductive systems can reveal important information to aid both the diagnosis of sexually transmitted infections (STIs) and other significant gynecological conditions, such as endometriosis. Unlike the male, the urinary and reproductive systems in females are anatomically separate. However, for convenience in this description, they are referred to collectively as the "female urogenital tract." The female urogenital tract is less accessible than that of the male. This fact influences the facilities, the equipment, and the time needed to perform an adequate urogenital tract examination in female patients.

The female urogenital tract is susceptible to a range of sexually transmitted pathogens. Many factors influence this susceptibility, including the type of epithelial cells that line the urogenital tract, the age of the woman, her hormonal status, the presence of cervical ectopy, and the integrity of the normal urogenital defense mechanisms. For example, bacterial pathogens, such as *Neisseria gonorrhoea* and *Chlamydia trachomatis*, have a particular affinity for the specific types of epithelial cells found in both the urethra and the cervix.

Another important consideration when examining the female patient is that while men frequently experience early symptoms and signs of STIs, prompting rapid diagnosis and treatment, women are far more likely to carry infections asymptomatically in the urogenital tract where they may remain undetected and untreated for years. This factor in turn contributes to the higher rate of major long-term consequences of STIs seen in women.

These consequences include upper genital tract infection, chronic pelvic pain, infertility, adverse pregnancy outcomes, and genital cancer. For instance, the majority of cervical cancer has now been linked to infection of the female urogenital tract with oncogenic types of human papillomavirus (HPV). Although HPV-related cancer is relatively rare in men, cervical cancer is the second most common cancer in women in areas of the world where routine screening is not readily available.

Although this chapter focuses on the examination of the female urogenital tract, a basic examination for STIs, as well as diagnosis of a range of other significant conditions that can affect the female urogenital tract, may need to include a more comprehensive examination of the patient. A careful and systematic clinical history along with assessment of risk factors and a review of presenting symptoms and signs are essential in guiding the subsequent examination. Other anatomical areas that are particularly important to consider in this context include the skin and hair, oral mucosa and pharynx, regional lymph nodes, abdominal organs, and the anorectal area.

To elicit the necessary information, interviewing the patient in a sensitive, nonjudgmental manner will help to develop rapport, encourage trust, and, most importantly, increase the patient's level of comfort during the subsequent examination. The examiner must be fully familiar with his or her equipment, including the vaginal speculums and proctoscopes, and with conducting a bimanual pelvic examination and rectal examination in female patients. Urogenital examinations are often daunting for female patients, and they need to feel confident that their examiner is both competent and caring. Opportunity for adequate preparation, training, assessment, and supervision for practitioners involved in this area are vital.

In this chapter, we briefly describe the anatomy of the female urogenital tract, outline techniques for examination, and discuss specimen collection and association of possible findings with some of the more common sexually transmitted pathogens.

ANATOMY OF THE FEMALE UROGENITAL TRACT

External Genitalia

Landmarks to note during examination of the female external genitalia include the following (see Figure 4-1):

The mons

Labia majora

Labia minora

Clitoris

Vestibule (the oval fossa between the labia minora and the vaginal opening)

The urethral orifice

The introitus (vaginal opening)

Skene's (paraurethral) glands

Bartholin's glands

The perineum (tissue between the introitus and the anus)

The mons is the hair-bearing fat pad that covers the pubic symphysis. Extending from the mons backward, the labia majora are folds of skin containing hair follicles and sebaceous and sweat glands. The labia minora lie medial to the labia majora and split anteriorly to form the prepuce and frenulum of the clitoris. Posteriorly, they extend to the perineum. The labia minora contain sebaceous glands, but no hair follicles or sweat glands. The clitoris is composed of erectile tissue and is located in the midline anterior to the urethral opening or urethral meatus. The oval-shaped vestibule lies between the labia minora and extends from the clitoris anteriorly to the posterior fourchette posteriorly.

The vaginal and urethral openings lie in the midline and open into the vestibule. Skene's glands (paraurethral glands) lie adjacent to the distal part of the urethra and have ducts that open into the distal urethra or just outside the urethral meatus. Bartholin's glands (greater vestibular glands) are paired glands that lie at 5 o'clock and 7 o'clock beneath the posterior lateral aspect of the vaginal orifice and open into a groove between the hymen (or its remnants) and the labia minora.

THE VAGINA AND CERVIX

The vagina is a fibromuscular tube that lies between the urethra anteriorly and the rectum posteriorly. The entrance to the vagina externally is called the introitus. The introitus lies just within the vestibule. Remnants

FIGURE 4-1 Female External Reproductive Organs

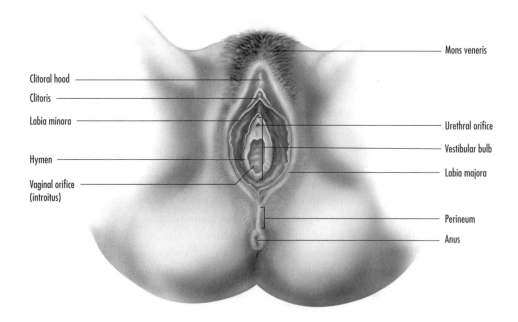

Clitoral hood

Clitoris

Labia minora

Hymen

Vaginal orifice (introitus)

Mons veneris

Urethral orifice

Vestibular bulb

Labia majora

Perineum

Anus

of the hymen, the membrane that originally covered the entrance to the vagina, may often be seen around the introitus and may be mistaken by patients for genital warts. The upper portion of the vagina forms a cup-shaped fornix around the cervix, the lower part of the uterus that protrudes into the upper part of the vagina. The fornix is divided into anterior, lateral, and posterior areas by the cervix.

The cervix is the narrow lower section of the uterus that can be seen on speculum examination at the top of the vagina. The cervix consists predominately of dense connective tissue. At the lower end of the cervix is a constricted opening called the external os. This provides a communication between the lumen of the cervix and the uterus above, and the vagina below. The external os may be small and round in the nulliparous women, but the shape is altered in women who have had vaginal deliveries and may range from round to slitlike or stellate appearance after childbirth.

The part of the cervix that extends into the vagina is called the ectocervix and is covered by nonkeratinized, stratified squamous epithelium. This stratified squamous epithelium has a junction with the simple columnar epithelium that lines the neck of the cervical canal. This junction is known as the transformation zone. The position of the squamocolumnar junction, or transformation zone, varies. In older women, it usually lies within the cervical canal. In adolescents and young women, the columnar epithelium may extend out beyond the external os on to the vaginal portion of the cervix where it is visible on speculum examination and is known as cervical ectopy, or ectropion. This normal appearance may be confused with changes due to infection or neoplastic changes. Inspection of the surface of the cervix often reveals small translucent or blue lumps just under the epithelium. These lumps are known as Nabothian follicles and are harmless, representing trapped mucous secretion.

■ UTERUS, FALLOPIAN TUBES, AND OVARIES

The uterus is a pear-shaped fibromuscular structure that lies between the bladder anteriorly and the rectum posteriorly. The upper two-thirds of the uterus is called the body, and the lower third is the cervix. The fallopian tubes extend from each side of the body of the uterus. The rounded part of the body above the attachment of the fallopian tubes is called the fundus. The isthmus is a short, slightly constricted portion of the uterus that joins the body and the cervix. The average size of the uterus is 5–7 centimeters in length and 4–5 centimeters in width.

The broad ligament is attached to each side of the uterus and is composed of a double layer of peritoneum enclosing neurovascular and lymphatic structures. The uterus is supported by the uterosacral and cardinal ligaments as well as a thin layer of investing connective tissue and the muscles and connective tissue of the pelvic floor.

The fallopian tubes extend from each side of the uterine fundus, curving towards the ovaries. The distal portion of the fallopian tubes are funnel shaped and open into the peritoneal cavity with fringed, finger-shaped fimbriae surrounding an ovary on each side of the uterus. The ovaries are almond-shaped organs attached to the fundus of the uterus medially on each side by the ovarian ligament. The ovaries receive their blood supply bilaterally through the infundibular pelvic ligament. The ovaries vary in size over the menstrual cycle, 3–5 centimeters long and 2–3 centimeters wide in childbearing years. They diminish in size by two-thirds after menopause and by that time should be nonpalpable.

■ THE EXAMINATION

At the beginning of the urogenital tract examination, there are some general considerations to keep in mind.

1. The patient should be invited to empty her bladder before the examination unless the history suggests that a urethral swab is indicated (for example, in a gonorrhea contact with urethral symptoms). A urine specimen should be obtained and kept in case it is needed for further analysis.

2. The examination couch and all other equipment should be prepared in advance. Appropriately designed examination couches and deep-cavity lighting should be used. Set the height and position of the examination couch, along with the lighting arrangement, to ease the examination and to maximize both the comfort of the patient and of the practitioner. Attention to getting these factors right can make the difference between a straightforward and comfortable examination and a traumatic experience for both the patient and the practitioner.

3. The speculum, especially metal ones, should always be warmed before use. Disposable plastic speculums can also be used.

4. Having an assistant available to help with the examination is strongly recommended (and essential if the examiner is male) to maximize the efficiency

of the examination, to avoid contamination of instruments, and to act as an advocate for the patient, as well as providing a chaperone for medicolegal reasons. (See Chapter 3 about the examination of the male patient for a more detailed discussion of chaperoning and trainee observers.)

5. Many patients are reluctant to tell the examiner when they feel uncomfortable or experience pain. It is helpful to specifically ask the patient at the beginning of the examination to report any undue discomfort immediately.

6. The patient should be draped appropriately with the drape extending over the knees, covering the legs and adjusted to ensure that the patient's dignity is maintained at all times. Some patients will prefer to be able to make eye contact with the examiner during the examination and some will prefer the drape to obscure eye contact.

7. The patient should be given adequate privacy and time to undress and position themselves on the couch.

External Genitalia

Using adequate lighting, the examination should begin with a thorough inspection of the external genitalia and inguinal region. Throughout the examination, the patient should be kept informed about what the examiner is doing and invited to comment if anything is painful or distressing. The inguinal lymph glands should be palpated and the location, mobility, number, size, and tenderness of any lymph glands recorded. The skin of the mons, inner thighs, perineum, and external labia majora should be carefully inspected. It is also important to inspect specifically the skin in the groin creases and the perianal area. Note should be made of the distribution of the hair in the area, plus any abnormalities of the skin, such as eczema, psoriasis, folliculitis as well as infective conditions such as warts, molluscum contagiosum, and pubic lice. There are marked individual differences in the characteristics and distribution of pubic hair. What might be considered hirsute in women from East Asia is often normal in women from southern Europe or the Middle East. Thinning of the pubic hair is normal in postmenopausal women, whereas patchy hair loss may be a feature of a range of diseases, such as syphilis and thyroid abnormalities. Pubic lice ("crab lice") can be identified from the appearance of small white eggs that adhere to the shaft of the pubic hair (and occasion-

ally the eye lashes). The pubic lice themselves may be seen moving within the hair-bearing area or occasionally fixed to the skin surface (see Chapter 13).

The labia should then be gently separated and the entire vulva carefully inspected. The inner aspects of the labia majora differ from the outer portions in that they are non–hair bearing.

Ulcers may occur on any part of the genitalia and have a range of causes, such as inflammatory, infective, and neoplastic conditions, including herpes simplex virus, syphilis, chancroid, aphthous ulceration, pemphigus, erosive lichen planus, pemphigoid, and Behçet's disease. All ulcerative lesions should be swabbed for herpes simplex virus (HSV), and venous blood for syphilis serology should be obtained. Additional investigations of genital ulcers will be dictated by the patient's age, past medical history, family history, travel history, and previous sexual contacts (see Chapter 17). Biopsy should be performed on all ulcers that appear atypical or fail to heal. Other significant lesions that affect the external genitalia include genital warts caused by human papillomavirus and molluscum contagiosum caused by a poxvirus. Genital warts may appear as typical cauliflower-like lesions, either singly or in groups, and may be flat or form continuous sheets. The posterior introitus is a common area for warts to develop, and this site should be carefully inspected as they can be easily overlooked (see Chapter 22). Visible warts are usually benign, but occasionally infection with oncogenic types of wart virus may cause atypical lesions to occur (vulval intraepithelial neoplasia, or VIN). These are usually flat lesions on the labia that may ulcerate and occasionally become invasive. Molluscum contagiosum are small, rounded umbilicated lesions with a central core of material that contain the poxvirus particles. They are usually transmitted by close contact and occur on the lower abdomen, inner thighs and outer aspects of the labia. Molluscum contagiosum are benign lesions that usually resolve spontaneously without treatment.

The greater vestibular glands (Bartholin's glands) are located at 5 o'clock and 7 o'clock in the vestibule. During the examination, the vestibular glands should be gently palpated by placing the thumb on the outer labia and the forefinger at the vaginal introitus. Each side should be evaluated for swelling and tenderness and any drainage from the duct noted. Normally, the gland should not be palpable; however, in some women, an asymptomatic ductal cyst may be present that does not require further treatment. Bartholin's glands may be involved in a number of pathological processes. An infected gland is enlarged and exquisitely tender. An abscess (Bartholin's abscess) may form that requires incision and drainage if fluctuant. Such an abscess may be associated with sexually transmitted pathogens, and full screening for these is important.

The opening of the vestibular glands may become inflamed and tender to touch externally as part of a condition called "vulval vestibulitis," which is an important cause of genital pain (see Chapter 26). Any solid mass that is detected in this area in postmenopausal women requires excision biopsy.

Next, the labia minora should be separated to inspect the introitus for any signs of redness, swelling, fissures, ulceration, or discharge. Redness, swelling, and discharge visible at the introitus is commonly due to fungal infection (usually *Candida albicans*) or less commonly *Trichomonas vaginalis* infection (TV) (see Chapter 7). Fissuring between the labia is also commonly seen with fungal infection but may also represent an atypical herpetic infection, so this finding should prompt taking a swab for HSV culture from the area (see Chapter 18). With the labia still separated, it is possible to observe vaginal relaxation and to look for any stress incontinence by asking the patient to cough or bear down. Any bulging of the vaginal walls, for example, due to a rectocele or cystocele or leakage of urine can be noted.

The urethral meatus is located between the clitoris anteriorly and the vaginal introitus. Its position should be identified and any erythema or discharge noted. If urethritis is suspected, the urethral meatus can be milked for discharge by placing the index finger into the vagina and gently stroking the urethra from inside out. Skene's glands, which lie on either side of the urethral meatus, should also be examined at the same time for inflammation and discharge.

Speculum Examination

The speculums used for examining the vagina and cervix are available in metal and plastic both of which may be disposable (see Figure 4-2). They come in a range of sizes and lengths. The smallest size for adequate examination should be chosen. The size required depends on the patient's age, parity, and weight. A medium speculum is usually adequate to view the cervix and tolerated well by most women. Larger or longer speculums are available for women whose cervix is not accessible with a medium speculum. Virginal and pediatric speculums are also

FIGURE 4-2   Medical Examination with Speculum and Spatula in Place

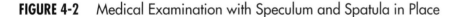
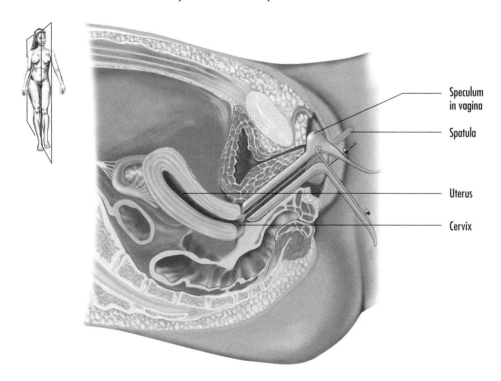

available for adolescents, women whose hymen is still intact, postmenopausal women with a narrowed introitus, and women who may have particular anxieties about speculum examinations. It should be remembered, however, that the view of the cervix offered by the smaller speculums may be slightly restricted so that their use should be use reserved for carefully selected cases.

The speculum should always be warmed before use and lubricated with water. Lubricating gels and oils should be avoided as they can interfere with interpretation of some samples such as Pap smears. At the beginning of the procedure, the patient should be touched gently on the inner thigh and informed that the speculum is going to be inserted. The patient should be asked to relax the perineal muscles to help with speculum insertion. The speculum is held at a 45° angle and, with the labia apart, introduced into the vaginal introitus. An alternative technique is to press two fingers posteriorly just inside the introitus, and the speculum slides over the fingers into the vagina. Once the speculum has been inserted into the vagina, it can be rotated into a flat position and then advanced farther into the vagina with gentle downward pressure to avoid pressing on the sensitive urethra. The speculum can then be opened until the cervix comes into view. This requires practice and should always be done as gently as possible as it can be uncomfortable for some women. If the cervix is difficult to locate it is preferable to remove the speculum and insert a finger into the vagina to locate the position of the cervix, reposition the patient if necessary, and reinsert the speculum, rather than trying to open the speculum wider and wider in an attempt to visualize the cervix. When the cervix is fully in view, the speculum can be locked into position. Once locked, the speculum will normally stay in place, freeing the examiner's hands to obtain specimens.

With the speculum in place the following should be noted:

1. The presence of any discharge. Its volume, color, and consistency. Try to establish whether the discharge is originating from the vaginal walls or the cervix. This will help to determine the cause of the discharge.

2. Characteristics of the vaginal wall. Presence of inflammation, ulceration, hemorrhage, or lesions such as warts should be identified. Ensure that the portions of the vagina in front of, behind, and to the sides of the cervix (fornices) of the vagina are also carefully inspected, as abnormalities in these areas can be overlooked. Occasionally, retained foreign bodies such as tampons or condoms can be concealed.

3. The cervix should be inspected. The cervical os should be identified. If discharge is present, whether it is arising from the ectocervix or coming through the cervical os should be noted. The characteristics of the discharge, including volume, color, and consistency and any blood should be recorded. A clear mucoid discharge may be present, and this is normal. Its volume and consistency varies throughout the menstrual cycle. The presence of purulent or blood stained discharge indicates an abnormality and it is often associated with infections such as chlamydia or gonorrhea. Inflammation of the cervix (cervicitis) needs to be distinguished from the condition of cervical ectropion, or ectopy. Cervical ectropion is a circumferential area around the cervical os where the cells of the transformation zone are clearly visible. Cervical ectopy can be associated with an increase in mucoid discharge. Cervical ectropion is commonly seen in younger women or women taking oral hormonal contraceptives.

The cervix may demonstrate several other characteristic appearances. "Strawberry cervix" is a name given to the appearance of the cervix caused by the protozoan parasite *T. vaginalis* (see Chapter 7). The strawberry appearance is caused by multiple small petechial lesions on the surface of the cervix, which may bleed easily. Single or multiple areas of ulceration may occur on the cervix and should prompt sampling for herpes simplex infection and screening for syphilis. Warty lesions may also be seen on the cervix (see Chapter 22). These lesions may range from typical exuberant exophytic warts to subtle flat areas of warty change. Any warty change visible on the cervix should be evaluated by a trained coloposcopist A common lesion found on the cervix is the Nabothian follicle, or Nabothian cyst, which is a benign condition caused by the transformation of mucus-producing columnar epithelial cells to squamous epithelial cells at the transformation zone of the cervix, trapping mucus and forming a cyst.

Having noted these features, and when the appropriate specimens have been taken, the speculum can be gently and carefully removed by unlocking the jaws and partially closing them to avoid trapping the cervix. The jaws can then be fully closed as the speculum is moved into the lower portion of the vagina, while taking care to avoid pinching the vaginal wall.

Bimanual Examination

The bimanual, pelvic examination is normally carried out after the speculum examination (see Figure 4-3).

FIGURE 4-3 Bimanual Examination

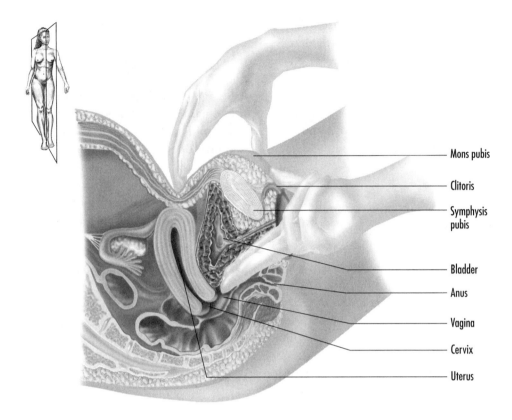

Mons pubis

Clitoris

Symphysis pubis

Bladder

Anus

Vagina

Cervix

Uterus

The operator usually stands to allow eye contact with the patient. Two hands are used, the vaginal hand and the abdominal hand. The aim is to evaluate the pelvic structures, including the uterus, fallopian tubes, ovaries, bladder, and supporting structures. With gloved hands, the middle and index fingers of the vaginal hand are lubricated. The labia are gently parted with the abdominal hand, and the middle and index fingers of the vaginal hand are slowly and gently inserted into the vagina with slight downward pressure. The cervix is located, noting its position, shape and consistency, mobility, and any tenderness. Moving the cervix from side to side is not normally painful, although it may be uncomfortable. Any cervical motion tenderness ("cervical excitation") during this part of the examination may be an important sign of pathology, including pelvic infection, pelvic inflammatory disease (PID), or ectopic pregnancy, which may be associated with the presence of an adnexal mass. The abdominal hand should be placed at the level of the umbilicus and gentle pressure applied, moving the abdominal hand toward the pelvis in the midline while applying pressure with the vaginal hand anteriorly, elevating the cervix until the uterus is felt. The operator may find resting the elbow on the hip or knee if seated may be useful in stabilizing the arm of the vaginal

hand. With the uterus trapped between the vaginal and the abdominal hand, the uterine fundus is palpated for size, shape, contour, mobility, and tenderness. The size of the uterus is variable but should not normally be greater than 9 cm by 6 cm in parous women. An enlarged uterus can be a sign of pregnancy or indicate the presence of uterine fibroids. A small uterus is found in postmenopausal women or in women on the oral contraceptive pill.

Next, the abdominal hand should be placed in the right lower quadrant of the abdomen and the finger of the vaginal hand in the right fornix, displacing the uterus to the opposite side. Gentle downward pressure should be applied with the abdominal hand while trying to identify the right ovary with the vaginal hand. The examination is then repeated on the left side so that both adnexae (which includes the fallopian tubes, ovaries, and their supporting structures) have been assessed. The ovaries in women of reproductive age should not be larger than 5 cm and should not be palpable at all in postmenopausal women. Fallopian tubes are not normally palpable in women of any age. The size, shape, mobility, and tenderness of any of these structures plus the presence of any masses should be carefully noted. A palpable ovary in a postmenopausal woman should always prompt suspicion of neoplasia and immediate evaluation is indicated. Tenderness, thickening, or palpable masses in the fallopian tubes likewise indicate the need for further investigation. Bilateral tenderness along with pain on movement of the uterus or cervix ("positive cervical excitation") is often a sign of an infective or inflammatory process. Ectopic pregnancy should always be considered if tenderness is more marked on one side of the pelvis than the other. That the appendix also extends into the pelvis and may become inflamed should also be remembered.

Examination of the Oropharynx, Rectum, and Rectovaginal Examination

Comprehensive examination of the female patient for sexually transmitted infections should include the oropharynx and rectum when indicated by clinical history or symptoms. When examining the oropharynx, the patient should be seated comfortably. The occipital, cervical, submaxillary, and submental lymph glands should be palpated for any tenderness and enlargement. The mouth and oropharynx should be carefully inspected with a suitable light and the presence of any abnormalities such as ulceration noted. Appropriate specimens should be obtained from any areas of ulceration and from the posterior pharynx, tonsils, and tonsillar crypts.

Examination of the rectum is usually carried out after the vaginal speculum examination. It should start with a thorough inspection of the perineal and perianal skin. The presence of any abnormalities of the skin, such as inflammation or fissuring, viral warts, or ulceration, should be noted and the anal canal inspected for any signs of discharge or bleeding. In patients without rectal symptoms, samples from the anorectal area may be obtained by placing a moist swab, 2–4 cm into the anal canal and using gentle lateral pressure to allow contact with the rectal mucosa. In symptomatic patients, anorectal specimens should be obtained under direct vision following the insertion of a proctoscope. The proctoscopes used in this situation are usually disposable plastic and require a suitable light source. The patient is positioned on the left side with her knees drawn up. The proctoscope is lubricated with a suitable lubricating jelly and inserted gently into the anus in the direction of the umbilicus. The introducer (central core portion of the proctoscope) is then removed to allow the rectal mucosa to be directly observed. The presence of any discharge, ulceration, bleeding, or other abnormalities such as

warts should be carefully noted and appropriate samples taken. The proctoscope can then be gently withdrawn noting any lesions of the anal canal as this is done.

The need for a digital rectovaginal examination may be indicated by either the patient's history or the findings on bimanual examination. A digital rectovaginal examination allows confirmation of the findings on the bimanual examination and enables evaluation of 1–2 cm higher in the pelvis than the bimanual pelvic examination alone. It also allows further assessment of the lower gastrointestinal tract. The procedure should be carefully explained to the patient before the examination. Gloves should be replaced and relubricated. The patient should be asked to bear down (Valsalva maneuver) while a lubricated middle finger is inserted slowly into the rectum and the index finger of the other hand is inserted into the vagina. The maneuvers undertaken during the bimanual pelvic examination should be repeated to ensure that all areas of the pelvis have been palpated. The characteristics of the rectal mucosa along with any masses should be noted and the posterior pelvis, posterior uterine fundus, and the rectovaginal septum should be palpated. Characteristics of the uterus, particularly if it is retroverted or retroflexed, are often easiest to ascertain with this examination. The presence of stool in the rectum should be noted. If indicated by the history, the stool may be tested for occult blood, although the sensitivity and specificity of this test is not optimal.

Specimen Collection

The specimens that should be obtained will depend on the patient's history, risk assessment, and findings on clinical examination. Criteria for selection of diagnostic tests for STIs should also account for whether the tests are used for individual diagnosis or for screening purposes. The costs, disease prevalence, test performance, and legal and social considerations are also important. Diagnostic laboratory tests for STIs and screening strategies will be discussed in future chapters.

Specimens obtained may include urethral and endocervical samples for Gram's staining and culture; samples, usually from the vagina, for bacterial, fungal, and trichomonal isolation; viral cultures from any ulcerated lesions; a wet mount (wet prep); measurement of the vaginal pH; and a Papanicolaou smear (Pap, or cervical smear). Venous blood samples will be necessary to screen for infections such as syphilis, and for diagnosis of the bloodborne viruses, including HIV, hepatitis B, and hepatitis C. Recent advances in laboratory detection techniques using amplification of specific nucleic acid sequences, including polymerase chain reaction (PCR), ligase chain reaction (LCR), and gene probe transcription-mediated amplification (TMA) have seen significant increases in the sensitivity of diagnostic tests for *Chlamydia trachomatis* and *Neisseria gonorrhoea* (see Chapter 19). These new techniques have also led to changes in the samples that are needed. In many cases, noninvasive samples using vulval or low vaginal swabs (which can be self-taken) or urine samples are proving to be as sensitive as urethral and cervical samples). It is therefore important to check with your local diagnostic laboratory to determine which techniques are available for the most effective samples to take in each case. It is with these considerations in mind that the following general guidance is given.

Recommended Specimens for Screening Asymptomatic Women

Current recommendations for screening in women without any symptoms include taking samples for syphilis, HIV antibodies, *N. gonorrhoea*, and *C. trachomatis* (www.bashh.org/guidelines). Syphilis and HIV are screened for using venous blood samples. Gonorrhea and chlamydia are currently tested for by obtaining swabs in women, although less invasive tests, including urine samples, and self-taking vaginal samples are also available, depending on local laboratories.

Site(s) of sampling will depend on the sexual history and whether a woman has had a hysterectomy. The endocervix is the currently recommended sampling site for screening for gonorrhea and chlamydia with the urethra being used if the woman has had a hysterectomy. Pharyngeal and rectal samples for gonorrhea may also be taken if the clinical history indicates exposure of these sites. Endocervical samples for gonorrhea are collected after the cervix has been visualized as part of the speculum examination. The sample is obtained by inserting a cotton-tipped swab into the cervical os and gently rotating it for about 5 seconds. If nonmolecular testing methods for gonorrhea are used, the swab is then placed in suitable transport media, or plated onto special gonococcal culture media and transferred to a CO_2 incubator. *Chlamydia trachomatis* is an obligate intracellular organism, and samples obtained from the endocervix should be taken in accordance with the manufacturer's instructions for each given sampling kit. In general, the swab is inserted into the cervical os and rotated to increase the collection of cellular material. If it is not possible to visualize the cervix (for example, in children, or women with vaginismus), it may be appropriate to obtain material from the lower part of the vagina. Urethral specimens are obtained with a fine-tipped cotton swab inserted into the urethral meatus for about 1 cm.

Rectal swabs for gonorrhea may be taken if the clinical history indicates exposure at this site. Swabs are obtained by passing a cotton-tipped swab moistened with saline through the anal canal and then asking the patient to bear down so as to bring the rectal mucosa into contact with the tip of the swab. Pharyngeal specimens for gonorrhea should be obtained if indicated by the history. The patient should be seated upright with a good light source and a tongue depressor used. Swabs are obtained by gently rolling a cotton-tipped swab over the tonsillar areas and posterior pharynx.

The Papanicolaou Smear

The Papanicolaou (Pap) smear is a screening tool used to examine the squamocolumnar junction within the cervical transformation zone for precancerous changes or cervical intraepithelial neoplasia (CIN). The age at which the first Pap smear examination is recommended and the frequency of screening vary from country to country. Local guidance and protocols should be followed. The Pap smear can be done as part of a general screen for other sexually transmitted infections. When taking a Pap smear it is important that the speculum is lubricated with warm water rather than lubricant jellies, as these can interfere with interpretation of the results. Most developed countries now use liquid-based cytology for cervical screening. Samples are obtained from the endocervix with a flexible plastic brush. It is important that the whole of the cervix is visualized and that the entire circumference of the squamocolumnar junction is sampled. The transformation zone may extend up into the endocervical canal.

Women should be warned that they may feel some discomfort as the Pap smear is taken, but women frequently feel no sensation at all. The degree of discomfort may be exaggerated if there is an infection of the cervix. The CDC has recommended collecting Pap smears before the swabs are taken. However, this may cause bleeding, which can interfere with the performance of some nonculture tests for STIs. In some clinics, therefore, the swabs are taken before the Pap smear is done. It is not known whether this decreases the performance of the pap test.

Summary of STI Screening Tests of Choice in Asymptomatic Women

Site of Specimen

Venous Blood	Syphilis (EIA or TPPA or cardiolipin test plus TPHA) HIV antibodies
Cervix	Culture for *N. gonorrhoea* NAAT test for chlamydia (NAAT = Nucleic acid amplification test)

Note. Self-taken vaginal/vulval swabs, urethral swabs, and urine (if urethral swab is not available) may be used as alternative to cervical sample for chlamydia NAATS testing.

Recommended Specimens for Screening in Women with Genital Discharge

In women with symptoms of genital discharge, the following samples, taken as part of the speculum examination, are currently recommended to allow an appropriate diagnosis. A speculum is inserted into the vagina and the cervix visualized as described earlier. The clinical appearance of the vulva, vaginal walls, and cervix should be carefully assessed. The presence of any discharge and bleeding along with its site of origin (i.e., vaginal wall or cervix) should be carefully established. It is worth noting that chlamydia and gonorrhea cause inflammation and discharge from the cervix while fungal infections and bacterial vaginosis usually affect the walls of the vagina.

The optimal site of sampling from the vagina will depend on the clinical findings. A swab from the lateral vaginal walls should be obtained if there is a discharge associated with the vaginal wall, and this can be used to prepare a slide for both Gram's staining and for microbiological culture. Swabs for fungal typing are also useful in cases of persistent or recurrent fungal infection With the speculum in place, a pool of discharge will often collect in the tip of the speculum and in the posterior fornix of the vagina. The pH of this discharge can be assessed by taking a cotton-tipped swab of the discharge and touching it onto narrow range pH paper, avoiding the cervical mucous. Normal vaginal pH is around 4.5. A pH greater than 4.5 is seen in bacterial vaginosis and trichomonas infection (see Chapter 7). A lower pH is often seen in candida infection. The pH can be difficult to interpret if there are mixed infections or in the presence of cervical mucus (high pH) water, blood or semen.

A sample of discharge from the posterior fornix is also traditionally used to prepare a wet mount slide or "wet prep." This is then used to look for *T. vaginalis* and as supplementary evidence for other conditions, such as bacterial vaginosis. A wet mount slide is prepared by placing a small drop of normal saline onto a glass microscope slide and adding a sample of discharge obtained from the posterior fornix using a cotton-tipped swab or plastic loop and covering this with a glass coverslip. This preparation is then viewed immediately by direct microscopy for the presence of trichomonads. These protozoan parasites are about twice the size of white blood cells, independently mobile with visible flagellae. It has been estimated that direct observation for *T. vaginalis* has a sensitivity of approximately 70% when compared with culture (Bickley et al. 1989). Culture techniques for trichomonas are also available as are nucleic acid amplification tests. The presence of white blood cells (polymorphs) is also significant. Normally, the wet preparation should show predominantly epithelial cells with only occasional white blood cells. Greater than 1:1 white cells to epithelial cells should prompt evaluation for the presence of infection. "Clue cells" may also be identified. These are vaginal epithelial cells covered with bacteria that obscure the borders of the cells and give them a speckled or "salt and pepper" appearance. The presence of greater than 20% of clue cells without an increase in polymorphs suggests bacterial vaginosis (see Chapter 7).

The Gram's stained sample from the vaginal walls is useful for detection of both fungal infection (sensitivity approximately 70%) (Zdolsek et al. 1995) and of bacterial vaginosis. Other approaches include grading the vaginal flora on Gram's staining have been described, but these require specialized training

Amsel's criteria for diagnosis of bacterial vaginosis require at least three of the four criteria to be present to confirm the diagnosis:

1. Thin, white, homogeneous discharge.

2. Clue cells on microscopy of wet mount.

3. pH of vaginal fluid >4.5.

4. Release of fishy odor on adding alkali (10% KOH).

The Hay/Ison criteria are used to evaluate a Gram's stained vaginal smear. The Hay/Ison criteria are defined as follows:

Grade 1 (normal): Lactobacillus morphotypes predominate.

Grade 2 (intermediate): Mixed flora with some lactobacilli present, but Gardnerella or Mobiluncus morphotypes also present.

Grade 3 (bacterial vaginosis): Predominantly Gardnerella and/or Mobiluncus morphotypes. Few or absent lactobacilli.

In women presenting with genital discharge, swabs should also be taken from the endocervix for Gram's staining and cultures for gonorrhea and for chlamydia as described earlier. The rectum and oropharynx should also be swabbed for gonorrhea if indicated by the sexual history or clinical symptoms and signs. It may be necessary to take swabs by using a proctoscope if women describe symptoms such as rectal pain, bleeding, or discharge. It is recommended that all women presenting with genital tract discharge should also be offered screening for syphilis and HIV infection.

Summary of Tests of Choice for Women with Vaginal Discharge

Site of Specimen

Urethra	Microscopy (Gram's stain) plus culture for gonorrhoea
Cervix	Microscopy (Gram's stain) plus culture for gonorrhoea
	NAATS test for chlamydia
Vagina	Microscopy (Gram's stain) for fungal infection plus culture
	Microscopy ("wet prep") for Trichomonas vaginalis
	± culture Trichomonas vaginalis
	Microscopy (Gram's stain ± "wet prep") for bacterial vaginosis

Note. Self-taken vaginal, vulval/introital swabs may be used for NAATS testing for gonorrhea or chlamydia depending on local guidance and availability.

Rectum*	Culture for gonorrhea
	Tissue culture (or NAATS test if tissue culture not available) for chlamydia
Oropharynx*	Culture for gonorrhea
	Tissue culture (or NAATS test if tissue culture not available) for chlamydia
Urine	NAATS testing for chlamydia if cervical/ vaginal sample not available

NAATS = nucleic acid amplification tests.
* If indicated by sexual history, symptoms, and signs.

Recommended Tests for Women Presenting with Genital Ulceration

Women presenting with genital ulceration will frequently require screening for other STIs as described previously. It is particularly important to take a detailed history, including a careful drug and travel history both from the woman and her partner. Tests recommended for women presenting with genital ulceration should include the following:

Screening for syphilis
Dark ground microscopy or NAATS testing of swabs from the ulcer (if available), plus blood testing (syphilis EIA, IgM + IgG, TPPA, and cardiolipin test).

Screening for herpes simplex virus
Swab base of ulcer for viral culture or NAATS testing if available.

Additional tests if indicated by sexual history/travel history or signs:-

Chancroid: Ulcer swab for culture or NAATS testing if available.

Donovanosis: Direct microscopy of tissue sample from ulcer.

Lymphogranuloma venereum: Ulcer swab for NAATs testing, immunofluorescence, microscopy or culture.

Proctoscopy with direct visualization of the ulcer may be necessary for anorectal symptoms.

Herpes simplex virus is the commonest cause of painful genital ulceration likely to present in women (see Chapters 17 and 18). A sample for viral isolation should be obtained from vesicles if present or from the base of any ulcerative lesion. Viral isolation diminishes with the time that the ulcer has been present and is influenced by whether it is a primary or recurrent episode. It is estimated that use of PCR increases HSV detection rates by two to three times compared with viral culture).

Completion of the Examination

When the examination has been completed and all samples taken, the drapes should be pulled down to cover the genitalia and the patient helped to the sitting position. A tissue should be offered to clean the perineum. Gloves should be removed and hands washed before leaving the room to allow the patient to dress. Discussion of findings should be done after the patient has dressed.

■ KEY POINTS

- The female genital examination is a key part of STI and general reproductive health care.

- The examination should be conducted in a comfortable setting in a nonjudgmental manner.

- The external exam should focus on identifying mucosal and epithelial abnormailitis, genital ulcerations, and similar lesions. Careful attention should be paid to examine all mucosal and skin folds.

- The internal exam should delineate vaginal pathology, alterations in the cervical mucosa, presence of discharge or other lesions and presence of tenderness during the direct or bimanual examination.

- A lower abdominal examination, including a rectal exam when indicated, is important for defining pelvic pathology

- Routine specimens obtained include testing for gonorrhea and chlamydia, vaginal wet mount for trichomonas, yeast and bacterial vaginosis, and Pap smear when indicated. Other exams include herpes testing, direct dark field exam for syphilis, and pregnancy tests when clinically necessary.

REFERENCES

Amsel R, Totten PA, Speigal CA, Chen KC, Eschenback D, Holmes KK. Non-specific vaginitis: diagnostic criteria and microbial and epidemiologic associations. *Am J Med*. 1983;74:14–22.

Bergeron S, Binik YM, Khilife S, Pagidas K. Vulvar vestibulitis syndrome: a critical review. *Clin J Pain*. 1997;13:27–42.

Bickley LS, Krisher KK, Punsalang A, Trupei MA, Reichman RC, Menegos MA. Comparison of direct fluorescent antibody, acridine orange, wet mount and culture for detection of *Trichomomas vaginali*s in women attending a public sexually transmitted disease clinic. *Sex Trans Dis*. 1989;16:127–131.

Centers for Disease Control and Prevention. Recommendations for the prevention and management of *Chlamydia trachomatis* infections. *MMWR Morb Mortal Wkly Rep*. 1993;42(No. RR-12):1–39.

Centers for Disease Control and Prevention. Screening tests to detect *Chlamydia trachomatis* and *Neisseria gonorrhoea* infections. *MMWR Morb Mortal Wkly Rep*. 2002;51(No. RR-15):1–48.

Gelbart SM, Thomason JL, Osypowski, et al. Growth of *Trichomonas vaginalis* in commercial culture media. *J Clin Microbiol*. 1990;28:962–964.

Holmes KK, Sparling PF, Mardh P, et al. *Sexually Transmitted Diseases*. 3rd ed. New York: McGraw-Hill, 1998;120–123.

Ison CA, Hay PE. Validation of a simplified grading of gram stained vaginal smears for use in genito-urinary medicine clinics. *Sex Trans Infect*. 2002;78:413–415.

Knox J, Tabriz SN, Miller P, et al. Evaluation of self-collected samples for *Chlamydia trachomatis, Neisseria gonorrhoea* and *Trichomomas vaginalis* by polymerase chain reaction among women living in remote areas. *Sexually Transm Dis*. 2002;29:697–654.

Kolator B, Rodin P. Comparison of anal and rectal swabs in the diagnosis of ano rectal gonorrhoea in women. *Br J Vener Dis*. 1979;55:186–187.

Koutsky LP. Epidemiology of general human papilloma virus. *Am J Med*. 1997;102(45):3–8.

Lee VH, Rankin JS, Alpert S, et al. Microbiological investigations of Bartholin's gland, abscesses, and cysts. *Am J Obst Gynecol*. 1997;129(2):150–153.

Murphy M, Fairley I, Wilson J. Exophylic cervical warts: an indication for colposcopy? *Genitourin Med*. 1993;69:81–82.

Odds FC, Webster CE, Riley VC, Fisk PG. Epidemiology of vaginal candida infection: significance of numbers of vaginal yeasts and their biotypes. *Eur J Obst Gynaecol Reprod Biol*. 1987;(1):53–66.

Palmer HM, Mallison H, Wood RL, Herring AJ. Evaluation of the specificities of five DNA amplification methods for detection of *Neisseria gonorrhoea*. *J Clin Microbiol*. 2003;41:835–837.

Screening Guidelines Committee of the BASHH Clinical Effectiveness Group. Sexually transmitted infection screening and testing guidelines. 2006 edition. www.bashh.org/guidelines.

Thomason JL, Gelbart SM, Anderson RJ, Walt AK, Osypowski PJ, Broekhuizen FF. Statistical evaluation of diagnostic criteria for bacterial vaginosis. *Am J Obstet Gynaecol*. 1990;162:155–160.

Wald A, Huang ML, Carrell D, Selke S, Corey L. Polymerase chain reaction for detection of herpes simplex virus (HSV) DNA on mucosal surfaces: Comparison with HSV isolation in cell culture. *J Infect Dis*. 2003;188:1345–1351.

Zdolsek B, Hellberg D, Froman G, Nilsson S, Mardh PA. Culture and wet smear microscopy in the diagnosis of low-symptomatic vulvovaginal candidosis. *Eur J Obst Gynaecol Reprod Biol*. 1995;58(1):47–51.

5

Gonorrhea and Chlamydia

Jonathan M. Zenilman

▦ INTRODUCTION

Chlamydia and gonorrhea are, respectively, the two most commonly reported bacterial infections. Although they initially present as localized mucosal infections, both have been implicated in the pathogenesis of pelvic inflammatory disease and both facilitate HIV transmission. Long-term complications include tubal infertility, ectopic pregnancy, and chronic pelvic pain.

▦ EPIDEMIOLOGY OVERVIEW

Chlamydia and gonorrhea are reportable infections in most countries, although underreporting of cases is a well-recognized limitation of estimates derived from surveillance. In general, publicly funded clinics, with relatively high proportions of economically disadvantaged persons, are generally more likely to submit reports than private clinicians.

In the United States and Western Europe, gonorrhea rates peaked in the early 1970s and then gradually decreased in response to gonorrhea control programs that focused on detection (see Figure 5-1). Gonorrhea rates are higher in ethnic minorities and in persons from lower socioeconomic status (SES). The ethnic disparity remains even after controlling for SES.

The epidemiology of chlamydia is markedly different. Chlamydial infections tend to be broader dispersed across society and are highest in adolescents and young adult populations. Overall trends are difficult to discern

because of major campaigns to increase chlamydia testing, which have resulted in increased detection.

Both chlamydia and gonococcal infection are appreciated as major threats to sexual health, which has prompted the development of major intervention and screening strategies.

Challenges to Clinical Assessment

Both gonorrhea and chlamydia are often asymptomatic, especially in women, which present major challenges in estimating disease burden. Clinic-based estimates and public reports are biased toward symptomatic infections presenting to clinicians. Population-based estimates provide the most accurate assessment of disease burden but are expensive and logistically intensive. In the United States, population-based surveys have been conducted in a variety of populations, such as military inductees, job training program applicants, adolescents, and studies in specific cities and urban venues. Similar studies have been performed in the United Kingdom, largely as part of preparing for and implementing the national chlamydia strategy. In the interests of brevity, only the U.S. examples will be presented.

National population-based studies of U.S. adolescents that have included chlamydia testing have consistently demonstrated that overall chlamydia prevalence was 4–7%, and gonorrhea prevalence at 1–3% (Forhan 2009). All studies show a consistent regional difference, with the south having the highest prevalence and with

FIGURE 5-1   Gonorrhea Incidence per 100,000 in the United States, 1941–2006

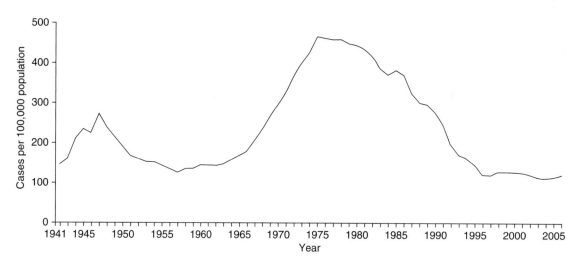

Note the peak in 1972.
Source: Division of STD Prevention, U.S. Centers for Disease Control.

rates in women higher than in men. There are substantial racial disparities that persist even after controlling for access to health care and socioeconomic status. For example, chlamydia rates in African Americans are three to four times higher than the overall population, and for gonorrhea, they are more than 20 times higher (Datta et al. 2007). These disparities are not limited to the United States. For example, surveillance data and directed studies in London and Leeds have shown similar racial disparities for gonococcal infections.

For both infections, the highest incidence rates are observed in women aged 15–19 years and men aged 20–24, probably reflecting sexual partnering patterns. However, the incidence curve for chlamydia dramatically drops after the mid-20s, and >90% of morbidity occurs in those younger than 25 years old (see Figure 5-2) (CDC 2010A). Hypotheses to explain this include the affect of sexual behavior as well as potentially important immunological correlates. For example, there are only a limited number of chlamydial serovars, and after infection, there is development of either partial or full immunity. Therefore, after exposure to multiple strains, there is the potential to become functionally immune. In contrast, gonococcal strains undergo a continual genetic recombination process, resulting in a nearly infinite number of potential strain populations. Therefore, immunity to gonococcal infection does not develop after exposure.

Military recruits are another population that highlights the importance of testing asymptomatic populations and provides insight into the prevalence of chlamydial infection. For example, among more than 13,000 female military recruits who were older than 17 years of age studied by Gaydos in the U.S. military, the prevalence of chlamydial infection varied dramatically by age, decreasing from 12% among 17-year-olds to less than 2.5% for women older than 33 years of age. In these female Army recruits, the prevalence was 14.9% in African Americans and 5.5% among whites. Among male recruits, the prevalence of chlamydial infection was considerably lower (5.3%). The prevalence was considerably higher among African Americans (11.9%) and whites (2.8%).

■ RISK FACTORS FOR GONOCOCCAL AND CHLAMYDIAL INFECTION

Epidemiological studies have identified behavioral risks associated with gonococcal and chlamydial infections. These include the following:

- *Adolescents and young adults.* Risk is inversely associated with age and is especially related to age at first sexual intercourse.

- *Multiple sex partners or a partner with other partners during the last three months or a recent new sex partner.* Partnering patterns are particularly important. Young

FIGURE 5-2 Age Distribution of Chlamydia Infection in the United States per 100,000

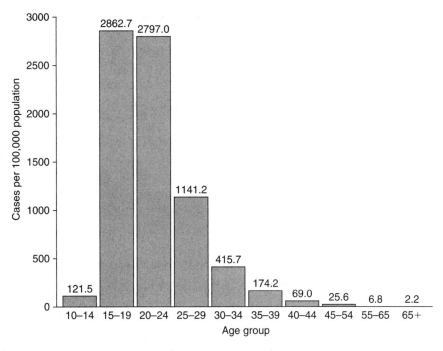

Source: Division of STD Prevention, U.S. Centers for Disease Control.

women with a partner who is substantially older are at particularly high risk. Homosexual men, especially young men who have sex with men who have multiple partners, are also at high risk for GC/CT.

- *Inconsistent use of barrier contraceptives.* Condoms have been demonstrated to be highly effective in preventing gonococcal and chlamydial transmission.

- *Socioeconomic factors.* Rates are typically higher in lower socioeconomic class groups, persons with lower education levels, and those with poorer healthcare access. In particular, there are significant racial disparities between blacks and whites that are not due to biological susceptibility and persist even when controlling for healthcare access. The reasons for these disparities are not particularly well understood. This is particularly the case for gonococcal infection.

- *Social networks.* Bacterial sexually transmitted infections, such as gonorrhea, chlamydia, and syphilis are highly dependent on the social network environment. Proxies for social network have included mapping studies of neighborhoods, which have demonstrated that extraordinarily high rates of disease are seen in certain geographically defined areas.

- *Proxies for high-risk behavior include incarceration* (see Chapter 43). Studies in juvenile detention centers and jails have found that these are high-yield venues for screening.

Risk factor analyses are useful for broad-brush epidemiological studies. However, risk-based assessments as tools for screening have not been that useful, largely because the sensitivity and specificity of risk-based assessment has been found to be low. Therefore, the intervention approaches used have been focused on increasing screening and ensuring access to effective treatment and partner management.

■ MICROBIOLOGY OVERVIEW

Both *Neisseria gonorrhoeae* and *Chlamydia trachomatis* are obligate human pathogens. These organisms do not live independently in the environment and have no other natural host. Although they cause syndromes that are often similar, they are microbiologically quite different.

Neisseria gonorrhoeae is a fastidious aerobic and facultatively anaerobic gram-negative diplococcus. Other Neisseriae are commensal organisms of the human mucosal surfaces. The organism grows best at 35–36°C on medium containing hemoglobin and a variety of other nutrients, in a moist atmosphere containing at least 3% CO_2, and has a replication time of approximately 40 minutes. These growth requirements actually made isolation difficult until easy-to-use transport media and microbiological techniques were developed in the 1970s. Characteristic colonies are small, rounded, and glistening gray (see Figure 5-3) after 24 hours of incubation and are nonhemolytic on blood agar, and the microbiological speciation is performed using either biochemical or immunological tests.

Chlamydia trachomatis (CT) is a bacteria that is morphologically much different and smaller than the gonococcus. It is an obligate intracellular pathogen, cannot produce its own ATP-derived metabolic energy, and therefore cannot be cultured on standard artificial media. It exists in two different forms during its life cycle. The extracellular form is metabolically inert and is known as an elementary body (see Figure 5-4). Once intracellular, chlamydia transforms into the reticulate body, which is the metabolically active, replicative form. *Chlamydia trachomatis* encompasses a number of subtypes, or serovars. These are divided into two groups. The L1, L2, L3 serovars are associated with lymphogranuloma venereum, which is an inflammatory genital ulcer disease (see Chapter 17). Serovars B through K are associated with mucosal chlamydial infection, such as urethritis and cervicitis. It has a complex life cycle, which requires 72 or more hours to complete, where replication occurs within a eukaryotic host cell. To survive and replicate,

the organism must attach and penetrate the host cell. It has evolved a series of complex strategies to accomplish this. This organism also generates a significant immune response, especially to a series of compounds termed heat shock proteins, which, in turn, appear to upregulate the host's immune system. The association between relatively asymptomatic chlamydial infection and the exuberant scarring often seen in pelvic inflammatory disease (PID) has been attributed to this complex immune response.

From the standpoint of pathogenesis, both organisms preferentially infect columnar epithelial cells, which is why the infected tissues are the male and female urethra, the endocervix, the anorectal canal, the pharyngeal pillars, and in cases of vertical transmission, the conjunctivae and respiratory tracts.

■ CLINICAL FEATURES

The clinical features of gonorrhea and chlamydia overlap, and therefore, they will be discussed in parallel.

Clinical Disease in Men

Urethritis in Men

Dysuria and purulent discharge are the most common symptoms (see Figure 5-5). For gonorrhea, most men have one or both symptoms within 1 week of infection, although 5–10% of cases remain asymptomatic. In chlamydia, the predominant symptom tends to be dysuria,

FIGURE 5-3 Colonies of *N. gonorrhoeae* on NYC Agar Plate

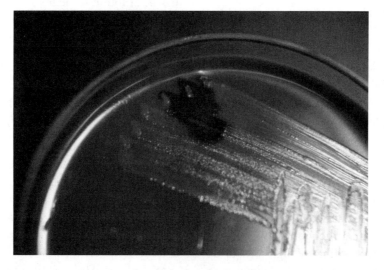

The dark stain represents a positive oxidase test that classifies these colonies as *Neisseria*.

FIGURE 5-4   Cervical Epithelial Cell Parasitized by a Multitude of Elementary Bodies

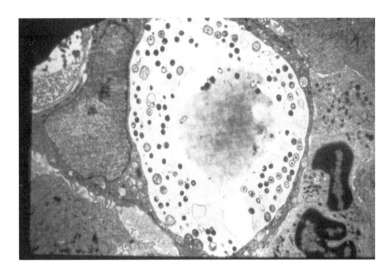

rather than discharge, the incubation period is longer, and up to a third of patients may be asymptomatic. The discharge in gonorrhea is more frequently purulent and in chlamydia may be watery or mucoid (see also Chapter 14), and is often termed "nongonococcal urethritis." However, clinical characteristics such as degree of pain or discharge cannot be accurately used to differentiate between the two disorders. Besides discharge and dysuria, there may be local inguinal lymphadenopathy. In gonococcal cases, especially those left untreated, local complications may occur including penile lymphangitis or edema, especially in uncircumcised men.

Besides chlamydia and gonorrhea, the differential diagnosis of urethritis includes a large number of agents which also cause nongonococcal urethritis including mycoplasma genitalium, ureaplasma species, trichmonas vaginalis, and viruses. Flowchart algorithms for the differential diagnosis of urethritis are presented in Chapter 14. In men who practice insertive rectal intercourse, enteric organisms also need to be considered. Untreated urethritis usually resolves within 6 months. Because the majority of symptomatic men seek early treatment, there are few current epidemiological data on the long-term sequelae of untreated gonococcal or chlamydial urethritis. In developing countries, where chronic untreated infections still occur, paraurethral and preputial abscesses, fistula formation, and urethral strictures occur frequently. Epididymitis (see Chapter 21) and prostatitis (see Chapter 27) are manifestations of ascending infections in men. In men younger than 35 years of age, who

FIGURE 5-5   Gonococcal Urethritis with Associated Lymphangitis and Satellite Lesions

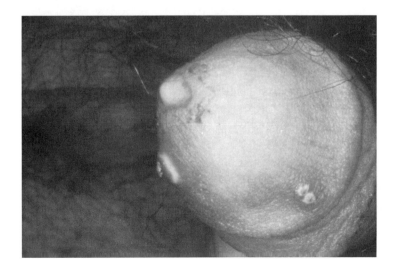

have no anatomical abnormalities and who have not had urethral instrumentation, epididymitis and prostatitis should be presumed to have a sexually transmitted etiology unless proved otherwise.

Cervical Infection in Women

Cervicitis is the primary genital manifestation in women. Cervical infection occurs in the columnar epithelial cells proximal to the squamocolimnar junction. Clinically, over half of women with gonococcal or chlamydial cervicitis are either asymptomatic or have very nonspecific complaints, which highlight the need for aggressive screening of women who are at risk. The most common symptom is discharge. Other symptoms include lower abdominal tenderness, vaginal pain, and dyspareunia (painful sexual intercourse), abnormal menses, or dysuria (see Chapter 24). Symptoms may be especially prominent at the time of menses. Because cervical discharge may alter the local vaginal flora, patients may develop a secondary bacterial vaginosis, which in turn will result in symptoms of malodor, vaginal discharge, and pruritis. Labial tenderness or swelling may occur in cases where the Bartholin's or Skene's gland is inflamed.

When a speculum examination is performed, in most women with gonococcal cervicitis, purulent endocervical exudates and cervical erythema and edema are seen (see Figure 5-6). Chlamydial cervicitis is more characterized by cervical friability. It is important in the examination to differentiate cervical discharge from vaginal discharge, as the etiologies of each syndrome can be quite different. Bimanual examination of the pelvis is strongly recommended in evaluating women with known or suspected gonococcal or chlamydia infection. For example, as many as half of women with endocervical gonorrhea and a quarter with documented chlamydia may at initial evaluation have upper-tract signs such as adnexal tenderness, if such signs are carefully sought. A negative examination does not rule out presence of either organism, as many women with these infections may have no clinical signs. The examination should include careful evaluation for signs of PID. As explained in Chapters 8 and 16, if PID is suspected, the clinician should have a very low threshold for treatment.

Besides gonorrhea and chlamydia, the differential diagnosis of cervicitis is broad and includes herpes simplex, mycoplasma genitalium, HPV, and cervical dysplasia, and, in some cases, inflammation due to vaginal disorders such as trichomoniasis.

Upper Genital Tract Infection and PID

PID is the most important complication of cervical infection (see also Chapter 15). Ascending infection from the endocervix through the uterine cavity to the fallopian tubes usually occurs within one to two menstrual cycles in 10–20% of women with untreated or undertreated gonococcal or chlamydial infection. PID is actually a spectrum of soft-tissue infections, including endometritis and salpingitis. Leakage of infected material can result in tubo-ovarian abscess and pelvis peritonitis. Tubal scarring, the major long-term sequelae of PID, leads to increased susceptibility to repeated episodes of PID, as well as to an increased incidence of tubal infertility and ectopic pregnancy.

FIGURE 5-6 Cervical Friability and Edema in a Patient with Documented Chlamydial Cervicitis

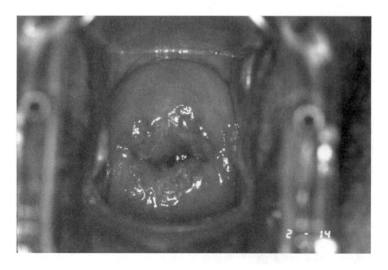

Clinical diagnosis of PID traditionally has been made on the basis of the triad of lower abdominal pain, abnormal cervical or vaginal discharge, and tenderness on bimanual examination. Fever occurs in only half the cases. Women with PID may have crampy, dull lower abdominal pain occurring with menses or irregular menses over several cycles before the disease becomes overt. On bimanual examination, the signs of PID are uterine traction tenderness, adnexal tenderness, or adnexal enlargement. Although adnexal abscesses are unusual in gonococcal PID, clinical suspicion should lead to further evaluation, such as sonography. The wide spectrum of disease, including mild cases, and the relative nonspecificity of clinical signs, make accurate diagnosis difficult. Laparoscopic studies have demonstrated clinicopathological correlation in only two-thirds of cases. Therefore, careful clinical observation of the patient is extremely important.

Because of the diagnostic problems and the profound sequelae of untreated or undertreated disease, the Centers for Disease Control and Prevention (CDC) and other authorities recommend an aggressive approach to PID diagnosis and treatment (see Chapter 8). Treatment regimens for PID are designed to include adequate antimicrobial coverage for *N. gonorrhoeae*, *C. trachomatis*, gram-negative organisms, and anaerobes. Hospitalization may be necessary in severe cases. In addition, if foreign bodies, such as IUDs, are present, they should be removed.

Anorectal Infections

Anorectal chlamydia and gonococcal infections occur in homosexual men or heterosexual women with a history of receptive rectal intercourse. A small proportion of women with endocervical gonorrhea have coexistent rectal infection. In women, anorectal gonorrhea is not related to rectal intercourse; infected perineal secretions are thought to secondarily infect the anorectal mucosa.

Most anorectal infections are asymptomatic. In those with infection due to receptive rectal intercourse, symptoms such as tenesmus, mucoid or bloody discharge, hematochezia, perianal irritation, and constipation are seen more frequently. Anoscopy in symptomatic cases may show erythema, exudates, and friable mucosa in the anal canal and terminal rectum. In asymptomatic cases, however, anoscopy is often normal. The differential diagnosis of anorectal gonorrhea, especially in homosexual men, includes rectal herpes, rectal syphilis, lymphogranuloma venereum, and *C. trachomatis*. Up to 85% of anorectal gonococcal and chlamydial infections may be asymptomatic. Because of increasing prevalence, especially in homosexual men, routine screening of all gay men with a history of receptive rectal intercourse is recommended.

Pharyngeal Infection

Pharyngeal infection occurs commonly with both gonorrhea and chlamydia. However, there has been controversy since the late 1970s whether chlamydia actually causes invasive disease in the throat and therefore has been largely discounted by clinical experts. Infection results from oral sexual exposure to an infected partner. Although exudative pharyngitis and sore throat may occur, pharyngeal gonorrhea is most commonly asymptomatic. Sore throat in some patients may be more related to a postfellatio syndrome than to an infectious process. Diagnosis of pharyngeal gonorrhea should be made by culture because of the high prevalence of commensal *Neisseria*, which cross-reacts with other diagnostic tests.

Ophthalmia

Ophthalmia due to either organism occurs in neonates born to women with endocervical disease. GC/CT ophthalmia is rarely seen in developed countries, because of implementation of prenatal screening programs and universal ophthalmic prophylaxis at birth with silver nitrate, erythromycin, or tetracycline drops.

Gonococcal ophthalmia can occur in adults and is either a result of autoinoculation or exposure to infected secretions during intercourse. Ophthalmia is an ophthalmological emergency and should be urgently referred to a specialty center.

It begins with a conjunctival inflammation that may rapidly progress to a purulent discharge, hyopion, and keratitis. Unless recognized and treated early, corneal blindness can rapidly occur. Chlamydial ophthalmia has a much slower course but is predominantly a hemorrhagic conjunctivitis that can result in scarring if not treated. Adult gonococcal ophthalmia is occasionally seen in young adults with anogenital gonorrhea. Accidental autoinoculation is thought to cause many cases. Purulent keratoconjunctivitis is seen clinically and should be considered an ophthalmological emergency.

Gonorrhea and Chlamydia in Children

Gonococcal or chlamydial infections in prepubertal children should be considered evidence of sexual abuse unless proved otherwise. Because of forensic implications, specific diagnosis is imperative and early consultation with appropriate legal and laboratory resources should be obtained. In young girls, either a symptomatic or an asymptomatic vulvovaginitis may be seen. Urethritis has been described in boys, and anorectal, rectal, and pharyngeal infection may be seen in both sexes. When this is suspected, the clinician is obligated to notify law enforcement and child protective service agencies. Testing in these situations should be performed in consultation with an expert reference laboratory.

■ SYSTEMIC SYNDROMES

Disseminated Gonococcal Infection

Rarely, mucosal gonococcal infection leads to disseminated gonococcal infection (DGI), which is gonococcal septicemia.

DGI rarely presents to sexual health services as these present as febrile illnesses, typically to primary care or urgent care practitioners. Symptoms and signs include fevers, chills, and joint pains. Symptoms referable to the genital or other sites of sexual exposure are typically absent, as the syndrome is predominantly caused by organism strains that tend to cause only minimal inflammation. The characteristic findings are either polyarthralgias, or tenosynovitis, or septic arthritis, which may be associated with skin lesions on the extensor surfaces (see Figure 5-7). These lesions can be petechial, papular, pustular, hemorrhagic, or necrotic, are usually seen on the distal extremities, and are asymmetrically distributed. Fingers, toes, hands, and wrists are commonly involved in an asymmetrical fashion. Blood cultures are positive for *N. gonorrhoeae* in about 50% of cases. DGI should be suspected in young adults who present with acute febrile illness associated with clinical signs of joint inflammation. Before antibiotic treatment, gonococcal testing should be performed from the genital, rectum, and pharynx. DGI generally responds rapidly to appropriate antibiotic therapy.

Reactive Arthritis Syndrome

Approximately 1% of men with urethritis develop reactive arthritis, and approximately one-third of these patients have the complete manifestations of this syndrome. Reactive arthritis typically manifests 2-weeks after the genital infection, although it may occur up to 3–6 months later. This syndrome is also caused by a variety of other pathogens, predominantly enteric organisms, such as *Salmonella*, *Shigella*, and *Campylobacter*. Patients will complain of systemic symptoms, primarily low-grade fever and symmetrical polyarthralgias. Typical manifestations (all do not have to be present) include uveitis, a macular rash on the trunk, a macular, sharply bordered penile circanate rash (circanate balanitis), and a desquamative rash on the plantar soles (keratoderma blenorrhagicum). Treatment of these patients typically requires primary treatment for chlamydia or the inciting pathogen, if identified, and courses of nonsteroidal anti-inflammatory agents for the rheumatologic symptoms.

■ DIAGNOSIS OF GONORRHEA AND CHLAMYDIA

Definitive diagnosis of cervical and gonococcal urethritis in males and cervicitis in women is made by culture or nucleic acid–based tests. Cultures for gonorrhea, which

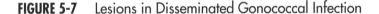

FIGURE 5-7 Lesions in Disseminated Gonococcal Infection

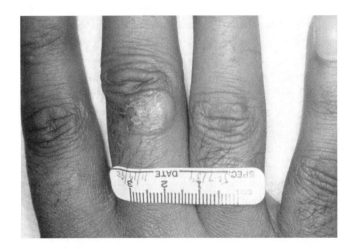

were once widely available, are increasingly supplanted by the easier-to-use nucleic acid tests. Chlamydial culture is available only in research settings and specialty centers.

Sensitivity and specificity of the NAAT testing methods are 95–99%. NAAT testing can be performed either on direct genital secretions (cervical or urethral swab), urine in either men or women, or self-administered vaginal swab. Specimens taken using modern collection techniques are stable at room temperature and can be easily transported, facilitating widespread screening implementation.

Posttreatment/therapy testing is not recommended. NAAT tests, because they assay for nucleic acid fragments of the organism, are often false positive after treatment, because organism DNA fragments can be present for up to 2 weeks posttreatment. In high-risk persons, recommendations are for rescreening 3–6 months after treatment for detection of reinfection.

Gram's stain of secretions may be useful in identifying gonococcal cases at the bedside and has sensitivity of 90% for gonococcal urethritis and 50% for cervicitis. However, Gram's stain requires easy access to microscopy, which is often not available.

Diagnosis of rectal and pharyngeal infections is difficult because most of the diagnostic tests have been developed primarily for genital infections. These tests have been increasingly used for rectal and pharyngeal infection, and recent studies have demonstrated equivalent sensitivity and specificity. However, before testing for rectal and pharyngeal infection with nonculture tests, it would be prudent to check with the local laboratory regarding the specific policies and procedures.

Coinfection

Gonorrhea and chlamydia coinfection is common. Up to 40% of persons with gonococcal infection have chlamydia coinfection. Rates are highest in poor urban areas. Therefore, treatment policy since 1985 has recommended that all patients infected with gonorrhea be treated for chlamydia as well. This policy is considered more cost-effective than presumptively testing patients, if chlamydia tests had not been performed. Conversely, in patients diagnosed with chlamydia, gonococcal infection is uncommon except for areas where gonorrhea is hyperendemic.

Treatment Issues

Effective treatment regimens are predicated on providing, when possible, single-dose oral regimens (CDC

2010B). A major challenge to treatment has been the increasing prevalence of resistant organisms. This has been primarily a problem with gonococcal infections.

Resistance to Antimicrobials

Chlamydia trachomatis has largely been spared the issues of antimicrobial resistance. Occasional tetracycline-resistant isolates have been described, but these have not disseminated and the public health importance of these strains is limited.

Neisseria gonorrhoeae has developed a multiplicity of antimicrobial resistance determinants and has demonstrated continual creativity in responding to new drugs. Plasmid-mediated resistance to penicillin has been described since the 1970s and plasmid-mediated resistance to tetracycline since 1985. Chromosomally mediated resistance to penicillins and the cephalosporins has been demonstrated since the 1980s. This mechanism is difficult to diagnose, because the organism gradually accumulates chromosomal mutations that increase the minimum inhibitory concentration (MIC) to the antimicrobial.

Quinolones were first recommended widely for gonococcal therapy in 1989. By the mid-1990s, resistant strains were being regularly identified in Southeast Asia, where widespread over-the-counter use of the drugs was believed to have been a key factor in inducing the development of resistant strains. These organisms quickly spread throughout the Pacific basin and began to be seen in the United States, Western Europe, and the United Kingdom, especially in homosexual men. Prevalence rates overall increased to >5% in the United States by 2005, and in 2004, the CDC recommended that quinolones not be used for treating gonorrhea in homosexual men, and this was extended as a general recommendation in 2006. Similar patterns were seen with azithromycin resistance. Gonococcal treatment options are therefore currently limited.

■ PUBLIC HEALTH MANAGEMENT

Treatment of Sexual Partners

Sexual partners are often asymptomatic and, unless treated, will reinfect the index patient or spread infection to other partners (see Chapter 30). A traditional approach of using members of the public health field team to notify exposed sex partners has been employed, but many health departments are no longer tracing these partners because of staffing shortages and lack of resources. In lieu of public health advocacy, patients are asked to notify their partners of the need for medical evaluation and treatment. This approach has been deemed a public health failure

Because of the perceived failure of traditional notification programs, several studies have been designed to determine whether gonococcal or chlamydial reinfection rates could be decreased through a new model of partner care. Expedited treatment policies include either providing the index patient with "treatment packs" that are given to the partner or providing local venues, such as pharmacies, where partners can confidentially obtain treatment. The advantages of this approach are clearly the expansion of providing therapy for partners. The disadvantages are that partners are not provided with a comprehensive STI evaluation, and therefore education is required to ensure that they seek care in case they develop symptoms.

Prevention

Prevention of GC and CT infection include the following principles:

1. Counseling patients on reducing high-risk behaviors. This is particularly challenging, especially for adolescents and those at high risk.

2. Consistent condom use. Consistent condom use has been shown to be highly protective in preventing incident GC and CT infection.

3. Treatment of partners. The most common reason for reinfection is contact with an untreated partner. This is more fully addressed in Chapter 30; however, patients should be intensively counseled on the need for partner therapy, as well as that many cases are asymptomatic and that the lack of symptoms does not rule out infection.

4. Engagement in screening programs. Periodic and regular screening for GC/CT reduces the associated complications of pelvic inflammatory disease and has the public health impact of reducing the overall population burden of infection.

Chlamydia Screening

Initial studies demonstrated that implementation of widespread chlamydia screening resulted in reduced incidence of PID. Clinical practice guidelines currently strongly recommend routine chlamydia screening for sexually active women younger than 25 years. These have been incorporated into quality assurance guidelines for managed care organizations in the United States and are the cornerstone of the UK National Chlamydia Strategy.

These interventions are restricted to patients who present for medical care, and many adolescents and young adults do not access the healthcare system, despite outreach efforts.

TABLE 5-1   Treatment Recommendations for Gonococcal and Chlamydial Infections

Treatment for Mucosal Gonorrhea (any anatomical site)

Ceftriaxone r 250 mg intramuscularly

or

Cefixime 400 mg orally

Provide either medicine as a single dose. Treatment for chlamydia (below) should also be provided. If patient is allergic to penicillin, then options are to treat with a quinolone regimen, but to perform a posttreatment clinical evaluation and to emphasize to the patient the importance of returning.

Treatment for Chlamydia

Azithromycin 1 g orally in a single dose

or

Doxycycline 100 mg orally twice a day for 7 days

Source: CDC, 2010B.

Current screening recommendations are for chlamydia testing of sexually active women younger than age of 25 years as part of routine annual testing. Gonorrhea testing is suggested if persons are in an area endemic for gonorrhea or have had recent exposures. In practice, many of the NAAT tests are offered in a multiplex format and both tests may be run on a single specimen. Initial screening efforts focused on women; however, many STI intervention programs are now screening men.

Specific populations may benefit from more frequent screening intervals. For example, screening every 6 months has been suggested for adolescents at high risk for reinfection. In addition the availability of NAAT tests, with their ease of administration (not requiring a genital examination to obtain specimens) and transport stability, has facilitated testing in a wide variety of field venues, such as in schools, in corrections facilities, and by mail over the Internet.

Relationship to HIV Transmission

Gonorrhea and chlamydia facilitate HIV transmission. This relationship has been established in studies performed both in sub-Saharan Africa and in the United States and have consistently found that the presence of either infection increases the risk of HIV transmission by approximately threefold. Mechanistic hypotheses for this relationship include increased genital inflammation, the recruitment of CD4 target cells in patients with chlamydia to the genital sites, and upregulating of HIV receptors on mucosal dendritic cells in response to inflammation. From a population perspective, gonorrhea and chlamydial infection may be more important than genital ulcer diseases, such as syphilis and chancroid, because they may be associated with a higher attributable fraction of HIV seroconversion cases. This issue has also become particularly important since the late 1990s, because of an upsurge in rectal gonorrhea and chlamydia in homosexual men who have high rates of HIV coinfection.

Despite these relationships, studies that have targeted STI treatment to reduce HIV transmission have failed to demonstrate reduction in HIV transmission events. However, all patients evaluated for GC/CT because of high-risk exposures, or who have GC/CT identified on screening, should be tested and counseled for HIV. The clinical manifestations of GC/CT and the therapy are not changed in the presence of HIV. Conversely, as discussed in Chapter 10, HIV providers caring

for sexually active patients should assess periodically for GC/CT infection as they would any other sexually active person.

■ KEY POINTS

- Gonorrhea and chlamydia are mucosal infections. Rarely each may cause systemic symptoms. Any exposed mucosal site can become infected. Asymptomatic infection is common in both males and females.

- Gonorrhea and chlamydia are the most frequently reported infectious diseases in many developed countries.

- The incubation period for gonorrhea is 24–48 hours, for chlamydia it is approximately a week. These short time periods make public health intervention difficult.

- Large scale screening programs are the primary public health approach to these infections. Screening should target sexually active persons at risk and all pregnant women.

- Gonorrhea and chlamydia testing is performed almost exclusively by high-sensitivity, DNA amplification tests which can be easily used in field settings.

- Treatment for gonorrhea is becoming increasingly a challenge because of the evolution of resistance. The primary treatment modality is third-generation cephalosporins.

- Preferred treatment approach for chlamydia is Azithromycin, 1 gram as a single dose, which improves compliance.

- Persons with gonorrhea have high coinfection rates with chlamydia; therefore, cotreatment is standard.

REFERENCES

Bernstein KT, Stephens SC, Barry PM, et al. *Chlamydia trachomatis* and *Neisseria gonorrhoeae* transmission from the oropharynx to the urethra among men who have sex with men. *Clin Infect Dis.* 2009;15;49(12):1793–1797.

Burstein GR, Eliscu A, Ford K, et al. Expedited partner therapy for adolescents diagnosed with chlamydia or gonorrhea: a position paper of the Society for Adolescent Medicine. *J Adolesc Health.* 2009;45(3):303–309.

Burstein GR, Gaydos CA, Diener-West M, Howell MR, Zenilman JM, Quinn TC. Incident *Chlamydia trachomatis* infections among inner-city adolescent females. *JAMA.* 1998;280(6):521–526.

Burstein GR, Snyder MH, Conley D, et al. Chlamydia screening in a health plan before and after a national performance measure introduction. *Obstet Gynecol.* 2005;106(2): 327–334.

Burstein GR, Zenilman JM, Gaydos CA, et al. Predictors of repeat *Chlamydia trachomatis* infections diagnosed by DNA amplification testing among inner city females. *Sex Transm Infect.* 2001;77(1):26–32.

Cecil JA, Howell MR, Tawes JJ, et al. Features of *Chlamydia trachomatis* and *Neisseria gonorrhoeae* infection in male Army recruits. *J Infect Dis.* 2001;184(9):1216–1219.

Centers for Disease Control and Prevention (CDC). Sexually transmitted disease surveillance 2009. Atlanta, GA: Department of Health and Human Services; 2010A.

Centers for Disease Control and Prevention (CDC). Sexually transmitted disease treatment guidelines, 2010. *Morb Mort Week Rep.* 2010; 59(RR-12):1–110.

Datta SD, Sternberg M, Johnson RE, et al. Gonorrhea and chlamydia in the United States among persons 14 to 39 years of age, 1999 to 2002. *Ann Intern Med.* 2007;147: 89–96.

Delpech V, Martin IM, Hughes G, Nichols T, James L, Ison CA; Gonococcal Resistance to Antimicrobials Surveillance Programme Steering Group. Epidemiology and clinical presentation of gonorrhoea in England and Wales: findings from the Gonococcal Resistance to Antimicrobials Surveillance Programme 2001–2006. *Sex Transm Infect.* 2009;85(5):317–321.

Fenton KA, Ward H. National chlamydia screening programme in England: making progress. *Sex Transm Infect.* 2004;80(5):331–333.

Forhan SE, Gottlieb SL, Sternberg MR, et al. Prevalence of sexually transmitted infections among female adolescents aged 14 to 19 in the United States. *Pediatrics.* 2009;124:1505–1512.

Gavin L, MacKay AP, Brown K, et al; Centers for Disease Control and Prevention (CDC). Sexual and reproductive health of persons aged 10–24 years—United States, 2002–2007. *MMWR Surveill Summ.* 2009;58(6):1–58.

Gaydos CA, Howell MR, Pare B, et al. *Chlamydia trachomatis* infections in female military recruits. *N Engl J Med.* 1998 10;339(11):739–744.

Hosenfeld CB, Workowski KA, Berman S, et al. Repeat infection with chlamydia and gonorrhea among females: a systematic review of the literature. *Sex Transm Dis.* 2009;36(8):478–489.

LaMontagne DS, Fenton KA, Randall S, Anderson S, Carter P. Establishing the National Chlamydia Screening Programme in England: results from the first full year of screening. *Sex Transm Infect.* 2004;80(5):335–341.

Risley CL, Ward H, Choudhury B, et al. Geographical and demographic clustering of gonorrhoea in London. *Sex Transm Infect.* 2007;83(6):481–487.

Rompalo AM, Gaydos CA, Shah N, et al. Evaluation of use of a single intravaginal swab to detect multiple sexually transmitted infections in active-duty military women. *Clin Infect Dis.* 2001;33(9):1455–1461.

Wang SA, Harvey AB, Conner SM, et al. Antimicrobial resistance for *Neisseria gonorrhoeae* in the United States, 1988 to 2003: the spread of fluoroquinolone resistance. *Ann Intern Med.* 2007;147(2):81–88.

6

Human Papillomaviruses

Deblina Datta, Eileen F. Dunne, Mona Saraiya, and Lauri Markowitz

■ INTRODUCTION

Human papillomaviruses (HPVs) are a group of over 100 viruses, of which approximately 40 types are transmitted via genital contact. HPV is the most common sexually transmitted infection in the United States (Weinstock 2004). While most HPV infections are transient and cause no clinical sequelae, some infections can cause genital warts, anogenital cancers, oropharyngeal cancers, cervical cancer, and recurrent respiratory papillomatosis. This chapter will primarily focus on HPV epidemiology, genital warts epidemiology and treatment, cervical cancer prevention, and HPV vaccine.

■ HPV OVERVIEW

HPV Infection and Clinical Sequelae

HPVs are nonenveloped, double-stranded DNA viruses in the family Papillomaviridae. HPV infection targets the basal layer of epithelial cells, where infection may evade detection by host immune systems. HPV types are numbered and categorized as "nononcogenic" or "oncogenic" based on their associations with cancers.

Nononcogenic types cause genital warts and recurrent respiratory papillomatosis, a rare condition affecting the respiratory tract of children born to mothers infected with nononcogenic HPV. Among the nononcogenic types, types 6 and 11 are responsible for 90% of all genital wart lesions.

Persistent infection with oncogenic HPV types are associated with the development of cervical, vulvar, vaginal, penile, and anal cancers. There have been reports of association between oncogenic HPV types and a subset of oropharyngeal cancers as well. HPV types 16 and 18 have been associated with 70% of all cervical cancers worldwide. Newly licensed HPV vaccines have been developed to prevent infection with these two important HPV types.

HPV Epidemiology and Natural History

Since genital HPV infection is primarily transmitted through sexual intercourse, the most consistently reported predictors of infection have been age of sexual debut and number of sex partners (lifetime and recent). HPV is acquired rapidly after sexual debut.

Most HPV infections are transient and cause no clinical problems; 70% of new HPV infections clear within 1 year, and approximately 90% clear within 2 years, with a median duration of 8 months (Ho 1998). Persistent infection with high-risk types of HPV is the most important risk factor for cervical cancer precursors and invasive cervical cancer and risk for persistence and progression to precancerous lesions varies by HPV type, with HPV 16 having the highest oncogenic potential. Factors associated with cervical cancer in epidemiologic studies include cigarette smoking, increased parity, increased age, other sexually transmitted infections, immune suppression, long-term oral contraceptive use, and other host factors. The time between initial HPV infection and development of cervical cancer is usually decades. Many aspects of the natural history of HPV are poorly understood, including the role and duration of naturally acquired immunity after HPV infection.

Burden of HPV

Although HPV infection is not a reportable condition, there have been several large-scale, national surveys of HPV infection (based on DNA detection) in the United States. In a nationally representative sample of the U.S. general population aged 14–59 years, overall prevalence of any HPV was 26.8%. Prevalence was highest among women aged 20–24 years (44.8%). Prevalence of HPV 6, 11, 16, or 18 was 6.4% among those aged 14–24 years (Dinh 2008). Clinic-based studies among sexually active women have demonstrated highest prevalence among those aged 14–19 years (Datta 2008). Studies from the United Kingdom and Nordic countries are similar.

HPV infection also is common among men. Among heterosexual men in clinic-based studies, prevalence of genital HPV infection often is greater than 20% and is highly dependent on the anatomic sites sampled and method of specimen collection.

■ GENITAL WARTS

Epidemiology and Burden of Disease

Genital warts are one of the most common sexually transmitted infections diagnoses and the vast majority are caused by infection with HPV types 6 and 11. In the United States, 5.6% of men and women aged 18–59 years have had ever been diagnosed with genital warts (Datta 2008). A study from four Nordic countries found that 10.6% of women aged 18–45 years had ever been clinically diagnosed with genital warts (Kruger 2007).

Data on prevalence and incidence of genital warts are primarily from evaluations of large claims databases; in these studies, genital warts occur most commonly among young persons in their early to late 20s, and rates are higher in females than in males.

The burden of genital warts must also consider recurrences, as repeat visits for genital warts are common. Observational studies have generally found that the mean duration is 3 months, and that patients have an average of slightly more than 3 follow-up visits for management. The facility burden of HPV disease is also high. Studies in STI clinics have estimated that HPV management accounts for between one-sixth and one-quarter of all STI clinic visits. Direct economic impact of genital warts is difficult to ascertain, but estimates are in the hundreds of millions of dollars annually.

Men who have sex with men (MSM) have a higher burden of genital and anal warts. Persons with compro-

mised immune function (including HIV infection or posttransplant) are more likely to develop genital warts than those with normal immunity. HIV-infected persons have a 2.5–3 time increased incidence. In addition, this population is likely to have more debilitating disease (larger warts, disease that lasts longer, and disease that is less responsive to treatment).

Genital warts typically occur months to years after incident HPV 6 or 11 infection. One study found that about two-thirds of persons who acquired infection developed genital warts. Genital warts are believed to be highly transmissible, but there are few studies. In one study from the 1970s, 64% of sexual partners of patients with genital warts subsequently acquired genital warts 3 weeks to 8 months after sexual contact (average 2.8 months) (Oriel 1971). The most common risk factors for genital warts are age (younger age groups > older age groups) and sexual behavior (increased numbers of lifetime/recent sex partners).

■ CLINICAL DETECTION AND TREATMENT

Anogenital warts are diagnosed by physical examination. Genital warts appear as small papules, or flat, smooth, or pedunculated lesions. Sometimes they can be soft, pink, or white cauliflower-like sessile growths on moist mucosal surfaces (condyloma accuminatum), or keratotic lesions on squamous epithelium of the skin or surface with a thick, horny layer (see Figure 6-1). Acetic acid is used but some providers, but it is not specific for genital warts and may result in unnecessary interventions. Biopsy of suspicious lesions may be important in some settings (e.g., if the diagnosis is uncertain; the lesions do not respond to standard therapy; the disease worsens during therapy; the patient is immunocompromised; or warts are pigmented, indurated, fixed, bleeding, or ulcerated). Squamous cell carcinomas arising in or resembling genital warts might occur more frequently among immunosuppressed persons requiring biopsy for confirmation of diagnosis, so for suspicious cases providers should consider biopsy (CDC 2010).

If anogenital warts are detected, some experts recommend that clinicians conduct a complete anogenital exam and screen for chlamydia, gonorrhea, syphilis, hepatitis B, and HIV infection. Detection of genital warts is not a reason to recommend more frequent cervical cancer screening, as the HPV types that cause genital warts are different from those that cause cancer. However, women should receive routine cervical cancer screening as recommended.

Treatment is directed to the clinical manifestations of HPV infection but not infection itself. No single treatment is ideal for all patients or all lesions. Genital warts may remain the same, grow in size and number, or regress on their own. Patients and providers may decide on a specific treatment based on convenience, cost, availability, methods of administering therapy, or location of the wart(s); some patients elect to wait to see whether genital warts regress on their own. Treatment can induce wart-free periods, but the underlying viral infection can persist and may result in recurrence (in about 30% of cases). No data suggest that treatment modalities for external genital warts should be different in the setting of HIV infection. Extensive genital warts, warts that have not responded to treatment, or warts that are located in specific locations (e.g., rectal or cervical), should be managed by a specialist. Treatment options for genital warts include patient-applied and provider-administered therapies (CDC 2010). Treatment is also summarized in Table 6-1 and Chapter 22.

Patient-applied therapies are optimal for some patients because of the convenience of administering at home but should only be used when the warts can be identified and accessed for treatment, and the likelihood of compliance is high. A follow-up appointment several weeks into therapy to determine appropriateness of medication use and response to treatment may be useful. Patient-applied therapies include podofilox 0.5% solution or gel; imiquimod 5% cream; and a new therapeutic, sinecatechins 15% ointment. Sinecatechins 15% ointment (Veregen®) is a botanical product that is a mixture of eight catechins, which are the major polyphenols found in green tea leaves, with epigallacatechin gallate (EGCG) as the primary catechin.

Patients should apply podofilox solution with a cotton swab, or podofilox gel with a finger, to visible genital warts twice a day for 3 days, followed by 4 days of no therapy. This cycle may be repeated, as necessary, for up to four cycles. Patients should apply imiquimod cream once daily at bedtime, three times a week for up to 16 weeks. The treatment area should be washed with soap and water 6 to 10 hours after the application. Sinecatechins 15% ointment should be applied three times a day for up to 16 weeks.

Provider-applied therapies include cryotherapy with liquid nitrogen or cryoprobe, trichloroacetic acid (TCA) or bichloroacetic acid (BCA) 80–90%, podophyllin resin 10–25% in a compound tincture of benzoin and surgical removal. There are also other provider-applied therapies with less data available and/or more reported side effects. Cryotherapy should be reapplied every 1–2 weeks. Podophyllin resin should be applied to each wart in small amounts and allowed to air dry. To reduce local irritation, the preparation may be thoroughly washed off 1–4 hours following application. Both TCA and BCA should be applied sparingly and allowed to dry before the patient sits or stands. If pain is intense, the acid can be neutralized with soap or sodium bicarbonate. A white "frosting" will develop on the wart after the TCA or BCA dries. Both podophyllin and TCA or BCA treatments can be repeated weekly. Anogenital warts may be surgically removed by tangential scissor excision, tangential shave excision, curettage, electrosurgery, or other methods.

Genital warts are generally benign and resolve with time; most genital warts resolve within 6 months (with or without treatment). However, a large proportion (~30%) of genital warts recur, which can result in

FIGURE 6-1   (a) Gingival Wart; (b) Multiple Penial Warts

(a)
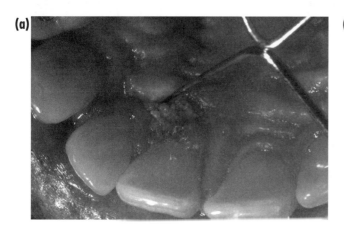

(b)
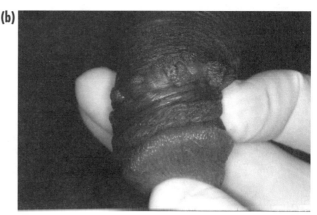

frequent office visits, sometimes costly and debilitating treatment, and substantial psychosocial burden. There are rare cases of giant condyloma of Bushke and Lowenstein, a slow-growing, highly destructive condyloma caused by HPV 6 or 11 infection, that may have a foci of squamous cell carcinoma. This tumor does not metastasize but causes severe and local destruction; this unusual condition most commonly occurs among immunocompromised individuals.

■ CERVICAL CANCER AND CERVICAL SCREENING GUIDELINES

Cervical Cancer and Precursor Lesions Epidemiology and Burden

In the United States, cases of cervical cancer are routinely reported to cancer registries supported by the Surveillance, Epidemiology, and End Results program (administered by the National Cancer Institute), and the National Program of Cancer Registries (administered by the Centers for Disease Control and Prevention), which together cover approximately 100% of the U.S. population. In 2007, the last year in which data were available, 12,280 cases of cervical cancers were diagnosed with an incidence rate of 7.9 per 100,000 women. The number of deaths was approximately 4,000 with a mortality rate of 2.4 per 100,000. Cervical cancer incidence rates have decreased approximately 75% and death rates approximately 70% since the 1950s, largely because of the introduction of Pap testing. Adenocarcinomas have been thought to be more difficult to detect because they are found higher in the endocervix; they account for approximately 20% of cervical cancer cases in the United States. HPV 16 and 18 account for approximately 70–80% of both of these types, and adenocarcinoma incidence is thought to be increasing.

The incidence of cervical cancer increases with age. The median age of cervical cancer diagnosis is 47. In 2007, the U.S. incidence rate was 0.2 per 100,000 among females ages 15–19 (or 19 cases), 1.3 among females 20–24 years of age, 5.1 among females 26–29, and peaked at almost triple that rate (14.7) in women 40–44 years old. Cervical cancer cases are rare among women younger than 30 years of age.

Cervical cancer incidence and mortality varies by racial/ethnic group. These findings have been observed in multiple locales, but are most extensively described in the United States (see Figure 6-2).

FIGURE 6-2 Cervical Cancer Incidence and Mortality by Race/Ethnicity, United States, 2006.

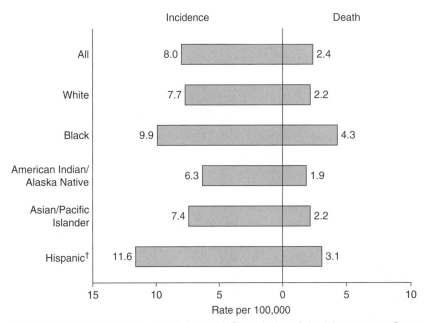

Rates are per 100,000 and age-adjusted to the 2000 U.S. standard population (19 age groups–Census P25–1130).
Incidence data are from NPCR and SEER registries that met USCS publication criteria in 2006 and cover~96.1% of the U.S. population.
Underlying mortality data are provided by National Center for Health Statistics (NCHS) (www.cdc.gov/nchs).
†Hispanic ethnicity is not mutually exclusive from race (white, black, American Indian/Alaska Native, Asian/Pacific Islander).

Source: CDC.

Traditional risk factors for cervical cancer now need to be examined in the context of HPV infection given the etiological role of HPV infection (see Box 6-1). For example, lifetime number of sexual partners and age of first intercourse have become more risk factors for HPV infection, and when HPV infection is taken into account, these factors are no longer considered as important. Infection with two sexually transmitted infections can increase the risk of cervical cancer: *Chlamydia trachomatis* and *Herpes simplex* virus (HSV-2). Both have been associated with twofold increased risk, but exact mechanisms have not been identified. Women infected with HIV and other immunosuppressive conditions, such as renal transplant recipients, are at increased risk of HPV infection, cervical precancer, and invasive cervical cancer. In HIV-infected persons, it is unclear if highly active antiretroviral therapy (HAART) reduces risk of cervical cancer. HAART therapy appears to increase life expectancy and may increase the opportunity for persistent HPV infection to lead to invasive cervical cancer.

Smoking is a known risk factor for squamous cell cervical cancer, showing a dose response by number of cigarettes and younger age of initiation. However, the exact mechanisms of this increased risk remain unclear (i.e., direct toxicity or indirect immunosuppression). The relationship between smoking and HPV is considered one of the classic situations where tobacco is a tumor promoter. Among current users of oral contraceptives, the risk of invasive cervical cancer increased with longer duration of use, but risk rapidly declines after discontinuation.

Although HPV infection is usually asymptomatic, cervical infection can result in histologic changes classified as cervical intraepithelial neoplasias (CIN) grades 1, 2, or 3, on the basis of increasing degree of abnormality in the cervical epithelium or adenocarcinoma in situ (AIS). Spontaneous clearance or progression to cancer in the absence of treatment varies for CIN 1, CIN 2, and CIN 3. CIN 1 usually clears spontaneously (60% of cases) and rarely progresses to cancer (1%); a lower percentage of CIN 2 and 3 spontaneously clear (30–40%), and a higher percentage progress to cancer if not treated (>12%) (Ostor 1993).

Persistent HPV infection can result in precancerous cervical lesions as well as invasive cervical cancer. With regular Pap testing, almost all abnormal cervical cells can be identified and further evaluated at colposcopy. Precancerous cervical lesions and invasive cancer are diagnosed specifically by biopsy (obtained with colpos-copy). Treatment decisions are based on cervical biopsy results (e.g., obtained with colposcopy) not on the Pap test result.

For mild precancerous cervical biopsy lesions (mild dysplasia, i.e., CIN 1), the recommended management is follow-up with further evaluation. For more severe precancerous cervical lesions such as CIN 2 or CIN3, a woman has several treatment options, including observation (especially for CIN2), removal of the area of abnormality (laser, loop electrosurgical excisional procedure, or LEEP, cold-knife conization) or destruction of the area of abnormality (cryotherapy, laser vaporization). Treatment is highly dependent on the woman's

---

BOX 6-1 Etiology of Cervical Cancer

ESTABLISHED

HPV
Persistent presence of any of at least 15 HPV-DNA types in cervical cells

Exogenous hormones
Long-term use of oral contraceptives (5+ years)

Smoking
Dose response unproven
Likely role of cancer promoter

Parity
High parity (5+ pregnancies)

Sexual Partners

POSSIBLE (REQUIRING FURTHER RESEARCH)
Other STIs
Chlamydia trachomatis
HSV-2

Other environmental factors
Low socioeconomic status
Dietary factors

Host factors
Early age at infection
Genetic background (HLA, p53 . . .)
Susceptibility of the transitional zone
Viral integration
Immune response to HPV and determinants of viral clearance
Nonspecific cervical inflammation

Adapted from Bosch, de Sanjose 2003

FIGURE 6-3a Papanicolaou Stain, Atypical Cells of Undetermined Significance

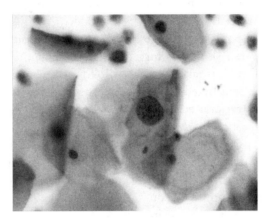

Note epithelial cell with large nucleus, which can be either due to neoplastic or inflammatory.

FIGURE 6-3b Papanicolaou Stain, Low Grade Squamous Intepithelial Lesion (LSIL)

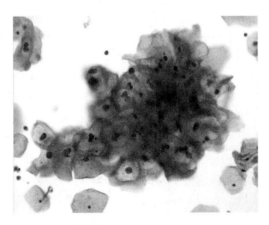

Note larger nuclei, heterogeneous nuclei, and occasional nucleoli. Nuclei still account for < 25% of the cellular volume.

FIGURE 6-3c Papanicolaou Stain, High Grade Squamous Intraepithelial Lesion (HSIL)

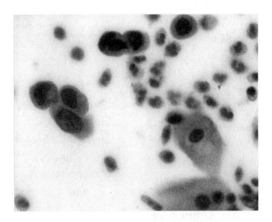

Note large nuclei (accounting for > 50% of cell volume), substantial heterogeneity, nucleoli, changes in cellular shape.

age, fertility preservation, and other risk factors. Each of those has its indications, advantages, and disadvantages, but, importantly, cure rates are comparable.

For invasive cervical cancer, a woman also has several treatment options, including surgery, radiation therapy, and chemotherapy, alone or in combination, depending on stage of disease. Even with a cervical cancer diagnosis and depending on the stage of disease at diagnosis, a woman may have the option to preserve her fertility or keep her ovaries. The survival rate 5 years after diagnosis of cervical cancer varies, depending on the stage of cervical cancer. The risk increases with higher stages of disease.

There are usually no symptoms associated with cancer of the cervix, so routine screening tests to look for changes in the cervical cells are important. By the time a woman experiences symptoms, such as malodorous vaginal or watery discharge, postpareunia bleeding, dyspareunia, or metrorrhagia, cervical cancer has progressed beyond the early stages and prompt referral is warranted.

Anal Cancer Epidemiology and Burden

Anal cancer is rare but occurs primarily in heterosexual women and MSM. Women at high risk for anal cancer include those with high-grade cervical lesions and cervical and vulvar cancers. Men who have sex with men and persons who have HIV are also at high risk for anal cancer. In specific subgroups of men, such as men with an AIDS diagnosis, the incidence of both in situ and invasive anal cancer is significantly increased. The elevated risk of anal cancer observed among persons with AIDS most likely reflects the increased incidence, prevalence, and persistence of HPV infections as well as a high prevalence of cofactors for such cancers, such as cigarette smoking, among persons infected with HIV. HPV 16 is associated with the majority of anal cancers. Anal intraepithelial neoplasia (AIN) is recognized as a precursor of anal cancer, although the natural history of these lesions (i.e., rate of progression and regression) is less clear than for CIN, and there are currently no national recommendations for anal cytological screening.

Cervical Cancer Screening Guidelines

Cervical cancer screening with the Pap test can detect cytologic changes that reflect the underlying tissue changes. However, cytologic abnormalities detected by the Pap test can be ambiguous or equivocal. Abnormalities include ASC-US, atypical glandular cells of undetermined significance (AGUS), low- and high-grade

squamous intraepithelial lesions (LSIL, HSIL), and AIS. HPV types 16 and 18 are more commonly found in association with higher-grade lesions (see Figure 6-3).

No routine reporting or registry exists for abnormal Pap tests or cervical cancer precursor lesions in the United States; however, data are available from managed care organizations and administrative data sets. Each year, at least 30 million women undergo Pap testing, and approximately 1.4 million of these Pap tests are considered abnormal (Saraiya 2010).

Cervical cancer screening using cervical cytology (Pap test) is an effective, low-cost screening test for preventing invasive cervical cancer. Current guidelines from the American College of Obstetricians and Gynecologists (ACOG) recommend that cervical screening should begin at age 21 years. This is based on the low incidence of cervical cancer and limited utility of screening below this age. The U.S. Preventive Services Task Force and American Cancer Society (ACS) recommend that women start cervical screening with cervical cytology tests after or within 3 years of initiating sexual activity but by no later than age 21 years of age. Recommended screening intervals (see Table 6-1) should continue through 65 years (USPSTF) or 70 years (ACS).

Diagnostic HPV Testing

HPV tests are available for clinical use in women undergoing cervical cancer screening. These tests should not be used for women <20 years of age, or for STI "screening" apart from use as indicated in cervical cancer screening. HPV tests detect viral nucleic acid (i.e., DNA or RNA) or capsid protein. There are two tests approved by the Food and Drug Administration for high-risk HPV testing: (1) the digene HC2 High-Risk HPV DNA test (Qiagen, Gaithersburg, MD) and (2) the Cervista™ High-Risk HPV test (Hologics, Bedford, MA), which detect the presence of any of 13-14 high-risk HPV types. There is one FDA-approved test for type-specific high-risk HPV testing, the Cervista™ 16/18 HPV test, which detects and reports type-specific infection with HPV 16 or 18. It is the only test that provides information on the actual HPV type(s) present; others report a positive result if any of the types is positive. There is one FDA-approved test on the market, the digene HC2 HPV DNA test (Qiagen, Gaithersburg, MD), which detects the presence of any of 13 high-risk or 5 low-risk HPV types. There are no clinical indications and use of this test is highly discouraged by all major guidelines, especially in the STI clinic setting as

TABLE 6-1   Recommended Screening Intervals

	American Cancer Society (ACS)[1,2] 2002	U.S. Preventive Services Task Force (USPSTF)[3] 2003	American College of Obstetricians and Gynecologists (ACOG)[4] 2009
When to start screening	Approximately 3 years after onset of vaginal intercourse, but no later than age 21.^	Within 3 years of onset of sexual activity or age 21, whichever comes first. (A recommendation)	Age 21 regardless of the age of onset of sexual activity. Should be avoided before age 21. (Level A evidence)
Screening Method & Intervals			
Conventional Cytology	Annually; every 2-3 years for women age ≥30 years with a history of 3 negative cytology tests.* Sexual history should not be used as a rationale for more frequent screening.	At least every 3 years (A recommendation)	Every 2 years from age 21-29 years (Level A evidence); every 3 years for women age ≥30 years with a history of 3 negative cytology tests. * (Level A evidence)
Liquid-based cytology	Every 2 years; every 2-3 years for women age ≥30 years with a history of 3 negative cytology tests* Sexual history should not be used as a rationale for more frequent screening.	Insufficient evidence (I recommendation)	Every 2 years from age 21-29 years (Level A evidence); every 3 years for women age ≥30 years with a history of 3 negative cytology tests. * (Level A evidence)
HPV co-test (cytology + HPV test)	Not recommend under age 30. Age ≥30 years, no more than every 3 years if HPV negative, cytology normal. Sexual history should not be used as a rationale for more frequent screening.	Insufficient evidence (I recommendation)	Age ≥30 years, no more than every 3 years if HPV negative, cytology normal (Level A evidence), even with new sexual partners. Not recommended for women younger than 30 years.
Primary HPV testing[§]	Not FDA approved	Not FDA approved	Not FDA approved
When to stop screening	Women age ≥70 years with ≥3 recent, consecutive negative tests and no abnormal tests in prior 10 years. * At risk women* should continue screening as long as they are in reasonable health.	Women age >65 years with adequate recent screening with normal Pap tests, who are not otherwise at high risk for cervical cancer. (D recommendation)	Between age 65-70 years with 3 consecutive normal cytology tests and no abnormal tests in the past 10 years (Level B evidence); an older woman who is sexually active and has multiple partners should continue to have routine screening.

(continues)

TABLE 6-1   Recommended Screening Intervals *(continued)*

	American Cancer Society (ACS)[1,2] 2002	U.S. Preventive Services Task Force (USPSTF)[3] 2003	American College of Obstetricians and Gynecologists (ACOG)[4] 2009
Screening post-total hysterectomy	If removal for benign disease and no history of high-grade CIN or worse, may discontinue screening. Women with an undocumented history should be screened until 3 consecutive normal tests, and no abnormal tests within a 10-year period are achieved.	Discontinue if removal for benign disease. *(D recommendation)*	If removal for benign disease and no history or high-grade CIN of worse, may discontinue screening. *(Level A evidence)* Women for who a negative history cannot be documented should continue to be screened. *(Level B evidence)*
The need for a pelvic exam	The ACS and others should educate women, particularly teens and young women, that a pelvic exam does not equate to a cytology and that women who may not need a cytology test still need regular health care visits including gynecologic care. Women should discuss the need for pelvic exams with their providers	Not addressed	Physicians should inform their patients that annual gynecologic examinations may be appropriate. *(Level C evidence)*[‡]
Screening among those immunized against HPV 16/18	It is critical that women, whether vaccinated or not, continue screening according to current ACS early detection guidelines.	Not addressed	Recommendations remain the same regardless of vaccination status. *(Level C evidence)*

[1] Saslow D, et. al. American Cancer Society Guideline for the Early Detection of Cervical Neoplasia and Cancer. *CA Cancer J Clin* 2002; 52: 342-362.

[2] D. Saslow et. al. American Cancer Society guideline for HPV vaccine use to prevent cervical cancer and its precursors CA Cancer J Clin 2007 Jan-Feb;57(1):7-28

[3] USPSTF. Screening for Cervical Cancer. Jan 2003. Available at: http://www.ahrq.gov/clinic/3rduspstf/cervcan/cervacanr.pdf

[4] ACOG Practice Bulletin no. 109: Cervical cytology screening. ACOG Committee on Practice Bulletins-Gynecology. *Obstet Gynecol.* 2009 Dec;114(6):1409-20

^ Provider discretion and patient choice should be used to guide initiation of screening in women aged 21 years and older who have never had vaginal intercourse and for whom the absence of a history of sexual abuse is certain.

* Some exceptions apply (e.g., women who are immunocompromised, have a history of prenatal exposure to DES, HIV positive, women previously treated for CIN 2 or 3, or cancer etc.).

CIN = cervical intraepithelial neoplasia

§ Primary HPV testing is defined as conducting the HPV test as the first screening test. It may be followed by other tests (like a Pap) for triage.

‡ More specific guidance from 2003 states an annual pelvic examination is a routines part of preventive care for all women age ≥21 years even if they don not need cervical cytology screening. (level C evidence)

low-risk HPV type testing is not clinically useful, only high-risk HPV DNA testing is indicated.

High-risk HPV DNA tests are licensed and recommended for triage of women aged 21 years or older who have ASC-US (atypical squamous cells of undetermined significance) cytology results and for routine adjunctive testing (along with cervical cytology) for screening of women aged 30 years or older.

HPV DNA testing (including HR HPV and HPV 16/18 tests) is not recommended for deciding about HPV vaccination, STI screening for HPV, triage of LSIL (low-grade squamous intraepithelial lesion) or higher, testing of adolescents <21 years of age, or primary cervical cancer screening as a stand-alone test (i.e., without a cervical cytology test).

If the results of the cervical cytology test are abnormal, follow-up care should be provided according to the *ASCCP 2006 Consensus Guidelines for Management of Abnormal Cervical Cytology*; information regarding management and follow-up care is available at http://www.asccp.org.

When it is necessary to repeat the Pap test because the report interpretation was "unsatisfactory," the repeat test must be determined by the laboratory to be "satisfactory" and "negative" before screening can be resumed at regularly scheduled intervals.

Liquid-based cytology is an acceptable alternative to conventional Pap tests with similar test-performance characteristics.

■ SPECIAL CONSIDERATIONS FOR CERVICAL SCREENING

Pregnancy

Pregnant women are screened at the same frequency as nonpregnant women; however, recommendations for management differ.

HIV Infection

HIV-positive women are recommended to have cervical cytology screening twice (every 6 months) within the first year after initial HIV diagnosis and, if both tests are normal, to resume annual screening thereafter. HIV-positive women with ASC-H, LSIL, or HSIL on cytologic screening are recommended to have colposcopic evaluation. Recommendations for management of HIV-positive women with ASC-US vary from more conservative management (immediate colposcopy) as recommended by the U.S. Department of Health

and Human Services to the same management as HIV-negative women with ASC-US, which may include HR HPV DNA testing as recommended by ASCCP.

Adolescents (Younger Than 21 Years)

Prevalence of high-risk HPV is very high in this group. These infections tend to clear rapidly and lesions due to these infections also have high rates of regression to normal. ASCCP and ACOG therefore recommend that adolescents with ASC-US or low-grade SIL be managed with repeat cytologic testing at 12 months and 24 months. Only those with HSIL at either follow-up visit or persistence of ASC-US or LSIL at 24 months should be referred for colposcopic evaluation.

Hysterectomy

Women who have had a total hysterectomy do not require a routine Pap test unless the hysterectomy was performed because of cervical cancer or its precursor lesions. For women with hysterectomy due to CIN 2 or worse, cervical or vaginal cuff screening can be discontinued once three normal Pap tests have been documented (ACOG). In these situations, women should be advised to continue follow-up with the physician(s) who provided health care at the time of the hysterectomy, if possible. If the cervix remains after a hysterectomy, a woman should receive regularly scheduled Pap tests as indicated.

■ PROPHYLACTIC HPV VACCINES

In June 2006, the FDA approved the first prophylactic vaccine in the United States. The quadrivalent vaccine, manufactured by Merck (Gardasil™, Merck and Co, Inc.) protects against oncogenic and nononcogenic types and is composed of virus-like particles from the L1 capsid protein of the HPV 6, 11, 16, and 18 viruses. The quadrivalent vaccine was licensed for use among females aged 9–26 years and in October 2009 was licensed for use among 9- to 26-year-old males.

In clinical trials, almost all vaccines developed antibody after vaccination with mean geometric antibody titers higher than those observed after natural infection with HPV. The vaccine demonstrated high efficacy for prevention of external genital lesions (including genital warts) and cervical cancer precursor lesions (CIN2/3 or AIS) in phases II and III, randomized, double-blind, placebo-controlled trials among women aged 16–26 years. In a combined analysis of these trials with a follow-up period of about 41 months, efficacy against HPV 16 or 18 related CIN2/3 or AIS among women naïve for infection with vaccine HPV types was 98% (95% CI 93–100%). The quadrivalent vaccine also had 100% efficacy in preventing precursors to vaginal and vulvar cancers (VaIN 2/3 and VIN 2/3). Efficacy against genital warts due to types 6 and 11 was 99% (Kjaer 2009). The quadrivalent vaccine has also been studied in males and high efficacy against HPV 6, 11 related genital warts was found in this population (CDC–ACIP 2010).

A bivalent vaccine, manufactured by GlaxoSmith-Kline (Cervarix™) was approved by the FDA for use among 10- to 25-year-old females. The bivalent vaccine is also based on the L1 capsid protein and is directed against HPV 16 and 18. Randomized, multicenter, double-blind, placebo-controlled trials of women were also conducted with bivalent vaccine. The bivalent vaccine demonstrated excellent immunogenicity and efficacy in preventing CIN 2/3 or AIS among women naïve for infection with vaccine HPV types, 93%. Efficacy against VaIN and VIN was not measured.

Both vaccines also demonstrated good safety profiles and were recommended for use in the United States and have been adopted in many other countries.

HPV Vaccine Recommendations

Currently, the Advisory Committee on Immunization Practices (ACIP) has recommended routine vaccination of females aged 11 or 12 years with three doses of either quadrivalent or bivalent HPV vaccine. Vaccination can be given beginning at 9 years of age. Catch-up vaccination is recommended for females aged 13–26 years. Among females naïve for infection with vaccine HPV types, the quadrivalent vaccine prevents against infection with four HPV types: two oncogenic types, 16 and 18, and two nononcogenic types, 6 and 11, preventing against both cervical cancer and genital warts. The bivalent vaccine prevents infection with HPV types 16 and 18 and therefore provides protection against cervical cancer only. Both vaccines are likely to prevent other HPV 16 and 18 related cancers as well (see Table 6-2).

ACIP states that males aged 9–26 years may be vaccinated with the quadrivalent vaccine but has not included the vaccine in the routine vaccination schedule. Vaccination for both males and females before exposure to HPV (i.e., before sexual debut) will provide maximum benefit. However, vaccination after sexual debut

may provide protection against infection with HPV types not already acquired.

History of HPV infection, abnormal cervical cytology, genital warts, or treatments on the cervix are not reasons to withhold vaccine from eligible persons, since vaccination may provide protection against HPV types not already acquired. Providers should not perform any prevaccination testing with HPV tests or cervical cytology to determine whether vaccine should be administered.

While HPV vaccines have not been causally associated with adverse outcomes of pregnancy or adverse events in the developing fetus, they are not recommended for use during pregnancy. If a woman is found to be pregnant after initiating the vaccination series, the remainder of the three-dose regimen should be delayed until after completion of the pregnancy. If a vaccine dose has been administered during pregnancy, no intervention is needed. Pregnancy testing is not needed before vaccination.

Two separate vaccines in pregnancy registries have been established for persons who receive HPV vaccine during pregnancy. Patients and healthcare providers should report:

- Any exposure to quadrivalent HPV vaccine during pregnancy to Merck at telephone: 1-800-986-8999.

- Any exposure to bivalent HPV vaccine during pregnancy to GlaxoSmithKline at telephone: 1-888-452-9622.

Vaccine can be given to lactating women, immunocompromised persons, or persons with minor acute illnesses. Vaccine is contraindicated among persons with hypersensitivity to any vaccine components or to yeast.

Immunized women should continue to receive ongoing regular cervical screening as HPV vaccine only protects against the HPV types responsible for 70% of cervical cancers.

Safety of HPV Vaccines

The most common adverse events reported after HPV vaccination in clinical trials were local reactions. Post licensure vaccine safety monitoring has found reports of vasovagal syncope, which is common among adolescents receiving vaccines. To avoid serious injury related to a syncopal episode, vaccine providers should consider observing patients for 15 minutes after they are vaccinated.

Providers and patients are recommended to report any clinically significant adverse events after receipt of

TABLE 6-2   Quadrivalent and Bivalent Human Papilomavirus (HPV) Vaccines

Vaccine (Manufacturer) Brand name	Quadrivalent HPV Vaccine (Merck & Co., Inc.) Gardasil	Bivalent HPV Vaccine (GlaxoSmithKline) Cervarix
Year licensed in United States	2006 (females) 2009 (males)	2009 (females)
ACIP Recommendations/Guidance	Routine vaccination: 11- or 12-year-old girls* May be given to 9–26 year old males for prevention of genital warts	Routine vaccination: 11- or 12-year-old girls*
VLP types	HPV 6/11/16/18	HPV 16/18
Adjuvant	AAHS: 225 µg amorphous aluminum hydroxyphosphate sulfate	AS04: 500 µg aluminum hydroxide 50 µg 3-O-desacy-4'-monophosphoryl lipid A
Efficacy against HPV 16/18 related CIN2+	>98%	>93%
Efficacy against HPV 6/11 related genital lesions	~99%	—
Seroconversion to vaccine types	>99%	>99%
Duration of protection	Unknown, follow-up has occurred up to 5 or 7 years with excellent duration of projection	

Source: Adapted from ACIP Presentation, October 21, 2009. Available at http://www.cdc.gov/vaccines/recs/acip/downloads/mtg-slides-oct09/02-2-hpv.pdf

*Either vaccine is recommended for 11 or 12 year old girls; vaccine is recommended for 13 through 26 year olds who have not started or completed the vaccine series. Vaccine can be started at 9 years of age.

either the quadrivalent or bivalent HPV vaccine to the Vaccine Adverse Events Reporting System (VAERS) at http://vaers.hhs.gov, even if causal relation to vaccination is not certain. VAERS reporting forms and information are available electronically at http://www.vaers.hhs.gov or by telephone (800-822-7967). Web-based reporting is available and providers are encouraged to report electronically at https://secure.vaers.org/VaersDataEntryintro.htm to promote better timeliness and quality of safety data.

Vaccine safety data are continually monitored through VAERS, the Vaccine Safety Datalink, and pregnancy registries. A summary of HPV vaccine safety reports are found at www.cdc.gov/vaccinesafety/vaccines/HPV/Index.html.

■ **KEY POINTS**

• HPV is the most common sexually transmitted infection.

• HPV infection is often acquired soon after initiation of sexual intercourse and is often asymptomatic.

• The majority of HPV infections, even those associated with cancers, spontaneously clear without causing clinical disease.

• The major viral types that cause genital warts are types 6 and 11; the viral types that are associated with cervical cancer are types 16, 18, 31, 45, and others.

- Pap smears are a major public health intervention for prevention of cervical cancer. This does not prevent infection, but identifies persons who require excision and follow-up.

- The HPV vaccines provide primary prevention of cervical precancers, cancers, and other conditions and are highly effective in preventing infection with the vaccine associated types.

REFERENCES

Bosch FX, de Sanjose S. Human Papillomavirus and Cervical Cancer—Burden and Assessment of Causality. *J Natl Cancer Inst Monogr.* 2003;31: 3–13 .

CDC. Quadrivalent Human Papillomavirus Vaccine Recommendations. Recommendations of the Advisory Committee on Immunization Practices (ACIP). *Morb Mortal Wkly Rep.* 2007;56 (RR-2) 1–24.

CDC. FDA licensure of quadrivalent human papillomavirus vaccine (HPV4, Gardasil) for use in males and guidance from the Advisory Committee on Immunization Practices (ACIP). *Morb Mortal Wkly Rep.* 2010;59:630–632.

CDC. Sexually transmitted disease treatment guidelines, 2010. *Morbid Mortal Week Rep.* 2010;59(RR-12).

Datta SD, Koutsky LA, Ratelle S, et al. Human papillomavirus infection and cervical cytology in women screened for cervical cancer in the United States, 2003–2005. *Ann Intern Med.* 2008 Apr 1;148(7):493–500.

Dempsey AF, Koutsky LA, Golden M. Potential impact of human papillomavirus vaccines on public STD clinic workloads and on opportunities to diagnose and treat other sexually transmitted diseases. *Sex Transm Dis.* 2007;34:503–507.

De Vuyst H, Lillo F, Broutet N, Smith JS. HIV, human papillomavirus, and cervical neoplasia and cancer in the era of highly active antiretroviral therapy. *Eur J Cancer Prev.* 2008 Nov;17(6):545–554.

Dinh TH, Sternberg M, Dunne EF, Markowitz LE. Genital warts among 18- to 59-year-olds in the United States, National Health and Nutritional Examination Survey, 1999-2004. *Sex Transm Dis.* 2008;35:357–360.

Dunne EF, Unger ER, Sternberg M, et al. Prevalence of HPV infection among females in the United States. *JAMA.* 2007 Feb 28;297(8):813–819.

Ho GY, Bierman R, Beardsley L, et al. Natural history of cervicovaginal papillomavirus infection in young women. *N Engl J Med.* 1998;338(7):423–428.

Jin F, Prestage GP, Kippax SC, et al. Risk factors for genital and anal warts in a prospective cohort of HIV-negative homosexual men: the HIM study. *Sex Transm Dis.* 2007; 34:488–493.

Kjaer SK, Sigurdsson K, Iversen OE, et al. A pooled analysis of continued prophylactic efficacy of quadrivalent human papillomavirus (Types 6/11/16/18) vaccine against high-grade cervical and external genital lesions. *Cancer Prev Res.* 2009;2:868–878.

Kliewer EV, Demers AA, Elliott L, et al. Twenty-year trends in the incidence and prevalence of diagnosed anogenital warts in Canada. *Sex Transm Dis.* 2009;36:380–386.

Koshiol JE, Laurent SA, Pimenta JM. Rate and predictors of new genital warts claims and genital warts-related healthcare utilization among privately insured patients in the United States. *Sex Transm Dis.* 2004;31:748–752.

Kruger Kjaer S, Tran TN, Sparen P, et al. The burden of genital warts: a study of nearly 70,000 women from the general female population in the 4 Nordic Countries. *J Infect Dis.* 2007;196:1447–1454.

Oriel JD. Natural History of genital warts. *Br J Vener Dis.* 1971;47:1–13. *Am J Epidemiol.* 2003 Feb 1;157(3): 218–226.

Ostor AG. Natural history of cervical intraepithelial neoplasia: a critical review. *Int J Gynecol Pathol.* 1993 Apr; 12(2):186–192.

Pirotta M, Stein AN, Conway EL, et al. Genital Warts Incidence and Health Care Resource Utilisation in Australia. *Sex Transm Infect.* 2010;86:181–186.

Saraiya M, McCaig L, Ekwueme DU. Ambulatory Care Visits for Pap tests, abnormal Pap test results, and cervical cancer procedures in the United States. *Am J Managed Care.* 2010;16:e137–144.

Schiffman, MH and Hildesheim. Cervical cancer. In Schottenfeld D and Fraumeni JF Jr. (Eds.) *Cancer Epidemiology and Prevention.* New York: Oxford University Press, 2006, 1044–1067.

Weinstock H, Berman S, Cates W Jr. Sexually transmitted diseases among American youth: incidence and prevalence estimates, 2000. *Perspect Sex Reprod Health.* 2004 Jan-Feb;36(1):6–10.

Winer RL, Lee SK, Hughes JP, et al. Genital human papillomavirus infection: incidence and risk factors in a cohort of female university students. *Am J Epi.* 2003;157(3): 218–226.

Winer RL, Kiviat NB, Hughes JP, et al. Development and duration of human papillomavirus lesions, after initial infection. *J Infect Dis.* 2005;191:731–738.

7

Vaginitis

Jane R. Schwebke

◼ INTRODUCTION

Vaginal infections are a major cause of morbidity among women of reproductive age. Despite their population-based impact, these infections are still considered to be minor problems and are frequently overlooked, or incorrectly diagnosed and treated.

The three major causes of infectious vaginitis are candidiasis, trichomoniasis and bacterial vaginosis (BV). Of these, trichomoniasis is sexually transmitted and BV is sexually associated. Although vulvovaginal candidiasis occurs primarily in women of reproductive age and may possibly be associated with sexual intercourse, its epidemiology does not suggest sexual transmission.

◼ TRICHOMONIASIS

The annual incidence of trichomoniasis in the United States is estimated at 3 million cases. This infection is frequently seen concomitantly with other sexually transmitted infections (STIs), particularly gonorrhea. Most women with trichomoniasis also have changes in their vaginal bacterial flora, which are consistent with BV.

Unlike other STIs that have higher prevalences among adolescents and young adults, rates of trichomoniasis are more evenly distributed among sexually active women of all age groups.

Trichomonas vaginalis, a flagellated parasite, is the causative agent of this infection. Although there are two additional species of *Trichomonas* that infect humans, *T. vaginalis* is the only one that infects the urogenital

tract. Trichomoniasis is almost exclusively a sexually transmitted infection; however, the organism can survive on fomites for a short period. The incubation period of this infection is unknown; however, in vitro studies suggest an incubation period of 4–28 days.

Symptoms of trichomoniasis in women include vaginal discharge, irritation, and pruritus. Occasionally, women complain of vague abdominal discomfort, the etiology of which is unclear. *Trichomonas vaginalis* has not been documented to cause upper genital tract infection. About half of all women infected with *T. vaginalis* are asymptomatic. Signs of infection in women include vaginal discharge (42%), odor (50%), and edema or erythema (22–37%). The color of the discharge may vary. Colpitis macularis, also known as, strawberry cervix (see Figure 7-1), is a specific clinical sign for this infection but is only detected reliably by colposcopy and not during routine examination. The urethra is also infected in most cases. In males, the infection is usually asymptomatic; however, it can cause nongonococcal urethritis (NGU) (see Chapter 14).

◼ DIAGNOSIS

Diagnosis of trichomoniasis in the female currently relies on evaluation of symptoms, visualization of the organism by microscopy of vaginal secretions (see Figure 7-2), a rapid dipstick technique, or a DNA probe technique. Despite the availability of diagnostic tests, many clinicians still rely on syndromic diagnosis based on signs, symptoms, or both. A complaint of vaginal discharge has

FIGURE 7-1   Colpitis Macularis (Strawberry Cervix) in the Setting of Trichomonas Vaginitis.

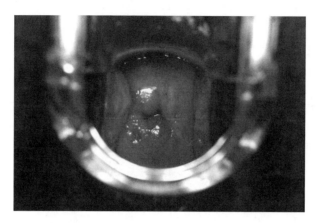

Note incidental bifurcated cervix.

been shown to correlate most often with the diagnosis of trichomoniasis, or BV, whereas a complaint of vulvovaginal itching most often correlates with candidiasis. However, the use of syndromic management has several inherent problems, including misdiagnosis, failure to diagnose asymptomatic infections, inability to counsel the patient regarding appropriate referral of sexual partners, and failure to screen for other STIs. Thus, this approach should only be undertaken when diagnostic resources are lacking.

■ VAGINAL WET MOUNT DIAGNOSIS

The most commonly used laboratory diagnostic test is examination of the vaginal fluid using light microscopy. A sample of fluid is mixed with normal saline and examined at 400× for motile trichomonads (see

Figure 7-2). In preparing and examining the sample for microscopy, obtain a sufficient amount of the specimen so that it will not be too dilute when mixed with the saline. White blood cells may also be seen, as well as findings consistent with BV as this is frequently a coinfection. The vaginal pH in patients with trichomoniasis is variable. The whiff test (mixing vaginal secretions with 10% potassium hydroxide to detect a fishy odor) is variable. Although direct microscopic examination of the vaginal fluid for motile trichomonads is the fastest, least inexpensive diagnostic method, the sensitivity of this test compared with culture is limited and at best is 70% (Schwebke 2004).

Currently, the gold standard for the diagnosis of trichomoniasis is culture. Culture is usually a reference method and is performed by cultivation in Diamond's medium. There are also newer, commercially available

FIGURE 7-2   Microscopy of Vaginal Secretions in Trichomonas Vaginitis

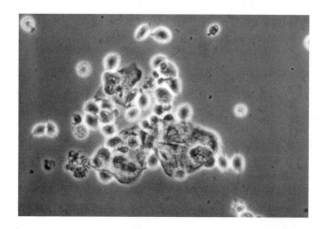

culture methods. For example, the *InPouch*, composed of liquid media in a clear pouch, is easily transportable and has been used successfully with both clinician-obtained and self-obtained specimens. Self-obtained specimens are useful in situations in which pelvic examination is not possible or desirable (e.g., screening in adolescents, developing countries). Results from culture are available in 2 to 5 days.

Other tests for the diagnosis of trichomoniasis in women include an office-based oligonucleotide probe test (Affirm VPIII, Becton Dickinson, Sparks, MD) or an office-based "dipstick" technique (OSOM Trichomonas Rapid Test, Genzyme Diagnostics). Trichomonads may be seen on Pap smears, with a sensitivity of about 60% and a specificity of 95% and may be identified as part of a routine urinalysis (Schwebke 2004). Polymerase chain reaction techniques are being developed.

Trichomoniasis is one of the few STIs that is more difficult to diagnose in males than in females. Most often, the syndromic approach is used in this setting, or males are treated because they are sexual contacts to an infected female. Direct microscopic examination of urethral discharge or of the sediment of a first morning urine may reveal trichomonads but has limited sensitivity. Culture of both the urethra and urine sediment is currently the best approach. PCR or other nucleic acid approaches may be available soon.

■ TREATMENT

Treatment is either with metronidazole or tinidazole, both 2 grams orally in a single dose (CDC 2010). Sexual partners should also be treated. Metronidazole intravaginal gel has limited efficacy and is not recommended; likewise, topical antifungal preparations are of no value. Metronidazole is safe in pregnancy. Occasionally, patients are allergic to metronidazole. Since there is no effective alternative outside this class of drugs, desensitization is the only option. Another therapeutic dilemma is metronidazole resistance in *T. vaginalis*. This resistance is relative and usually can be overcome with higher doses of oral metronidazole or by using tinidazole, which has greater activity against *T. vaginalis* and superior phamacokinetics to metronidazole. In various doses, tinidazole has been shown to be effective against resistant strains of *T. vaginalis*. If the patient fails prolonged therapy with tinidazole, they should be referred to a center where susceptibility results can be performed. There are limited anecdotal reports of success with intravaginal paromomycin

cream. This can be ordered through local compounding pharmacies. Caution should be exercised, however, as paramomycin can cause significant vaginal irritation. Women with asymptomatic infection should be treated. If left untreated, about one-third will eventually become symptomatic and, without treatment, they continue to transmit the infection. Males may also be treated with either metronidazole or tinidazole, and these antibiotics are recommended as part of the treatment regimen of the male with persistent NGU.

Infection with *T. vaginalis* has been implicated as a cause of preterm delivery in a multicenter study of vaginal infections in pregnancy, suggesting that treatment of the pregnant woman should not be postponed. A more recent prospective study of treatment of women with asymptomatic trichomonas in pregnancy to prevent preterm birth was halted prematurely because of a trend in increased preterm birth in the treatment group compared with the placebo. However, there were several methodological problems with the study, including an unusually high dose of metronidazole for treatment and that women in the placebo arm may have been treated off study by their primary care physician. Thus, recommendations for routine screening and treatment of trichomonas in pregnancy are unclear. Acquisition of the human immunodeficiency virus (HIV) has also been associated with trichomoniasis in several international studies possibly as a result of local inflammation often caused by the parasite.

■ BACTERIAL VAGINOSIS

The most prevalent cause of vaginal discharge worldwide is bacterial vaginosis. In the United States, the prevalence of BV in the general population is about 25%, but in populations at high risk for STIs, the prevalence may exceed 50%. Although not proven to be sexually transmitted, the epidemiology of BV suggests that it is sexually associated. It is primarily seen in sexually active women, and epidemiological risk factors associated with BV include multiple or new sexual partners and a history of STI. Douching has also been associated with BV in retrospective studies. BV frequently occurs as a coinfection with other STIs.

The etiology of BV is unknown. The condition can best be described as a stable alteration in the vaginal ecosystem. The healthy vagina is primarily inhabited by moderate numbers of lactobacilli, particularly hydrogen peroxide–producing strains (see Figure 7-3). These bacteria are thought to act as a natural barrier to infection by

FIGURE 7-3   Normal Vaginal Gram Stain Showing Healthy Epithelial Cell and Predominance of Gram-Positive Lactobacilli

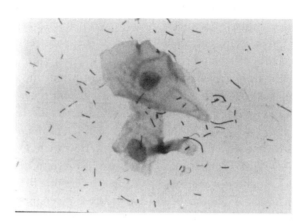

successfully competing with potential invaders. In vitro studies have demonstrated their ability to kill pathogens, including HIV. In BV, there is a decrease in the lactobacilli and a marked increase in the anaerobic and facultatively anaerobic bacteria. These bacteria include anaerobic cocci, *Bacteroides, Porphyromonas, Prevotella, Mobiluncus,* and genital mycoplasmas, as well as newly recognized bacteria such as *Atopobium vaginae.* The total concentration of bacteria in the vagina is also greatly increased (see Figure 7-4).

This change in flora is accompanied by an increase in the vaginal pH and by the production of amines by the bacteria.

One-half of women with BV are symptomatic; most complain of vaginal discharge and a fishy odor. Women may also note an odor after sexual intercourse due to mixing alkaline semen with vaginal secretions. Among women with asymptomatic BV, it is unclear whether the symptoms are poorly recognized or truly absent.

■ DIAGNOSIS FOR BV

The diagnosis of BV is complicated because a specific etiologic agent has not been identified. Several approaches to the diagnosis of BV exist. The syndromic approach is based on the patient's history alone or the history combined with observation of the discharge. Symptoms such as odor, discharge, and odor after intercourse are suggestive of BV, but they are not confirmatory nor do they rule out the presence of concurrent infections such as trichomoniasis. Vaginal discharge complaints are more likely due to BV or trichomoniasis, whereas vaginal yeast infections are more often associated with the pruritus.

FIGURE 7-4   Bacterial Vaginosis, Gram Stain

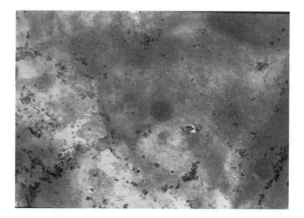

Note increased number of bacteria, large number of Gram-negative pleomorphs, and epithelial cells without clear borders.

Nonetheless, the syndromic approach should be reserved for those situations in which resources are too limited to derive a specific diagnosis. A specific diagnosis should be sought whenever possible so that appropriate therapy and counseling can be provided.

Culture of vaginal secretions is not helpful and is not recommended especially since Garnerella may be present in lower concentrations in many women without the syndrome (Sobel 1997).

Clinical diagnosis is most commonly used and is based on the Amsel criteria. This is a composite criteria consisting of the presence of a homogeneous vaginal discharge, a vaginal pH of >4.5, a positive whiff (fishy odor) test, and the presence of clue cells (see Figure 7-5) in the vaginal fluid wet prep. Clue cells are epithelial cells that have a ground glass appearance due to numerous adherent bacteria. A diagnosis of BV requires presence of three of the four criteria. In clinical practice, these individual parameters may be influenced by recent behavior and may be subjectively interpreted. The sample for pH measurement should be obtained from the vagina directly and should not be contaminated with cervical secretions that are normally more alkaline. The most common method is to use narrow range pH paper (pH range 4–7). Blood, semen, and recent douching may also interfere with the pH test, and therefore, this may not be valid in menstruating women. The whiff test, which detects an amine (fishy) odor, is subject to interobserver variability and experience. Clue cells, defined as squamous epithelial cells covered with bacteria to the extent that the edges of the cell are obscured, are also subject to the interpretation of the microscopist.

The careful observer, however, will go beyond the Amsel criteria and will note the amount and morphotypes of the vaginal bacteria in the wet prep. In BV, there will be many coccobacillary morphotypes and a paucity of large rods that represent the lactobacilli. Motile curved rods, which represent *Mobiluncus*, are pathognomonic for BV. Although white blood cells are not associated with this syndrome, they may be present in the vaginal fluid as a result of a concurrent lower genital tract infection and thus their presence does not rule out the diagnosis of BV. In preparing and examining the sample for microscopy, obtain a sufficient amount of the specimen so that it will not be too dilute when mixed with the saline. A modification to the original Amsel criteria, which requires that clue cells represent at least 20% of all epithelial cells present, has been suggested to improve the specificity of the criteria; however, this may be too rigid for clinical practice.

Use of Gram's stain of the vaginal secretions for the diagnosis of BV, using the Nugent's criteria, has been widely used in the research setting but are not clinically used.

Timing of specimen collection may have an important influence on the diagnosis of BV, especially if the Gram's stain method is used. Although the normal vaginal flora is described as consisting primarily of lactobacilli, variability in the day-to-day composition of the flora as detected by Gram's stain is common. Studies suggest that only 20% of women maintain a lactobacillus-predominant flora consistently throughout the menstrual cycle. Others exhibit transient changes, sometimes dramatic, throughout the cycle with the majority of changes occurring around the time of menses. Thus, interpreting a single Gram's stain specimen could lead to an erroneous diagnosis of BV.

FIGURE 7-5   Bacterial Vaginosis

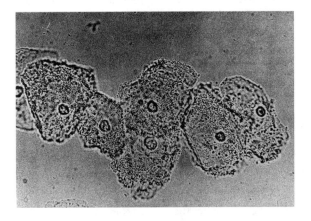

Light microscopy demonstrating clue cells, epithelial cells with ground glass appearance.

Additional tests are commercially available for the diagnosis of BV. A rapid card test detects proline aminopeptidase, an enzyme found in the vaginal secretions of women with BV (PIP Activity TestCard™, Quidel, San Diego, CA). A second rapid card test, which detects elevated pH and amines (QuickVue Advance, Quidel, San Diego, CA), may be a useful screening tool for determining which patients should be more fully evaluated. A semiautomated test for vaginitis, which includes BV, is also available (Affirm VPIII, Becton Dickinson, Sparks, MD). This test detects high concentrations of *Gardnerella* by use of a DNA probe and compares favorably to reference methods.

■ TREATMENT FOR BV

Recommended treatment regimens for BV include metronidazole or clindamycin both of which are available in oral and topical intravaginal preparations (CDC 2010. Cure rates of 70–80% are the norm, but recurrences are common. For metronidazole, the recommended oral regimen is 500 mg orally twice a day for 7 days. The 2 gram one-time oral dose should not be used for BV. Clindamycin is dosed at 300 mg twice a day for 7 days but is used much less frequently than metronidazole. Tinidazole is also approved for treating BV. Topicals are as efficacious for treating BV as oral agents and avoid systemic side effects although local side effects such as vaginal yeast infections may occur. Available products include intravaginal metronidazole gel, clindamycin 2% cream, and clindamycin ovules. Many clinicians are reluctant to use metronidazole during pregnancy; however, there is no data to support these concerns. For women with recurrent BV, twice weekly prophylaxis with intravaginal metronidazole gel has been shown to be effective. Earlier studies failed to show a benefit from treating male sexual partners of women with recurrent BV but used single-dose therapy, which is likely to be ineffective. Condoms have been shown to be effective in preventing recurrent BV. Reconstitution of the vaginal flora with exogenous lactobacilli has been suggested as an adjunct to antibiotic therapy but has not been shown to be effective.

■ ASYMPTOMATIC BV AND THE PREGNANCY CONTROVERSY

Treatment of asymptomatic BV is controversial. Some data suggest a benefit of treatment in certain situations. Among women at high risk for preterm delivery because

of a prior preterm delivery, combination therapy with erythromycin and metronidazole was found to be associated with a decrease in preterm births, especially among those women who had BV. Treatment of BV before elective first-trimester abortion has been shown to decrease the rate of postabortal pelvic inflammatory disease (PID). Also, BV has been associated with endometritis, PID, and vaginal cuff cellulitis in women undergoing hysterectomy; however, no prospective treatment data are available.

It appears that BV-associated bacteria are able to ascend into the upper genital tract. In the pregnant patient, organisms have been demonstrated in the chorioamnion of women who delivered preterm. Histologic evidence of subclinical chorioamnionitis may also be present in this setting and may act as the rigger for the initiation of labor. BV has also been associated with low-birth-weight infants. As mentioned earlier, there is good prospective data to link BV with postabortal PID. In the nonpregnant patient, BV has been retrospectively associated with infectious complications following hysterectomy as well as with PID. BV-associated bacteria and histologic evidence of endometritis have been demonstrated in the endometria of patients with BV, with or without clinical signs of upper tract infection. Tubal cultures of women with PID frequently yield anaerobic organisms, often in the absence of gonorrhea or chlamydia. However, prospective studies of the prevention of PID by treatment of BV are lacking.

BV has also been associated with acquisition of HIV. In several international studies, BV has been shown to be independently associated with HIV prevalence and incidence. In vitro hydrogen peroxide–producing lactobacilli have been shown to be inhibitory to HIV. BV has also been shown to be associated with other STIs, including PID, trichomoniasis, and cervicitis and with urinary tract infections. Thus, it may be that the lack of protective lactobacilli among women with BV increases the risk of acquisition of a pathogen if exposed.

Recurrence of bacterial vaginosis is common and may occur in as many as 60% of patients. If an underlying cause can be identified, such as antimicrobial use or other STI infections, these issues should be resolved. In most cases, recurrences can be managed symptomatically. In cases where recurrences occur often, or affect a patient's lifestyle, then suppressive therapy with either intravaginal metronidazole or tinidazole can be considered.

■ VAGINAL YEAST INFECTION (CANDIDIASIS)

Vaginal candidiasis is one of the most common causes of vaginitis and occurs throughout the life span and is not associated with sexual activity. Candida species, especially *Candida albicans*, are found in low numbers in most women. Alterations of vaginal ecology may induce overgrowth of the organisms, with concomitant development of symptoms. Inducing factors for vaginal candidiasis are myriad and include:

- Systemic antimicrobial use, which eradicates the normal flora allowing overgrowth

- Systemic diseases, such as diabetes mellitus and autoimmune diseases

- Vaginal atrophy

- Systemic steroid use

■ DIAGNOSIS AND CLINICAL PRESENTATION

Symptoms of vaginal candidiasis include vaginal irritation, erythema of the vaginal introitus and external genitalia, dyspareunia, and discharge that has a classic cheeselike consistency. The vaginal fluid pH is typically acidic and does not demonstrate clue cells. Light microscopy of vaginal fluid after addition of 10% KOH will demonstrate budding yeast or mycelia forms (see Figure 7-6). In the presence of symptoms, a negative KOH smear has high sensitivity of ruling out candidiasis

Management usually includes attempting to identify an underlying cause, if possible (e.g., antibiotic use) as well as pharmacotherapy. There are a large number of options for treatment. The 2010 CDC STD treatment guidelines include the following recommendations:

- Oral therapy: Fluconazole 150 mg as a single dose

- Intravaginal short-course options:
  - Butoconazole 2% cream 5 g intravaginally for 3 days
  - Clotrimazole 2% cream 5 g intravaginally for 3 days
  - Miconazole 200 mg vaginal suppository, one suppository for 3 days
  - Miconazole 1,200 mg vaginal suppository, one suppository for 1 day

■ FURTHER CLINICAL CONSIDERATIONS

- It is not necessary to treat sexual partners of patients with vaginal candidiasis.

- Some persons may have recurrent or persistent yeast vaginitis. The most common etiology is the presence of underlying chronic disease, and therefore periodic symptomatic treatment with one of the previous regimens may be indicated.

- Colonization with nonalbicans *Candida* (such as *C. tropicalis* or *C. parasilosis*) may be associated with some cases of recurrent infections. Nonalbicans *Candida* are often resistant to first-line therapies such as fluconazole. If this is suspected, a vaginal culture may be obtained, with specific requests for speciation and susceptibility testing. This is one of the few situations when cultures are actually recommended.

FIGURE 7-6   Yeast Vaginitis, KOH Showing Budding Yeast and Mycelia

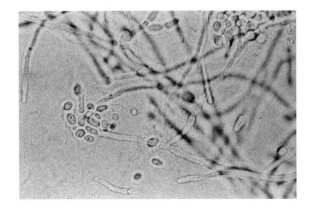

- Some alternative medicine providers and many Internet Web sites have suggested that recurrent *Candida*, in the setting of a negative workup, may be associated with altered immune status or nutritional deficiencies. These assertions are not evidence-based; however, practitioners should be aware that patients may be pursuing these alternative approaches. Therapies such as probiotics, yogurt douches, and megavitamins have not been shown to be effective.

■ AN APPROACH TO THE DIFFERENTIAL DIAGNOSIS OF VAGINITIS

- Women who present with vaginal symptoms may have either cervical disease or vaginitis. Since vaginal discharge may also be a result of unrecognized cervical inflammation (from the patient's perspective), an initial full evaluation should include cervical inspection and testing for gonococcal and chlamydial infection. Clinicians should also be aware that cervical inflammation may also induce changes in the vaginal flora that cause bacterial vaginosis; antibiotic therapy for gonorrhea or chlamydia may induce yeast vaginitis, and trichomonas may be epidemiologically associated with other STIs, such as gonorrhea. Herpes simplex infection, especially primary disease, may result in vaginal discharge and prurititis.

- Under the ideal circumstance, patients evaluated for vaginitis should have a full examination and wet mount examination. A flowchart for interpretation of signs and symptoms, summarizing the differential diagnosis of all three entities, is presented in Table 7-1.

- With the exception of trichomoniasis, partner therapy is not currently recommended.

- Recurrences are not infrequent and are usually managed symptomatically.

TABLE 7-1   Differential Diagnosis of Vaginitis

	Normal	Candidiasis	Bacterial Vaginosis	Trichomoniasis
pH	<4.5	Variable; may be normal	>4.5	4.5
Discharge Quality	White, clear, small amount	Cheeselike	Homogeneous, increased quantity; whitish gray	Frothy, increased, yellow green
Microscopic	Epithelial cells with clear borders, predominance of gram-positive lactobacilli	Budding yeast on Gram's stain or KOH light prep. Increased WBCs Epithelial cells with clear borders	Epithelial cells with ground glass appearance ("clue cells"), Gram's stain shows gram-negative organisms, overall bacterial counts increased	Increased WBCs; motile trichomonads present
KOH "Whiff"	Negative	Negative	Positive	Variable
Symptoms	None	Vaginal itching, irritation, discharge; "feeling raw"	Vaginal discharge, fishy odor, dyspareunia, may have some lower abdominal pain	Vaginal discharge, vulvar pruritis

WBC = white blood cell.

■ SUMMARY

Trichomoniasis and BV are sexually associated infections that remain very prevalent and are responsible for morbidity associated with local symptomatology and more serious complications, such as preterm birth and susceptibility to other STIs, including HIV. Although currently not considered public health priorities, accumulating information on the possible consequences of these infections may lead to greater interest in their control.

■ KEY POINTS

- Trichomonas is a sexually transmitted infection, thus sex partners should be treated.

- Single-dose metronidazole or tinidazole may be used to treat trichomoniasis.

- Tinidazole is the drug of choice for treating metrondiazole-resistant trichomonas.

- Bacterial vaginosis (BV) behaves like a sexually transmitted infection but has not been proven to be sexually transmitted.

- The microbiologic cause of BV remains unknown.

- Many women may exhibit changes in their vaginal flora patterns throughout their cycle.

- BV can be treated with either oral or intravaginal metronidazole or clindamycin.

- Recurrent BV may be managed with prophylactic intravaginal metronidazole and use of condoms.

- Vaginal candidiasis is extremely common and is not associated with sexual intercourse.

REFERENCES

Amsel R, Totten PA, Spiegel CA, Chen KCS, Eschenbach D, Holmes KK. Non-specific vaginitis: diagnostic and microbial and epidemiological associations. *Am J Med*. 1983;74:14–22.

Centers for Disease Control and Prevention. Sexually transmitted disease treatment guidelines 2010. *Morb Mortal Week Rep* 2010;59(RR-12):1–110.

Cohen MS. Trichomonas vaginalis infection in male sexual partners: implications for diagnosis, treatment, and prevention. *Clin Infect Dis*. 2007;44(1):13–22.

Eschenbach DA. Bacterial vaginosis and anaerobes in obstetric-gynecologic infection. *Clin Infect Dis*. 1993;16:S282–S287.

Eschenbach DA, Hillier S, Critchlow C, Stevens C, DeRouen T, Holmes KK. Diagnosis and clinical manifestations of bacterial vaginosis. *Am J Obstet Gynecol*. 1988;158:819–828.

Fredricks DN, Fiedler TL, Marrazzo JM. Molecular identification of bacteria associated with bacterial vaginosis. *N Engl J Med*. 2005;353(18):1899–1911.

Hillier SL. Diagnostic microbiology of bacterial vaginosis. *Am J Obstet Gynecol*. 1993;169:455–459.

Hillier SL, Nugent RP, Eschenbach DA, et al.. Association between bacterial vaginosis and preterm delivery of a low-birth weight infant. *N Engl J Med*. 1995;333:1737–1742.

Klebanoff MA, Carey JC, Hauth JC, et al. Failure of metronidazole to prevent preterm delivery among pregnant women with asymptomatic *Trichomonas vaginalis* infection. *N Engl J Med*. 2001;345:487–493.

Pappas PG, Kauffman CA, Andes D, et al; Infectious Diseases Society of America. Clinical practice guidelines for the management of candidiasis: 2009 update by the Infectious Diseases Society of America. *Clin Infect Dis*. 2009;48(5):503–535.

Schwebke JR. New concepts in the etiology of bacterial vaginosis. *Curr Infect Dis Rep*. 2009;11(2):143–147.

Schwebke JR, Burgess D. Trichomoniasis. *Clin Microbiol Rev*. 2004;17(4):794–803.

Schwebke JR, Desmond R. Natural history of asymptomatic bacterial vaginosis in a high-risk group of women. *Sex Transm Dis*. 2007;34(11):876–877.

Schwebke JR, Desmond R. Risk factors for bacterial vaginosis in women at high risk for sexually transmitted diseases. *Sex Transm Dis*. 2005;32(11):654–658.

Seña AC, Miller WC, Hobbs MM, et al. Reduced fluconazole susceptibility of *Candida albicans* isolates in women with recurrent vulvovaginal candidiasis: effects of long-term fluconazole therapy. *Diagn Microbiol Infect Dis*. 2009;64(3):354–356.

Sobel JD. Vaginitis. *N Engl J Med*. 1997;337:1896–1903.

Sobel JD. *Vulvovaginal candidosis* [review]. Lancet. 2007;369(9577):1961–1971.

Sobel JD, Ferris D, Schwebke J, et al. Suppressive maintenance antibacterial therapy with 0.75% metronidazole vaginal gel to prevent recurrent bacterial vaginosis. *Am J Obstet Gynecol*. 2006;194:1283–1289.

8

Pelvic Inflammatory Disease

Mark H. Yudin and Jonathan D. C. Ross

▪ INTRODUCTION

Pelvic inflammatory disease (PID) is an infection of the female upper genital tract and describes a spectrum of infectious inflammatory disorders. It may involve any combination of the endometrium, fallopian tubes, pelvic peritoneum, and contiguous structures. It is a serious and important public health problem, with millions of dollars spent each year in the United States on diagnosis and treatment. It is also one of the most commonly seen infectious disorders in women, with both short- and long-term consequences. In this chapter, we will discuss several important aspects of PID, including epidemiology and risk factors, etiologic agents, pathogenesis, diagnosis and treatment, short- and long-term sequelae, and strategies for prevention.

▪ EPIDEMIOLOGY AND RISK FACTORS

PID is a significant public health problem. Unfortunately, diagnosis is often difficult, and patients may be asymptomatic or have atypical presentations. It has been estimated that up to two-thirds of cases are unrecognized, and underreporting is common. For these reasons, and because PID is not generally a reportable disease, exact figures of incidence and prevalence are unknown and must be estimated. Currently, approximately 1 million cases of symptomatic PID are identified annually in the United States. It is estimated that

10–15% of women of reproductive age have had one episode of PID and that PID accounts for around 2% of consultations made by young women in primary care (Simms 1999).

The epidemiology of PID is complex, and many variables have been identified that impact the risk of its acquisition. A list of these risk factors is presented in Table 8-1.

Age

Age is an independent risk factor for PID and is inversely related to the rate of PID. PID rates are highest for women aged 15 to 25 years, and are low for women older than 35 years. Adolescents are at particular risk, and are three times as likely as women aged 25 to 29 years to develop PID.

Adolescents possess both biologic and behavioral characteristics that place them at greater risk for acquiring PID. Biologic factors include a lower prevalence of potentially protective chlamydial antibodies, a higher likelihood of anovulatory cycles with cervical mucus that is easier to penetrate, and larger zones of cervical ectopy with more columnar cells for which bacterial and viral infectious agents have a greater affinity. In terms of sexual behavior, sexually active teenagers are more likely than older women to have multiple and concurrent partners and may be more likely to have unprotected intercourse.

TABLE 8-1 Risk Factors for Pelvic Inflammatory Disease

Patient Characteristics
- young patient age
- low socioeconomic status
- single marital status
- urban residence

Sexual Behavior
- multiple sexual partners
- concurrent sexual partners
- number of new sexual partners in previous 30 days
- high frequency of sexual intercourse
- young age at first intercourse

Prior and Present Infection
- PID
- gonorrhea
- chlamydia
- bacterial vaginosis

Contraception
- IUD

Cigarette Smoking

Substance Abuse

Menstruation

PID = pelvic inflammatory disease
IUD = intrauterine device

Other Demographic Factors

In addition to age, other demographic factors have been suggested as risk factors for developing PID. Socioeconomic measures such as low levels of education, unemployment, and low income have been associated with an increased risk. It has also been suggested that women who live in urban areas are at a higher risk for PID than those living in rural areas. Each of these risk factors may be markers for sexual behavior, and this is likely the basis for the association.

Sexual Behavior

Sexual behaviors associated with increased PID risk include multiple sexual partners, number of new sexual partners in the previous 30 days, high frequency of sexual intercourse, and young age at first intercourse. The number of sexual partners is one of the most important risk factors for the development of PID. Multiple sexual partners or a new partner may increase the risk of exposure to infectious agents. The frequency of intercourse has been associated with the development of PID in some studies. Increased frequency can increase exposure to both sexually transmitted pathogens and nonsexually transmitted organisms, such as group B streptococci.

Male sexual partners of women with PID are a source of both initial and recurrent infections. In earlier studies, gonorrhea in male partners of women was as high as 60%, and nearly half of the males were asymptomatic. In partners of women with nongonococcal PID, only about 10% of the men have clinical nongonococcal urethritis (NGU), but subclinical inflammation with chlamydia is probably higher. Asymptomatic partners, if not treated, pose substantial risk for reinfection and may contribute to the high rate of recurrence in women treated for PID. This highlights the integral role of partner treatment in the management of PID.

Prior and Present Infection—Past PID Episodes Increase the Risk

Women with a previous episode of PID are at an increased risk for developing subsequent infection. Patients with PID are two to three times more likely than those without PID to have a history of prior infection. Roughly, one-fourth of women with acute PID will have a subsequent episode. Factors that may be important in developing future PID include untreated male sexual partners, sexual behavior, inadequate antibiotic therapy, or disease severity. Women with a history of cervical gonococcal infection without PID are at increased risk. This may be related to a high rate of reinfection in these patients or to subclinical tubal infection at the time of cervical gonorrhea. Because gonorrhea does not confer immunity against subsequent infections, repeat gonococcal infections are seen commonly—up to 15% within one year in some studies.

Recent data have suggested an association between bacterial vaginosis (BV) and upper genital tract infection, endometritis, and PID. A prospective study did not, however, suggest that BV is a direct cause of PID, although it may increase the risk of upper genital infection when superinfection with *Neisseria gonorrhoeae* or *Chlamydia trachomatis* occurs.

Contraception

Contraceptive choice has a large impact on the risk of developing sexually transmitted infections (STIs) and PID. Women who use no method of contraception are at an increased risk for STIs and PID, while the proper use of barrier methods can decrease this risk. The use of condoms, diaphragms, and spermicides all decrease the risk of cervical infection with *N. gonorrhoeae* and *C. trachomatis* and PID. Latex condoms provide greater protection than natural membrane condoms.

The use of the combined oral contraceptive pill (OCP) has been shown to reduce the risk of PID by 40–60% (Wolner-Hanssen 1990). Hypotheses for the protection provided by the OCP include maintenance of cervical mucus throughout the entire menstrual cycle, light menstrual flow from an inactive endometrium, and decreased myometrial contractile activity.

In contrast to women using the OCP, women who use an intrauterine device (IUD) are at an increased risk for the development of PID. IUD users have two to four times the likelihood of developing PID compared with nonusers, and the risk is higher for nulliparous compared with multiparous women. In contrast to much popular belief, the increased risk is, however, limited to the first 1 to 3 months after insertion. In a large study of more than 22,000 users, the risk was six times greater in the first 20 days after insertion than at all other times, during which the risk was low for up to 8 years of use. The mechanism of the increased risk is unknown but thought to be due to a transient bacterial contamination of the endometrial cavity following insertion.

Douching

Vaginal douching is associated with PID, but prospective studies do not suggest a causal link. The symptoms of discharge, odor, and intermenstrual bleeding associated with PID may themselves increase the likelihood of douching, rather than douching causing PID (Ness et al. 2005; Rothman et al. 2003). Nevertheless, some clinicians discourage douching because of the potential for increased PID risk and increased rate of bacterial vaginosis.

Other Risk Factors

Other proposed risk factors for developing PID include cigarette smoking, substance abuse, and menstruation. Current and previous smokers have twice the risk of de-

veloping PID than women who do not smoke. Similarly, alcohol and illicit drug use, especially cocaine, are associated with PID. Finally, there is an association between the development of PID and the timing of the menstrual cycle. Studies have shown that women with gonococcal or chlamydial PID are most likely to develop symptoms within the first seven days of menses (Eckert et al. 2002). For women with PID caused by other organisms, symptoms are least likely to develop at this time.

■ MICROBIAL ETIOLOGY

PID is a polymicrobial infection, and several different organisms have been implicated as etiologic agents. Many cases of PID are associated with more than one organism. It is customary to divide the pathogens into sexually transmitted and endogenous organisms. The sexually transmitted organisms include *N. gonorrhoeae*, *C. trachomatis*, genital tract mycoplasmas, and perhaps viruses and protozoa. Endogenous organisms include various anaerobic and facultative (aerobic) bacteria. Table 8-2 presents the microbial etiology and classification of acute PID.

Sexually Transmitted Organisms

The most common sexually transmitted organisms causing acute PID are *N. gonorrhoeae* and *C. trachomatis*. The proportion of women with PID infected with one of these pathogens varies widely and depends on their endemic rates in the populations studied. *Neisseria gonorrhoeae* has been recovered from the cervix in 27–81% and from the fallopian tubes in 13–18% of women with acute PID. *Chlamydia trachomatis* has been recovered from the cervix in 5–39% and from the fallopian tubes in up to 10% of women with acute PID. Chlamydia has also been implicated as a contributor to tubal infertility and ectopic pregnancy, two major sequelae of PID.

The genital tract mycoplasmas, *Mycoplasma hominis*, *Ureaplasma urealyticum*, and *Mycoplasma genitalium*, have also been suggested as potential causes of acute PID (Anagrius et al. 2005). They have been isolated from the fallopian tubes or abdomen in some women with acute PID and not in those without PID. At present, their role remains controversial. Finally, the role of viruses and protozoa, such as herpes simplex virus, cytomegalovirus, and *Trichomonas vaginalis* in acute PID, is still under study.

TABLE 8-2   Microbial Etiology and Classification of Acute PID

Sexually-Transmitted Organisms

Neisseria gonorrhoeae

Chlamydia trachomatis

Genital Tract Mycoplasmas
- *Mycoplasma genitalium*
- *Mycoplasma hominis*
- *Ureaplasma urealyticum*

Viruses and Protozoa
- Herpes Simplex
- Cytomegalovirus
- *Trichomonas vaginalis*

Endogenous Organisms

Anaerobic Bacteria
- *Bacteroides (Prevotella)* species
- *Peptostreptococcus* species
- *Peptococcus* species
- *Atopobium* species
- *Leptotrichia* species

Facultative (Aerobic) Bacteria
- *Gardnerella vaginalis*
- *Streptococcus* species
- *Escherichia coli*
- *Haemophilus influenzae*

Endogenous Organisms

In addition to the sexually transmitted organisms, a number of anaerobic and facultative (aerobic) bacteria have been identified as causative agents in PID. Anaerobic bacteria include *Bacteroides* (*Prevotella*), *Peptostreptococcus,* and *Peptococcus* species. Facultative bacteria include *Gardnerella vaginalis, Streptococcus* species, *Escherichia coli,* and *Haemophilus influenzae.* In recent studies, these were the only organisms identified in one-third of hospitalized cases of acute PID. In the other two-thirds of cases, they coexisted with *N. gonorrhoeae* or *C. trachomatis* 50% of the time. It is hypothesized that in women with cervical gonorrhea and PID, these bacteria act as secondary invaders and follow the initial gonococcal infection of the upper tract. It has also been observed that endogenous organisms are a more frequent cause of PID than sexually transmitted organisms in older PID patients. Outside

of the research setting, specific culture or diagnostics for PID-related organisms is not performed.

■ PATHOGENESIS

PID results from direct canalicular spread of organisms from the endocervix upward to the upper genital tract. Untreated, 10–17% of women with gonorrhea and 1–10% of women with chlamydia develop PID. Four pathophysiological cofactors have been proposed: (1) uterine instrumentation, (2) hormonal changes during menses and menses itself, (3) retrograde menstruation, and (4) virulence factors of individual organisms.

With uterine instrumentation, the cervical canal must be opened, thereby disrupting the barrier between the lower and upper genital tracts. Procedures in which this occurs include cervical dilatation, curettage, abortion, tubal insufflation, hysterosalpingography, and IUD insertion. This barrier is also disrupted during menses, when the cervical mucus plug is lost. Menstruation is a time of increased PID risk for several reasons. In addition to losing the mucus plug, the mucus that remains has a low bacteriostatic effect. The endometrium is sloughed, which decreases local protection against bacteria. Menstrual blood is a good culture medium. Finally, retrograde menstruation may carry pathogens to the fallopian tubes or peritoneum.

Virulence factors, the host immune response, and the natural history of individual organisms also play a role in the pathogenesis of PID. In the fallopian tube, gonococci attach to and penetrate mucosal epithelial cells, resulting in cell destruction. Virulent gonococci contain pili, fine hairlike projections, which promote attachment to epithelial cells. They also produce an endotoxin that damages tubal mucosa in the absence of live organisms. In contrast to the gonococcus, after *C. trachomatis* reaches the fallopian tube, it attaches to the epithelium and is engulfed by endocytosis. Bacterial replication then occurs within the cell. With this organism, tissue damage and scarring result from the host immune response to the infection, with the production of a variety of cytokines. The inflammatory response is mediated by a chlamydial heat-shock protein (hsp 60).

The final common pathway in PID is inflammation, regardless of the inciting organism. The inflammatory reaction leads to vasodilatation, transudation of plasma, and migration of cellular elements into tissue. Mucosal cell destruction occurs, leading to the production of purulent material that can exude from the fimbria of the fallopian tube and cause peritonitis. Contiguous structures may then be affected , which can lead to the formation of a tubo-ovarian abscess (TOA).

■ DIAGNOSIS

The clinical diagnosis of PID is often difficult to make. Women present with a wide variety of symptoms and signs that often overlap with other disorders. Women with PID can be misdiagnosed with other gynecologic disorders but also with disorders of the gastrointestinal, urinary, and musculoskeletal systems. Unfortunately, the clinical diagnosis of PID is imprecise. There is no single historical, physical, or laboratory finding that is both sensitive and specific for the diagnosis of PID. Therefore, because of the implications of potential infertility, PID is often treated based on minimal findings (CDC 2010).

The first step in the evaluation of a woman with suspected PID is the history. Table 8-3 presents the essential components of the history. Lower abdominal pain is the most consistent symptom in confirmed PID and is usually continuous, bilateral, and present for <3 weeks duration. Pain localized to the right lower quadrant is more likely to be due to appendicitis. Right upper quadrant pain can occur when there is spread of infection to the liver capsule (Fitz-Hugh-Curtis syndrome). Most patients with acute PID have had pelvic pain for less than 3 weeks. Other nonspecific symptoms include nausea and vomiting, vaginal discharge and bleeding, and diarrhea. A critical differential diagnosis is appendicitis. In studies comparing PID and appendicitis, nausea and vomiting were usually present in patients with appendicitis but only in roughly half of those with PID. Clues from the menstrual, contraceptive, and sexual histories need to be integrated with the clinical findings. For example, recent insertion of an IUD, prior STI history, multiple sexual partners, and unprotected intercourse, especially in the previous 30 days, raise the probability of a PID diagnosis.

The physical examination is the next step in the evaluation. Fever is not present in most cases. On abdominal and pelvic examination, it is common to find bilateral lower abdominal, uterine, adnexal, and cervical motion tenderness (CMT). The Centers for Disease Control and Prevention (CDC) recommend that empiric treatment should be given to any sexually active woman who presents with pelvic or abdominal pain if they also have CMT, uterine tenderness, or adnexal tenderness with no other cause apparent. A number of supporting and more specific criteria can also help confirm the diagnosis (see Table 8-4). When interpreting the pelvic examination, remember that movement of the pelvic organs will be

TABLE 8-3   Historic Data Useful in Patients with Suspected Pelvic Inflammatory Disease

Patient Age

Pain Characteristics
- onset
- position
- quality
- radiation
- severity
- aggravating/alleviating factors
- associated symptoms
- urinary symptoms
- gastrointestinal symptoms
- fever/chills
- vaginal bleeding
- vaginal discharge
- treatment tried

Obstetric History

Gynecologic History
- Menstrual History
- Contraceptive History
- barrier methods
- OCPs
- IUD
- sexual history
- last exposure
- number of partners in previous 30 days
- number of lifetime partners
- age at first intercourse
- history of STIs/PID
- symptoms in sexual partner(s)

Medical/Surgical History

Social History
- marital status

OCP = oral contraceptive pill
IUD = intrauterine device
STI = sexually transmitted infection
PID = pelvic inflammatory disease

TABLE 8-4   2010 CDC Criteria for the Diagnosis of Pelvic Inflammatory Disease

Minimum Diagnostic Criteria

- pelvic or lower abdominal pain, and one or more of the following:
  - cervical motion tenderness OR
  - uterine tenderness OR
  - adnexal tenderness

Additional Diagnostic Criteria

- oral temperature >101°F (>38.3°C)
- abnormal cervical or vaginal mucopurulent discharge
- presence of abundant numbers of WBC on saline microscopy of vaginal secretions
- elevated erythrocyte sedimentation rate
- elevated C-reactive protein
- laboratory documentation of cervical infection with *N. gonorrhoeae* or *C. trachomatis*

Definitive Diagnostic Criteria

- endometrial biopsy with histopathologic evidence of endometritis
- transvaginal sonography or magnetic resonance imaging techniques showing thickened, fluid-filled tubes with or without free pelvic fluid or tubo-ovarian complex, or Doppler studies suggesting pelvic infection (e.g., tubal hyperemia)
- laparoscopic abnormalities consistent with PID

painful if peritoneal irritation is present, regardless of the cause. Therefore, CMT and adnexal tenderness may be found with a variety of disorders, especially appendicitis.

There are a variety of diagnostic tests that may be useful in cases of suspected PID. The most clinically useful blood tests are C-reactive protein (CRP) and erythrocyte sedimentation rate (ESR), both of which may be elevated in cases of moderate or severe PID. The sensitivities of CRP and ESR range from 74% to 93% and 75% to 81%, respectively. The specificities range from 67% to 81% and 25% to 68%, respectively, and therefore cannot be used in practice to definitively rule in or rule out the diagnosis. Similarly, the white blood cell count (WBC) is nonspecific and is only elevated in 44%

of women with acute chlamydial PID. Vaginal fluid wet mounts and cervical Gram's stains may be helpful and should be obtained if available. In PID, an increased number of leukocytes are often seen, and the absence of mucopurulent cervicitis or inflammatory cells in the wet mount has a good negative predictive value for excluding PID. A pregnancy test to help exclude ectopic pregnancy is indicated in all sexually active women presenting with recent onset lower abdominal pain.

In difficult diagnostic cases, endometrial biopsy may be useful, is easily performed, and does not require anesthesia. Endometritis, measured by the presence of leukocytes and plasma cells, has a good sensitivity (70–89%) and specificity (67–89%) for diagnosing PID. Good local antiseptic technique is required to ensure that infection is not introduced into the uterine cavity while performing the biopsy. The biggest obstacle to using endometrial biopsy to diagnose PID is that results are often not available for 2 to 3 days. Ultrasound may aid in the diagnosis if grossly abnormal fallopian tubes or a TOA are visualized, but a normal ultrasound does not rule out PID.

Since the 1960s, laparoscopy has been the gold standard for PID diagnosis but is rarely performed because of the need for general anesthesia, skilled operators, and expense. For a diagnosis of PID, the fallopian tubes should be erythematous and edematous, and should have at least one of the following signs: pus present inside the tube or coming from the distal end (pyosalpinx), fresh (easily breakable) periadnexal adhesions, or sticky exudate on the tubal surface. Compared with laparoscopy, the sensitivity and specificity of clinical criteria at reference centers is only 65%. Furthermore, inter- and intraobserver variation in the interpretation of laparoscopy can be substantial. Laparoscopy should be used in conjunction with other tests, especially in cases where the diagnosis is unclear.

■ TREATMENT

The goals of PID treatment are to control the acute infection and to prevent long-term sequelae such as infertility, ectopic pregnancy, and chronic pelvic pain. Early diagnosis and treatment are crucial for maintaining fertility. Several studies have shown that therapeutic efficacy in the prevention of infertility is directly related to the interval between the onset of symptoms and the initiation of treatment. If women are treated early in the course of infection, tubal damage is minimized and fertility is unimpaired.

Antibiotic therapy for PID can be administered orally or parenterally and in inpatient or outpatient settings. For women with PID of mild to moderate severity, outpatient management provides equal efficacy compared with inpatient care. Table 8-5 presents the criteria for hospitalization suggested by the CDC in their 2006 guidelines for treatment. Careful follow-up is imperative, and pain and tenderness resulting from acute PID should begin to resolve within 48 to 72 hours of initiating antibiotics. Patients starting oral therapy, especially those with moderate to severe PID, should be reevaluated within 2 to 3 days, and if no clinical improvement has occurred, then hospital admission for parenteral therapy and observation is required.

PID treatment must provide empiric broad-spectrum coverage of likely etiologic pathogens to account the polymicrobial nature of PID. Whichever regimen is used, it must provide coverage for *N. gonorrhoeae*, *C. trachomatis*, anaerobes, gram-negative facultative bacteria, and streptococci. Table 8-6 presents the parenteral treatment regimens recommended for inpatient care by the CDC in the 2010 guidelines. It is suggested that parenteral therapy may be discontinued 24 hours after a patient improves clinically and that oral therapy should then continue for 14 days of treatment. Regimen A (cefotetan or

cefoxitin plus doxycycline) provides good coverage against all the major pathogens. Regimen B (clindamycin plus gentamicin) provides good coverage against anaerobes and aerobes, but its coverage against *N. gonorrhoeae* and *C. trachomatis* is not as good as that of Regimen A. These parenteral regimens have each been investigated in at least one clinical trial and provide broad-spectrum coverage with high short-term response rates (Ness 2002).

TABLE 8-5   2010 CDC Criteria for Hospitalization in Patients with PID

- Surgical emergencies, such as appendicitis, cannot be excluded.
- The patient is pregnant.
- The patient does not respond clinically to oral antimicrobial therapy.
- The patient is unable to follow or to tolerate an outpatient oral regimen.
- The patient has severe illness, nausea and vomiting, or high fever.
- The patient has a tubo-ovarian abscess.

TABLE 8-6   2010 CDC Recommended Treatment Regimens for Parenteral Treatment of PID

A. Cefotetan 2 g IV every 12 hours or Cefoxitin 2 g IV every 6 hours
PLUS
Doxycycline 100 mg IV or orally every 12 hours (can be given orally if tolerated)

- Parenteral therapy may be discontinued 24 hours after a patient improves clinically, and oral therapy with doxycycline (100 mg twice daily) should continue for a total of 14 days.

B. Clindamycin 900 mg IV every 8 hours
PLUS
Gentamicin loading dose IV or IM (2 mg/kg of body weight), followed by a maintenance dose (1.5 mg/kg) every 8 hours. Single daily dosing may be substituted.

- Parental therapy may be discontinued 24 hours after a patient improves clinically, and oral therapy with doxycycline (100 mg twice daily) or clindamycin (450 mg orally 4 times daily) should continue for 14 days.

Alternative Parenteral Regimen
Ampicillin/Sulbactam 3 g IV every 6 hours
PLUS
Doxycycline 100 mg IV or orally every 12 hours

Table 8-7 presents the outpatient treatment regimens recommended for outpatient care by the CDC in the 2010 guidelines.

The management of women with PID is considered inadequate unless their sexual partners are also evaluated and treated. This is crucial because without appropriate evaluation and treatment, there is a high risk of reinfection. Sexual partners should be screened for sexually transmitted infections and treated empirically with regimens effective against both gonorrhea and chlamydia.

■ SEQUELAE

One of the main goals in the treatment of PID is the prevention of sequelae. Women with PID may experience both short- and long-term consequences as a result of upper genital tract infection. Short-term sequelae include perihepatitis (Fitz-Hugh-Curtis syndrome), TOA,

TABLE 8-7 2010 CDC Recommended Treatment Regimens for Oral Treatment of PID

Regimen
Ceftriaxone 250 mg IM in a single dose
PLUS
Doxycycline 100 mg orally twice a day for 14 days
WITH OR WITHOUT
Metronidazole 500 mg orally twice a day for 14 days
OR
Cefoxitin 2 g IM in a single dose and Probenecid, 1 g orally administered concurrently in a single dose
PLUS
Doxycycline 100 mg orally twice a day for 14 days
WITH OR WITHOUT
Metronidazole 500 mg orally twice a day for 14 days
OR
Other parenteral third-generation cephalosporin (e.g., ceftizoxime or cefotaxime)
PLUS
Doxycycline 100 mg orally twice a day for 14 days
WITH OR WITHOUT
Metronidazole 500 mg orally twice a day for 14 days

and mortality. Long-term sequelae include infertility, ectopic pregnancy, and chronic pelvic pain.

Short-Term Sequelae

Fitz-Hugh-Curtis Syndrome

Perihepatitis occurs in 15–30% of women with acute PID, and clinically manifests as right upper quadrant pain. It involves inflammation of the liver capsule, and classically consists of "violin string" adhesions between the liver capsule and the diaphragm or anterior peritoneum.

Tubo-Ovarian Abscess (TOA)

TOA occurs in 15–34% of women with acute PID. The most common pathogens isolated from TOAs are anaerobic organisms, such as *Bacteroides* and *Prevotella* species, and *E. coli*, aerobic streptococci, and *Peptostreptococcus* species. It is relatively uncommon to isolate *N. gonorrhoeae* or *C. trachomatis*. The abscess may remain localized and only involve the tube and ovary or spread to involve other contiguous structures such as bowel, bladder, or the opposite adnexa. With the presence of a TOA, there is always the risk of rupture. Currently, the diagnosis of TOA is most accurately made with ultrasound. The typical appearance is a complex or cystic adnexal mass with multiple internal echoes.

Most TOAs are treated with a combination of antimicrobial therapy and drainage although medical therapy alone is reasonable for small TOAs that are amenable to close observation. The choice of antibiotics is based on the likely organisms present. Both clindamycin and metronidazole have excellent anaerobic coverage and ability to penetrate and remain active inside abscesses. The gold standard for the treatment of TOA is a combination of clindamycin and an aminoglycoside such as gentamicin, although multiple antimicrobial regimens are effective. Surgical drainage is indicated if medical therapy fails or if there is rupture of the abscess. Rupture has been reported to occur in 3–15% of TOAs and represents a surgical emergency. Delay in management can lead to sepsis, shock, or death.

Mortality

Mortality associated with PID is very low in developed countries. However, in developing countries, or in rural areas with poor healthcare access, death can occur and is usually due to rupture of a TOA with generalized peritonitis and septic shock.

Long-Term Sequelae

Infertility

One of the most important long-term complications of acute PID is tubal factor infertility (TFI). This occurs as a result of tubal damage following PID. It has been shown that the rate of TFI is directly related to the number of episodes of PID. Each repeat episode approximately doubles the rate, such that roughly 12% of women are infertile after a single episode, almost 25% after two episodes, and more than 50% after three or more episodes. Among women with only one episode of PID, the rate of TFI is proportional to the severity of the infection. *Chlamydia trachomatis* is the most consistently associated with TFI and is thought to be related to endogenous inflammation induced by the chlamydia heat-shock protein.

While there is substantial evidence to implicate chlamydia as a risk factor for TFI, the role of other organisms has been infrequently studied.

Ectopic Pregnancy

Ectopic pregnancy results from tubal functional impairment as a consequence of scarring following PID. Similar to TFI, the rate of ectopic pregnancy is related to the number of episodes of PID. Overall, there is a 7- to 10-fold increase in risk for women with a history of PID compared with women without such a history. Among women with only one episode of PID, like TFI, the rate of ectopic pregnancy is proportional to the severity of infection, and *C. trachomatis* is most often implicated.

Chronic Pelvic Pain

Chronic pelvic pain may be seen following PID and is usually a result of pelvic adhesions caused by the inflammatory response to the infection. It is estimated to occur in 17–24% of women following acute PID. Similar to other sequelae, the rate of chronic pelvic pain is proportional to the number and severity of episodes of PID.

■ PID AND HUMAN IMMUNODEFICIENCY VIRUS (HIV) INFECTION

Women with PID have a higher prevalence of HIV infection than those without PID. The reported seroprevalence of HIV infection in women diagnosed with acute PID ranges from 2.7% to 22%. HIV infection is associated with clinically more severe PID, but existing treatment regimens have a high efficacy and should continue to be used as guided by the clinical severity.

■ PREVENTION

Strategies for preventing PID and its sequelae must be aimed at different levels: the community at large, the healthcare provider, and the individual. Community health promotion and education programs and the provision of appropriate clinical services are essential. Healthcare providers must play a leading role in preventing PID and its sequelae. Clinicians need to assume responsibility for primary prevention activities such as counseling, patient education, and community awareness. Current knowledge is essential to provide appropriate preventive services and management of disease. Risk reduction counseling is an important component of prevention. Finally, individuals must assume an active role in disease prevention. The maintenance of healthy sexual behavior and the use of barrier methods are two key components to this.

■ CONCLUSION

PID is a serious and commonly seen infectious disorder in women. By gaining a better insight into the risk factors, disease prevention strategies can become more effective, resulting in a reduction in the incidence of both short- and long-term sequelae.

■ KEY POINTS

- Pelvic infection is one of the most common causes of morbidity in young women.

- PID results in short-term physical pain and psychological distress and, in the long term, causes chronic pelvic pain, infertility, and ectopic pregnancy.

- Sexual behavior linked with the acquisition of sexually transmitted infections is strongly associated with PID.

- *Chlamydia trachomatis* and *Neisseria gonorrhoeae* are the two most commonly identified bacteria initiating PID.

- Numerous other pathogens can also be isolated in the genital tract of women with pelvic infection, including anaerobes, mycoplasmas, gram-negative bacteria, and viruses.

- The clinical diagnosis of PID is imprecise.

- Measuring markers of inflammation (WBC, ESR, CRP) increase diagnostic specificity but reduce sensitivity.

- Laparoscopy and endometrial biopsy are more sensitive diagnostic tests but are not recommended routinely because of cost, time delay, and potential morbidity associated with the test.

- Antimicrobial therapy should include coverage for chlamydia, gonorrhea, anaerobes, gram-negative bacteria, and streptococci.

- Early diagnosis and treatment is required to optimize long-term outcomes.

REFERENCES

Anagrius C, Lore B, Jensen JS. *Mycoplasma genitalium*: prevalence, clinical significance and transmission. *Sex Transm Infect.* 2005;81:458–462.

Centers for Disease Control and Prevention. Sexually Transmitted Diseases Treatment Guidelines 2010. *MMWR Morb Mort Wkly Rep.* 2010;59(RR-12):63–67.

Eckert LO, Hawes SE, Wolner-Hanssen PK, et al. Endometritis: The clinical-pathologic syndrome. *Am J Obstet Gynecol.* 2002;186(4):690–695.

Haggerty CL, Ness RB. Diagnosis and treatment of pelvic inflammatory disease. *Women's Health* (London). 2008 July; 4(4):383–397.

Haggerty CL, Ness RB. Newest approaches to treatment of pelvic inflammatory disease: a review of recent randomized clinical trials. *Clin Infect Dis.* 2007 Apr 1;44:953–960.

Hillis SD, Joesoef R, Marchbanks PA, et al. Delayed care of pelvic inflammatory disease as a risk factor for impaired fertility. *Am J Obstet Gynecol.* 1993;168(5):1503–1509.

Molander P, Sjoberg J, Paavonen J, Cacciatore B. Transvaginal power Doppler findings in laparoscopically proven acute pelvic inflammatory disease. *Ultrasound Obst Gynecol.* 2001;17(3):233–238.

Ness RB, Hillier SL, Kip KE, et al. Douching, pelvic inflammatory disease, and incident gonococcal and chlamydial genital infection in a cohort of high-risk women. *Am J Epidemiol.* 2005;161(2):186–195.

Ness RB, Hillier SL, Kip KE, et al. Bacterial vaginosis and risk of pelvic inflammatory disease. *Obstet Gynecol.* 2004; 104(4):761–769.

Ness RB, Smith KJ, Chang CC, Schisterman EF, Bass DC; Gynecologic Infection Follow-Through GI. Prediction of pelvic inflammatory disease among young, single, sexually active women. *Sex Transm Dis.* 2006;33(3):137–142.

Ness RB, Soper DE, Holley RL, et al. Effectiveness of inpatient and outpatient treatment strategies for women with pelvic inflammatory disease: results from the Pelvic Inflammatory Disease Evaluation and Clinical Health (PEACH) Randomized Trial. *Am J Obstet Gynecol.* 2002;186(5):929–937.

Rein DB, Gift TL. A refined estimate of the lifetime cost of pelvic inflammatory disease. *Sex Transm Dis.* 2004;31(5):325.

Rothman KJ, Funch DP, Alfredson T, Brady J, Dreyer NA. Randomized field trial of vaginal douching, pelvic inflammatory disease and pregnancy. *Epidemiology.* 2003;14(3):340–348.

Simms I, Rogers P, Charlett A. The rate of diagnosis and demography of pelvic inflammatory disease in general practice: England and Wales. *Int J STD AIDS.* 1999;10:448–451.

Walker CK, Wiesenfeld HC. Antibiotic therapy for acute pelvic inflammatory disease: the 2006 Centers for Disease Control and Prevention sexually transmitted diseases treatment guidelines. *Clin Infect Dis.* 2007 Apr 1;44 Suppl 3:S111–122.

Wolner-Hanssen P. Oral contraceptive use modifies the manifestations of pelvic inflammatory disease. *Brit J Obst Gynaecol.* 1986;93(6):619–624.

Wolner-Hanssen P, Eschenbach DA, Paavonen J, Kiviat N, Stevens CE, Critchlow C, et al. Decreased risk of symptomatic chlamydial pelvic inflammatory disease associated with oral contraceptive use. *JAMA.* 1990;263(1):54–59.

9

Infectious Syphilis

Kevin A. Fenton and Patrick French

INTRODUCTION

Syphilis is a chronic, systemic infection characterized by periods of active clinical disease interrupted by periods of latency. Despite the existence of simple, validated screening tests, effective prevention measures and cheap treatment options, syphilis remains a major global problem, with an estimated 12 million people becoming infected every year. Congenital syphilis, a consequence of infection during pregnancy, results in serious adverse outcomes in up to 80% of the cases and is estimated to affect more than 1 million pregnancies annually. Approximately 35% of these pregnancies will end in fetal or perinatal death, 20% in low-birth-weight babies, and 20% in babies born with congenital syphilis. This chapter reviews the biology, recent epidemiology, diagnosis, prevention, and control of infectious syphilis in developing and developed country settings.

BIOLOGY AND CLINICAL PRESENTATION

Globally, syphilis is most commonly transmitted through sexual intercourse or from an infected mother by transplacental passage of treponemes to the fetus. Bloodborne, nonsexual personal contact and accidental direct inoculation are less common modes of transmission. The disease is caused by the spirochete *Treponema pallidum* subsp. *pallidum*, which belongs to a family of spiral-shaped bacteria, the *Spirochaetaceae* (spirochetes), and is related to other pathogenic treponemes that cause nonvenereal diseases.

Transmission mainly occurs via sexual exposure. After inoculation and penetration of the mucosal surfaces or abraded skin, *T. pallidum* subsp. *pallidum* attaches to host cells and initiates multiplication. A primary lesion develops at the site of inoculation 2 to 6 weeks after infection. Typically, it begins as a painless indurated papule whose surface necroses to form a hard-based, well-circumscribed ulcerated lesion (chancre) teeming with treponemes. However, it may present as multiple ulcers, and occasionally the ulcer is painful.

Traditionally, syphilis has been divided into three clinical stages: primary, secondary, and late (including tertiary and late benign syphilis). Latent syphilis is a serological diagnosis where symptoms are not apparent and which is differentiated into early (infection duration < 1 year) or late (infection duration > 1 year) (see Figure 9-1). In the United Kingdom and World Health Organization definitions, the differentiation between early and late latent infection is 2 years.

EPIDEMIOLOGY

Syphilis in Developed Country Settings

In developed country settings, the social determinants of syphilis among low socioeconomic status minority subpopulations have been studied best in the United States. Unsurprisingly, similar epidemic drivers to those found in developing countries are often observed, including poverty, youthful age composition, relative scarcity of men, relative low status of women, lower access to acceptable health services, and minority race-ethnicity. However, in many western industrialized countries, the recent resurgence of syphilis among men who have sex

FIGURE 9-1   Time Course of Syphilis

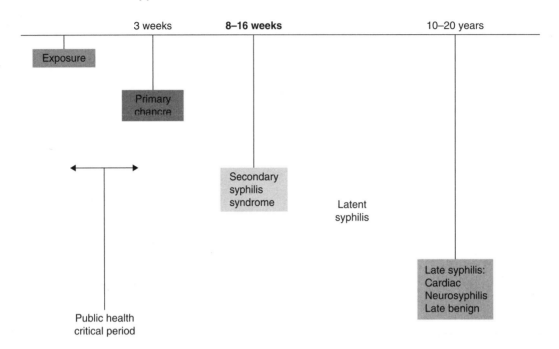

with men (MSM) highlights the continued evolution of the epidemic among population subgroups with high rates of partner change or poor access to screening and treatment services.

Recent increases in infectious syphilis have been reported in the United States, Western Europe, and many other industrialized settings although the magnitude of the increases and the affected populations vary. In Western Europe, rates of infectious syphilis fell to their lowest levels in many EU countries by the early 1990s, despite near concomitant and substantial increases in syphilis incidence in the former USSR. The decreases in Western Europe were accompanied by marked reductions in the incidence of congenital syphilis and tertiary disease. By 1995, rates had reached a nadir in most of the reporting EU countries, with the majority of infections diagnosed among migrants from high prevalence countries or among EU nationals who had sexual contact with infected individuals outside of the region. Since that time, syphilis has again been on the increase across the EU, initially affecting MSM and subsequently heterosexual men and women, newborns, commercial sex workers, and drug users. Among MSM, the resurgence of syphilis has been associated with increasing high-risk sexual behavior, expanding and new sexual networks, and use of recreational drugs. Among heterosexuals, risk factors have included sexual activity overseas, migration from high-prevalence countries, commercial sex work contact, and drug use.

In the United States, disease rates rapidly declined in the late 1940s after the introduction of penicillin therapy and broad-based public health programs. The resurgence of primary and secondary (P&S) syphilis in the United States began in 2000 and has continued unabated. (see Figure 9-2). In 2007, P&S syphilis cases increased to 11,466 from 9,756 in 2006, an increase of 17.5%. The rate of P&S syphilis in the United States was 15.2% higher in 2007 than in 2006 (3.8 vs. 3.3 cases per 100,000 population), and during this time period, the rate of P&S syphilis increased 17.9% among men (to 6.6 cases per 100,000 men) and increased 10.0% among women (to 1.1 cases per 100,000 women). Marked differences are seen by racial/ethnic groups, and in 2007, 46.0% of reported P&S cases occurred among African Americans, and rates of P&S syphilis for both men and women were highest in African American men and African American women. In 2006 and 2007, the rate of P&S syphilis was 5.9 and 7.0 times higher among African Americans than among non-Hispanic whites, respectively, in contrast to 1992 when the African American rate was 62 times that of the non-Hispanic white rate (CDC 2007).

Syphilis in Developing Country Settings

Syphilis is distributed worldwide, but it is particularly problematic in developing countries, where it is a leading

FIGURE 9-2 Primary and Secondary Syphilis Rates, United States, 1989–2008. Total, by Sex, and Male-to-Female Rate Ratios

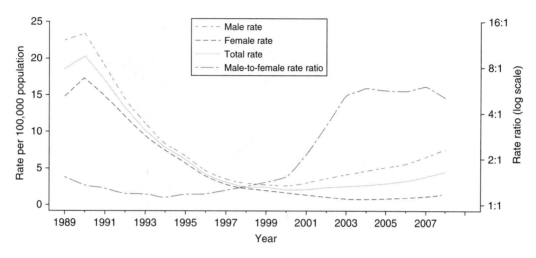

Source: CDC.

cause of genital ulcer disease. In these settings, the predominant mode of transmission is through heterosexual sexual intercourse, although vertical transmission of infection remains a major concern. In developing countries, increased incidence and prevalence of syphilis have been associated with increases in poverty, unemployment, inequality, large-scale migration, political and economic upheaval, war, and lack of established health infrastructure.

In the absence of active surveillance, it is difficult to accurately assess the annual number of pregnant women with syphilis. Seroprevalence studies from the 1970s and 1980s demonstrated a wide range of seroprevalence values among pregnant women, from 0.03% in Scotland to 16.0% in Brazil, with rates particularly high in sub-Saharan Africa, where maternal syphilis continues to contribute to substantial perinatal morbidity and mortality (Saloojee 2004). Consequently, there is an urgent need for scaling up syphilis screening and treatment in high-prevalence areas. Cost-effectiveness studies have shown that syphilis screening is highly cost effective, yet irregularly implemented. Furthermore, the relationship between syphilis and HIV transmission is well established, which is particularly important in areas of Africa and Asia that have been impacted by both epidemics.

The newly proposed World Health Organization Strategy for the Global Elimination of Congenital Syphilis aims to mobilize resources and provide a plan to address this underrecognized health problem. The strategy is based on accelerating progress in four key areas: (1) ensuring sustained political commitment and advocacy; (2) increasing access to, and quality of, maternal and newborn health services; (3) screening and treating pregnant women and their partners; and (4) establishing surveillance, monitoring, and evaluation systems.

■ CLINICAL COURSE

Primary Syphilis

Initial infection with *T. pallidum* usually occurs through sexual contact at a mucosal membrane. The incubation period ranges between 10 and 30 days. Typically, 3 weeks (range 2 to 6 weeks) after the initial exposure, a chancre develops at the site of contact. Most chancres are genital, but extra genital lesions occur in 12–14% of individuals. Anal canal, vaginal, and cervical chancres occur but are usually subclinical and undiagnosed in most individuals. The chancre starts as a macule, which becomes a papule and then ulcerates. The ulcer is a usually a painless lesion with an indurated border and has associated painless lymphadenopathy (see Figure 9-3). However, a third of HIV-antibody-negative and up to two-thirds of HIV-positive individuals with primary syphilis have multiple ulcers. Although the ulcer of primary syphilis is characteristically painless, a significant minority of primary chancres are painful. In our clinical experience, superinfection with other organisms, such as *Staphylococcus* and *Streptococcus*, may cause a purulent discharge or painful lesions, and up to 10-15% of patients in some studies have co-incident herpes. Coinfection with *Haemophilus ducreyi* is also common in some resource-poor countries. The great majority of patients with primary syphilis

FIGURE 9-3   Penile Chancre

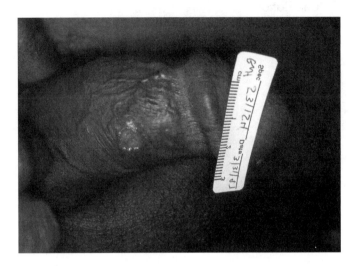

present with mucosal or skin ulceration; however, there are other less typical presentations that include balanitis and proctitis.

The differential diagnosis of primary syphilis includes other STIs that cause ulceration, particularly herpes, chancroid, donovanosis, and lymphogranuloma venereum. Non-STI causes of genital ulceration include erosive lichen planus, Crohn's disease, Behçet's disease, squamous cell carcinoma, and fixed drug eruption (see Chapter 17). A dark-field microscopic examination of the ulcer reveals characteristic motile treponemes (see Chapter 20). Syphilis is a systemic disease. Even in primary syphilis, systemic dissemination may occur. Ten to fifteen percent of patients in some studies with early primary syphilis will have cerebrospinal fluid abnormalities.

Secondary Syphilis

Left untreated, the chancre will heal spontaneously within 2–3 weeks and 10–40% of patients with secondary syphilis have a healed ulcer present when they are diagnosed. Secondary syphilis results from the multiplication and dissemination of treponemes throughout the body. *Treponema pallidum* subsp. *pallidum* is found in many different tissues despite the presence of high levels of antitreponemal antibodies. The secondary stage occurs typically 4–8 weeks after resolution of the primary lesion and lasts for several weeks or months and may reoccur in approximately 25% of untreated patients.

Secondary syphilis is a systemic vasculitis caused by high levels of *T. pallidum* in the blood and associated immunologic responses. The most characteristic feature of

FIGURE 9-4   Palmar Secondary Syphilis: (a) Macular; (b) Psoriaform

(a)

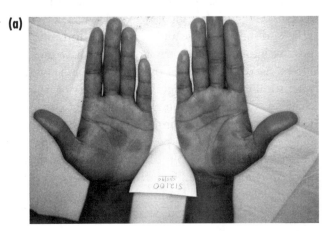

(b)

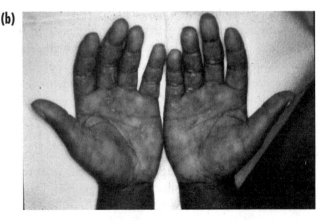

FIGURE 9-5 Secondary Syphilis, Mucus Patches: (a) On the Tongue; (b) On Hard Palate.

(a)

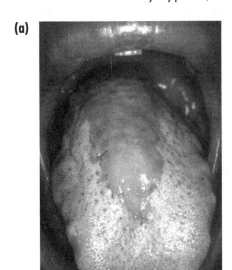

(b)

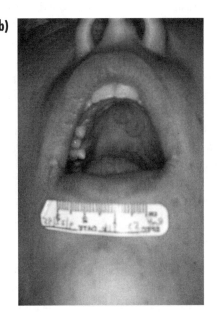

secondary syphilis is a rash that may be macular, papular, maculopapular, papulosquamous, or psoriasiform (see Figure 9-4). The rash often involves the palms and soles and is usually nonpuritic although it may be itchy particularly in individuals of black African and South Asian ethnicity. On the mucosal surfaces, superficial ulcers called mucus patches may form (see Figure 9-5). Where mucus patches oppose one another (perianally, in groin, mouth angle, etc.) warty lesions called condylomata lata may form (see Figure 9-6). Mucus patches and condylomata lata are both highly infectious.

Most patients with secondary syphilis developed generalized lymphadenopathy, and some patients de-velop flulike symptoms, including fever, myalgia, and arthralgia. Rarer manifestations of secondary syphilis include patchy alopecia and symptoms and signs of a visceral vasculitis. This vasculitis may cause a wide range of presentations, including hepatitis, nephritis, uveitis, and neurological involvement. This early meningovascular syphilis typically presents with headache and cranial nerve lesions, particularly eighth nerve involvement, causing high-frequency hearing loss. Left untreated, the secondary syphilis syndrome will spontaneously resolve, usually after one to two months.

The differential diagnosis of secondary syphilis is wide because there are a large number of causes for

FIGURE 9-6 Secondary Syphilis, Condyloma Lata on the Buttocks

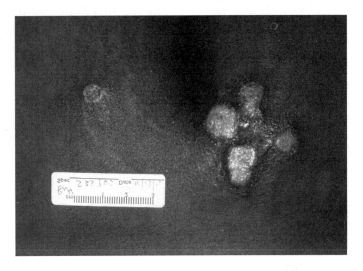

generalized rash. However, there are far fewer conditions in which the rash is associated with constitutional symptoms with or without generalized lymphadenopathy. The differential diagnosis includes acute infections that cause rash, lymphadenopathy, and constitutional symptoms, such as acute Epstein-Barr infection, primary HIV infection, measles, and toxoplasmosis. Generalized dermatoses, such as lichen planus, pityriasis rosea, and psoriasis, may mimic syphilis but are usually not associated with lymphadenopathy and constitutional symptoms. See Chapter 11 for an extensive description of nonsexually transmitted dermatoses in the differential diagnosis for secondary syphilis.

Other Clinical Manifestations

Early latent syphilis is a serologic diagnosis in which an individual with no symptoms or signs of syphilis has negative followed by positive syphilis serology or has a fourfold increase in nontreponemal test titer (i.e., two dilutions) within 1 year in the United States, 2 years in the United Kingdom, with previous documentation of the earlier serology. Late latent syphilis is a serologic diagnosis of asymptomatic syphilis occurring more than 1–2 years after baseline diagnosis. The late complications of syphilis, such as neurosyphilis, cardiovascular syphilis, and gummatous syphilis, do not develop until 10–20 years after the resolution of early syphilis. In HIV patients, case reports have suggested that late complications may occur earlier. Latent syphilis is defined exclusively by serological evaluation. A flowchart algorithm for staging latent syphilis and determining treatment strategy is described in Figure 9-7. A comprehensive treatment of syphilis serology and diagnostic criteria is described in Chapter 20.

Neurosyphilis

Neurosyphilis is the late complication of syphilis, which is currently the cause of most concern, especially in HIV-infected patients. Neurosyphilis traditionally is divided into five categories: (1) asymptomatic neurosyphilis, (2) meningovascular syphilis, (3) parenchymal syphilis (which includes spinal cord disease—tabes dorsalis, general paresis), (4) gummatous syphilis, and (5) syphilitic meningitis. Asymptomatic neurosyphilis is the most commonly encountered clinical problem. Asymptomatic neurosyphilis should be considered in patients who do not respond appropriately (from a serological standpoint) to therapy.

The pathophysiology of neurosyphilis may be related to early dissemination of treponemes into the spinal fluid. As indicated previously, approximately 15% of patients with primary syphilis and 40–60% of patients with secondary syphilis have associated CSF abnormalities. Nevertheless, these patients resolve these abnormalities with appropriate therapy. Over the past few years, there has been concern about increased incidence of neurosyphilis in HIV-infected patients because of the associated immunosuppression. Prospective studies have not documented the need for early aggressive therapy in these patients. Rather, close, frequent follow-up and vigilance for complications is recommended.

Congenital Syphilis

In women with untreated primary or secondary syphilis, the vertical transmission rate is an estimated 75–95%. Transmission occurs transplacentally. Late congenital syphilis is rarely seen in the antibiotic era. Signs and symptoms of congenital syphilis may mimic those of adults (and may be similar to that of acute secondary syphilis). Screening and treatment for congenital syphilis during pregnancy effectively prevents this disorder. Therefore, a case of congenital syphilis is considered a public health sentinel event because it is completely preventable.

The diagnosis of congenital syphilis is complex because of the passively acquired antibody in the immediate postpartum period. For example, infants whose mothers have had successfully treated syphilis may often have positive syphilis serologies. The development of surveillance definitions for congenital syphilis is based on the importance of, and need to, differentiate those with active infection from those with inactive infection.

Syphilis and HIV Interactions

The resurgence of syphilis in the context of high-HIV-prevalence populations in developed and developing countries has increased interest in the clinical interactions between these two infections. With minor differences, syphilis generally presents similarly in HIV-infected and HIV-uninfected patients. In primary syphilis, HIV-infected patients may present with more than one chancre (up to 70% of patients) and with larger and deeper lesions. About a quarter of HIV-infected patients present with concomitant lesions of both primary and secondary stages of syphilis at the time of diagnosis. Syphilis also causes transient increases in the viral load and decreases in the CD4 cell count that resolve after the infection is treated.

FIGURE 9-7   Treatment Strategy for Latent Syphilis

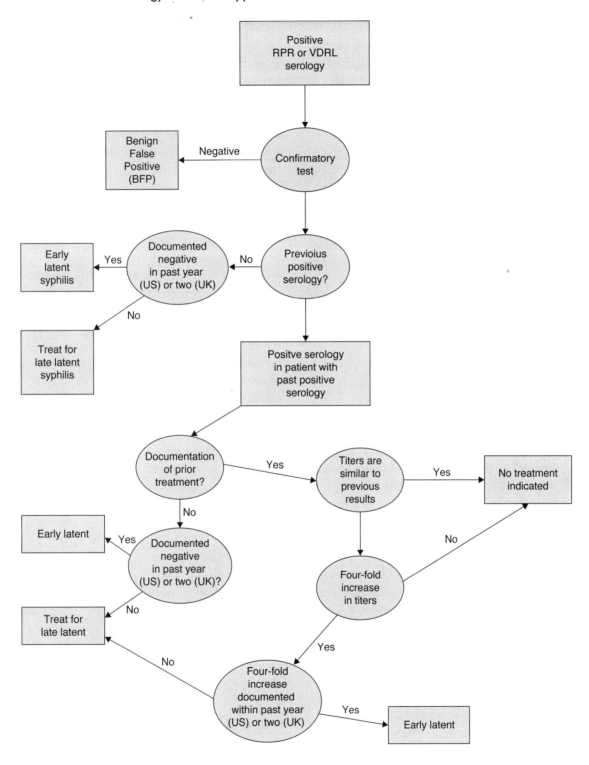

Symptomatic early neurosyphilis has garnered recent interest given its reemergence in the 1980s among HIV-infected persons and the suggestion that people with HIV infection progress more rapidly to neurosyphilis than those without infection although whether this is definitely the case remains uncertain. Most neurologic symptoms of early neurosyphilis result from acute or subacute meningitis, abnormalities in cranial nerve function, and inflammatory vasculitis leading to a cerebrovascular accident. Given that syphilis facilitates both the transmission and the acquisition of HIV infection, concomitant expansion in the HIV epidemic, especially among MSM population in developed country settings, has been a major concern. Studies in the United States and Europe suggest that there is limited evidence of increasing HIV incidence associated with the syphilis outbreaks.

■ DIAGNOSIS

Diagnosis of Primary Syphilis

Dark-field examination of the ulcer exudate establishes the diagnosis (see Chapter 20). Realistically, dark-field microscopy is not available in most settings. False negatives may occur if patients apply bactericidal creams to the lesions. Nucleic acid amplification tests for *T. pallidum* subsp. *pallidum* show promise as a highly sensitive and specific test for primary syphilis but are not yet widely used in clinical settings. Therefore, diagnosis is most often clinically established by the presence of a lesion associated with serological findings.

Serology

Serological diagnosis of syphilis is a two-step procedure. Initially, a nontreponemal screening test is performed. The most widely used tests are the venereal disease research laboratory (VDRL) and the rapid plasma reagin (RPR). Results for these tests are reported as titers, that is, the dilutions required to achieve a negative reaction using standard reagents. Patients with a positive nontreponemal test should have a confirmatory test such as the fluorescent treponomal antibody-absorbed (FTA-ABS) or microhemagglutination (MHATP or HATS) tests. Up to 20% of patients with positive nontreponemal tests will have negative confirmatory tests. These are termed *benign false positives* (BFP). Most frequently, these are seen in patients with past series of intravenous drug abuse, pregnancy, systemic disorders, such as lupus, and other infectious processes, such as Lyme disease. BFPs with titers >1:16 are extremely unusual.

In primary syphilis, the sensitivity of serologic testing is 85%. The false negative cases occur because seroconversion may occasionally take longer to develop than the genital ulcer. Patients with a genital ulcer and a negative serology should be retested approximately two weeks later, in which cases the serology will usually be positive if the patient had syphilis. Some authorities recommend performing a confirmatory test (such as the

FTA-ABS) in these cases because seroconversion occurs earlier then the nontreponemal tests. This is useful only if rapid turnaround time of test results is available.

In secondary syphilis, sensitivity of serological diagnosis is close to 100%. Titers in secondary syphilis may be extremely high. Occasionally, this may cause the "prozone phenomenon," in which the binding sites for *T. pallidum* antibody on the reagent-containing beads are saturated, leading to a false-negative result. If a prozone is suspected, diluting the serum before conducting the test solves the problem.

Use of Serology to Define Case Incidence and Treatment

Several ground rules apply in using serological diagnosis. First, longitudinal comparison should only be made of the same test. In other words, in individual patients, RPRs cannot be used as a comparison when an initial VDRL is performed. Second, there may be different laboratories in setting standard set points. Therefore, care should be taken in making comparisons when tests are done at different laboratories. Third, the benchmark used for serological definition of a cure is a fourfold decrease in titers. The time course for this transition is variable; however, three to six months is a useful benchmark. For example, a patient with secondary syphilis and a titer of 1:256 is effectively treated if titers drop below 1:64. This benchmark is considered the lower bounds of effective treatment. In a large study of more than 700 patients in Canada, 72% of patients with primary and secondary syphilis had complete sero-reversion after 3 years (Romanowski 1991). Finally, recurrent syphilis is diagnosed as a fourfold increase or twofold dilution increase in titer is observed during observation or screening.

The decline in titers after treatment does not begin immediately. For example, in cases of early syphilis with rapidly increasing titers, a paradoxical increase in titers is occasionally observed for 1–4 weeks after treatment. This increase is actually due to the immunological response due to the infection.

Management of the Patient with Serofast Serologies

If titers have not decreased appropriately by 6 months after treatment, most observers recommend evaluation for systemic disease. A physical examination should be performed, including careful evaluation of the cranial nerves. A lumbar puncture should be performed with evaluation of CSF protein, cell count, and CSF-VDRL.

The CSF-VDRL is only 60–70% sensitive for the diagnosis of neurosyphilis but is highly specific. Therefore, most experts recommend presumptive treatment for neurosyphilis if an otherwise unexplained increase in CSF protein or lymphocytes is seen even in the presence of a negative CSF-VDRL.

Rapid, cheap point-of-care tests for syphilis are increasingly used in resource-poor settings. These may have a particularly important role to play in congenital syphilis prevention as it allows diagnosis and treatment at the first antenatal visit.

Evaluation for Neurosyphilis

In general, patients with latent syphilis and a reactive serology of greater than 1:32, or patients of any stage who have not had appropriate serologic response, should have CSF evaluation, including CSF protein, cell count, and CSF-VDRL. In neurosyphilis, the protein is elevated and there is often a lymphocytic pleocytosis. A positive CSF-VDRL is seen in approximately 70–80% of patients. In approximately one quarter of patients the CSF-VDRL may be negative. In these patients, if an unexplained cell count and protein are observed with a peripherally elevated serology, neurosyphilis should be a serious consideration. The treatment for neurosyphilis traditionally has been 18–24 million units of penicillin intravenously daily for 10–14 days. However, no control trials have ever been performed.

Syphilis in HIV-Infected Patients

All stages of syphilis are seen more commonly in HIV-infected patients. Studies in STI clinics have demonstrated that HIV prevalence in patients with syphilis is up to three times higher then nonsyphilis patients in these settings. Because of initial reports of treatment failure, many experts believed that all patients with syphilis and especially patients with coexistent HIV infection should be aggressively treated. Prospective studies presented by Centers for Disease Control and Prevention (CDC) investigators have demonstrated that in most cases this is not necessary (Zetola 2010).

When Is a Lumbar Puncture Indicated?

Lumbar puncture is indicated in the following situations:

- Patients who have not had an appropriate serological response to treatment.

- Individuals with latent syphilis at initial presentation who have one of the following:
  - Evidence of central nervous system involvement, such as cranial nerve signs, optic neuritis, or meningeal symptoms.
  - HIV infection. (Some authorities use a 1:32 serology threshold.)
  - Infants with congenital syphilis.

- Routine lumbar puncture is not indicated in the evaluation of hospitalized patients with reactive serologies.

TREATMENT

The efficacy of penicillin for the treatment of syphilis is well established based on a long history of expert opinions, reinforced by case series and clinical trials (CDC 2010). Penicillin G, administered parenterally, is the preferred drug for treatment of all stages of syphilis, including syphilis during pregnancy (see Table 9-1). The preparation(s) used (i.e., benzathine, aqueous procaine, or aqueous crystalline), the dosage, and the length of treatment depend on the stage and clinical manifestations of disease and by geographic region. In the United States, benzathine penicillin is the recommended preparation, while the procaine salt of penicillin, 600,000 units intramuscularly for 10 to 14 days, is also recommended or preferred in many European countries. For patients who are allergic to penicillin, macrolides and cephalosporins may be used, with certain caveats. Although azithromycin was thought of as a promising alternative oral agent for the treatment of early syphilis, recent studies from San Francisco, California; Baltimore, Maryland; Seattle, Washington; and Dublin, Ireland, have identified macrolide-resistant strains among these populations. Treatment of primary, secondary, and early latent syphilis is recommended with benzathine penicillin. In patients who are allergic to penicillin, doxycycline may be used as per Table 9-1. Treatment for patients with late latent syphilis, late syphilis, or syphilis of unknown duration (serological syphilis in which an initial benchmark cannot be defined) should be with benzathine penicillin 2.4 million units intramuscularly for 3 weeks. Patients with neurosyphilis should be treated with high-dose intravenous penicillin, 24 million units for 10 days. Pregnant women with syphilis should be treated only with penicillin-based regimens.

TABLE 9-1   Treatment of Syphilis

Primary, Secondary Syphilis

Benzathine penicillin, 2.4 million units IM single dose.

> *For penicillin-allergic patients:*
> Doxycycline, 100 mg p.o. b.i.d. for 2 weeks

Early Latent Syphilis

Benzathine penicillin, 2.4 million units IM single dose.

> *For penicillin-allergic patients:*
> Doxycycline, 100 mg p.o. b.i.d. for 2 weeks

(HIV-infected patients should be treated as late latent syphilis)

Late Latent Syphilis or Late Syphilis (Non-CNS)

Benzathine penicillin, 2.4 million units IM weekly for 3 weeks

> *For penicillin-allergic patients:*
> Doxycycline, 100 mg p.o. b.i.d. for 4 weeks

Neurosyphilis

Penicillin G, 18-24 million units IV daily, for 10–14 days.

■ PUBLIC HEALTH INTERVENTIONS

Strong case finding and robust disease surveillance are the cornerstone of an effective public health response to syphilis epidemics. Identifying key populations to screen are critical. For example, in the United States, screening has been particularly effective in programs that target homosexual men and heterosexual individuals at high risk, such as jail and prison inmates and intravenous drug users. Syphilis screening is routine for persons attending STI clinics. Care has to be taken to ensure that stigmatization does not occur. Early diagnosis is essential both to link patients to effective care and to prevent the spread of infection. This is particularly the case in areas experiencing outbreaks of syphilis, and among individuals who may, by virtue of sexual behavior or HIV status, may have atypical disease presentations.

Partner notification (PN; see Chapter 30) remains an important tool for ensuring that partners of those newly diagnosed with syphilis are informed of their exposure risk and offered the opportunity for testing and care. Syphilis is unique among infectious diseases in that there is a well-documented public health "critical period" (see Figure 9-1). This is defined as the interval between infection and the development of the primary lesion. During this phase, which averages 2–3 weeks, the patient is *infected* but is not *infectious*. This therefore provides a window for disease interventions such as partner notification and treatment to occur and to prevent a potential "next generation" of infections.

Current CDC guidelines suggest that persons who were exposed within the 90 days preceding the diagnosis of primary, secondary, or early latent syphilis in a sex partner might be infected even if seronegative; therefore, such persons should be treated presumptively. Long-term sex partners of patients who have latent syphilis should be evaluated clinically and serologically for syphilis and treated on the basis of the evaluation findings. Marked variations in PN practice and standards of syphilis exist across Europe and have become more challenging within the context of the recent MSM epidemics.

For perinatal transmission of syphilis, the application of universal and then targeted screening and treatment has all but eliminated this condition in many developed settings. To prevent congenital syphilis, most screening programs recommend serological screening in both the first and last trimester of pregnancy. Nevertheless, continued vigilance is needed as disparities in access to, and uptake of, effective and high-quality antenatal services, especially among socioeconomically deprived and migrant communities, may threaten the recent gains made in this arena. Indeed, the recent increases in syphilis in women in the United States and in Western Europe may well presage a resurgence of congenital syphilis.

Other proven interventions, such as mass-media education campaigns; interventions to change high-risk behavior in groups with a high prevalence of syphilis infection; distribution and use of condoms; expanded screening, especially in outreach settings; and linkage to care, are all useful tools to prevent syphilis in community settings. Involving affected communities in finding solutions to local outbreaks and epidemics has been a key strategy for enhancing syphilis prevention.

■ CONCLUSION

Syphilis remains a major global public health challenge. While traditional public health approaches to disease control should remain the cornerstone of our response, efforts must be made to incorporate and evaluate new diagnostic tools and social network approaches for improved early case ascertainment and cluster identification. The evidence currently suggests that a large reduction in congenital syphilis is feasible with relatively simple interventions focused on maternal and newborn care. However, despite all these factors, congenital syphilis still causes a high burden of disease. As we look to the future, a combination of culturally competent, evidence-based prevention interventions, robust disease surveillance, monitoring and evaluation of prevention, treatment, and care activities must form the cornerstone of our prevention efforts.

■ KEY POINTS

- Syphilis is a chronic, systemic infection characterized by periods of active clinical disease interrupted by periods of latency. Every year, an estimated 12 million people are infected. Congenital syphilis results in serious adverse outcomes in up to 80% of the cases and is estimated to affect more than 1 million pregnancies annually.

- Syphilis infection in pregnancy is highly prevalent in many areas of the world. In developing country settings, maternal syphilis continues to contribute to substantial perinatal morbidity and mortality, even though antenatal syphilis screening can avert these adverse pregnancy outcomes and is cost effective.

- Syphilis screening during pregnancy has been shown to be at least as cost effective as prevention of mother to child transmission (PMTCT) of HIV infection and more cost effective than many widely implemented interventions. Current PMTCT interventions present an opportunity to integrate, to reinforce, and to improve syphilis screening.

- In Western Europe, rates of infectious syphilis fell to their lowest levels in many European Union (EU) countries by the early 1990s. The decreases in Western Europe were accompanied by marked reductions in the incidence of congenital syphilis and tertiary disease.

- Congenital syphilis had continued to decline in the United States throughout the 1990s and early 2000s. However, between 2005 and 2006, the overall rate of congenital syphilis increased 3.7% in the United States to 8.5 cases per 100,000 live births.

- The resurgence of syphilis in the context of high-HIV-prevalence populations in developed and developing countries has increased interest in the clinical interactions between these two infections. With minor differences, syphilis generally presents similarly in HIV-infected and HIV-uninfected patients. About a quarter of HIV-infected patients present with concomitant lesions of both primary and secondary stages of syphilis at the time of diagnosis.

- Penicillin G, administered parenterally, is the preferred drug for treatment of all stages of syphilis, including syphilis during pregnancy.

- Strong case finding and robust disease surveillance are the cornerstone of an effective public health response to syphilis epidemics.

- Other proven interventions, such as mass-media education campaigns; interventions to change high-risk behavior in groups with a high prevalence of syphilis infection; distribution and use of condoms; expanded screening, especially in outreach settings; and linkage to care, are all useful tools to prevent syphilis in community settings.

REFERENCES

Centers for Disease Control and Prevention. *Sexually Transmitted Disease Surveillance 2007*. Atlanta, GA: U.S. Department of Health and Human Services, Centers for Disease Control and Prevention; 2009.

Center for Disease Control and Prevention (CDC). Sexually transmitted diseases treatment guidelines, 2010. *Morb Mort Week Rep.* 2010;(RR-12):26–39.

Centers for Disease Control and Prevention. Trends in primary and secondary syphilis and HIV infections in men who have sex with men—San Francisco and Los Angeles, California, 1998–2002. *MMWR Morb Mortal Wkly Rep.* 2004;53:575–578.

Doherty L, Fenton KA, Jones J, et al. Syphilis: old problem, new strategy. *BMJ.* 2002;325(7356):153–156.

Fenton KA, Breban R, Vardavas R,. Infectious syphilis in high-income settings in the 21st century. *Lancet Infect Dis.* 2008;8(4):244–253.

Fenton KA, Lowndes CM. Recent trends in the epidemiology of sexually transmitted infections in the European Union. *Sex Transm Infect.* 2004;80(4):255–263.

Larsen SA, Steiner BM, Rudolf AH. Laboratory diagnosis and interpretation of tests for syphilis. *Clin Microb Rev.* 1995;8:1–21.

Lewis DA, Young H. Syphilis. *Sex Transm Infect.* 2006; 82(suppl 4).15–15.

Low N, Broutet N, Adu-Sarkodie Y, Barton P, Hossain M, Hawkes S. Global control of sexually transmitted infections. *Lancet.* 2006;368(9551):2001–2016.

Lukehart SA, Hook EW III, Baker-Zander SA, Collier AC, Critchlow CW, Handsfield HH. Invasion of the central nervous system by *Treponema pallidum*: implications for diagnosis and treatment. *Ann Int Med.* 1988;109: 855–862.

Rolfs RT. Treatment of syphilis, 1993. *Clin Infect Dis.* 1995; 20(suppl 1):S23–S38.

Romanowski B, Sutherland R, Fick GH, et al. Serologic response to treatment of infectious syphilis. *Ann Intern Med.* 1991;114:1005–1009.

Saloojee H, Velaphi S, Goga Y, Afadapa N, Steen R, Lincetto O. The prevention and management of congenital syphilis: an overview and recommendations. *Bull World Health Organ.* 2004;82(6):424–430.

Schmid G. Economic and programmatic aspects of congenital syphilis prevention. *Bull World Health Organ.* 2004; 82(6):402–409.

Stamm LV. Biology of *Treponema pallidum*. In: Holmes KK, Sparling PR, Mardh P-A, et al., eds. *Sexually Transmitted Diseases.* 3rd ed. New York: McGraw-Hill, 1999: 467–472.

St. Louis ME, Farley TA, Aral SO. Untangling the persistence of syphilis in the South. *Sex Transm Dis.* 1996;23(1): 1–4.

Zetola NM, Klausner JD. Syphilis and HIV infection: an update. *Clin Infect Dis.* 2007;44(9):1222–1228.

10

HIV

Robyn Neblett and Emily J. Erbelding

HIV infection occurs concurrently with many other sexually transmitted infections (STIs) and has a complex interaction with them. Immunologic suppression induced by HIV infection may influence the natural history and transmissibility of other sexually transmitted infections, particularly those in which cell-mediated immunity plays a primary role in response to infection. In turn, an HIV-infected individual also infected with another STI is more likely to transmit HIV through sexual contact than other HIV-infected persons. The term "epidemiologic synergy" has been applied to this complex relationship among intersecting epidemics. Available data indicate that most individuals infected with HIV who engage in medical care remain sexually active. Accordingly, early STI detection and treatment in this population has great implications, both for health outcomes in the infected individual and for the community at large. This chapter will summarize the effect of HIV on the natural history, clinical presentation, and treatment response of the more common STIs and will also address issues related to STI screening and sexual risk behavior in HIV clinical practice.

■ GENITAL ULCER DISEASE

There is consensus that genital ulcer disease (GUD) is highly associated with HIV acquisition and transmission. Genital ulcers result in breaks in the genital tract lining or skin that may create a portal of entry for HIV. Prospective and retrospective studies have established that the risk is increased two- to fivefold. In an HIV-infected person, the presence of a genital ulcer increases

the probability of HIV transmission to an uninfected sex partner. In general, genital ulcers in patients coinfected with HIV tend to be larger, persist longer, and multiple. In the United States, genital ulcers among sexually active individuals are most often caused by genital herpes, syphilis, or chancroid.

Genital Herpes

The interaction of the herpes viruses with HIV has been the subject of extensive research. Cross-sectional studies using serologic testing have documented a very high prevalence of coinfection with HSV-1, HSV-2, or both, in persons infected with HIV. In HIV-infected individuals, the seroprevalence of HSV-2 in the United States is 70%; for HSV-1 or HSV-2 it is 95%. Because of the importance of cell-mediated immunity in the host immune response to chronic herpes infections, more frequent and severe herpes recurrences would be predicted as immunodeficiency progresses over time. Early in the AIDS epidemic, persistent and severe mucocutaneous ulcerations due to HSV-2 were described in HIV-infected homosexual men. As a result of this clinical observation, the persistence of mucocutaneous herpes for greater than 1 month meets the clinical case definition for AIDS.

Both HIV-infected men and women in longitudinal follow-up have been shown to have higher rates of both clinically evident (symptomatic) shedding of HSV-2 from anogenital sites, as well as asymptomatic shedding of HSV. HSV shedding is also inversely related to CD4-counts and in persons with dual HSV2/HIV who have CD4 < 200, a quarter of patients have cultivable HSV-2 in their genital secretions. HAART therapy reduces the frequency of genital lesions but has little effect on reducing subclinical HSV reactivation as measured by either HSV culture or PCR. Accordingly, HSV reactivation is still frequent among HAART-treated patients and the interaction between HSV-2 and HIV remains of concern even if patient is on HAART.

Subclinical HSV-2 reactivation influences mucosal HIV-1 replication. Analysis of swabs from the base of the herpes lesion in coinfected individuals indicates that HIV-RNA can be consistently detected from herpetic lesions and that the HIV titer present is independent of plasma HIV-1 viral load. This suggests that herpetic lesions make an HIV-infected person more infectious (with respect to HIV) at the time of clinically evident herpes outbreaks. HSV-2 has been shown in vitro to stimulate HIV replication. HSV has also been shown to amplify HIV replication in genital ulcers. Studies from sub-Saharan Africa have conclusively shown that the presence of HSV results in enhanced HIV transmission in HIV-discordant couples, and this is amplified further when HSV-2-related genital lesions are present. Therefore, the HIV/HSV co-infected individual may be more likely to transmit HSV-2 or HIV in any given sexual encounter.

In the context of advanced AIDS, persistent and clinically atypical lesions of the skin and mucous membranes due to HSV-1 or HSV-2 are commonly encountered. HSV ulcers are often large, deep, slow to heal and appear in atypical areas of the body. Other clinical syndromes, such as disseminated HSV, herpes esophagitis, as well as central nervous system disease, have been reported but appear to be much less common.

Treatment of HSV

Consensus panel recommendations for HSV treatment are the same as in HIV-uninfected. Studies among HIV-1-infected individuals have shown that these medications are well tolerated in this population and demonstrate no interaction with antiretroviral medications used in the treatment of HIV-1. However, because recurrent herpes outbreaks tend to be more severe in the setting of advanced immunosuppression, many practitioners experienced in clinical HIV use higher doses of herpes antiviral therapy (acyclovir 800 mg five times daily; valacyclovir 1 gm three times daily; or famciclovir 500 mg three times daily) in persons with advanced HIV/AIDS than are recommended for the episodic treatment of genital herpes. Formal practice guidelines

related to higher antiviral dosing in the HIV-infected patient situation do not exist.

Resistance

Acyclovir-resistant genital herpes have emerged in HIV-infected immunocompromised individuals. These appear as genital ulcers that persist or recur in a patient receiving antiviral treatment. HSV resistance should be suspected and a viral isolate should be obtained for sensitivity testing. In addition, clinicians should take care to ensure that the diagnosis is correct. In persons with advanced HIV infection, nonhealing genital ulcers may also occur because of cytomegalovirus.

The most common mechanism of HSV resistance to acyclovir is deficiency of thymidine kinase, which renders acyclovir ineffective given the drug requires viral thymidine kinase for initial phosphorylation. All acyclovir-resistant strains are resistant to valacyclovir, and the majority is resistant to famciclovir. Effective treatment often requires intravenous foscarnet until clinical resolution is attained. Topical cidofovir gel or topical trifluridine has also indicated benefit.

Treatment of acyclovir-resistant herpes can prove very difficult and inconvenient. Accordingly, preventing the emergence of acyclovir-resistant HSV among HIV-infected patients with advanced immunosuppression is prudent. Acyclovir resistance tends to emerge when significant HSV viral replication occurs under the selective pressure of antiviral agents, suggesting that long-term effective suppression of HSV replication may be the management strategy most likely to prevent the emergence of resistant viral strains. However, the benefits of this approach compared with early and effective antiviral therapy at the onset of recurrences has not been evaluated in comparative trials.

HSV Treatment and Transmission

Early in the HIV epidemic, it was recognized that treatment with acyclovir in persons with dual infection resulted in decreased HIV viral load, and limited data suggest that treatment with antiherpes medications may result in improved HIV outcomes. This led to the hypothesis that, in highly HIV-endemic areas, anti-HSV treatment may provide benefit in reducing transmission. However, two randomized controlled trials have shown that chronic suppression with herpes antivirals does not prevent HIV transmission in couples with HSV-2/HIV who are HIV discordant. This is likely due to chronic immune activation around healing or subclinical genital ulcerations that occurs even with clinically effective chronic suppressive therapy.

Antiviral HSV chemotherapy provides clinical benefits both as episodic treatment of symptomatic patients and as suppressive therapy for prevention of recurrent disease. Daily suppressive acyclovir therapy among HSV-2/HIV-1 coinfected persons may be considered in light of data on the effect of suppressive therapy on HIV-1 levels and the established effect of suppressive therapy on the rate of symptomatic HSV-2. However, HSV antivirals and herpes suppression were associated with decrease in HIV replication, suggesting individual-level benefit beyond suppression of genital herpes.

Chancroid

Chancroid, caused by the bacteria *Haemophilus ducreyi*, is a common cause of genital ulcer disease (GUD) in developing countries. In the United States and Western Europe, there are low levels of endemic disease, punctuated periodically by outbreaks, which have been linked to using crack cocaine, trading sex for drugs or money, and sexual activity in homosexual men.

In patients coinfected with HIV and chancroid, HIV can be recovered from the base of the ulcers making an HIV-uninfected individual more susceptible to acquiring HIV should contact with HIV-infected genital secretions occur. Comparative studies indicate that ulcerations due to chancroid in persons coinfected with HIV are likely to be deeper and have a larger base than in those without HIV infection. Trials focusing on chancroid treatment indicate that chancroid ulcerations in those with concurrent HIV may be more refractory to effective antibiotic therapy, particularly single dose therapy, ceftriaxone (250 mg IM once), or azithromycin (1 gm orally once). Accordingly, some specialists prefer the erythromycin 7-day regimen (500 mg tablet three times a day × 7 days) for treating HIV-infected persons.

Syphilis

There has been substantial interest in the management of syphilis in HIV-infected patients since the late 1980s. The interaction of syphilis and HIV infection is complex and remains the subject of ongoing research.

HIV infection alters the epidemiology, natural history, and response to treatment of syphilis. As with the other GUDs, patients with syphilis have a two- to five-fold increased risk of acquiring HIV in observational cohort studies. Early (primary and secondary) syphilis also appears to stimulate HIV replication and therefore is suspected of increasing transmission efficiency to persons exposed to the dually infected individual. This is of particular concern given the rapid increase in the rate of syphilis among HIV-infected men who have sex with men over the past decade.

Clinical Presentation

Conventional staging of syphilis is unchanged by HIV coinfection. In primary syphilis, HIV-infected patients may present with chancres that are larger, deeper, or multiple. Approximately one-quarter of HIV-infected individuals presents with lesions of both primary and secondary syphilis at time of diagnosis. The rash of secondary syphilis may mimic various dermatologic conditions and in HIV-infected individuals on HAART has been misdiagnosed as a drug-eruption rash. Seronegative secondary syphilis has been described in HIV infection, though routine serologic tests are felt to be reliable for diagnosis of nearly all cases of syphilis in HIV-infected persons.

In both HIV-infected and HIV-uninfected persons, dissemination of *Treponema pallidum* to the central nervous system occurs early. Studies conducted in the 1920s and confirmed in the 1980s demonstrated that up to 20% of persons with primary syphilis and >40% of secondary syphilis had demonstrable spirochetes in the cerebrospinal fluid. A large case series evaluating CSF in syphilis patients demonstrated that those who were HIV infected were more likely to meet diagnostic criteria for neurosyphilis especially if CD4 < 350/mm^3. Other reports have suggested that coexistent neurosyphilis with early stage syphilis has become a more common presentation in the HIV/AIDS era. Furthermore, the degree to which CNS invasion occurs does not seem to differ among HIV-infected and HIV-uninfected hosts. Whether neurologic complications of syphilis occur more frequently and earlier in HIV-infected patients has not been evaluated definitively. Although most experts believe that HIV-infected patients with early syphilis (primary, secondary, or early latent) have an increased risk of neurologic complications the magnitude of any such risk is uncertain.

Diagnosis

Standard serological testing for syphilis in HIV-infected persons is generally reliable and should be the same as in the general population. Atypical presentations are uncommon but have been observed. There have been reports of false-negative serologic syphilis tests, but many of these appear to be due to prozone phenomena in persons with extremely high titers. HIV infection in syphilis patients may also be associated with unusually high titer reactivity in nontreponemal serologic testing, in some cases being over 1:1,000,000. Direct testing methods, such as dark-field microscopic examination, direct fluorescent antibody-treponemal pallidum (DFA-TP), and PCR, should be considered when the diagnosis of syphilis cannot be confirmed.

Both HIV-negative and positive individuals should have examination of the cerebrospinal fluid if treatment failure is documented by serologic follow-up, or if the patient has neurologic signs or symptoms at the time of staging. In addition, HIV-infected individuals with a diagnosis of late latent syphilis or syphilis of unknown duration should have CSF examination performed to evaluate for neurosyphilis. Some experts recommend CSF examinations in HIV-infected persons with nontreponemal serum titer $\geq$ 1:32, regardless of syphilis stage, or those with early stage infection and a CD4 cell count <350 cells/μL regardless of titer.

Treatment

Treatment trials of early syphilis have clearly indicated that both HIV-infected and HIV-uninfected patients treated with standard regimens for early syphilis have CNS outcomes that are not significantly different. HIV-positive patients who have early syphilis might be at increased risk for neurologic complications, but the magnitude of these risks is likely minimal. No treatment regimens of enhanced therapy for syphilis have been demonstrated to be more effective in preventing neurosyphilis in HIV-infected persons. HIV-positive patients should be treated in accordance with the same recommendations as HIV-negative patients. Benzathine penicillin G continues to be the treatment of choice for all stages of syphilis in HIV-infected persons. Individuals who are penicillin allergic may be treated with alternative regimens, including doxycycline or tetracycline. Alternatives to penicillin have not been well studied in HIV-infected patients, but available data do not indicate inferior response to this class of drugs. Careful follow-up after therapy is essential given individuals with HIV infection are more likely to have serologic treatment failure at 1-year follow-up. CDC and other authorities recommend serologic follow-up at closer intervals (3, 6, 9, 12, 24 months) in individuals with HIV infec-

tion than recommended for those without HIV infection (6, 12 months).

◼ NONULCERATIVE SEXUALLY TRANSMITTED INFECTIONS

Gonorrhea/Chlamydia

Though gonorrhea and chlamydia are distinct bacterial infections, given they infect the same mucosal surfaces and cause the same clinical syndromes, they will be grouped together for this discussion. Gonorrhea (GC) and chlamydia (CT) have both been conclusively linked to increased HIV transmissibility and susceptibility. Nonulcerative STIs increase the concentration of cells in genital secretions that can serve as targets for HIV. Studies have shown that HIV-infected individuals who are also infected with other STIs are particularly likely to shed HIV in their genital secretions. This has been demonstrated at both urethral and cervical sites, where local HIV viral load in the setting of CT/GC-mediated inflammation is potentiated to three or four times the level of plasma viral load. Because the incidence of gonorrhea and chlamydia greatly exceeds rates for curable genital ulcer disease in most communities, inflammatory nonulcerative STIs may actually be quantitatively more important, in terms of attributable fraction of HIV transmission. The increase in HIV shedding from the genital mucosal sites observed with either cervical or urethral gonorrhea or chlamydial infection reverses with effective antimicrobial therapy, though it is unclear how long it takes for HIV-RNA levels to return to their "baseline." Thus, an HIV-infected individual coinfected with either GC or CT may be more "infectious" with respect to HIV for some time after their bacterial STI has been cured.

Treatment

Available data indicate that HIV-infected individuals respond as well to standard antibiotic therapy for uncomplicated GC or CT as do those who have not been diagnosed with HIV infection. Antibiotic therapies and recommended clinical follow-up are the same with or without concurrent HIV infection. In terms of systemic complications, there is no increased susceptibility to disseminated gonococcal infection. For chlamydia, there have been a number of case series reporting reactive arthritis (Reiter's syndrome) in patients with HIV, but no conclusive evidence exists that this relatively rare chlamydial complication occurs more readily with HIV infection.

Pelvic Inflammatory Disease

Pelvic inflammatory disease (PID) is a common complication of infection with either GC or CT in women. In general, it is estimated that as many as a third of women with untreated gonorrhea or chlamydia will develop PID. Upper tract infection is usually polymicrobial, often involving gram-negative enteric bacteria and anaerobes. There are no data to conclusively show that HIV-infected women are more susceptible to develop PID as a result of gonorrhea or chlamydia. However, there are very clear data from case series and prospective studies that, when PID occurs, it is more likely to be asymptomatic or subsymptomatic but is paradoxically more severe among HIV-positive women. Tubo-ovarian abscesses are substantially more common in these patients, and in one study, surgical intervention is more frequently required. Compared with HIV-seronegative women, women with concurrent HIV who present with PID have a lower total white blood cell count and a higher temperature, a longer febrile course during treatment, and require a longer hospital stay. These differences in PID complications may be attributable to impaired immunity conferred by HIV infection, but a delayed clinical presentation in HIV-infected women may also explain this apparent increase in PID-related morbidity. Therefore, physicians caring for patients at risk should have a lower threshold for laparoscopy or gynecological intervention particularly if other opportunities pathogens might be playing a role. HIV-infected women with PID respond equally well to standard parenteral and oral antibiotic regimens when compared with HIV-negative women. Given the range of opportunistic pathogens that may lead to a clinical presentation compatible with PID, more aggressive diagnostic evaluation and intervention should be considered in HIV-infected women who do not respond to routine therapy for PID, particularly if she is immunocompromised.

Trichomonas

Infection with *Trichomonas vaginalis* is the most common curable STI in young, sexually active women. Cohorts of HIV-infected women have not been shown to have increased incidence of trichomonal vaginitis in longitudinal follow-up when compared with women of similar behavioral profiles who are HIV-uninfected. *Trichomonas vaginalis* infection of the male urethra is also a relatively common cause of nongonococcal urethritis in both HIV-infected and HIV-uninfected men. Infection with *T. vaginalis*, either isolated from the male urethra or the female vagina, has been associated with increased HIV-RNA shedding in genital secretions. Antibiotic regimens for the treatment of trichomoniasis do not differ according to HIV serostatus.

Bacterial Vaginosis

Bacterial vaginosis (BV) is caused by altered vaginal microbial ecology, with loss of the hydrogen peroxide–producing *Lactobacillus* sp. and overgrowth of anaerobes and other gram-negative bacilli. In several large epidemiologic studies focusing on populations with a high prevalence of HIV, BV has been associated with increased risk of HIV seroconversion among women. The specific mechanism by which altered vaginal ecology enhances the risk of HIV acquisition if exposure occurs is unknown. BV is often a highly refractory condition, frequently recurring after standard antibiotic therapy. BV appears to be more persistent in HIV-positive women though there is no evidence that BV is refractory to standard antibiotic therapy in women with concurrent HIV infection. Patients who have BV and are infected with HIV should receive the same treatment regimen as those who are HIV negative. The influence of BV on HIV viral shedding in the genital tract of HIV-infected woman is unknown.

Vulvovaginal Candidiasis (VVC)

Candidal infection of the mucosal surfaces occurs commonly in persons with HIV infection and is often an early indicator of disease progression. Candidal infection of the esophagus or lower airways meets criteria for the 1997 case definition of AIDS. Recurrent VVC meets "B" clinical criteria in those with HIV infection as suggestive of symptoms of HIV. Well-controlled cohorts comparing women with HIV infection to those who are HIV-uninfected but have similar risk profiles show increased rates of vaginal mucosal colonization with *Candida* sp. in those who are HIV infected and colonization rates correlate with increasing severity of immunosuppression. Therapy for HIV-infected women with VVC does not differ from recommended therapy for women without HIV infection. However, episodic fluconazole treatment in patients with AIDS is associated with the development of azole-resistant esophageal candidiasis, a serious infection requiring intravenous antifungal therapy. Thus, topical azoles rather than systemic therapy may be preferable in managing VVC in HIV-infected women.

Human Papilloma Virus

Human papilloma virus (HPV), the causative agent of anogenital warts and cervical cancer, is an extremely common STI in the general population and also highly prevalent among those with HIV infection. The prevalence of HPV infection among HIV-infected women is higher than it is among uninfected women and is associated with a degree of immune suppression. Surveillance data collected by the Centers for Disease Control and Prevention in 2003–2005 found that nearly half of HIV-infected women followed in longitudinal care settings had cervical infection with high-risk, oncogenic-HPV types (types 16, 18). Similarly, the incidence of genital warts in many HIV-infected cohorts has been shown to be higher compared with HIV-seronegative controls, even among those with CD4 cell counts greater than 500/mm³ who have preserved immune function.

HIV infection, particularly in those with more advanced CD4 cell depletion, is associated with a much greater risk of oncogenic outcomes linked to infection with specific HPV subtypes (13, 16, 31, 33, 35, 58). These outcomes include cervical intraepithelial neoplasia (CIN) most commonly, but also vulvar intraepithelial neoplasia (VIN) and vaginal intraepithelial neoplasia (VAIN) as well as anal intraepithelial neoplasia (AIN) in men who have had sex with other men. In women, persistent infection with high-risk HPV subtypes is strongly associated with an elevated risk of CIN as well as with invasive cervical cancer. Women with HIV infection are more likely to have persistent infection with high-risk HPV subtypes compared with HIV-seronegative controls, even when adjustments are made for a number of sexual partners. Similarly, HIV-infected gay or bisexual men are more likely to demonstrate persistence of high-risk HPV subtypes and a higher incidence of AIN than HIV-seronegative men with similar behavioral profiles. In women, VIN and VAIN lesions occur much less frequently overall than CIN lesions, but unusual cases have been described in women with HIV infection, underscoring the need for routine cytologic surveillance of the vaginal wall, even in women who have undergone hysterectomy. Immune reconstitution with successful antiretroviral therapy has been associated with resolution of low-grade cervical cytologic abnormalities.

Screening

HIV-infected women require more frequent Papanicolaou smear screening then HIV-negative women. At time of HIV diagnosis, women should have a thorough gynecologic examination, including a Pap smear. If the initial smear result is normal, a second screening should be done in 6 months. If both results are normal, then HIV-infected women should have a Pap smear annually. More frequent screening may be considered in women with known HPV infection, prior treatment for dysplasia, or CD4 count < 200 cells/μL. Many authorities also recommend anorectal Pap smears in men and women who participate in anoreceptive intercourse. However, recommendations for anal Pap smear screening are currently not included in standard guidelines. Some clinicians follow the cervical cancer screening guidelines and perform anal Pap smear at initial visit, repeated at 6 months, and then annually if results are normal. Most practice currently applied algorithms lead to patients with ASCUS or higher cytologic changes being referred for high-resolution anoscopy. The benefits to cytologic screening for anal intraepithelial neoplasia are unproven.

■ STIs and Risk Behavior in HIV Primary Care

Early diagnosis and medical intervention for those with HIV infection is clearly indicated to improve health outcomes for the infected individual. Early care has been strongly promoted as a public good as well, based on the premise that medical care for those with HIV infection will decrease the chance that they will transmit HIV infection to others, either through behavior change or through biomedical interventions.

Counseling targeting risk behavior reduction, entry into drug treatment, and referral for mental health services all support individual behavior change to reduce HIV transmission within the community. Provider-delivered brief interventions have been shown to reduce HIV transmission behavior. In addition, screening for bacterial STIs at 6- to 12-month intervals improves STI detection and allows for early institution of therapy to reduce transmission to others. The identification of a new STI though screening an HIV-infected person may help a clinician identify ongoing risky sexual behavior that might otherwise have gone undetected. As such, STIs may be useful as "biomarkers" to identify those in need of more specialized risk reduction counseling.

■ Summary

Nonulcerative and ulcerative STIs increase susceptibility and transmission of HIV (see Figure 10-1). Infection with HIV alters the natural history of other STIs, particularly

FIGURE 10-1 Infection with STIs

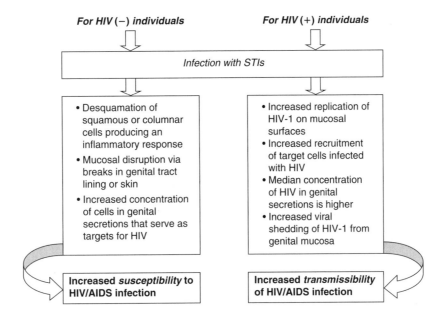

those in which the cell-mediated immunity plays a large role in host response to infection. Early detection and treatment of concurrent STIs in HIV clinical practice promotes improved health, both for the infected individual and for the community at large.

■ KEY POINTS

- Persons with HIV are at higher risk for STIs. All persons with STIs should be routinely tested for HIV. Similarly, persons with HIV should be assessed for STI infection routinely.

- The clinical presentation and management of gonorrhea and chlamydia is similar in HIV-infected and uninfected patients.

- The presentation of genital ulcer diseases (herpes, syphilis, and chancroid) in HIV patients may present with larger and more difficult to heal ulcerations; this is generally correlated with lower CD4 counts. However, treatment protocols are not different.

- Syphilis is a complex disease that may present with more advanced complications in persons with HIV, but does not require a different treatment approach, unless neurosyphilis is strongly suspected. These patients, however, do require more frequent monitoring.

- HIV increases the expression of HPV disease, including larger genital warts and abnormalities on Pap smear.

REFERENCES

Bartlett J, Gallant J, Pham P. *2009–2010 Medical Management of HIV Infection*. Baltimore: Johns Hopkins University, Knowledge Source Solutions; 2009.

Centers of Disease Control and Prevention. Sexually transmitted diseases treatment guidelines. *MMWR Morb Mortal Wkly Rep*. 2010;59(RR-12):1–110.

Corey L, Wald A, Celum C, Quinn T. The effects of herpes simplex virus-2 on HIV-1 acquisition and transmission: a review of two overlapping epidemics. *J Acquir Immune Defic Syndr*. 2004;35(5):435–445.

Fisher JD, Fisher WA, Cornman DH, et al. Clinician-delivered intervention during routine clinical care reduces unprotected sexual behavior among HIV-infected patients. *J Acquir Immune Defic Syndr*. 2006;41(1):44–52.

Ghanem K, Erbelding E, Cheng W, et al. Doxycycline compared with benzathine penicillin for the treatment of early syphilis. *Clin Infect Dis*. 2006;42:e45–e49.

Marra CM, Maxwell CL, Smith SL, et al. Cerebrospinal fluid abnormalities in patients with syphilis: association with clinical and laboratory features. *J Infect Dis*. 2004;189(3):369–376.

Richardson JL, Milam J, McCutchan A, et al. Effect of brief safer-sex counseling by medical providers to HIV-1 seropositive patients: a multi-clinic assessment. *AIDS*. 2004; 18(8):1179–1786.

UCSF HIV InSite. Homepage. http://www.hivinsite.org/InSite. Accessed January 21, 2010.

Zetola N, Klausner J. Syphilis and HIV infection: an update. *Clin Infect Dis*. 2007;44:1222–1228.

11

Rashes and Genital Dermatoses

Doshi Hemendra Kumar

■ INTRODUCTION

In clinical practice, patients are always disturbed when something unusual crops up in the groin or anogenital area. Because of the possibility of sexually transmitted infection (STI), clinicians must be nonjudgmental and compassionate but also cognizant of the wide variety of both sexually transmitted and nonsexually transmitted dermatological conditions that may be present. Besides STIs, the possibilities include non-STI infections, neoplastic, inflammatory, papulosquamous, and autoimmune conditions.

A simple basic knowledge of skin lesions with particular emphasis on the anogenital and groin area is essential. In this chapter, I will provide a simple overview of genital dermatology, followed by the common genital dermatoses and their differential diagnosis. The genital skin is often moist, and parts of it are highly sensitive and endowed with a plethora of sensory nerves. The perineal area is endowed with numerous types of functional and nonfunctional glands, namely, eccrine, sebaceous, and apocrine and pilosebaceous glands with the hair follicles.

■ APPROACHING BASIC RASHES

In assessing a genital rash, the following seven cardinal features should be addressed (see Figure 11-1):

1. Presenting subjective symptoms, like pain, burning sensation, irritation, numbness, and, the most important symptom of skin, pruritus.

2. Shape of the lesion.

3. The color and consistency compared with the normal surrounding skin.

4. Number and arrangement whether single, multiple, linear in alignment, circular, irregular in arrangement, or well circumscribed.

5. Distribution in relation with skin of other parts.

6. Are the lesions totally localized primary to the genitalia or secondary to skin lesions elsewhere, for example, psoriasis, pemphigus.

7. The general condition of the patient, including the examination for lymphadenitis.

FIGURE 11-1 Evaluation of Skin Lesions

- Subjective symptoms—pain, numbness, pruritis
- Shape
- The color and consistency
- Number and arrangement of lesions
- Distribution of lesions
- Genital or nongenital localization
- Consideration of other comorbidities

Symptoms

- Irritation and discomfort are the most prominent symptoms.

- Pain and burning on urination, movements, sexual intercourse, as in lichen sclerosus.

- Itchiness or pruritus is a cardinal feature of majority of skin conditions, including over the vulva, perineum, prepuce, glans, or the shaft of the penis, anogenital area, like in scabies, or candidiasis or tenia cruris. It results in excoriations, lichenification, and infections.

- Numbness may occur as in herpes zoster. Hence a detailed history needs to be taken.

Type of Primary Lesions

Describing the skin lesion is key to establishing the differential diagnosis. The classic dermatological classifications are described.

- **Macule:** is a flat circumscribed lesion of <1 to 1.5 centimeters with different texture and can be pigmented or even hypopigmented.

- **Patch:** is >2 cm and may be regular or irregular, for example, in vitiligo.

- **Plaque:** is an elevated 1–1.5 cm regular, irregular, generally bordered lesion larger than 2 cm. The surface is usually scaly, crusted, or macerated. It can be a coalescence of papules as in psoriasis or thickening and enlarging of existing patch as in granuloma annulare.

- **Papule:** is a small, firm elevated palpable lesion of 0.5 to 1 cm in diameter. It can be an epidermal or dermal or combination of both and of normal color, for example, scabies. The surface can be usually smooth.

- **Nodule:** is a firm palpable elevated lesion of 0.5 to 1 cm. It may be dome shaped, oval, or elliptical.

- **Vesicle:** small, elevated well-circumscribed lesion of <0.5 cm containing a clear to opaque fluid. Usually vesicles are superficial, thin walled, and easily ruptured, as in herpes simplex, forming superficial ulcers. It can be discrete or grouped. When numerous, they can be arranged in various formations. For example, in herpes zoster vesicles are arranged in a linear fashion while in herpes genitalia they are grouped.

- **Bulla:** is larger than a vesicle, v >0.5 cm. The walls can be thin or thick and usually tense. The fluid can be clear or hemorrhagic; crusting and scab formations occur after they rupture. Usually, they are painful.

- **Pustule:** is the same as a vesicle, but the clear fluid is replaced by pus. Generally, it denotes infections but can also be sterile. Pricking it will produce pus.

The Shape of the Lesion

The following are a guidance to describe shapes of the lesion:

- Sessile: are elevated but with a flat top like a plateau, for example, common skin warts on the shaft of the penis and lichen planus.

- Pedunculated: a small but elongated pedicle and the main lesion can dangle from it, for example, achondron.

- Cauliflower-like, like broccoli. Numerous tentacles protrude from the base lesion. Usually, these protrusions are friable, such as viral warts on the corona of penis.

- They can be round, oval rhomboidal shape, or even irregular.

Secondary Changes: When there is loss of the epidermis causing **erosions,** healing without scarring, while **ulcers** form when there is loss of full thickness of epidermis and part of the dermis, resulting in scar formation on healing. Sometimes **atrophy** occurs as a result of thinning of epidermis and the dermis. There is wrinkling with loss of skin margins. **Lichenification** is a result of persistent and prolonged scratching causing thickening of the skin and exaggerated creases.

Color and Consistency

The **color** of the lesions in dermatology gives numerous clues about what is going on beneath the epidermis. However, the color of the lesions varies with the skin type. On fair skin, most of lesions are obvious except those with hypopigmentation. In many lesions, there is excess, reduction, loss of, presence of, or alteration of melanin (brown), reduced hemoglobin (bluish red), oxyhemoglobin (bright red), and beta carotene (yellowish). Psoriasis is red, papules of lichen planus are violaceous, and eczemas are generally pinkish.

The **consistency** can be firm, hard, or soft. The margins or the pattern of lesion give important clues. In tinia cruris, the margins are clear, advancing with central clearance, while in psoriasis, it maybe polygonal. In basal cell carcinoma, it is raised and rolled in contrast to notched, irregular malignant melanomas.

The **arrangement** may be linear as in herpes zoster, grouped and circular as in herpes simplex, reticulate as in lichen planus with the lacelike arrangement of the surface (**Wickham's striae**). It can be annular as in granuloma annulare. A **Köbner** phenomenon occurs in psoriasis, lichen planus, and few other conditions where linear lesions appear along scratch marks or in scars.

The **distribution** is equally important as in herpes simplex or syphilis chancre of syphilis at the site of primary inoculation; herpes zoster follows the lines of dermatome.

Many lesions are primarily in the perineum and genitalia as is erythroplasia of Queyrat, lichen sclerosis, or secondary to lesions on the other parts of the body like psoriasis or pemphigus. Psoriasis, though, follows a classical pattern and is smooth and shiny on the genitalia and not scaly as on other parts.

Thus, it is the combinations of many factors that make a visual diagnosis of basic skin lesions possible. The recognition of lesions confidently requires years of experience. It can be stressed that even the experienced dermatologist quite often needs a second opinion.

Investigations

Most dermatological diagnoses can be made clinically with a high predictive value. Investigations are done to process a differential diagnosis or to rule out other conditions, taking into account that nonclassical presentations may occur. For optimal dermatological diagnosis, the following should be available:

1. Hand lens with good illumination, preferably with good light source

2. Small ruler or measuring caliper

3. Blunt scalpel blade for scraping scaly lesions

4. KOH 20–40% and access to stains like methylene blue, Gram's stain, and so forth

5. Wood's (UV) light

6. Microscope

7. Biopsy punches, if the clinician is qualified to do skin biopsies

▪ GENITAL DERMATOSES

Genital dermatoses may be syndromes that are unique to genitalia or may be a presentation of a systemic skin disorder. Among the latter, some disorders may present with signs and symptoms similar to those seen in other skin regions (e.g., herpes zoster, psoriasis), whereas some systemic disorders may present with a unique appearance specific to the genitalia. In either case, genitalia may be the first site on which these lesions appear. Hence, ensure a proper history to find out the following:

- First episode or recurrence and the duration and the nature of the complaint

- Prophylactic measures taken to overcome, such as use of oral or topical medications

- Dysuria, allergies, any systemic involvement, the presence of any inflammation, edema, urethral discharge erosion ulcers, and any change of color such as hyperpigmentation and hypopigmentation

Genital dermatoses can broadly be divided into the following groups:

- Fixed drug eruption

- Allergic or irritant contact dermatitis

- Infection

- Papulosquamous systemic disease

- Balanitidis

- Tumors

- Neoplasm

- Autoimmune conditions

- Normal variants

- Trauma

- Miscellaneous

▪ FIXED DRUG LESIONS

Fixed drug eruptions are lesions that occur on the genital skin as a reaction to systemic drugs after sensitization (see Figure 11-2). The history is key to making the diagnosis. Similar to other hypersensitivity reactions, there is no reaction at time of the initial (sensitizing) exposure. The lesions may appear after 7–10 days of treatment or

FIGURE 11-2 Fixed Drug Eruption After Taking Trimethoprim/Sulfamethoxazole

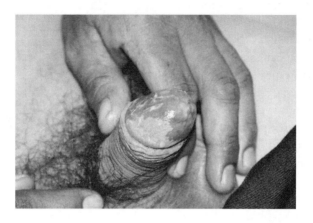

upon rechallenge. The lesion is a well-defined erythematous patch, plaque, and at times bulla. Initially, there is itchiness and or burning sensation within hours of taking the drugs. Eventually, it leaves a residual dark hyperpigmentation patch or plaque on healing. Recurrence is at the same site, genitalia being the typical area, though the lips and paraumbilical region are other common sites. Common drugs involved are tetracycline, sulfonamides, dapsone, penicillins, and paracetamol (acetaminophen).

Treat with local applications of mild steroidal creams and identifying and avoiding the responsible medication is essential.

ALLERGIC, IRRITANT, AND CONTACT DERMATITIS

Irritant or contact dermatitis often occurs after using deodorants or scented soaps (see Figure 11-3). The clinical presentation is a highly pruritic and erythematous lesion, which is limited to the area of contract.

Contact dermatitis of genitalia may result from use of contraceptive, medication, or passive transfer of allergens from the other sites. Lubricants from condoms, feminine hygiene deodorant spray, and douches can produce allergic dermatitis of the genitalia. For example, K-Y Jelly contains propylene glycol, which is known to cause allergic dermatitis of the penis and the vulva. Patients often present with marked edema (see Chapter 12).

Contact dermatitis from condoms or rubber diaphragms is suggested by the history and the presence of a sharply delineated dermatitis at the base of the penile shaft or tip of the glans penis or even the vulva, mons, or clitoris. If indicated, patch testing will find the offending agent. At times, secondary infections make the condition more challenging to diagnose as the intense itch, acute inflammation, and severe erythema cause more confusion. Intercourse with a female partner with vaginal candidiasis may result in irritant balanitis in the male partner.

Patients with contact urticaria from latex condoms may present with local swelling or pruritus during intercourse. This is type 1 IgE-mediated allergic reaction.

FIGURE 11-3 Irritative Dermatitis—Scrotum

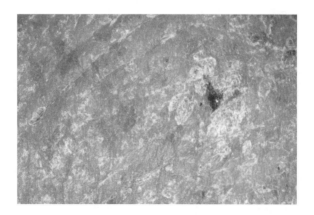

Bullous Erythema Multiforme

Erythema multiforme presents as maculopapular target lesions that appear rapidly (see Figure 11-4). It is associated with herpes simplex infections, where antigens have been isolated from the base of the lesions, and also drugs (such as sulphonamides) collagen vascular diseases and systemic vasculitis. In >50% of cases, there is no detectable precipitating factor.

Cutaneous lesions may be macular, papular, commonly seen in HSV as erythema multiforme minor and vesicular to bullous in severe cases due to drugs. Bullae develop suddenly on the oral and genital mucosa, ulcerate, and become covered with a grayish white to yellowish membrane; hemorrhagic crusting is common. There may be a marked conjunctival suffusion. Skin lesions though not always present are dull red maculopapules that may develop into target lesions; cropping at intervals of a few days is usual. This is a systemic disorder and will typically involve multiple regions. The rash is often found on the hands, wrists, forearms, elbows, and knees. In persons with risk exposures, syphilis serologies should be performed to rule out secondary syphilis.

Treatment is symptomatic, but prednisolone may be needed in severe cases. Recurrences can occur, particularly with herpetic infections. In severe cases, hospitalization is needed.

■ INFECTIONS

Infection and inflammation of the glans is known as balanitis, prepuce as posthitis, and combination as in uncircumcised male is known as balano-posthitis. Likewise, in the female, vulval involvement is known as vulvitis while combination with vagina is known as vulvovaginitis. Nonsexually transmitted genital dermatoses can be due to fungal, viral, bacterial, or parasitic causes.

Fungal

The most common are candida and tinea infections, which are superficial. Deep fungal infections occur exclusively in the profoundly immunocompromised.

Candida albicans

Occurs on moist surfaces, typically in the skin folds and intertriginous areas (see Figures 11-5 and 11-6). The intertriginous area is their favorite site because of the heat, humidity, and constant friction that results in macerating effect on the stratum corneum.

Higher rates are seen in patients with diabetes, malignancy, steroid use, HIV, pregnancy broad-spectrum antibiotic use, oral contraceptive use, and tight-fitting clothing. The causative organism is the oval yeast in the commensal state, but in its pathogenic state, it divides by budding and produces pseudohyphae.

In the female, candida usually originates in the vagina, spreading to the vulva and the groin and may present as a dermatoses, a vaginitis (see Chapter 7), or both. In males, it presents as balanitis. The glans penis is usually red and inflamed and is more severe in the uncircumcised male who presents as balano-posthitis.

Candida intertrigo is very common in all ages and has to be distinguished from other causes of intertrigo. The lesion begins as pustules and erythema with the rupture and merger of multiple pustules that leaves raw and macerated sodden skin. In severe cases, inflammation and erythema can extend deep into the roof of the folds of the groin, Satellite lesions in a centrifugal pattern should be looked for as a hallmark of candida infection.

FIGURE 11-4 Erythema Multiforme Secondary to Herpes Simplex

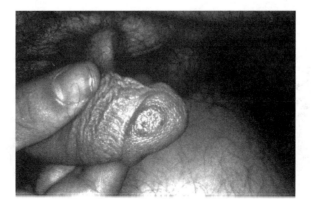

FIGURE 11-5 Penial *Candida Balanitis* in an Uncircumcised Male

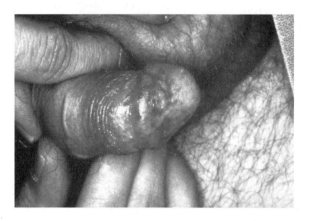

Treatment is simple, though at times frustrating in recalcitrant patients. All efforts must be made to keep the area dry. Clotrimazole cream application twice a day will suffice in most cases. Use of oral ketoconazole 100 mg or itraconazole 100–200 mg daily for 1–2 weeks will suffice. In recalcitrant cases, especially in HIV patients, fluconazole, 100–150 mg daily, may need to be used. At times, pulse therapy may be needed.

Tinea cruris (**Jock Itch, or Dhobi Itch**)

Tinea cruris is used to describe superficial fungal infection of the groin and genitalia (see Figures 11-7 and 11-8). It is usually pruritic, sparing the scrotum and the depth of the folds of the groin. The lesions are scaly with marginated usually circular active borders and central clearing; they expand downward to the thighs, backward to the buttocks and intergluteal area, and upward to the suprapubic area, at times up to the natal clefts. In HIV or other immunosuppressed persons, the lesions may be extensive and are severe.

One of the three genera of the anthrophilic dermatophyte affects the groin. By far *Trichophyton uubrum* is the commonest followed by *Epidermophton floccosum* and *T. mentagrophytes*.

It is diagnosed by examining the scrapings for hyphae to distinguish it or to rule out candida and erythrasma. Culture to identify the specific organism is not required. Wood's light will not show how any definite classical feature except to rule out erythrasma and rare mycotic infections.

Systemic use of 7–14 days of itraconazole, 100–200 mg daily, will suffice. Washing twice daily with polytar and local application of mild emollients with mild steroid in combination with antifungal creams may be needed.

FIGURE 11-6 Genital Candidiasis in a Child

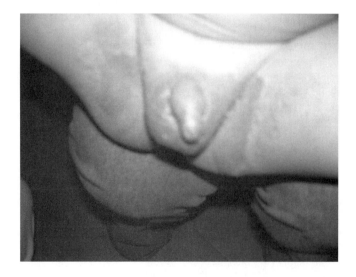

FIGURE 11-7 Tinea Cruris A

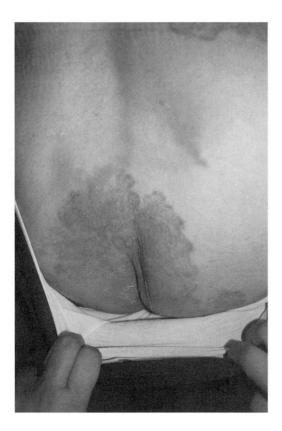

FIGURE 11-8 Tinea Cruris B

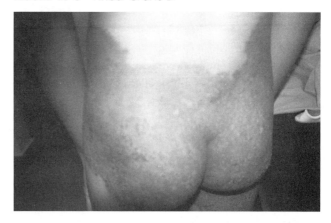

FIGURE 11-9 Local Genital Penicilliosis

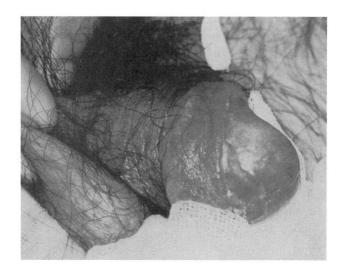

Deep Fungal Infections

These lesions present as poxlike with central umbilication (see Figures 11-9 and 11-10). Occasionally, lesions with necrotic centers may appear. The color ranges from pale to pinkish to red nodules and may be umbilicated. This occurs exclusively in patients with advanced HIV disease or profoundly immunosuppression due to steroids or chemotherapy. Fungi that may be involved depend on the endemic area, and include histoplasma, dermatophytes, *Penicillium marneffei*, *Cryptococcus neoformans*. Biopsy will confirm the diagnosis as well as rule out the other fungal causes. Hospitalization and systemic therapy is typically required.

Seborrheic Dermatitis

This eczematous condition is thought to be hypersensitivity to commensal yeast *Pitrosporum ovale*. It commonly affects the face over the nasolabial folds, scalp, upper trunk, and flexures. In HIV patients, it is often more severe, especially in advanced immunosuppression.

Itchiness may be minimal, scaly erythema, which is mild with folliculitis over the nasolabial area. It can be a confusing factor in a patient with psoriasis, particularly

FIGURE 11-10 Disseminated Fungal Infection (Penicilliosis)

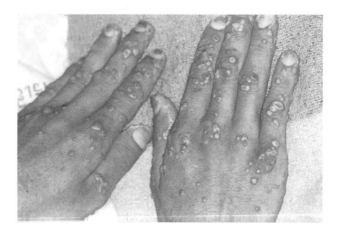

in the groin, in which it is termed as inverse psoriasis and sebopsoriasis. The genital and perianal regions are also common sites. If seen in isolation it needs to be differentiated from tinea, candidiasis, and intertrigo. Sometimes it may present as severe symmetrical erythematous inflammation over the vulva, called intertriginous seborrheic eczema.

Microscopic examination of scrapping of the scaly lesions is necessary to rule out other fungal infection and to show the presence of pitrosporum. Management is with topical ketoconazole or other imidazole.

■ VIRAL INFECTIONS

Herpes Zoster (*Varicella Zoster* Virus)

Herpes zoster (shingles) can have genital dermatomal presentations if the recurrence is in the L5, S1 dermatomes. This can be indistinguishable from genital herpes and is suspected when there is a classical presentation with negative HSV cultures, or if there is a distinct unilaterality to the lesions. It is estimated that 1–2% of clinical genital herpes is actually herpes zoster. Varicella Zoster virus (VZV) disease is more common in older adults and in persons with AIDS or other causes of immunosuppression. In HIV patients, with low CD4 count, the vesicles will be larger and can be bullous and hemorrhagic (see Figure 11-11).

Molluscum Contagiosum

This condition is caused by large DNA poxvirus and may be acquired by intimate contact (Figure 11-12).

FIGURE 11-11   Genital Varicella Zoster with Hemhorragic Bullae

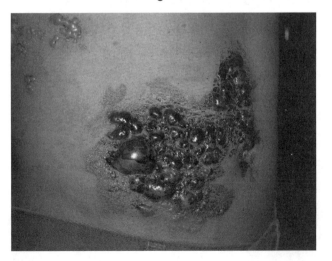

FIGURE 11-12   Mollucsum Contagiosum Lesion Showing Characteristic Central Umbilication

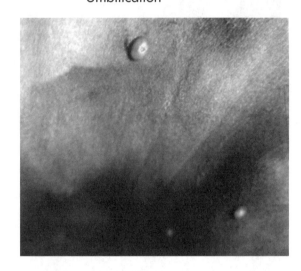

In immunocompromised persons, there can be a large number of genital lesions, which may also be seen on the limbs, trunk, and face. Lesions are large painless papules, or vesicles, characterized by a central depression (umbilication) at the center. Treatment is by simple curettage or by liquid nitrogen cryotherapy.

Condyloma Acuminata

Classic condyloma acuminata may appear anywhere on the epithelial surfaces of the skin and have a cauliflower-reticulated appearance (see Figure 11-13). Management is detailed in Chapter 22.

FIGURE 11-13   Condyloma Acuminate A

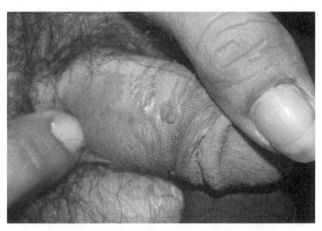

■ BACTERIAL INFECTIONS

Erythrasma

Erythrasma (see Figure 11-14) is a common cause of intertrigo and is caused by *Corynebactrium minutissimus*. The typical appearance is superficial, red, scaly plaques with symmetrical lesions on the thighs, which can macerate. Differentiation from tinea and other superficial dermatoses is by Wood's light, as erythrasma produces a coral red to pink fluorescence. Treatment is with topical or systemic (in severe cases) erythromycin or clindamycin.

Pyogenic Infections

Streptococci or staphylococci are the major causes of folliculitis, furunculitis, and abscesses. In particular, infection due to methicillin-resistant *Staphylococcus aureus* has been a major concern and is highly prevalent in homosexual men, drug users, persons recently incarcerated, or those involved in contact sports. When suspected, cultures should be obtained and treatment provided with appropriate systemic antimicrobials.

Genital Tuberculosis

Genital tuberculosis is primarily of historic interest. In most cases, superficial infections occurred as a result of autoinoculation with sputum in a patient with active tuberculosis. Rare cases may occur in systemic (miliary) disease.

■ PARASITIC INFESTATIONS

Pediculosis Pubis

Pubic lice (see Figure 11-15) is transmitted by close contact and is caused by *Pthirus pubis*, which infests pubic hair, perianal area, and axillae. The parasite can survive

FIGURE 11-14 Erythrasma

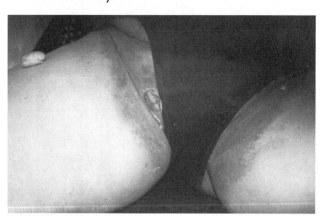

FIGURE 11-15 Pediculosis

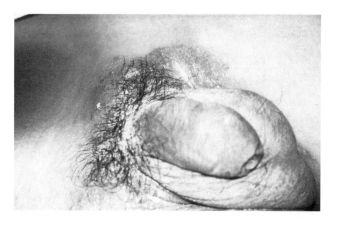

outside up to 44 hours, hence the possibility of transmission without direct human-to-human contact. The parasite has three pairs of strong claws that allow it to attach to the pubic hair. Clinical presentation is intense pruritis, small bluish macules, and small punctuate lesions may be seen on the skin. Management is described in Chapter 13.

Scabies

Scabies is particularly found in children and in patients with HIV, caused by *Sarcoptes scabies* (see Figures 11–16 and 11–17). The mite burrows down into stratum corneum and lays eggs. The mite's fecal matter induces intense itching, and the inflammation and pruritis lead to characteristic excoriating and tracking of the burrows. Reddish brown nodules may persist for months even after treatment. Management is described in Chapter 13.

FIGURE 11-16 Scabies A

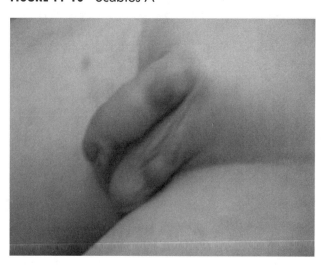

FIGURE 11-17 Scabies B

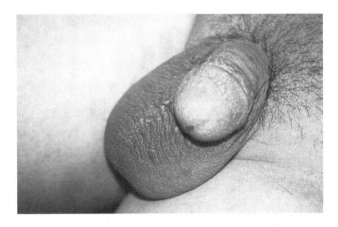

scales are absent, and lesion can appear as sharply marginated, inflamed, reddened, occasionally glazed papule or plaques. When lesions occur only on the genitalia, the diagnosis is difficult to make. When only genital lesions are seen, other sites should be closely inspected, around the sacral and perineal areas. The presence of concomitant fungal infection needs to be ruled out; scraping for candida or tinea is needed.

Genital psoriasis should be confirmed by biopsy, as there are other entities that should be ruled out, including Bowen's disease, erythroplasia of Queyrat, Zoon's balanitis, or even circanate balanitis of reactive arthritis. Psoriasis cases should be referred to a dermatologist for management.

◼ PAPULOSQUAMOUS SYSTEMIC DISEASE

Two of the most common papulosquamous diseases that affect genitalia are psoriasis and lichen planus. Less common causes are lichen nitidus, Crohn's disease, ulcerative colitis, sarcoidosis, Behçet's disease, and erythema multiformis. Since secondary syphilis can mimic any of these disorders, all patients should be evaluated with syphilis serology.

Psoriasis

Psoriasis (see Figure 11-18) is a chronic, hyperproliferative condition of the epidermis. On the trunk and extremities, the lesions are pruritic, scaly erythematous plaques, or patches of various sizes and shapes. On the penis and intertriginous areas, the characteristic silvery

Lichen Planus

Lichen planus presents as violaceous, polygonal shiny, flat-topped papules, often arranged in annular pattern, with lacelike white streaks on the surface (see Figure 11-19). Linear lesions often appear along scratch marks or in scars (Köbner phenomenon). Penile and vulval lesions are common, presenting as erythematous erosions, resulting in pain and burning. It is thought to be immunomodulated and occurs in families; there is increased HLA-B7 in the affected individuals.

Genitalia are frequently involved in lichen planus, but occasionally genital lesions may be the only manifestation of the disease. It is common for the oral cavity to be involved. It can be described as a "VVG" syndrome with the involvement of the vulva, vagina, and the gingival area and lips. "Wickham's striae" is a term used in

FIGURE 11-18 Psoriasis of the Glans Penis

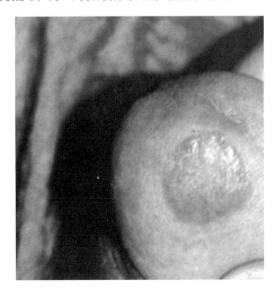

FIGURE 11-19 Lichen Planus

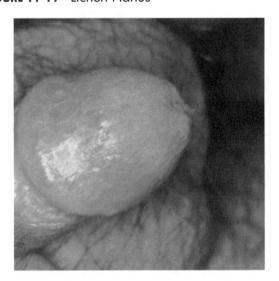

lichen planus to denote fine, lacy, whitened streaks, or striae, on the surface and periphery interlacing on moist, erythematous-glazed lesions of vulva or the gingival area.

Eventually, the papule flattens, persisting for few months and gradually changing from pinkish to blue and black. Finally, they may end up with atrophic cicatricial changes. This can be especially disabling if there is major vulval involvement.

Diagnosis is confirmed by biopsy. The condition often runs a variable course, and many cases are self-limited. Management is with the application of moderate to high potent steroid ointments or creams. Oral antihistamines are given at night, preferably the nonsedating types or even the immunomodulators. In cases that are refractory to topical therapy, systemic immuno-modulating approaches can be used.

Lichen Simplex et Chronicus

Lichen simplex et chronicus is a condition occurring as a result of vicious pruritis cycle, which is promoted by humidity, sweat, and tight-fitting clothing (see Figure 11-20). Severe pruritus ensues for no apparent reason (trigger factor), persisting for minutes to hours. It can be a form of neurodermatitis. One should look for other areas like ankles, elbows, forearms, and neck for similar lesions. As a result, the affected areas become lichenified and excoriated, resulting in abrasions and fissuring that heals by hyperpigmentation and thickening.

Treatment is by applications of mild to moderate or even stronger steroid creams with emollients. Antihistamines, like cetrizine or desloratidine can be taken in the morning and perhaps sedating antihistamines at night will suffice.

Lichen Nitidus

Lichen nitidus is a variant of lichen planus with numerous closely grouped small, minute pinhead-sized whitish, shiny flat or dome-shaped papules occurring on the shaft of penis. It is asymptomatic and transient requiring reassuring the patient. The patients are young adults or children. The condition is self-limiting, sometimes requiring moderate steroid creams.

Lichen Scleroses or BXO

Lichen scleroses are a progressive, sclerosing, inflammatory dermatosis of uncertain causes and are premalignant with a tendency to squamous cell carcinoma (see Figures 11-21 and 11-22). Hence, long-term observation and follow-up is essential.

In males, the major signs and symptoms are pruritus, burning, phimosis, dysuria, and painful erection of penis. In females, the condition can present in adolescents with dyspareunia or vaginismus. Therefore, a careful history is critical.

The lesions present as single or multiple erythematous papules, macules, or plaques that progress to sclerotic or atrophic white or ivory, coalescent flat-topped papule and plaques. Lesions commonly involves glans, prepuce, and vulva. At times, it may be mistaken for vitiligo. Occasionally the lesions in males may be bluish red with telangiectasia, or ulcers, small blisters, or bulla. This can lead to paraphimosis or phimosis, which may be the first presenting feature. In females, lesions appear as white shiny plaques, with erythema, blisters, and excoriations due to scratching. The lesions can involve the

FIGURE 11-20 Lichen Simplex Chronicus

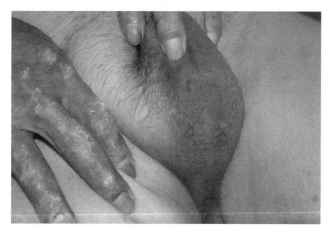

FIGURE 11-21 Lichen Sclerosis in a 10-Year-Old Girl

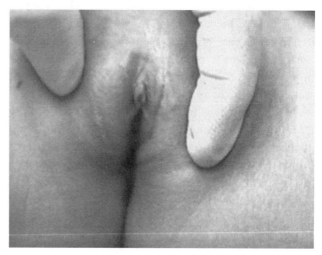

FIGURE 11-22   Lichen Sclerosis—Penile Lesion

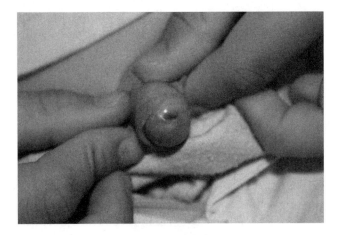

FIGURE 11-23   Plasma Cell Balanitis of Zoon

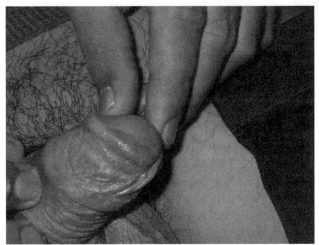

mons pubes, the vulva, occasionally burying the clitoris due to midline fusion.

Other sites can be over the area where there is constant rubbing or scratching resulting in microtrauma or chronic contact dermatitis due to friction, for example, over the shoulders. Occasionally the angle of lips can be involved. Squamous cell malignant changes can occur in later years and have been recorded in 5% of patients.

Referral for an initial biopsy is thus warranted and close follow-up over the years is a norm. Treat with topical steroids, and long-term follow-up and observation are essential.

■ BALANITIDIS

Plasma Cell Balanitis of Zoon

Plasma cell balanitis is a benign idiopathic condition that presents as a solitary, smooth, shiny, red orange to brownish red nonpalpable plaque of the glans and prepuce of an uncircumcised man, that is, preputial space affecting mainly in the middle-aged to older man. Under hand lens, one can see punctate petechial hemorrhagic spots. Though it is common in men, it can occur in females on the vulva. It is a chronic condition, though not a precancerous inflammation. Diagnosis is always by biopsy to differentiate from erythroplasia of Queyrat, secondary syphilis, and Kaposi's sarcoma.

Management is by improved hygiene, with daily cleaning of smegma. Moderate to strong steroid cream application will suffice. Occasionally, antibiotics or antifungal may be needed to clear secondary infection.

Circinate Balanitis

Circinate balanitis occurs as part of the reactive arthritis syndrome (see Figure 11-24). (See Chapters 5 and 14.)

There is an association with the HLA B27 gene in 60–80%, with the male-to-female ratio of 9:1. *Chlamydia trachomatis* is implicated in 70%. Other organisms implicated include enteric pathogens, such as *Salmonella, Shigella, Yersinia, and Campylobacter.*

The main clinical presenting features are conjunctivitis, iritis, tenosynovitis, arthritis of major joints like sacroiliac, and the ankles. There is a psoriatic type of lesion on the knees, elbows, ankles, and soles called keratoderma blenorrhagica. The most significant changes are lesions on the glans penis called balanitis circinate and occasionally on the vulva. The actual lesion consists of round, bizarre

FIGURE 11-24   Circinate Balanitis in the Reactive Arthritis Syndrome

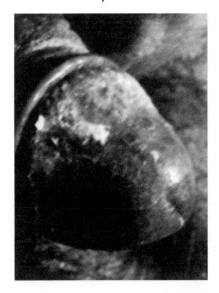

maplike eroded surface studded with small flesh red erosions surrounded by grayish white epithelial border. In some case, lesions may spread over the corona and preputial space. The lesions can be confused with psoriasis.

Treatment is with mild to moderate topical steroids and calcipatrol for the mucous and skin condition. Systemic treatment for reactive arthritis is nonsteroidal anti-inflammatory agents. Recurrence is common.

Erythroplasia of Queyrat

Erythroplasia of Queyrat is also known as Bowen's disease (see Figure 11-25). This is a premalignant condition, mainly in the uncircumcised male patient or on the vulva in females. The lesions are well-defined, slightly raised red plaque, which may have velvety texture and are often sore or itchy. In females, there are two clinical varieties: single intractably itchy and sore red plaque on the vulva and labia majora or multiple, well-defined pigmented plaques on the labia. In the males slightly elevated, soft, well-demarcated, bright red velvety plaque that occurs on the glans penis. Diagnosis is made by biopsy. Treatment is by cryotherapy or topical 5-fluorouracil.

Behçet's Syndrome

Behçet's syndrome (see Figure 11-26) is a multisystem condition affecting the mouth, genital, and eyes and is highly prevalent in parts of Asia and the Middle East, but occurs elsewhere as well. Mucocutaneous recurrent multiple, painful ulcers of genitalia and mucous lining

FIGURE 11-25 Erythroplasia of Queyrat (Bowen's Diseases)

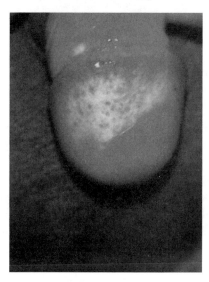

FIGURE 11-26 Behçet's Disease of the Scrotum

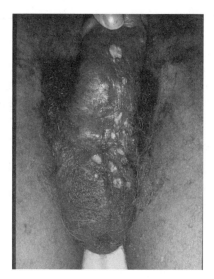

in the oral cavity occurs. Pustules, erythema nodosum, and erythema multiforme on the skin area is common. There is arthralgia of the knees. Healing occurs with scarring if the lesions do not clear within 2 weeks.

Bowenoid Genital Papulosis

Bowenoid genital papulosis is also known as pigmented penile papulosis, or bowenoid papules; this condition occurs in younger males and is considered to be carcinoma in situ with HPV 16 and 18 indicated. They can also occur in the females.

On the vulva, the lesion may appear as pigmented papules or plaques, while in males, the shaft and the glans penis will show grouped pale brown papules becoming darker on the shaft penis.

Seborrheic dermatitis and epidermal nevus maybe confused, thus requiring a biopsy to confirm diagnosis.

Management is by 5-fluorouracil, excision, or laser ablation may be the line of treatment.

■ TUMORS

There are few types of tumors that occur in the genital area. The vast majority are benign.

Epidermoid Cyst

Usually multiple, though single cysts can occur, with males occurring as asymptomatic pale whitish yellow nodules on the scrotum. They can be left alone, unless they cause disfigurement. These need to be differentiated from nodules due to scabies.

Campbell de Morgan Angiokeratoma

These reddish- to purplish-colored lesions occur usually in older subjects that commonly occur on the arms or trunk (see Figure 11-27). Occasionally, they can occur on the scrotum and penis or the vulva. They are benign but can become secondarily infected. In such cases, ablation with combined pigment and CO_2 lasers will be helpful.

Achrochordon

Achrochordon, also known as skin tags, and are common in flexural area. In the perineal region, they may grow slowly to a large size and can be multiple; they are soft-pigmented papules. They are basically asymptomatic, but the pedicle gets caught in the hair and causes pain and bleeding with secondary infection.

Seborrheic Keratoses

Seborrheic keratoses are benign brown blackish papules or plaques with stuck-on appearance. They are most common on sun-exposed areas, though occasionally they can occur in the flexural area, and they need to be differentiated from genital warts.

◼ NEOPLASMS

Verrucous Carcinoma

Verrucous carcinoma is a low-grade squamous cell carcinoma that occurs almost exclusively in uncircumcised men (see Figure 11-28). The presentation is balanitis

FIGURE 11-27 Angiokeratoma Fordyce of Scrotum

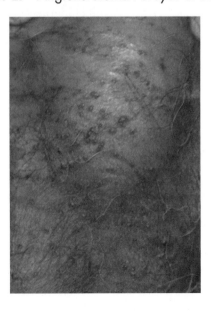

FIGURE 11-28 Verrucouls Penile Carcinoma

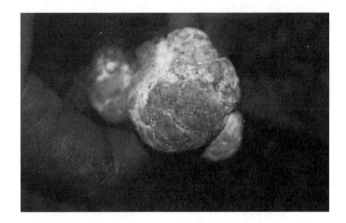

or phimosis. The lesions are dry, cauliflower-like on glans or anogenital mucosa with a tendency to infiltrate deeply locally and laterally but not beyond. These are also known as Buschke Löwenstein tumors, or giant condylomata. Treatment requires surgical excision and appropriate staging to ensure that the malignancy has not spread.

Squamous Cell Carcinoma

Squamous cell carcinoma may occur in uncircumcised of middle-aged male usually in the context of previous genital warts. The disease is more common in Asia and in tropical areas. The earliest symptoms include pruritus or burning under the foreskin.

Melanoma

Melanoma and other malignancies are rare but can occur on the glans penis and the shaft or prepuce in males and on the vulva in females.

◼ AUTOIMMUNE CONDITIONS

Pemphigus Vulgaris or Vegetans

Pemphigus is an autoimmune condition affecting mainly the epidermal part of the skin (see Figure 11-29). The desmosomes are gradually destroyed with loosening up of the epidermal keratinocytes by acantholysis. Pemphigus vulgaris and vegetans are the most common type. It is a disease of middle age, seen rarely in children, affecting both sexes, and is a common autoimmune disease in India, Malaysia, and China.

Clinically, the blisters are thin walled containing serous fluids over the scalp, trunk, mouth, axillae, and the groin, leaving no area unaffected in serious cases.

FIGURE 11-29 Pemphigus Vulgaris

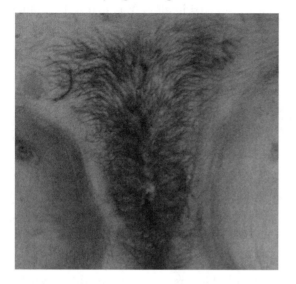

FIGURE 11-30 Pemphigoid

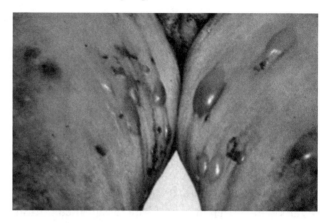

The blisters can be numerous, small to large bullae, and are surrounded by an inflammatory halo. They easily burst, resulting in painful erosions that heal by crusting; meantime, new ones develop nearby. The blisters can be rolled over one another and commonly involves mucous membranes of the mouth and genitalia.

Erosions on the genitalia may be the first sign and can be mistaken for streptococcal balanitis or fixed drug eruptions. The major other differential is bullous pemphigoid.

Diagnosis is made by biopsy, and direct immunofluorescence will show antibodies (IgG) deposited on the keratinocytes in and around the lesion, within the epidermis cells and the blister margins. A Tzanck stain will show acantholysis and grouping of epidermal cells within a round shape of separated intracellular connections.

Bullous Pemphigoid

Bullous is a benign autoimmune condition that affects the elderly (see Figure 11-30); it starts with itchy, urticarial erythematous lesions. This is followed by tense thick blisters that affect the epidermis and dermis area on the normal skin, mucosal area, and inner thighs. It is common in Western Europe and India. Several drugs are implicated as inducers, particularly the penicillins, captopril, and sulfa drugs.

The blisters are epidermal with the epidermis forming the intact roof. Clinically, the neck, axillae, inguinal folds, and inner aspects of thighs are affected. Tense dome-shaped vesicles, or bullae, with clear content arise spontaneously on a normal skin with a bizarre pattern.

The bullae do not burst easily. Itchiness is the main feature, the erosions are painful, however.

The diagnosis is made by biopsy. It is critical to differentiate from pemphigus as the prognosis and treatment are markedly different.

Genital Vitiligo

This is common and world-wide. In fair-skinned subjects, it may not be obvious; however, but may be disfiguring in pigmented skin. It occurs in associations with other parts of the body, especially the acral area, elbow, knees, and so forth. It is a pigmentary disorder with the possibility of an autoimmune component. The normal skin can be differentiated from vitiligo by shining the Wood's light.

Hypopigmentation can be induced by cryosurgery or laser surgery, especially in the darker subjects. Certain medications can induce it. The differential diagnosis is with lichen sclerosis.

■ FOREIGN BODIES AND TATTOOS

The practice of inserting inert foreign bodies in the preputial skin is common, especially in Southeast Asia. Beads, metal balls, silicon balls, and rings are implanted, which can lead to abrasions with resultant infections and pain.

■ TRAUMA

This common problem may result from multiple causes. The most common is zipper entrapment, or entrapment of pubic hair in tight-fitting clothing. Another potential etiology is human bites that may accidentally occur during oral sex. Local measures are usually sufficient.

PARAPHIMOSIS

Paraphimosis can occur as a result of many causes, such as infection and injury resulting in edema (see Figure 11-31). The prepuce is retracted, swollen, and inflamed; an attempt to reduce it maybe painful. Local measures are usually sufficient to reduce swelling. However, if this recurs, circumcision should be recommended.

CONCLUSION

The anogenital area is susceptible to local and systemic skin diseases. Clinicians should be observant and consider a wide differential of dermatological conditions when evaluating a patient in with an STI.

KEY POINTS

- Not all lesions on genitalia are due to sexually transmitted infections.

- Most lesions on the genitalia irrespectively due to STIs or non-STIs look alike in description, with similar symptoms and signs, and combinations of lesions occur.

- Patients with genital lesions are anxious; some lesions are peculiar to the genitalia. Thus, the onus falls on the attending physician to confirm or rule out STIs and HIV and come to a correct diagnosis and allay the fears of the patient. Offer an STI screen and HIV test for all patients. Lesions are severe, prolonged in all HIV patients, depending on the immune status.

- In doubt, refer to a consultant dermatologist for a biopsy under a local and get a histopathology opinion; the dermatopathologist is the best friend to keep.

- Lesions of psoriasis and seborrheic dermatitis on the genitalia look different from lesions from the rest of the body and may mimic other balanitidis.

- Sometimes patients with psoriasis and autoimmune conditions may present with genital complaints; do not forget to look for similar lesions on other parts of the body.

- All scaly, itchy conditions of genitalia must be examined with skin scrapes; these should be treated with KOH 10–20%, stained with methylene blue and examined for fungi.

- Having a Wood's light will help in differentiating many flexural conditions by the different color emitted peculiar to that condition, for example, coral red in erythrasma.

- Tumors need to be differentiated clinically as well by histopathology. Seventy percent of tumors are benign. However, some benign-looking lesions may change to malignancy.

- Do not overtreat normal variants. Reassuring the patient is sufficient.

FIGURE 11-31 Paraphymosis

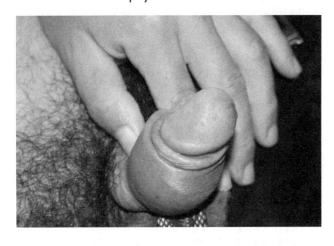

REFERENCES

Du Vivier A, McKee PH. *Atlas of Clinical Dermatology*. Edinburgh: Churchill Livingstone; 2002.

Edwards L. *Genital Dermatology Atlas*. Philadelphia: Lippincott Williams & Wilkins; 2004.

Fitzpatrick TB, Freedberg IM. *Fitzpatrick's Dermatology in General Medicine*. New York: McGraw-Hill, Medical Pub. Division; 2003.

Korman NJ. Pemphigus. *Dermatologic Clinics*. 1990; 8:689–700.

Korman NJ. Bullous pemphigoid. *Dermatologic Clinics*. 1993;11:483–498.

12

Genital Allergy

C. Sonnex

■ INTRODUCTION

Various conditions affect the genital area that appear to be precipitated or aggravated by sexual activity. This may be a recurrent problem and lead some patients to believe that they are in some way "allergic" to their sexual partner. "Hypersensitivity to sex," in the nonimmunological sense of the term, is well recognized, whereas true immunological hypersensitivity reactions associated with sexual activity are uncommon. Allergic reactions to a specific sexual partner are extremely rare. However, contact allergy may occur after exposure to a variety of exogenous antigens, including latex, spermicides, medical or nonmedical topical creams, or contact allergy to common allergens, such as laundry detergents, cosmetics, and deodorants. Genital allergy should be considered in patients presenting with genital soreness and irritation for which no infective or dermatological cause can be identified.

There are a variety of sexually transmitted infections (STI) and non-STI conditions that do not represent hypersensitivity but may lead patients to consider themselves allergic or hypersensitive to sex. The following entities should be considered and ruled out.

Cystitis

Postcoital urinary tract infection ("honeymoon cystitis") is a well recognized but poorly understood condition. Introital and vestibular bacteria are thought to be forced into the urethra during intercourse, and there is some evidence to suggest that a more posteriorly placed and almost intravaginal urethral meatus may predispose to this condition. An increased intraurethral resistance leading to ineffective bladder emptying may also contribute to some cases (see Chapter 24).

Genital Herpes

Sexual intercourse may trigger recurrences of genital herpes. If the outbreak presentation is nonclassical, that is, without the typical grouped vesicular lesions, it may present as genital irritation and erythema. In women with introital recurrences, genital pruritis and irritation are the presenting symptoms. The "skin trigger" theory of herpes recrudescence postulates that virus made in latently infected ganglion cells frequently travels via the nerves to the epithelium and that local immunity eliminates the virus. Minor skin trauma brought about by coitus could theoretically alter local immunity, as has been suggested for epilation and ultraviolet light-induced trauma and thus allow viral replication.

Bacterial Vaginosis

Some women are prone to recurrences of bacterial vaginosis after intercourse, although the reason for this is uncertain (see Chapter 7). Malodor, a common symptom of bacterial vaginosis, may only be noticeable after intercourse owing to the release of volatile amines, such as trimethylamine, by alkaline seminal fluid. This may

Adapted from Sonnex C. Review: Genital allergy. *Sex Transm Inf.* 2004;80:4–7.

give the false impression to both partners that they are somehow "allergic" to each other. Bacterial vaginosis may also be misdiagnosed in women with hypersensitivity to spermicides.

De-epithelialization of the Glans Penis

Prolonged or forceful coitus, with perhaps inadequate lubrication, may occasionally produce mild abrasion of the epithelium of the glans penis. This presents as a generalized erythema with punctuation, thought to be due to freshly exposed capillaries or capillary loops. The appearance may be very similar to a true hypersensitivity reaction.

■ HYPERSENSITIVITY REACTIONS

True genital allergic reactions should be more accurately considered as hypersensitivity reactions. There are four recognized types of immunological hypersensitivity reaction and types I, III, and IV have been reported to affect the genitalia or genital tract (see Table 12-1). When considering genital skin reactions, it is important to distinguish between true contact dermatitis (type IV hypersensitivity) and irritant problems. The latter result from a direct effect of the substance concerned with the genital epithelium in the absence of an allergic mechanism. Irritants may cause more intense reactions on the vulval epithelium compared with nongenital skin, probably as a result of a higher transepidermal water loss, capacitance, and blood flow in the vulva. Genital hypersensitivity reactions may be subdivided into those that are related to sexual activity (e.g., kissing, foreplay, coitus) and those that may occur in the absence of sexual contact.

■ SEXUALLY RELATED HYPERSENSITIVITY

Seminal fluid

Allergy to seminal fluid is extremely rare but there have been several reported cases in the literature. In 1958, J. L. H. Specken reported the case of a 65-year-old woman who suffered postcoital generalized urticaria at times accompanied by bronchospasm. This was the first description of hypersensitivity to semen, and, over subsequent years, a number of cases and a series of cases have appeared in the medical literature. Symptoms may occur with first exposure to seminal fluid or after years of "uneventful" sexual intercourse and range from purely local to generalized systemic reactions. Local responses consist of genital swelling, burning, irritation, or soreness that may occur during or soon after intercourse, usually becoming maximal at 24 hours and lasting 2–3 days. Semen contact with nongenital skin may also cause localized itching and urticaria. Generalized reactions associated with semen allergy include angioedema of the lips and eyelids, laryngeal edema, bronchospasm, and

TABLE 12-1   Summary of the Four Types of Hypersensitivity Reaction

Type 1: Immediate hypersensitivity

Dependent on the specific triggering of IgE sensitized mast cells by antigen.

Examples: asthma, hay fever, urticaria, anaphylaxis

Type II

Antibody is directed against antigens on specific host cells and tissues.

Examples: graft rejection, autoimmune hemolytic anemia, and myasthenia gravis

Type III

Antigen-antibody complexes are deposited in tissues.

Examples: rheumatoid arthritis, systemic lupus erythematosis (SLE), serum sickness, infective endocarditis, malaria

Type IV: Delayed hypersensitivity

Antigen-sensitized T cells release cytokines following secondary contact with the same antigen.

Examples: contact dermatitis, tuberculosis, leprosy

anaphylaxis, but, to date, death has not been reported. Semen allergy mainly affects younger women although postmenopausal cases are documented (Kint, Degreef, & Dooms-Goossens 1994; Mumford et al. 1978). An increasing intensity of reaction with subsequent episodes of coitus is a common feature. Levine et al. (1973) described a married woman with a 15-year history of hay fever who initially presented with swollen eyes, nasal congestion, and sneezing one hour after coitus. Ten days later, she developed similar symptoms together with diffuse urticaria and a sensation of throat swelling five minutes postejaculation. During the next year, her symptoms were prevented by using a condom or coitus interruptus. On four occasions, these precautions failed and symptoms developed.

Most affected women have a personal or family history of atopy, although this is not always the case, and familial "allergic seminal vulvovaginitis" has been described affecting a mother and three daughters (Chang 1976).

The specific allergen(s) within semen responsible for triggering type I hypersensitivity is still unknown. Mumford et al. (1978) described a woman with postcoital wheezing and dyspnea who, for three months before these symptoms, had complained of perineal irritation. Seminal plasma separated from sperm produced a positive intradermal skin test but a negative patch test. Both tests were negative with sperm only. Further analysis of the seminal plasma suggested that the sensitizing agent had a molecular weight of between 14,000 and 30,000 daltons. Other studies have confirmed that the potential allergens are glycoproteins of molecular weight between 12,000 and 75,000, and are probably derived from the prostate or seminal vesicles since vasectomy fails to prevent symptoms.

A number of studies have found an association between the onset of seminal fluid allergy and genital tract "procedures" such as tubal ligation, hysterectomy, intrauterine contraceptive device insertion, and pregnancy. It has been suggested that these events may in some way disrupt normal immunomodulation in the female genital tract (Jones 1991; Mathias et al. 1980), although the precise mechanism by which this may occur has not been elucidated.

Hypersensitivity reactions to seminal fluid other than type I are less common. Type III (immune complex) hypersensitivity to seminal fluid has been reported in a young woman who developed nasal congestion and urticaria eight hours after intercourse on her honeymoon (Mike, Bird, & Asquith 1990). She subsequently developed migratory arthralgia, periorbital edema, dyspnea

secondary to a restrictive ventilatory defect, and a hemorrhagic proctitis. Investigations showed the presence of circulating immune complexes in the serum and evidence of complement activation.

There are no reports of pure delayed-type hypersensitivity (DTH) reactions (type IV hypersensitivity) to seminal fluid although DTH reactions involving other factors may accompany type I hypersensitivity to seminal fluid. An experimental model of contact sensitivity for the murine oral mucosa does at least provide some theoretical basis for DTH reactions affecting the genital tract mucosa (Ahlfors & Czerkinsky 1991).

■ CONTACT SKIN AND MUCOSAL DERMATITIS EXPOSURES

A variety of compounds have been associated with genital dermatitis, mucositis, and local and systemic hypersensitivity reactions. The diagnosis depends on obtaining a comprehensive history.

Spermicides

Contact dermatitis to spermicidal preparations is an uncommon but well-recognized condition. Reactions are more frequently reported in men, probably because the skin component is more easily recognized. Reactions in women may be mucositis and therefore may present a vaginitis-type reaction. The sensitizing agent may an active compound (e.g., benzocaine), monophenoxypolyethoxy derivatives, hexyl resorcinol, chloramine, quinine, or an associated fragrance. Nonoxynol-9 may cause genital soreness and irritation secondary to the compound's irritant properties or as a result of contact dermatitis. Vaginal hypersensitivity to spermicide has been reported to present with clinical features similar to bacterial vaginosis.

Latex

Both type I and type IV hypersensitivity reactions have been reported to rubber products, including condoms. Commonly reported presentations include contact dermatitis, contact urticaria, and, more rarely, anaphylaxis. As with most natural allergens, the allergenic fraction of natural rubber latex varies in amount (due to factors such as climate, season, etc.) and in polypeptide content. Latex allergy may be associated with fruit allergy, in particular avocado, banana, kiwi fruit, melon, peach, and less commonly, fig, plum, chestnut, peanut, potato, papaya, and tomato. Other potential allergens used during condom manufacture include carbamates and thiurams, although the latter are no longer commonly used. "Hypoallergenic" condoms may contain lower amounts of additives but are not totally free of latex proteins and therefore should be used with caution in patients with documented rubber latex sensitivity. Individuals with latex sensitivity should be advised to use condoms made from synthetic materials, such as polyurethane. There have been no published reports to date of hypersensitivity reactions to the recently developed male polyurethane condom.

Contraceptive Jelly

Contact dermatitis has been reported following the use of contraceptive jelly and is due to propylene glycol sensitivity. Propylene glycol is widely used as a vehicle for cosmetics, body lotions, antiperspirants, and topical medicines and should be considered as a possible sensitizing agent in patients with genital dermatitis without an obvious cause.

Oral Medications

Ingested antigens may pass into seminal fluid and may therefore produce a hypersensitivity reaction in the sexual partner. In one case report, a woman allergic to walnuts developed an anaphylactic reaction after intercourse with her husband (Haddad 1978). He had eaten walnuts before coitus and walnut protein was subsequently detected in his seminal fluid. Postcoital hypersensitivity reactions have also been described in association with penicillin, vinblastine, and thioridazine ingestion.

Topical Preparations

Fisher (1979) reported the case of a young woman who repeatedly developed an eczematous eruption on her face, neck, and occasionally arms after sexual intercourse with her boyfriend. Patch tests to commonly encountered allergens, including cosmetics, were negative. Further investigation revealed that her boyfriend used 5% benzoyl peroxide for facial acne. Subsequent patch testing showed her to be sensitive to this preparation and her eczema subsided after her partner changed to a topical antibiotic cream. A similar case of consort dermatitis affecting the neck and chest due to oak moss present in a partner's aftershave has also been described (Held, Ruszkowski, & Deleo 1988).

Massage linament has been reported to cause a contact dermatitis and could therefore potentially cause problems in the male, although to date this has not described.

Exercise

Exercise-induced urticaria and anaphylaxis are well documented. Symptoms may be intermittent and often require an additional factor, such as food sensitivity. Although exercise-induced hypersensitivity secondary to sexual intercourse has not been reported to date, the theoretical possibility remains.

Butyl Nitrate

The use of inhaled nitrites ("poppers") by men who have sex with men is well recognized and reports of facial dermatitis associated with the use of butyl nitrite have been reported (Fisher, Brancaccio, & Jelinek 1981).

Newsprint

The importance of taking a full medical history is highlighted by the report of three women with persistent pruritis vulvae due to newspaper printer's ink sensitivity (Adno 1985). Their sexual partners were in the habit of reading newspapers in bed at night, which was "often followed by sexual relations including manual manipulation of the vulva."

■ NONSEXUALLY RELATED HYPERSENSITIVITY

Topical Medications

Medicaments are well-recognized causes of contact dermatitis in patients with leg ulcers and otitis externa but possibly less well appreciated as causes of vulval disease. Marren et al. (1992) found that just under a third of women with vulval symptoms failing to respond to standard therapy had evidence of contact hypersensitivity as diagnosed by patch testing. Medicaments are more common sensitizers than cosmetics and include ethylenediamine (present in Triadcortyl), framycetin, neomycin, clobetasol propionate, and crotamiton (Eurax). The possibility of contact dermatitis should be considered in patients experiencing a worsening of vulval symptoms while using topical steroids. This may be due to the steroid preparation itself, the vehicle, or additives such as an aminoglycoside, preservative, or biocide (e.g., chlorocresol).

Topical anesthetics vary in their ability to cause a contact dermatitis and cross-sensitization between preparations is uncommon. Lignocaine is considered to have low allergenic properties and is less likely to sensitize than other related preparations, such as benzocaine.

Topical imidazoles are frequently used in clinical practice but infrequently produce contact sensitivity. The imidazoles most commonly reported to cause sensitivity are miconazole, econazole, and tioconazole (treatment for onychomycosis). Cross-reactivity between preparations is well recognized. Although clotrimazole only occasionally cause problems, added preservatives, such as benzyl alcohol or octyldodecamole, may cause contact sensitivity and should be considered.

Other preparations used topically on the genitals and reported to cause contact dermatitis, albeit rarely, include clindamycin and acyclovir, although in the latter case other cream constituents, such as propylene glycol, were considered to be the most likely sensitisers.

Feminine Hygiene Sprays

Feminine hygiene sprays often comprise a perfume, an emollient, and a propellant. Irritant reactions from fluorinated hydrocarbon propellants sprayed too close to the genitals are more common than allergic reactions. Allergic reactions to the perfume component may be more likely to occur if there is preexistent skin damage, for example, secondary to candidiasis or dermatitis.

Sexual partners may also be affected, as in the case of a man who developed dermatitis of the penis, scrotum, and lower abdomen following sexual intercourse with his girlfriend. Patch testing showed a positive reaction to balsam of Peru. Further questioning revealed that his girlfriend used a hygiene spray before intercourse, which was found to contain balsam of Peru (Fisher 1979).

Bubble Baths and Scented Soaps

Children are prone to develop an irritant vulvitis, particularly after prolonged immersion in baths containing perfumes.

Cosmetics

Potential causes of a genital dermatitis include nail polish, particularly if the vulval skin is touched before the polish is dry, and perfumed toilet tissue. Lipstick-induced balanitis and penile dermatitis has not been reported but remains a theoretical possibility for men sensitive to octylgallate.

Self-Adhesive Pads

Some women with excessive vaginal secretions use self-adhesive pads for comfort and hygiene. A fragrance and disinfecting agent are commonly incorporated into the pad, and both may produce contact dermatitis. Sterry

and Schmoll (1985) reported the case of a woman with genital pruritis who had been using self-adhesive pads for several months. Patch testing was positive to the layer of the pad, which contained the fragrance and the disinfecting agent (CuII-acetyl acetonate and acetyl acetonate). A similar case has also been described of sensitivity to cinnamic alcohol and cinnamic aldehyde present as a perfume in a deodorant sanitary napkin (Larsen 1979).

Urine

Irritant ammoniacal dermatitis should be considered in incontinent patients with genital soreness, particularly if there is a preexistent genital dermatosis that fails to improve or worsens with treatment.

Candida

Candida is a well-recognized allergen (see Chapter 7). In vitro tests have documented the release of histamine from rat mast cells by Candida antigens (Lewis 1994) and bronchial hypersensitivity to aerosols of *Candida albicans* correlates well with type 1 but not type IV hypersensitivity. Clinically, Candida has been reported to induce asthma and "tea tasters' cough." Genital hypersensitivity to Candida has been implicated in some cases of vulvovaginal candidiasis (VVC). Anti-Candida IgE antibodies are often present in the vaginal secretions of women with recurrent VVC but not in control women. In addition, there have been reports of partially successful treatment of recurrent VVC by hyposensitization using subcutaneous injection of increasing doses of Candida antigen. Male genital hypersensitivity to Candida has been described and presents as soreness of the glans penis appearing 6–24 hours after intercourse with women with vaginal candidiasis (Catterrall 1966).

■ DIAGNOSIS

Most cases of vulvitis and balanitis are the result of infection or a dermatosis and respond to the appropriate treatment. The possibility of an irritant dermatitis or hypersensitivity reaction should be considered in those patients whose symptoms fail to improve. This may be suggested by a history of past or present allergies or a family history of atopy. A history of contact with possible allergens should be ascertained. This often requires direct questioning about the use of lubricants or scented sprays before sexual intercourse as patients may feel too embarrassed to volunteer this information. The temporal relationship between the onset of symptoms and intercourse may provide useful clues. Condom use prevents symptoms in cases of seminal fluid hypersensitivity and is a useful diagnostic test. Sensitivity to both latex and seminal fluid is likely to be a rare occurrence but has been reported. Some patients with mild allergic rhinitis have negative skin prick tests and radioallergosorbent test (RAST) but produce a local antibody response together with symptoms on nasal provocation. Vulval or vaginal provocation with allergen followed by colposcopic examination of the epithelium has not been assessed but could theoretically provide a useful means of assessing allergic vulvovaginitis.

Contact dermatitis should be assessed by patch testing and is considered a valuable investigative tool for patients with protracted vulval symptoms, particularly if there is no response or a worsening of symptoms while applying topical steroids. Patch testing on the mucosa is disappointing since mucous membranes react less clearly to allergens than the skin. In addition, patch testing in this area would prove difficult to perform.

In cases of suspected type 1 hypersensitivity reactions (e.g., latex, seminal fluid), a RAST and skin prick test should be performed. Skin prick tests are considered more sensitive than RASTs, but the systemic reaction rate is significant. Neither of these tests is appropriate for assessing contact dermatitis.

Performing and interpreting both skin prick tests and patch tests requires special training and should be only be undertaken in close collaboration with clinicians with appropriate expertise (e.g., dermatologists, allergologists).

MANAGEMENT

Guidance on the treatment of contact dermatitis and the management of steroid sensitivity is beyond the remit of this chapter. Once a potential sensitizer has been identified, avoidance is obviously the optimal approach to management. Condoms should be used in cases of seminal fluid hypersensitivity. Hyposensitization injection has been reported to provide partial therapeutic benefit. The role of genital biopsy is usually limited; however, this may provide histological confirmation of dermatitis and may also help to exclude other pathologies.

CONCLUSION

Genital allergy is an uncommon cause of genital soreness or irritation but should be considered as a possible diagnosis in all patients with persisting symptoms in whom there is no obvious dermatosis and investigations fail to show evidence of infection. Obtaining an accurate "allergy history" may prove difficult and will often require direct questioning regarding possible sensitisers. Type 1 and type IV hypersensitivity reactions are most commonly encountered and can be assessed by performing skin prick testing/RAST, or patch testing, respectively. This may require collaboration with an appropriately trained clinician in dermatology or allergology. Once an allergen has been identified, avoidance is the optimal approach to management.

KEY POINTS

- Genital allergy should be considered in patients presenting with genital soreness and irritation for which no infective or dermatological cause can be identified.

- True hypersensitivity reactions affecting the genitalia are uncommon.

- The diagnosis of genital allergy should be considered particularly in patients with a past or present history of allergies or a family history of atopy.

- Female genital burning and swelling occurring soon after ejaculation should raise the suspicion of seminal fluid allergy.

- The worsening of genital symptoms with subsequent acts of intercourse and the alleviation of symptoms with condom use are highly suggestive of seminal fluid allergy.

- Ingested antigens may pass into seminal fluid and produce a hypersensitivity reaction in the sexual partner.

- Individuals allergic to condoms may give a history of previous latex allergy (e.g., to rubber gloves) and fruit allergy.

- Direct questioning is often required to obtain information about contact with possible allergens in lubricants or sprays used prior to or during intercourse.

- Contact dermatitis should be considered in women with protracted vulval symptoms, particularly if there is no response or a worsening of symptoms while applying topical steroids.

- Contact dermatitis should be assessed by patch testing and a RAST and/or skin prick test performed in cases of suspected type 1 hypersensitivity reactions (e.g., latex, seminal fluid).

REFERENCES

Adno J. Pruritis vulvae, sex and printer's ink. *S Afr Med J*. 1985; 67:486.

Ahlfors E, Czerkinsky C. Contact sensitivity in the murine oral mucosa. I. An experimental model of delayed-type hypersensitivity reactions at mucosal surfaces. *Clin Exp Immunol*. 1991;86:449–56.

Catterrall RD. Urethritis and balanitis due to Candida. In: Winner HI, Hurley R, eds. *Symposium on candida infection*. London: Livingstone; 1966:113–8.

Chang T-W. Familial allergic seminal vulvovaginitis. *Am J Obstet Gynecol*. 1976;126:442–444.

Fisher AA. Consort contact dermatitis. *Cutis*. 1979;24:595–668.

Fisher AA, Brancaccio RR, Jelinek JE. Facial dermatitis in men due to inhalation of butyl nitrite. *Cutis*. 1981;271:146.

Haddad ZH. Clearer picture of food and allergy is still needed. *Persp Allergy*. 1978;1:2–3.

Held JL, Ruszkowski AM, Deleo VA. Consort contact dermatitis due to oak moss. *Arch Derm*. 1988;124:261–2.

Jones WR. Allergy to coitus. *Aust N Z J Obstet Gynaecol*. 1991; 31:137–141.

Kint B, Degreef H, Dooms-Goossens A. Combined allergy to human seminal plasma and latex: a case report and review of the literature. *Contact Dermatitis*. 1994;30:7–11.

Larsen WG. Sanitary napkin dermatitis due to the perfume. *Arch Dermatol*. 1979;115:363.

Levine BB, Siraganian RP, Shenkein I. Allergy to human seminal plasma. *N Engl J Med*. 1973;288:894–896.

Lewis FM, Gawkrodger DJ, Harrington CI. Colophony: an unusual factor in pruritis vulvae. *Contact Dermatitis*. 1994; 31:119.

Liccardi G, Senna G, Rotiroti G, D'Amato G, Passalacqua G. Intimate behavior and allergy: a narrative review. *Ann Allergy Asthma Immunol*. 2007;99(5):394–400.

Ludman BG. Human seminal plasma protein allergy: a diagnosis rarely considered. *J Obstet Gynecol Neonatal Nurs*. 1999;28(4):359–363.

Mathias TG, Frick OL, Caldwell TM, et al. Immediate hypersensitivity to seminal fluid and atopic dermatitis. *Arch Dermatol*. 1980;116:209–212.

Marren P, Wojnarowska F, Powell S. Allergic contact dermatitis and vulvar dermatoses. *Br J Dermatol*. 1992;126:52–56.

Mike N, Bird G, Asquith P. A new manifestation of seminal fluid hypersensitivity. *Q J Med*. 1990;75:371–376.

Mumford DM, Haywood TJ, Daily LJ Jr, McLerran CJ, McGovern JP. Female allergy to seminal plasma. *Ann Allergy*. 1978;40:40–43.

Nardelli A, Degreef H, Goossens A. Contact allergic reactions of the vulva: a 14-year review. *Dermatitis*. 2004;15(3):131–136.

Sterry W, Schmoll M. Contact urticaria and dermatitis from self-adhesive pads. *Contact Dermatitis*. 1985;13:284–285.

13

Scabies and Pediculosis

T. Thirumoorthy and Harneet Ranu Eriksson

■ INTRODUCTION

Scabies and pediculosis are ubiquitous, contagious parasitic dermatoses. Both are caused by ectoparasites, and patients usually present with itchiness. In addition to the unbearable itch, resistance to medication, secondary infection, and high risk of spreading the parasite to their close contacts, patients also must battle many myths, prejudice, and guilt connected to these infections.

■ SCABIES

Etiology

Scabies is a skin disease caused by the *Sarcoptes* mite. It has afflicted human societies for at least 2500 years. *Sarcoptes scabiei* plays an important role in the history of medicine because it is the first organism to be specially identified as the causative agent of a clinical condition by Giovanni Cosimo Bonomo in 1687. It is estimated there are about 300 million cases of scabies in the world each year.

The Parasite

The *Sarcoptes scabiei* adult female measures 0.4 mm by 0.3 mm, while the adult male measures 0.2 mm by 0.15 mm. The mite is white, oval with transverse corrugation, with four pairs of short legs (see Figure 13-1). The mite is too small to be noticed by the naked eye. The scabies mite needs no protection against enemies and can live in continuous 100% humidity, has no armor, no trachea, and no eyes unlike its nonparasitic relative mites. Female mites are able to move at 2.5 cm/min directed by host odor and thermal stimuli and complete their entire life cycles on humans.

Life Cycle and Pathogenesis

The life cycle begins with the mating of adult male and female mites. Afterward, the adult male dies while the female lays eggs in the skin burrow. She lives for 4–6 weeks during which she does not leave the burrow and produces eggs at a rate of 1–3 eggs/day. The tunnel is usually 1 cm long in the stratum corneum to the boundaries of the stratum granulosum of the epidermis. After 3–4 days, the eggs hatch and six-legged larvae are produced. Less than 10% of the eggs laid result in mature mites. The larvae then dig burrows and pass through two further developmental stages, protonymphs and tritonymphs, before molting into either females or males. All life cycle stages can penetrate intact epidermis by secreting enzymes that dissolve keratin.

During the first month of infection, the mite populations on an infected host increases to reach a parasite burden of up to 25 adult females after 50 days and up to 500 mites by 100 days. After this, the mite number decreases rapidly.

The incubation period before symptoms develop can range from days to months. In first-time infestations, it may take 2–6 weeks before the host's immune system becomes sensitized to the mite or its by-products, resulting in pruritis and cutaneous lesions. The subsequent infestation is usually recognized within 24–48 hours.

Transmission

Scabies is transmitted from person to person by direct skin contact. Transmission among household members is common. In crusted scabies, also known as Norwegian scabies, a patient can be infected with millions of mites and is therefore far more contagious. Fomite transmission is possible and can be contracted by wearing or handling heavily contaminated clothing or sleeping in contaminated bed. In adults, venereal transmission occurs.

Epidemiology

Scabies usually spreads in households and neighborhoods by way of frequent intimate personal contact and possibly inanimate objects surrounding the index patient. Crowded and poor living conditions, lack of good water supply, and long-term care institutions are known to increase the risk of transmission.

Sexual intercourse normally leads to close skin-to-skin contact, which enables transmission of scabies. Scabies is seen in patients attending sexually transmitted disease clinics and may coexist with gonorrhea, syphilis, pediculosis pubis, genital herpes, and other sexually transmitted infections (STIs). The diseases may have been contracted during the same or previous exposure.

In most parts of the world, scabies, especially in children and the elderly, is not a sexually transmitted infection. Social intimacy rather than sexual intimacy is the major route of transmission. However, in the sexually active population (16–55 years) it is prudent to take a sexual history in patients with scabies. Where there is a risk factor of changing sexual partners, it is important to offer screening for other sexually transmitted infections.

Clinical Features

Cutaneous manifestation of scabies is polymorphous. Classical scabies is manifested as nocturnal pruritis with characteristic symmetrical distribution of burrows, papules, pustules, nodules, and excoriations. The essential lesion is a nondescript, tiny papule often excoriated and tipped with blood crusts. The burrow is pathognomonic when correctly identified. The burrow is a thin grayish line that is straight, sinuous, or zigzag, about 2 to 15 mm long. Burrows may be completely absent or obscured by eczematization or secondary infection. Miniature wheals, vesicles, pustules, and, rarely, bullae may also be present.

Figure 13-2 illustrates the papules and burrows of scabies mite infestation. The distribution of the scabies

FIGURE 13-1 Low Magnification Scanning Electron Micrograph of Scabies Mite on Hair Shaft

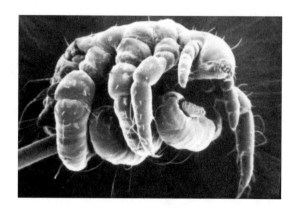

eruption is characteristic. It involves the sides and webs of the fingers, flexor aspects of wrists, extensor aspects of the elbows, anterior and posterior axillary folds, skin adjacent to the nipples in women, periumbilical areas, waist, penis (shaft and glans), scrotum, the extensor surfaces of knees, lower half of buttocks, and the lateral aspects of feet. The back is relatively free of involvement. The scalp, face, and soles are spared in adults. In infants, there is commonly a heavy involvement of palms and soles with spread to the face and scalp.

Nodular lesions are reddish brown and pruritic, occur in covered parts, and are encountered in the groin, axillae, and male genitalia. Lesions like these tend

FIGURE 13-2 Scabies on Penis and Scrotum

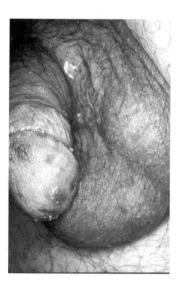

Note Circular Burrows at the Coronal Area.

to persist for weeks after adequate treatment. Secondary pyodermas of impetigo and ecthyma commonly complicate scabies. Secondary bacterial infection is most commonly due to *Staphylococcus aureus* or group A beta hemolytic streptococci. Constant scratching and the application of irritant topical scabicidal agents may result in extensive contact dermatitis.

Use of corticosteroids (topical or systemic) may ameliorate symptoms and signs of scabies infestation while transmissibility persists (scabies incognito).

In the elderly who are immobile or bedridden, the reaction to the mite is relatively muted, and the vivid inflammatory reactions seen in younger patients are usually reduced. Scabies is frequently not recognized unless there is a high index of suspicion. Elderly patients with scabies in nursing homes may be mistakenly treated for xerotic eczema.

Crusted scabies is a scaly dermatosis of the hands and feet, with subungal hyperkeratosis and an erythematous scaly eruption on the face, neck, scalp, nipples, sacrum, and trunk. Disseminated crusted scabies occurs in immunocompromised patients, such as those with HIV, organ-transplant recipients, and those on steroids. It is also common among institutionalized persons with disabilities.

There are millions of mites on patients with crusted scabies. Skin samples can contain up to 4700 mites per gram of skin. Crusted scabies is highly contagious even on casual contact. Pruritis is minimal because of the lack of host immune response to the mite.

Diagnosis

Once the diagnosis is suspected it should be confirmed by demonstration of the mite, the eggs, or the feces (scybala) from scrapings from burrows and papules if practically feasible.

Martin and Wheeler (1979) have described a simple epidermal shave biopsy technique to demonstrate the mite and its artifacts. The operator pinches a burrow or early papule between the thumb and forefinger and using a No. 15 scalpel blade with a gentle back-and-forth motion parallel to the skin, saws the top off the lesion and transfers it to a glass slide for microscopic examination.

Alternatively, a pin can be used to perforate an undamaged burrow at the dark point (site of mite). The needle is moved tangential to the skin from side to side. The mite will grip the end of the needle after which it can be transferred to the slide.

Burrows or unexcoriated papules are located with a hand lens. Mineral oil is placed on a sterile scalpel blade and allowed to flow onto lesions. Vigorous scraping with the blade removes the top of burrows or papules. The oil and scraped material are transferred onto a glass slide and a coverslip applied. Diagnosis is confirmed by the presence of any stage of the mite or the typical fecal pellets.

The burrow ink test may also be performed. A scabietic papule is rubbed and covered with ink, which is immediately wiped off with an alcohol pad. In the positive lesion, the ink will track down the burrow created by the mite and a zigzag line running across and away from the papule is formed.

In infants and children, a cellophane tape test can be done. A clear cellophane adhesive tape is applied to the lesion and removed with a brisk movement. Strips of adhesive tape are stuck on the slide and the slide examined microscopically.

Currently, there is no practical diagnostic immunologic test, and the diagnosis is made on history, epidemiology, and clinical features.

Treatment

The choice of drug for treating scabies must consider efficacy and potential toxicity. Treatment regimens should also be tailored to the patients needs. Problems with topical therapy include emerging resistance. Mites share biochemical pathways with humans; many of the therapeutic options impose a risk of toxicity to the patients, especially in infants.

Antiscabietic lotion or cream should be applied to all areas of the body, sparing only the head in adults and not only on the areas of clinical lesions.

In infants, young children, elderly patients with crusted scabies, the topical scabicide should be applied to the neck, scalp, and face. Contact with eyes and mouth should be avoided.

The scabicide may be washed off after 12–24 hours. Counseling and written instructions are recommended for good compliance to therapy. Clothing, bed linen, and towels should be washed in hot water.

All household members and sexual contacts in the last 30 days should be treated at the same time. Patients should be informed that the rash and pruritus of scabies may persist but at a significantly lower intensity after treatment. Where symptoms and signs persist, careful clinical assessment for reinfection, treatment failure, faulty application, and secondary allergic contact dermatitis needs to be carried out.

Topical Scabicides (Recommendations listed with an asterisk are also recommended in the CDC's U.S. 2010 STD Treatment Guidelines)

Permethrin 5% cream*

Permethrin 5% cream, a synthetic pyrethroid, is the preferred topical therapy for scabies. Permethrin acts by disrupting the sodium channels, resulting in the paralysis and death of the parasite. It is effective in all stages of the mite's life cycle. This preparation should not be confused with 1% solution for head lice, which is not effective in treating scabies.

It should be applied to the whole body; neck down to the feet (including the soles) and left on for 10 hours. It is used as a single application. It has low toxicity, minimal absorption, and is rapidly metabolized in the skin. The average daily adult dose is 30 g.

Adverse reactions consist of burning and stinging. To date, there are no clinically documented cases of Permethrin-resistant scabies with use of the 5% cream. It is safe for infants, pregnant, and breast-feeding women.

Gamma Benzene Hexachloride 1% (Lindane)*

Gamma benzene hexachloride kills the scabies mite by stimulating its central nervous system, causing paralysis and eventually death. Although it acts on the nervous system unlike the organophosphate insecticides, it is not a cholinesterase inhibitor. Cases of resistance and rare systemic toxicity have led to its withdrawal in several countries.

It is best avoided in infants and pregnant women because of the potential neurotoxic (seizures) and hematological (aplastic anemia) side effects. A single application is left on for 12 hours.

Malathion 0.5% Lotion

Inside the mite, malathion is converted into mala-oxon, which inhibits the neurotransmitter acetylcholinesterase and "jams" the transmission system, resulting in paralysis and death.

Malathion should be left in place for 8–12 hours before being washed off. It is considered safe and has no significant side effects. It provides residual protection. However, its strong odor makes it less favorable to patients. There is limited documented data on its efficacy and safety in large population studies.

Benzylbenzoate 25% Emulsion

Benzylbenzoate been used as an antiscabietic therapy since 1937. Like Lindane and malathion it too has neu-

rotoxic effects on the nervous system of mites. It is applied and left on for 24 hours on three to five successive days. It has a potential to cause irritant contact dermatitis. In children, the 10% emulsion is preferred.

10% Sulfur in Petrolatum

Various preparation of precipitated sulfur has been used, which includes 3–6% lotion or 5%, 10%, or 40% in petrolatum. It is left on for 24 hours, and the application is repeated for 3 days. This is often used in children under 6 months of age, in pregnancy, and in breast-feeding women. There is limited data on documented efficacy and safety.

Crotamiton 10% Lotion or Cream

Crotamiton is usually used for five successive daily applications. It is left on for 24 hours. Data on efficacy and safety are scanty but is generally considered safer for use in elderly and young children.

Systemic Treatment

Oral Ivermectin*

Ivermectin is administered orally. Ivermectin (Stromectol) interrupts GABA-induced neurotransmission of the scabies mite thus paralyzing them. It has been used widely since 1987 to control endemic onchocerciasis and filariasis. Millions of patients have received ivermectin worldwide with good tolerance. The preferred dose of ivermectin is oral 200 μg/kg to 250 μg/kg. A second dose in 7 to 10 days is recommended to reduce the risk of developing resistance. Several studies have demonstrated a cure after a single administration of 200 μg/kg of oral ivermectin, even in patients with HIV/AIDS in which infestation is difficult to cure. In crusted scabies, a single administration may not be enough.

Ivermectin has great value for managing scabies epidemics within healthcare institutions. Better results have been reported when used in combination with 5% Permethrin cream in crusted scabies. In addition to scabicides, patients should also be prescribed antihistamines, emollients, and topical steroids for postscabietic itch, which may persist for up to 2 weeks after treatment.

■ PEDICULOSIS PUBIS

Etiology

Three species that infest humans are *Pediculus humanus capitis* (head louse), *Phthirus pubis* (crab louse), and

Pediculus humanus corpus (body louse). Only *Phthirus pubis* shall be covered in this chapter.

The Parasite and Life Cycle

Lice are wingless insects that are obligate parasites. The pubic or crab louse has greater breadth than length, which ranges from 0.8 to 1.2 mm in length. The second and third pairs of legs are equipped with powerful claws that permit the louse to hold firmly to the pubic hair. The adult female lays up to 300 eggs that adhere to hair at the hair–skin junction. Nits hatch in 6–10 days and mature to adults in 10 days. The life cycle of the pubic louse egg to egg is 25 days. The louse inserts its mouth parts into a cutaneous capillary of the human host and sucks blood at frequent intervals. There is approximately a 30-day incubation period from exposure to onset of pruritis. The louse usually infests pubic hair but is known to infest chest hair, eyebrows, and eyelashes.

Epidemiology

Pediculosis pubis is primarily a disease of adults. It is spread by direct skin-to-skin contact and sexual contact. Condom use does not prevent pubic lice infestation. Nonsexual transmission has been reported in children and homeless populations.

Clinical Features

Itching is the primary symptom of pediculosis pubis. It is the result of an immune-mediated reaction to the louse saliva and may take 2 to 3 weeks to develop.

Lice and nits can be found on the pubic hair. Up to 60% of patients may have lice on other areas, such as beards and short hairs of the thigh, trunk, and perineal area. Infestation of the eyelashes must be assessed as it may often be overlooked.

Small, flat light brown to black flecks mark the presence of the parasite at the base of the hair shaft. The shiny oval nits cemented to the hair shafts are usually easily noticed. Purpuric and excoriated papules are often seen in the surrounding skin with blood stains on the underclothes.

Diagnosis

Pediculosis pubis can be diagnosed by physical examination alone. Diagnosis is confirmed by low-power microscopic examination of a plucked hair bearing a nit or by demonstration of a louse. Secondary pyodermas are common. Differential diagnosis includes impetigo, folliculitis, infected eczema, and seborrheic dermatitis.

Treatment

Ovicidal and pediculocidal activities of the pharmacological formulations, duration and quantity of the preparation applied, frequency of application, resistance to topical agents, and reinfestation influence the outcome of antilice treatments. A second application of topical therapy 3–7 days after initial treatment to ensure killing of mites missed in the egg stage is usually recommended.

Sexual contacts should be treated simultaneously and told to abstain from sexual intercourse for 10 days to 2 weeks. All bedding, towels, and clothing should also be washed. Causes of treatment failure include poor compliance, inadequate quantity of pediculide applied, reinfestation, and resistance. Hairy individuals may consider cutting short or shaving the hairy areas on the body.

Permethrin*

Permethrin (5% cream rinse) is a more potent pediculocide than pyrethrum. It is preferred as the first-line treatment. It has a residual activity of 2 weeks, which may be helpful in killing newly emerged young lice. It is applied to affected hair, left on for 10 minutes, and then washed off. Side effects include burning, tingling, numbness, and erythema. Higher cure rates have been shown after a second application 7–10 days later.

Malathion*

The 0.5% malathion lotion is highly effective in the treatment of pediculosis pubis. It is an organophosphate insecticide that should be left in place for 8 to 12 hours before washing it off. It is considered safe and has no significant side effects. Nevertheless its strong odor makes it less favorable.

Gamma Benzene Hexachloride 1%

Gamma benzene hexachloride (1% shampoo or lotion as Lindane, Kwell, Kwellada, and Scabene) is an organochlorine insecticide that is left on for 8 to 12 hours and then washed off. It has poor pediculocidal activity and growing resistance has been reported. Two applications 1 week apart is recommended for better results. The remaining nits may be removed with a fine-toothed comb or forceps.

▪ KEY POINTS

- The female mite *Sarcoptes scabiei* var. *hominis* causes human scabies. Infestation by this host-specific, eight-legged mite has a worldwide distribution although they are more predominant in tropical countries.

- The scabies mite lives its entire life cycle within the epidermis of the skin. It is not a known vector for disease. It may be acquired during sexual contact.

- Classical scabies is manifested as nocturnal pruritis with characteristic symmetrical distribution of burrows, papules, pustules, and excoriations.

- Diagnosis is confirmed by demonstration of the mite, the eggs, or the feces (scybala) from skin scrapings.

- Secondary bacterial infection is most commonly due to *Staphylococcus aureus*, group A beta hemolytic streptococci, or peptostreptococci.

- Crusted scabies (Norwegian scabies) is a psoriasiform dermatosis of the hands and feet, with subungal hyperkeratosis and an erythematous scaly eruption on the face, neck, scalp, and trunk. Generalized crusted scabies occurs in immunocompromised patients and requires treatment with oral ivermectin.

- Permethrin 5% cream a synthetic pyrethroid is the preferred scabicide. It has low toxicity.

- Pediculosis pubis is caused by *Phthirus pubis*, a wingless insect that is an obligate parasite. The crab louse is 0.8-1.2 mm in length and has second and third pairs of legs equipped with powerful claws that permit it to hold firmly to the pubic hair.

- Pediculosis pubis can be diagnosed by physical examination alone. Diagnosis is confirmed by low-power microscopic examination of a plucked hair bearing a nit attached by a cementing substance or by demonstrating a louse.

- Causes of treatment failure include misdiagnosis, failure to comply with treatment instructions, reinfestation, and resistance.

REFERENCES

Burgess IF. Biology and epidemiology of scabies. *Curr Opin Infect Dis.* 1999;12:177–180.

CDC. Sexually transmitted disease treatment guidelines, 2010. *Morb Mortal Week Rep.* 2010;59(RR-12):1–110.

Chosidow O. Scabies and pediculosis. *Lancet.* 2000;355:819–826.

Chosidow O. Scabies. *N Engl J Med.* 2006;354:1718–1827.

Clinical Effectiveness Group (Association of Genitourinary Medicine and Medical Society for the Study of Venereal Diseases). National guideline for the management of *Phthirus pubis* infestation. *Sex Transm Infect.* 1999;75(suppl 1):S78–S79. Updated http://www.bashh.org/documents/28/28.pdf.

Develoux M. Ivermectin. *Ann Dermatol Venereol.* 2004;131:561–570.

Fisher L, Morton RS. Phtirus pubis infestations. *Br J Vener Dis.* 1970;45:326–329.

Martin WE, Wheeler CE. Diagnosis of human scabies by epidermal shave biopsy. *J Am Acad Dermatol.* 1979;1:355–357.

McCarthy JS, Kemp DJ, Walton SF, Currie BJ. Scabies: more than just an irritation. *Postgrad Med J.* 2004;80:382–387.

Meinking TL, Taplin D, Hermida JL, Pardo R, Kerdel FA. The treatment of scabies with ivermectin. *N Eng J Med.* 1995;333:26–30.

Orkin M. Scabies: what's new? *Curr Probl Dermatol.* 1995;22:105–111.

Schultz MW, Gomez M, Hansen RC, et al. Comparative study of 5% permethrin cream and 1% Lindane lotion for the treatment of scabies. *Arch Dermatol.* 1990;126:167–170.

Wolf R, Avigad J, Brenner S. Scabies: the diagnosis of atypical cases. *Cutis.* 1995;55:370–371.

▪ WEBSITES

Scabies

http://www.bashh.org/documents/27/27.pdf

http://www.cdc.gov/STD/treatment/2006/ectoparasitic.htm#ecto2

Pediculosis Pubis

http://www.bashh.org/documents/28/28.pdf

14

Nongonococcal Urethritis

Mohsen Shahmanesh and Jonathan M. Zenilman

■ INTRODUCTION

Urethritis, or inflammation of the urethra, is a multifactorial condition that can be sexually acquired. It is classically characterized by the presence of discharge or dysuria. However, it can also be asymptomatic if inflammation is diagnosed by microscopic examination.

The diagnosis of urethritis is confirmed by demonstrating either an excess of polymorphonuclear leucocytes (PMNLs) in the anterior urethra (defined as >5 polymorphonuclear leukocytes per high-power field), or isolating a urethral pathogen. Urethritis is described as either gonococcal, when *Neisseria gonorrhoeae* is detected, or nongonococcal (NGU), when it is not (see Figure 14-1). Admittedly, the definition of gonococcal urethritis versus NGU is antiquated and largely reflects the limited diagnostic capabilities of clinical settings more than 40 years ago. Nevertheless, the criterion still has utility because differentiating gonococcal and nongonococcal urethritis has implications for both treatment and public health management. In women, the equivalent syndrome is mucopurulent cervicitis with approximately 40% of cases due to infection with *Chlamydia trachomatis*.

The conceptualization of NGU is riddled with uncertainties. Uncertainty begins with the diagnostic criteria used, which rather illogically equates the presence of PMNLs in either the urethral exudates or first voided urine (FVU) with a sexually transmitted pathogen. *Chlamydia trachomatis* has been most often associated with NGU, yet accounts for only 30–40% of cases. In chlamydia-negative cases, a known urethral pathogen is isolated in only 20–40%, even when highly sensitive detection methods are used, such as DNA amplification techniques. Most cases do not have an etiological diagnosis, even after careful search for additional pathogens, such as *Mycoplasma genitalium*, *Trichomonas vaginalis*, herpes simplex, and even adenoviruses. Moreover, the inflammatory exudates may persist for weeks after the successful eradication of *C. trachomatis* or other identified pathogens.

Limiting tests to men with discharge or dysuria only increases isolation of *C. trachomatis* or *M. genitalium* to a maximum of 50%. In a further 10%, an undiagnosed microbiological cause is found if the partner is tested for chlamydia or *M. genitalium*, and a urinary tract infection may be the cause of up to 10%. In the absence of

FIGURE 14-1 Non-Gonococcal Urethritis—Inflammatory Cells on Gram Stain, No Organisms Present

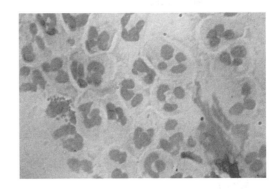

symptoms and signs, however, known NGU pathogens are isolated in less than one quarter of patients.

Conversely, using the criteria of the presence of PMNL in the urethra as a diagnostic criterion, between 20% and 40% of men with a known sexually transmitted pathogen in their urethra, such as chlamydia or gonococcal infection, will not have urethritis. Finally, interobserver, and even intraobserver error, especially in samples with low-grade inflammation (5–20 PMNL/hpf), make diagnostic consistency difficult. The tendency among clinicians has increasingly been to define urethritis in terms of urethral pathogens rather than the urethral inflammatory response.

Defining the epidemiology of NGU is also problematic. For example, gonorrhea and chlamydia are reportable infections, which include a case definition based on laboratory findings. NGU, in contrast, is a clinical diagnosis and subject to numerous biases in terms of ascertainment. Therefore, trend analyses are difficult, if not impossible, without performing careful clinic audits.

■ ETIOLOGY

The prevalence of the common organisms associated with NGU is listed in Table 14-1. Despite better and more sensitive microbiological tests, prevalence of known pathogens has fallen in more recent studies, which tend toward the lower part of the range shown in Table 14-1. Moreover, the contribution of viruses and urinary pathogens has been increasingly recognized. The commonest organisms implicated are *C. trachomatis* and *M. genitalium* with the latter perhaps causing more symptoms.

Chlamydia trachomatis is an obligate intracellular bacteria, which was first identified as a cause of conjunctivitis.

TABLE 14-1 Prevalence of the Most Common Pathogens Isolated from Patients with NGU

Microorganism	Prevalence
Chlamydia trachomatis	11–43%
Mycoplasma genitalium	9–25%
Trichomonas vaginalis	0–17%
Ureaplasma urealyticum (biovar 2)	0–5%
Herpes and adenovirus	6
Others	<5
No organism	30–80%

Its role as a major sexually transmitted pathogen was soon recognized. In men, it causes urethritis and epididymo-orchitis (Chapter 21) and in women is a common cause of cervicitis (Chapter 15) and pelvic inflammatory disease (Chapter 8). Because of the asymptomatic nature of most chlamydial infection, ongoing sexual transmission is common. Recent availability of accurate and sensitive nucleic acid amplification (NAATS) tests has allowed population screening studies showing prevalence rates of 8–12% in the those younger than 25 years old. More recently, a small bacterium, *Mycoplasma genitalium*, has been identified as an important pathogen in both males and females. The study of *M. genitalium* has been hampered by the fastidious nature of the organism, which makes it difficult to culture, and the absence of commercially available NATS tests. It was first shown to be associated with NGU, and accumulating evidence also links it to cervicitis, urethritis, and pelvic inflammatory disease in women.

Chlamydia is more likely to be isolated in younger patients than *M. genitalium*, and the two organisms rarely coexist in the same individual. These observations suggest a negative interaction between the two organisms. Patients with nonchlamydial NGU are older than those with chlamydial NGU but, otherwise, similar in ethnic mix and socioeconomic status.

The isolation of *Trichomonas vaginalis* varies enormously between different studies and depends on the prevalence of the organism in the community, which is more common in nonwhite ethnic groups and greatly increased with the use of more sensitive polymerase chain reaction assays. For example, trichomonas infections are more common in men with partners who have the infection, and studies in the United States have demonstrated trichomonas urethritis more frequently in persons who attend sexually transmitted infection (STI) clinics compared with those who attend non-STI clinic attendees.

The presence of *Ureaplasma urealyticum* organisms does not correlate with symptoms or signs of urethritis, and its exact role in NGU remains unclear, partly due to the ubiquitous presence of these organisms. However, certain biovars of *U. urealyticum* may be more likely to cause symptoms and probably account for a small proportion of NGU. Earlier studies suggested that this organism may be associated with NGU; however, later work suggested that it may be as likely to be commensal flora.

A urinary tract infection (UTI) may account for up to 10% of cases, although there is only one study evaluating this. UTIs accounting for NGU have been found to be more frequent in men reporting insertive rectal intercourse. Herpes simplex virus and adenoviruses account for up to 10% of symptomatic urethritis. HSV urethritis is found frequently (50–60%) in cases of primary genital herpes due to either HSV-1 or HSV-2. Adenoviruses are often associated with conjunctivitis. *N. meningitidis*, *Candida* sp., urethral stricture, and foreign bodies probably account for only a small proportion of cases (<10%).

In 30–80% of men with NGU, no organism is detected. Urethritis is associated with reactive arthritis. While this condition may follow chlamydial urethritis, it is also associated with a variety of other pathogens in which a "reactive" urethritis may also be observed, without any known pathogen isolated. Asymptomatic urethritis, without an observable discharge, may have a different etiology from symptomatic urethritis, with *C. trachomatis* being detected less frequently and at lower quantities. There is also a possible association of asymptomatic NGU with bacterial vaginosis—a condition associated with a wide range of microorganisms and often follows fellatio. As the mouth is colonized by more than 400 species of microorganisms, oral pathogens may contribute in an as yet undefined way to NGU. Many microbes may initiate an inflammatory response in the urethra that may be asymptomatic or self-limiting.

Urethritis may also be caused by insertion of foreign bodies into the penis. This includes using urethral rings, or self-catheterization or other sexual practices. Finally, there is the entity of "psychological urethritis" with symptoms of urethritis but either without evidence of urethral inflammation or due to an obsession with the "sexually transmissible nature" of an adequately treated persistent urethritis. Often these monosymptomatic obsessional conditions are signs of an underlying depressive or other psychotic conditions.

It is assumed that the etiological agents of sexually acquired male NGU could potentially cause genital tract inflammation in women, in particular pelvic inflammatory disease (PID). This is undoubted with chlamydial and gonococcal infection and likely with *M. genitalium* but remains to be substantiated for pathogen-negative NGU. Asymptomatic chlamydia-negative NGU is common in male partners of women with PID. However, because *M. genitalium* was not tested in earlier studies, the absolute risk for a women developing PID as a result of having a male partner with chlamydia-negative NGU is unknown.

▇ CLINICAL FEATURES

The usual symptoms are urethral discharge (Figure 14-2), dysuria, or penile irritation. However, up to 50% of men with chlamydial and the majority with *T. vaginalis*

FIGURE 14-2 Non-Gonococcal Urethritis— Classic Presentation of Mucoid Discharge

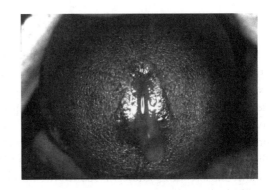

infection of the urethra will be asymptomatic. Symptoms appear to be more common with *M. genitalium*.

Examination may be entirely normal, or there may be a urethral discharge. The patient may not have been noticed the discharge or it was only present on urethral massage. The discharge may be mucoid or mucopurulent. A frankly purulent discharge is unusual and suggests gonococcal infection. The discharge from *T. vaginalis* often has a milky consistency. The meatus or subpreputial area may demonstrate erythema or mild edema.

Complications

Epididymo-orchitis and sexually acquired arthritis (reactive arthritis) may be associated with urethritis and is covered elsewhere. These are infrequent, occurring in fewer than 1% of cases though incomplete forms may be more common.

Diagnosis

The diagnosis of urethritis was traditionally based by demonstrating PMNLs in the anterior urethra. A flowchart is presented in Figure 14-3. This was made by means of either:

1. A Gram's stained urethral smear containing greater than or equal to 5 PMNL per high-power ($\times$1000) microscopic field (averaged over five fields with greatest concentration of PMNLs). Either a 5-mm plastic loop or cotton-tipped swab can be used. In the case of urethritis associated with herpes and other viral conditions, there may be a predominance of lymphocytes.

2. A Gram's stained preparation from a first voided urine (FVU) specimen, containing greater than or equal to 10 PMNL per high-power microscopic field.

Either test can be used. Patients should have held their urine for more than 2 hours to allow accumulation of inflammatory cells. The quality of the smear heavily depends on how the smear is taken, and there is both inter- and intraobserver variation. Positive leucocyte esterase activity (LEA) on FVU does not have adequate sensitivity to be considered a reliable rapid diagnostic test for NGU. A negative LEA, however, has a greater than 90% predictive value and can be used in population chlamydia screening studies to reduce the number needing *C. trachomatis* assay.

Eliminating urethral smear in asymptomatic patients without a demonstrable discharge will miss a maximum of 3% of cases of *C. trachomatis* and approximately 5% with *M. genitalium*. It will also delay the diagnosis of chlamydia in up to 30%. However, it would prevent 70–80% of people from being wrongly labeled as having an STI with all its social and psychological implications. Hence, most authorities believe that the urethral smear can be eliminated in asymptomatic patients without a demonstrable discharge.

Although in symptomatic patients urethral smear is more likely to be associated with the isolation of a urethral pathogen, a positive smear does not predict such a pathogen. Hence, it could be argued that the Gram's stained urethral smears can be completely dispensed with in the diagnosis of NGU once commercial testing kits for *M. genitalium* becomes available, although they may still be helpful for the immediate diagnosis of gonorrhea (see appropriate section).

FIGURE 14-3 Non-Gonococcal Urethritis—Gram Stain

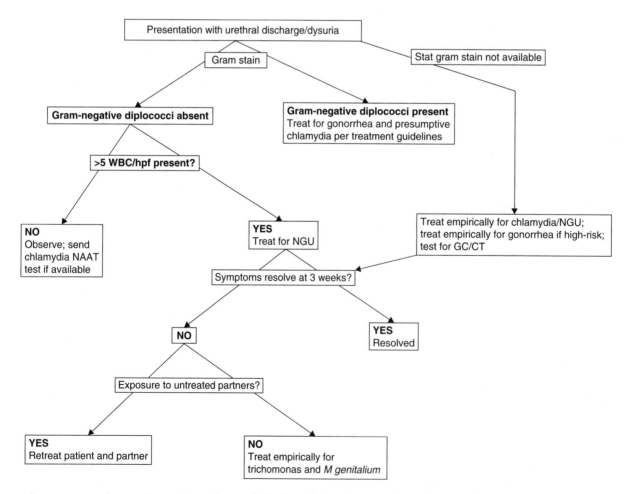

Note the presence of >5 polymorphonuclear cells/hpf, and the absence of stainable organisms.

Symptomatic patients, in whom no discharge or urethritis is detected, could be retested. They can hold their urine overnight, or they can be given empirical treatment if they are at high risk of infection or are unlikely to return for repeat evaluation.

Regardless of the presence of symptoms and signs, all patients at risk of urethritis should have a urethral culture for *N. gonorrhoea* and be tested for *C. trachomatis*. Even newer nucleic acid amplification tests will, however, miss approximately 10% of positive chlamydial infections. Commercial testing for *M. genitalium* is not available, and the place of such tests in routine clinical practice, once they become available, need to be determined. A midstream urine sample (MSU) should be obtained if a urinary tract infection is suspected. In one study using a dipstick, incorporating a nitrite and leucocyte esterase test has a sensitivity and specificity for urinary tract infection of 83% and 90%. The traditional two-glass test adds little to the diagnosis.

When Microscopy Is Not Available.

In the absence of microscopy, a diagnosis of urethritis can be made clinically by the presence of symptoms with or without the signs of a urethral discharge. While urethritis caused by *N. gonorrhoeae* produces a greater inflammatory response and is more likely to be purulent than *C. trachomatis* and *M. genitalium*, great overlap makes it difficult to predict the nature of the organism. Therefore, depending on the prevalence of the various microorganisms in the population being served, the clinician may choose to treat syndromically (see Chapter 42). This type of approach may be more practical in some urgent care– or emergency department–type settings, where microscopy is not available and follow-up cannot be assured. Alternatively, if the clinical picture is more in keeping with NGU, and there is good follow-up, the clinician may choose to treat for this condition, while awaiting results of gonococcal culture.

MANAGEMENT

The various treatments are summarized in Table 14-2 and comply with the CDC's 2010 STD Treatment Guidelines. Treatment should be initiated as soon as the diagnosis is made. However, assessing treatment efficacy is problematic, not least as no pathogen is identifiable in more than half the cases, and the inflammatory exudate may persist for an unknown length of time even when the putative organism has been eliminated. Therefore, treatment is often empiric.

Tetracycline and doxycycline are generally effective against *C. trachomatis* though sporadic cases of treatment failure have been reported. Azithromycin is equally effective and has the advantage of single-dose therapy but is more expensive. While, in general, effective treatments against *C. trachomatis* appear also to be effective in NGU, tetracyclines in the doses used, and a single 1-g dose of azithromycin, do not consistently eradicate *M. genitalium* and have no effect on *T. vaginalis*.

Patients should be given general explanation of the causes NGU and possible short-term and long-term implications for the health of the patient and his partner. The importance of evaluating and treating sex partner(s) should be emphasized. Patients and their partners should be advised to abstain from sexual intercourse, or use condoms consistently, until they have completed therapy and partners have been treated. Give advice about safer sex. All sexual partners at risk should be assessed and offered epidemiological treatment, maintaining patient confidentiality. The duration of "look back" is arbitrary; 4 weeks

TABLE 14-2 Recommended Regimes for the Treatment of Acute NGU

	Dosage	Length of time
Recommended		
Doxycycline	100 mg twice daily	7 days
Azithromycin	1 g	Single dose
Alternative regimens		
Erythromycin	500 mg twice daily	14 days
Ofloxacin	200 mg twice daily	7 days
Ofloxacin	400 mg daily	7 days

is customary for symptomatic men (up to 6 months for asymptomatic men). If *C. trachomatis* or *N. gonorrhoeae* are detected, ensure that all potential at-risk sexual partner have been notified. It is best to obtain details of contacts and arrange for contact tracing at the first clinic visit. Female contacts of men with chlamydial urethritis should be treated regardless of the results of chlamydia isolation because of potential effects on fertility of undiagnosed chlamydia. This has, however, not been evaluated in randomized prospective studies. Concurrent treatment of female sexual partners of men with chlamydia negative NGU is also recommended because *M. genitalium*, a probable cause of pelvic inflammatory disease, is not routinely tested, and there is some discordance in the isolation of chlamydia and *M. genitalium* between couples. However, as discussed earlier, current treatments for uncomplicated NGU does not always eradicate *M. genitalium*.

Follow-up of the patient is not usually necessary with doxycycline and azithromycin regimens, provided some provision is made to ensure compliance with medication, as well as absence of reinfection. This can be done by telephone, text messaging, or other means. Patients who are still symptomatic, who have not completed their medication, or who had unprotected sexual intercourse with an untreated partner should be asked to return to the clinic.

■ PERSISTENT/RECURRENT NGU

Persisting dysuria or discharge, despite apparent adequate treatment, occurs in up to 20% of patients. There is no consensus of opinion in either diagnosis or management of this condition. Chronic NGU has been arbitrarily defined as persistent or recurrent urethritis occurring 30–90 days following treatment of acute NGU. There is also some evidence of an immunological basis for the persistent inflammation. The diagnostic criteria are the same as for acute NGU, but a repeat urethral smear and microbiological investigation should *only* be performed with persistent symptoms, in which the possibility of reinfection has been excluded. This will avoid overdiagnosing chronic NGU and creating unnecessary anxiety.

Treatment should cover the two main organisms not adequately treated with the standard treatment regimens for acute urethritis. There is only one randomized treatment trial of chronic NGU using erythromycin for 3 weeks. An easier regimen would be to use azithromycin in a dose shown in a small study to eradicate *M. genitalium* (500 mg stat followed by 250 mg daily for 4–6 days), given concurrently with metronidazole 400 mg b.d. (or 2

g in a stat dose) to eradicate possible *T. vaginalis*. There is no evidence that female partners of men with persistent/ recurrent NGU are at increased risk of pelvic inflammatory disease. However, until we have a better understanding of the etiology of pathogen-negative NGU of female partners of such patients, it would be prudent to treat them as for NGU (see previous discussion).

The choice of further referral or investigation depends on the severity of symptoms. Urological investigation is usually normal unless the patient has urinary flow problems. Chronic abacterial prostatitis (see guideline on prostatitis) and psychosexual causes should be considered in the differential diagnosis. Patients with microscopic urethritis but who have no signs or symptoms after two courses of treatment should be strongly reassured that they do not harbor a sexually transmissible pathogen. There is no evidence that retreatment of an appropriately treated sexual partner prevents persistence of urethritis.

Chronic Therapy

In a subset of patients, symptoms, especially pain, may recur. If microbiological workup is negative and they have not been reexposed, chronic therapy is not indicated.

■ KEY POINTS

- Urethritis is characterised by the presence of discharge and/or dysuria, but can also be asymptomatic if inflammation is diagnosed by microscopic examination or on screening for *Chlamydia trachomatis*.

- The commonest organisms implicated are *C. trachomatis* and *Mycoplasma genitalium* with the latter perhaps causing more symptoms. In 30-80% no known pathogen is identified.

- Prevalence of *Trichomonas vaginalis* varies enormously in different settings. Viruses such as herpes and adenovirus are increasingly implicated.

- Epididymo-orchitis and sexually acquired arthritis (reactive arthritis) may infrequently be associated with urethritis

- In women, the equivalent syndrome is mucopurulent cervicitis with approximately 40% of cases being due to infection with *C trachomatis*.

- Examination may be normal, or there may be a urethral discharge which may be mucoid or mucopurulent. A frankly purulent discharge is unusual and suggests gonococcal infection.

- The diagnosis is confirmed by demonstrating either an excess of polymorphonuclear leucocytes (PMNs) in the anterior urethra (defined as >5 PMNs per high-power field), or isolating a urethral pathogen.

- All patients at risk of urethritis should have a urethral culture for *N. gonorrhoea* and also be tested for *C trachomatis*. A urethral smear need not be performed in asymptomatic patients without a demonstrable discharge.

- Treatment should be initiated as soon as the diagnosis is made with either Azithromycin or a tetracycline

- Sexual partners should be treated and sexual intercourse avoided until all partners complete treatment.

- Persistent urethritis should be distinguished from reinfection

SELECTED REFERENCES

Diagnosis of Acute NGU

Bradshaw CS, Tabrizi SN, Read TR, et al. Etiologies of nongonococcal urethritis: bacteria, viruses, and the association with orogenital exposure[comment]. *J Infect Dis.* 2006;193:336–345.

Falk L, Fredlund H, Jensen JS. Symptomatic urethritis is more prevalent in men infected with *Mycoplasma genitalium* than with *Chlamydia trachomatis*. *Sex Transm Infect.* 2004;80:289–293.

Geisler WM, Yu S, Hook EW III. Chlamydial and gonococcal infection in men without polymorphonuclear leukocytes on Gram stain: implications for diagnostic approach and management. *Sex Transm Dis.* 2005;32(10):630–634.

Horner P, Gilroy C, Thomas B, Naidoo R, Olof M, Taylor-Robinson D. Association of *Mycoplasma genitalium* with acute non-gonococcal urethritis. *Lancet.* 1993;342:582–585.

Horner PJ, Gilroy CB, Thomas BJ, Renton A, Taylor-Robinson D. The association of *Chlamydia trachomatis* and *Mycoplasma genitalium* with non-gonococcal urethritis. *Lancet.* 2000;342:582–585.

Marrazzo JM, Whittington WL, Celum CL, et al. Urine-based screening for *Chlamydia trachomatis* in men attending sexually transmitted disease clinics [published correction appears in *Sex Transm Dis.* 2001;28(7):429]. *Sex Transm Dis.* 2001;28:219–225.

Mena L, Wang X, Mroczkowski TF, Martin DH. *Mycoplasma genitalium* infections in asymptomatic men and men with urethritis attending a sexually transmitted diseases clinic in New Orleans. *Clin Infect Dis.* 2002;35:1167–1173.

Schwebke JR, Hook EW III. High rates of *Trichomonas vaginalis* among men attending a sexually transmitted diseases clinic: implications for screening and urethritis management. *J Infect Dis.* 2003;188:465–468.

Soper D. Trichomoniasis: under control or undercontrolled [review]?. *Am J Obst Gynecol.* 2004;190:281–290.

Tait IA, Hart CA. *Chlamydia trachomatis* in non-gonococcal urethritis patients and their heterosexual partners: routine testing by polymerase chain reaction. *Sex Transm Infect.* 2002;78:286–288.

Mucopurulent Cervicitis

Marrazzo JM. Mucopurulent cervicitis: no longer ignored, but still misunderstood [review]. *Infect Dis Clin North Am.* 2005;19:333–349.

Mycoplama genitalium

Ross JDC, Jensen JS. *Mycoplasma genitalium* as a sexually transmitted infection: implications for screening, testing, and treatment. *Sex Transm Infect.* 2006;82:269–271. doi:10.1136/sti.2005.017368.

Chronic NGU

Horner P, Thomas B, Gilroy C, Egger M, Taylor-Robinson D. The role of *Mycoplasma genitalium* and *Ureaplasma urealyticum* in acute and chronic non-gonococcal urethritis. *Clin Infect Dis.* 2001;32:995–1003.

Krieger JN, Hooton TM, Brust PJ, Holmes KK, Stamm WE. Evaluation of chronic urethritis: defining the role for endoscopic procedures. *Arch Intern Med.* 1988;148:703–707.

Shahmanesh M. Problems with non-gonococcal urethritis [editorial/review]. *Int J STD AIDS.* 1994;5:390–399.

Treatment

Burstein GR, Zenilman JM. Nongonococcal urethritis—a new paradigm [review]. *Clin Infect Dis.* 1999;28(suppl 1):S66–S73.

CDC. Sexually transmitted disease treatment guidelines, 2010. *Morb Mortal Week Rep.* 2010;59(RR-12):1–110.

Schmid G. Evolving strategies for management of the nongonococcal urethritis syndrome. *J Acquir Immune Defic Syndr.* 1995;274(7):577–579.

Stamm WE, Hicks CB, Martin DH, et al. Azithromycin for empirical treatment of the nongonococcal urethral syndrome in men: a randomised double-blind study. *JAMA.* 1995;274:545–549.

Online Resources

BASHH guidelines for NGU. http://www.bashh.org/guidelines.asp

15
Cervicitis

Jeanne M. Marrazzo and Hillary Liss

INTRODUCTION

The last decade has produced considerable advances in the diagnosis of the common etiologies of cervicitis, including *Chlamydia trachomatis* and *Neisseria gonorrhoeae*, and in understanding their pathogenesis. Despite this, clear understanding of why these bacteria cause cervical inflammation in a minority of women infected with either organism remains very limited. Moreover, many women with cervicitis have neither of these infections detected, even when highly sensitive diagnostic tests are employed. The most important reasons to properly diagnose and treat cervicitis are to prevent upper genital tract infection, particularly pelvic inflammatory disease (PID) and the well-known associated sequelae, as well as possible perinatal complications, including gonococcal or chlamydial conjunctivitis or chlamydial pneumonia of the newborn; however, many women with cervicitis are asymptomatic and thus go untreated.

Cervicitis is an inflammatory condition of the cervix, typically viewed as a consequence of infection with the sexually acquired pathogens *C. trachomatis* and *N. gonorrhoeae* and, occasionally, *Trichomonas vaginalis* or herpes simplex virus (HSV). In practice, cervicitis is a clinical diagnosis made when either mucopurulent discharge or easily induced bleeding (friability) is present at the endocervical os; more subtle signs include edema of the cervical ectropion (edematous ectopy) and presence of an elevated number of polymorphonuclear (PMN) white blood cells detected by Gram's stain of a smear of endocervical secretions. As with many syndromes with no gold standard for diagnosis,

however, inflammation at the cervix is considerably more complex, as is the range of pathology seen in the clinical setting.

UPDATE IN TERMINOLOGY

An important change in the current understanding of cervicitis is that mucopurulent discharge and easily induced endocervical bleeding or friability are comparable in predicting the presence of cervicitis. Requiring the presence of mucopurulent discharge decreases the sensitivity in detecting disease, particularly *C. trachomatis*. The Centers for Disease Control and Prevention emphasize referring to this clinical entity as cervicitis rather than mucopurulent cervicitis (MPC). Although it is still common to see these terms used interchangeably, it is preferable to refer to this syndrome as cervicitis to reflect these liberalized diagnostic criteria.

ANATOMY AND PHYSIOLOGY

The cervix consists of an underlying connective tissue matrix overlaid by two types of distinct epithelium. The endocervical canal and ectropion, if present, are lined by columnar epithelial cells. These cells provide targets of entry for *C. trachomatis* and *N. gonorrhoeae*. In contrast, the ectocervix is lined by squamous epithelium contiguous with the vaginal mucosa and is susceptible to pathogens associated with vaginitis, including trichomoniasis, bacterial vaginosis (BV), and vulvovaginal candidiasis. The ectocervix may also be affected by genital ulcerative diseases that occur on the vaginal mucosa, such as HSV and syphilis. Both types of epithelium are responsive to sustained hormonal changes. Estrogen, either endogenous or exogenous, has numerous effects on the cervicovaginal mucosa, but two are most important. First, estrogen promotes formation and maintenance of cervical ectopy, which is present in adolescents, during pregnancy, and in women taking estrogen-containing contraceptives. Second, estrogen is critical for maintaining adequate thickness of the squamous cervicovaginal epithelium (>20 cell layers). Progesterone, in contrast, can cause relative thinning of this epithelium. These hormones also affect the quality of endocervical mucos. Relatively high levels of estrogen during the follicular phase leading up to ovulation, for example, thin the endocervical mucus plug, thus facilitating passage of spermatozoa through the endocervical canal. Progesterone dominates the luteal phase of the cycle and acts to increase viscosity and reduce volume of endocervical mucus, making it more tenacious, resistant to passage by sperm, and possibly by pathogens.

Physiologically, endocervical mucus has intrinsic antimicrobial activity mediated by lactic acid, low pH, and antimicrobial peptides.

■ DEFINITION AND EPIDEMIOLOGY

No consensus definition for cervicitis as a research or clinical outcome currently exists, nor is there a diagnostic gold standard. This has led to a body of literature that is difficult to interpret and to findings that may be less than generalizable. At the most basic level, many studies have not distinguished between the presence of signs at the endocervix, lined by the columnar epithelial cells that are the target for chlamydial and gonococcal infection, or the ectocervix, composed of the squamous epithelium that also lines the vagina. These epithelia differ not only in the target organisms they host but also in endogenous defense mechanisms, secretory capacity, and vulnerability to infection with HIV-1. Some studies have required the presence of inflammation detected by Gram's stain of endocervical secretions to substantiate the clinical diagnosis of cervicitis, while others have not collected information on endocervical friability. These inconsistencies make generalizing across studies difficult and point out the need for consistent definitions and protocols in clinical research.

The presence of easily induced bleeding and mucopurulent discharge from the endocervical canal is the most straightforward sign of the endocervical inflammation that defines cervicitis. These signs, along with the more subtle presence of edematous ectopy, confer a considerably higher likelihood of detecting *N. gonorrhoeae* and *C. trachomatis*. However, some important conceptions about these signs have changed over the past several years. First, use of nucleic acid amplified tests (NAAT) for both of these sexually transmitted infections (STIs), in particular *C. trachomatis*, have higher sensitivity relative to earlier generations of diagnostic tests, while maintaining excellent specificity (see Chapter 19). This has resulted in the identification of an increasing proportion of cervical chlamydial and gonococcal infections not associated with signs of cervicitis. The quantity of organisms in both endocervical and urethral chlamydial infections correlates directly with the presence of mucosal inflammatory signs and with the ability of any diagnostic test to detect infection. NAAT detects relatively more infections in women without signs of cervicitis than in women with obvious signs of cervicitis. In other words, with NAAT, women with a lesser burden of disease are more likely to be diagnosed with an STI, such as cervical chlamydia infection, even without signs or symptoms consistent with cervicitis. This finding has resulted in a decrease in the estimated proportion of cervical chlamydial infections thought to cause cervical signs to approximately 10–20%. Second, even seemingly obvious signs of endocervical inflammation may have variable precision for these STI, as the predictive value of individual cervical findings suggestive of cervicitis may vary with patients' age and other STI-related risk factors.

Two tests used to assess endocervical inflammation are cited in much of the literature on cervicitis and deserve comment, as they are of limited practical clinical value. The independent value of inflammation detected by Gram's stain of a smear of endocervical secretions or by Papanicolaou smear as a criterion for cervicitis, especially in predicting chlamydial infection, has been variable. The CDC Sexually Transmitted Disease Treatment Guidelines stopped including inflammation on endocervical Gram's stain as presumptive evidence and indication for empiric treatment of chlamydial infection in 1993, and the sensitivity of endocervical Gram's stain for detection of *N. gonorrhoeae* at the cervix is only 50%. Another practical issue is the requirement of licensed point-of-care laboratories. However, Gram's stain of endocervical secretions to diagnose cervicitis continues to be used in selected settings in the United States, particularly those that provide focused STI care (STI clinics) and is still recommended by some investigators.

Most guidelines recommend a threshold level of 10 to 30 PMN leukocytes per high power (1000×, oil immersion) field, with PMN counts above this level supporting a diagnosis of cervicitis. As expected, the sensitivity of this test increases and specificity decreases as the threshold cutoff is decreased. Although inflammatory changes on Papanicolaou smear are associated with an increased likelihood of detection of several STIs, including *C. trachomatis*, *N. gonorrhoeae*, trichomoniasis, and human papillomavirus, this test is neither specific enough to direct empiric therapy for these pathogens nor practical in delineating immediate etiologies of cervicitis for empiric therapy to recommend its use for this purpose.

ETIOLOGIES AND PATHOGENESIS

Chlamydia trachomatis and *N. gonorrhoeae* are well-described causes of cervicitis (Table 15-1). Other relatively common STI can also cause clinically evident cervical inflammation. *Trichomonas vaginalis* may cause an erosive inflammation of the ectocervical epithelium, termed *strawberry cervix*, or colpitis macularis (see Chapter 7). This organism may cause a range of epithelial disruption, from small, isolated petechiae to large punctuate hemorrhages with surrounding areas of pale mucosa. The pathogenesis of these lesions probably arises in part from the variety of cytotoxic factors that *T. vaginalis* can elaborate. Again, why only some women develop evident cervical changes with trichomoniasis is not clear. Possible reasons include a direct relationship between quantitative burden of *T. vaginalis*, strain of organism involved, or host factors that might increase susceptibility to cervical inflammation.

Genital infection with HSV types 1 and 2 can also cause cervicitis (also see Chapter 18). The most striking example occurs in women previously uninfected with HSV type 1 or 2 who experience severe clinical manifestations of primary infection with HSV-2. Although most primary HSV-2 infections are asymptomatic, some women experience a severe primary infection that may include cervicitis. Typically, cervicitis in this setting is characterized by diffuse erosive and hemorrhagic lesions, usually in the ectocervical epithelium, and often accompanied by frank ulceration. Cervicitis is thought to occur in approximately 15–20% of women experiencing clinically evident primary HSV-2 genital infection. When cervicitis occurs in this setting, other manifestations of primary HSV-2 genital infection are usually evident, including external herpetic lesions, neurologic manifestations (including aseptic meningitis, urinary retention, and lumbosacral radiculitis), fever, and inguinal lymphadenopathy. Any of these symptoms and signs, including cervicitis,

may reappear with clinical recurrences of genital HSV-2; however, they are typically less severe during recurrences. Subclinical shedding of HSV-2 does not appear to be directly related to cervicitis. HSV-1 may also cause cervicitis similar to those described for HSV-2; however, the manifestations are typically less severe and usually occur only during the primary genital infection with HSV-1.

Mycoplasma genitalium has recently been implicated as a sexually transmissible cause of cervicitis. Manhart and colleagues (2003) studied archived endocervical fluid samples collected from 779 women attending an STD clinic from 1984 to 1986. Of the 719 samples, which contained material that was able to be amplified by PCR, women with *M. genitalium* isolated were 3.3 times more likely to have cervicitis as defined by the presence of endocervical mucopurulent discharge, easily induced bleeding, and Gram's stain with ≥30 PMN/HPF. Detection of *M. genitalium* was associated with each of these individual findings. This association persisted even when multiple cofactors were accounted for, including chlamydial and gonococcal coinfection, proliferative phase of the menstrual cycle, and age. The authors concluded that *M. genitalium* was independently associated with cervicitis in this population, may cause cervical inflammation, and should be considered a potential etiology of cervicitis. More recent studies appear to confirm this finding. Like *Mycoplasma pneumoniae*, *M. genitalium* appears to be sensitive to macrolides and tetracyclines, but further study is required to confirm the efficacy of these antibiotics in curing lower genital tract infection with this organism. *Mycoplasma genitalium* is difficult to culture and to date, clinical studies have relied on PCR to detect it. Currently, there are no available commercial tests to identify infection with *M. genitalium*. In addition, both the CDC Sexually Transmitted Disease Treatment Guidelines and the UK National Guidelines acknowledge the potential role of this organism in the etiology of cervicitis but do not recommend any change in investigations or management. Other infectious agents have been invoked as causes of cervicitis. Cytomegalovirus (CMV), a herpes virus that can be sexually transmitted, has been isolated in some of the few studies of cervicitis that have looked for it. The small number of studies and subjects involved, as well as the limited descriptions of study design and subject selection, make it difficult to conclude how much CMV contributes to the incidence of nonchlamydial, nongonococcal cervicitis. CMV is shed in secretions at several mucosal sites, and its detection in the setting of cervicitis may represent an "epiphenomenon" of

TABLE 15-1 Etiologies of Cervicitis and Suggested Management

Etiology	Management	Comments
Chlamydia trachomatis	Azithromycin 1 gram PO (single dose) OR Doxycycline 100 mg PO twice daily for 7 days	Minority of infected women have signs of cervicitis Urine, endocervical or vaginal NAAT highly sensitive for diagnosis of endocervical chlamydial infection
Neisseria gonorrhoeae	**Preferred regimens** Cefixime 400 mg PO (single dose) OR Ceftriaxone 250 mg IM (single dose) **Alternative regimens** Spectinomycin 2 g IM (single dose) OR Other single-dose cephalosporins, including ceftizoxime, cefoxitin with probenecid, cefotaxime, cefuroxime axetil, or cefpodoxime PLUS Treatment for chlamydia if chlamydial infection is not ruled out	Oral cefixime has recently been made available in the United States. Alternatively, many experts advocate use of cefpodoxime, 400 mg PO in a single dose As of April 2007, the CDC no longer recommends use of fluoroquinolones because of resistance Minority of infected women have signs of cervicitis Urine, endocervical or vaginal NAAT highly sensitive for diagnosis of endocervical gonococcal infection
Trichomonas vaginalis	Metronidazole 2 g PO (single dose) OR Tinidazole 2 g PO (single dose) OR Metronidazole 400 –500 mg PO twice daily for 7 days	
Herpes simplex virus (HSV)	Any of the following given orally for 7-10 days: Acyclovir 400 mg three times daily Famciclovir 250 mg three times daily Valacyclovir 500–1000 mg twice daily	Primary infection with HSV-2 may cause an especially erosive, hemorrhagic cervicitis
Empiric therapy	Most women should be treated for chlamydial infection Consider therapy for gonococcal infection based on age, risk, and local or patient subgroup prevalence Treat concomitant causes of any vaginitis present appropriately	All women should have diagnostic tests for *Chlamydia trachomatis* and *Neisseria gonorrhoeae* using most sensitive assays available (ideally NAAT) Evaluate for history suggestive of genital herpes, vaginitis, and use of irritative intravaginal preparations (spermicides, deodorants, and chemical douches) Evaluate and treat sex partners appropriately

Abbreviations: IM, intramuscularly; NAAT, nucleic acid amplified test (including polymerase chain reaction, transcription-mediated amplification, strand displacement assay); PO, by mouth.

endocervical inflammation. Recently, cervical shedding of human T-cell lymphotrophic virus 1 (HTLV-1) was found to be associated with the presence of cervicitis as defined by Gram's stain of endocervical secretions or by visible endocervical secretions in a cohort of commercial sex workers in Peru. However, whether HTLV-1 plays an etiologic role in cervical inflammation, or is simply shed in greater quantity during episodes of cervicitis, is not known. Various case reports have attributed the presence of cervicitis in individual women to infection with certain *Streptococcus* species—most notably, *S. agalactiae* (Group B streptococcus) and *S. pyogenes*—but reliable estimates of how commonly this might occur and whether a causal relationship does, indeed, exist, are not available.

Apart from the infections discussed previously, a variety of noninfectious and infectious systemic inflammatory processes and local insults can induce endocervical inflammation that can result in clinically evident cervicitis. Among the former are Behçet's disease, sarcoidosis, ligneous conjunctivitis, and tuberculosis. In the latter group are substances that erode cervicovaginal mucosa or cause an irritant mucositis, usually through frequent use at relatively high concentrations. These substances include chemical douches, some spermicides (specifically those with surfactant properties; nonoxynol-9 [N-9] is the prototype), and chemical deodorants. In one large study in which commercial sex workers were randomized to use vaginal sponges impregnated with 1 g of N-9, cervical erosions as assessed by colposcopy were seen more commonly among N-9 users, who were also more likely to acquire HIV infection during the course of the study than were nonusers.

Other less common causes of cervicitis include inflammatory changes related to trauma from foreign body, such as tampons or pessaries. Some birth control devices, such as diaphragms or cervical caps, can also lead to cervicitis by this means. Allergic reactions to latex condoms or topical contraceptives should also be considered. Finally, radiation therapy and malignancy can lead to changes in the cervix consistent with cervicitis.

■ NONGONOCOCCAL, NONCHLAMYDIAL CERVICITIS: FURTHER CONSIDERATIONS

A vexing clinical problem is that in many cases of cervicitis, neither *C. trachomatis* nor *N. gonorrhoeae* is detected, even when highly sensitive diagnostic tests are used. In addition, many women with these STIs do not present with any signs or symptoms of cervi-

citis. Nonetheless, cervicitis occurring in the absence of detectable gonococcal or chlamydial infection may confer an increased risk of poor pregnancy outcome and predict upper genital tract disease. The etiology of the rather large proportion of cervicitis in which neither gonorrhea nor chlamydia is detected is not clear. An undefined local inflammatory process might be induced or maintained through several pathways, including the effects of a persistent undefined pathogen, persistently abnormal vaginal flora, or an inappropriately exuberant primary host immune response. Such processes are probably further modulated by the effect of endogenous and exogenous hormones, including those experienced throughout the menstrual cycle and with the use of contraceptive formulations.

A possible association between BV and cervicitis, independent of concomitant chlamydial and gonococcal infection, has emerged. BV is the most common cause of vaginitis in diverse clinical settings and is characterized by overgrowth of commensal anaerobic flora relative to the hydrogen peroxide (H_2O_2)-producing *Lactobacillus* species that predominate in the healthy vagina (see Chapter 7). The observation that BV is associated with acquisition of *C. trachomatis* and *N. gonorrhoeae* poses a challenge to definitively demonstrating an independent relationship between BV and cervicitis. However, BV is strongly associated with adverse outcomes related to the upper genital tract, and the vaginal bacteria that characterize BV must cross the endocervical mucous barrier, where they may conceivably elicit a local inflammatory response as a result. More persuasively, including intravaginal antibiotic therapy for BV in the treatment regimen for women with cervicitis was associated with enhanced cure of cervicitis in two small studies. Finally, cervical shedding of HIV increases in the setting of BV, suggesting that BV may have direct effects at the endocervical mucosa.

Emerging data suggest that the risk profile of women who develop cervicitis in the setting of BV is different from that of women at risk for chlamydial or gonococcal infection. In a study of 424 women with BV, cervicitis was relatively common, occurring in 15%, and of these cases, the overwhelming majority (87%) were not associated with chlamydial or gonococcal infection of the cervix. Increasing age, fewer years of formal education, report of a new male sex partner or of a current female sex partner, more recent receptive oral sex, and absence of H_2O_2-producing *Lactobacillus* species were independently associated with an increased likelihood of cervicitis among women with BV. Intriguingly, vaginal colonization with

H₂O₂-producing *Lactobacillus* species was associated with a 60% reduction in the likelihood of cervicitis.

It is increasingly clear that endogenous hormones have a role in maintaining the integrity of cervicovaginal mucosa. Estrogen likely up-regulates and progesterone down-regulates the local immune response to some pathogens. Women with relative estrogen deficiency have an inability to maintain a normal vaginal pH (<4.5), which causes gradual erosion of the endocervical mucous layer. In a large study, women who used depot progesterone as their primary source of contraception were more likely to be diagnosed with endocervical chlamydial and gonococcal infection, as well as clinically diagnosed cervicitis.

■ CLINICAL MANIFESTATIONS AND DIAGNOSIS

Many women with cervicitis experience no symptoms whatsoever, but abnormal vaginal bleeding (after intercourse, between menses, after menopause), dyspareunia, vaginal discharge, urinary symptoms (dysuria, urinary frequency), and vulvovaginal irritation may be presenting complaints. Pain and systemic symptoms such as fever are rarely present in cervicitis and suggest possible involvement of the upper genital tract. Questions in the history regarding cervicitis should include asking about a history of STI risk factors and previous STI, contraception type and use, and use of intravaginal douches or topical vaginal therapies. In women with suspected cervicitis, a careful speculum examination should be performed, as well as a bimanual examination to rule out PID (suggested by cervical motion, lower abdominal or adnexal tenderness) (see Chapter 8). Presence of endocervical purulent discharge or sustained endocervical bleeding easily induced by gentle passage of a cotton swab through the cervical os (see Figure 15-1) are comparably predictive and most specific for cervicitis, but pay attention to the presence of ulcerative lesions of the cervix or of vaginitis.

Clinical definition of cervicitis is syndromic. Most clinicians do not have access to endocervical Gram's stain, and even when this test is performed, its predictive value is highly variable. Because the association between cervicitis and cervical infection with *C. trachomatis* and *N. gonorrhoeae* is well established, the CDC recommends testing for both organisms if cervicitis is present. Use one of the most sensitive diagnostic tests, NAAT, if possible, particularly for chlamydial infections, given the enhanced sensitivity of these tests. Examination of

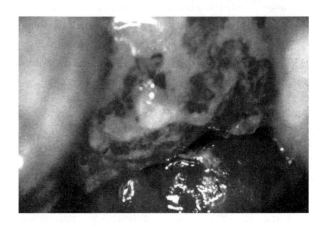

FIGURE 15-1   Cervical Edema, Friability, and Ectopy

vaginal fluid should be performed to look for the presence of bacterial vaginosis, trichomoniasis, or candidiasis, as treatment of concurrent vaginitis might enhance the resolution of cervicitis. Three of four Amsel criteria are sufficient to establish the diagnosis of BV, including presence of homogeneous vaginal discharge, vaginal fluid pH greater than 4.5, clue cells >20% of total vaginal epithelial cells seen on 100× magnification on saline microscopy, and amine (fishy) odor on addition of potassium hydroxide. Saline microscopy also offers the opportunity to look for motile trichomonads (although newer diagnostic tests may enhance clinicians' ability to make this diagnosis more readily and accurately), and for an elevated number of PMN (>10 per high power field), which may indicate a higher likelihood of cervical infection with *C. trachomatis* or *N. gonorrhoeae*.

■ MANAGEMENT

The 2010 CDC STD Treatment Guidelines recommend that empiric treatment of cervicitis directed at *C. trachomatis* and *N. gonorrhoeae* should be provided if the local prevalence of these infections is high, or if the likelihood of a woman's return for treatment based on a diagnostic test that turns out to be positive is judged to be low (see Chapters 5 and 42). Unfortunately, no specific prevalence parameters are provided to help guide clinicians regarding empiric treatment. Other factors that would support presumptive therapy for these infections include report of STI-related risk behavior (especially report of new or multiple sex partners in the prior 60 days, unprotected sex, or age ≤25 years), recent history of STI (especially chlamydial or gonococcal infection in the prior year), or use of a less sensitive diagnostic test (not NAAT). Recurrent infection with *C. trachomatis* is common among women, ranging from 8% to 25% in several studies and probably relates predominantly to resumption of unprotected sex with untreated partners. Although treatment for *C. trachomatis* should be a mainstay of presumptive therapy regimens, the approach involving possible infection with *N. gonorrhoeae* is less clear. Women with cervicitis who fall into subgroups with high prior likelihood of gonococcal infection should be empirically treated; these subgroups include adolescents in inner-city areas in many areas of the United States (prevalence rates >5%). In the United Kingdom, gonorrhea is also predominantly a disease of adolescents in inner-city areas (see Chapter 5).

Treating cervicitis, especially if it is caused by *C. trachomatis* or *N. gonorrhoeae*, is especially important among HIV-infected women, because cervicitis increases the amount of HIV-1 shed from the cervix. One small study demonstrated a decline for HIV-1 shed from the cervical mucosa after empiric treatment of cervicitis aimed at chlamydial and gonococcal infection, which likely reduces these women's risk of transmitting HIV-1 to sex partners. No change in therapy is required for women with HIV infection.

The limited available data suggest that antibiotics aimed at *C. trachomatis* and *N. gonorrhoeae* do not adequately treat nonchlamydial, nongonococcal cervicitis. Concomitant trichomoniasis, HSV, or symptomatic BV should be treated if detected. Further management of cervicitis for which neither identifiable STI nor BV plays a role is empiric and substantiated by little rigorous evidence; approaches include more extended courses of broad-spectrum antibiotics or ablative therapy. Current guidelines do not specify any alternative therapy if *M. genitalium* is suspected. However, many experts would recommend that women with persistent cervicitis and negative testing for *C. trachomatis* and *N. gonorrhoeae* receive a course of antibiotics with the best-proven efficacy against this pathogen

If diagnostic tests reveal infection with *C. trachomatis*, *N. gonorrhoeae*, or *T. vaginalis*, sex partners should be evaluated and treated for the appropriate STI. The CDC does not make any recommendations about treating partners of women without clearly identified etiology of their cervicitis. Women with cervicitis should be instructed to abstain from sexual intercourse for 7 days after a single-dose regimen or after completing a 7-day course of antibiotics to avoid reinfection or fur-

ther transmission. Test-of-cure 3 weeks after diagnosis and treatment of cervicitis is recommended only for pregnant women, women in whom symptoms persist, or in women whose compliance with therapy is questionable. NAAT may produce false-positive or false-negative results if used less than 3 weeks after the initial infection, because of the continued presence of dead organisms or persistent infection with a low burden of infectious organisms, respectively. Although test-of-cure is not routinely recommended, the CDC does encourage retesting all women with proven chlamydial or gonococcal infection 3–12 months after infection to assess for reinfection.

CONCLUSION

Many areas of uncertainty remain with cervicitis. Among the most critical is what should constitute appropriate empiric management of cervicitis in women at relatively low risk for chlamydial or gonococcal infection or in settings where gonococcal disease is relatively uncommon. From the perspective of etiology, it will be interesting to apply molecular methods to detect fastidious or uncultivated microorganisms to cases of nongonococcal, nonchlamydial cervicitis. Moreover, the ideal antibiotic regimen for eradicating *M. genitalium* remains to be determined. In men, a single dose of azithromycin has not been proven effective in treating many cases of *M. genitalium* (see Chapter 14). Because cervicitis increases risk of poor pregnancy outcome, predicts upper genital tract disease, and is associated with increased shedding of HIV-1 from the cervix, defining alternate etiologies and effective treatment for this condition should be a priority. Also, more investigation into whether effective treatment decreases the risks of these complications is imperative. Future research should focus on these issues, including clarification of the cervix's immune response to disruptions in the normal vaginal flora and to varying levels of sex hormones.

KEY POINTS

- Recognition and management of cervicitis is crucial for preventing upper genital tract infection and the accompanying sequelae, as well as neonatal complications.

- While gonococcal and chlamydial infections are commonly associated with cervicitis, other infectious and noninfectious etiologies are also frequently implicated and must be considered.

- Although the terms *mucopurulent cervicitis* and *cervicitis* have been used interchangeably, cervicitis is now considered more appropriate terminology, as mucopurulent cervical discharge or easily friable endocervical mucosa is equally predictive of the clinical syndrome.

- Endocervicitis is most commonly caused by *Chlamydia trachomatis* and *Neisseria gonorrhoeae*. In contrast, ectocervicitis can be caused by pathogens associated with vaginitis, including trichomoniasis, bacterial vaginosis, and vulvovaginal candidiasis, as well as genital ulcerative diseases that occur on the vaginal mucosa, such as HSV and syphilis.

- *Mycoplasma genitalium* is increasingly recognized as a cause of cervicitis; however, at this time, there is neither commercially available test for this infection, nor any specific changes in the recommendations for treatment when this organism is suspected.

- Work-up for cervicitis should include a careful history, physical exam, and the most sensitive laboratory evaluation available for *C. trachomatis* and *N. gonorrhoeae*. Microscopic evaluation of vaginal fluid with saline and potassium hydroxide can also help elucidate possible etiologies of cervicitis.

- It is essential to rule out pelvic inflammatory disease (PID) when making the diagnosis of cervicitis, as the management differs for the two syndromes, and failure to treat PID adequately can increase risk of infertility and ectopic pregnancy.

- Empiric therapy of cervicitis should be considered in women unlikely to return for follow-up, at high risk for sexually transmitted infections, or in high prevalence areas. Otherwise, it is reasonable to wait for the results of diagnostic tests before initiating therapy.

- Treatment of nonchlamydial, nongonococcal cervicitis, as well as recurrent cervicitis, may be challenging, and consultation with an expert should be sought.

- Sex partners of women with cervicitis should be evaluated and treated if an etiology for cervicitis is found. Otherwise, partner treatment is not generally recommended.

REFERENCES

Brunham RC, Paavonen J, Stevens CE, et al. Mucopurulent cervicitis—the ignored counterpart in women of urethritis in men. *N Engl J Med.* 1984;311:1–6.

Centers for Disease Control and Prevention. Sexually transmitted disease treatment guidelines, 2010. *Morb Mortal Week Rep.* 2010;59(RR-12):1–110.

Gaydos C, Maldeis NE, Hardick A, et al. *Mycoplasma genitalium* as a contributor to the multiple etiologies of cervicitis in women attending sexually transmitted disease clinics. *Sex Transm Dis.* 2009;36:598–606.

Geisler WM, Yu S, Venglarik M, Schwebke JR. Vaginal leucocyte counts in women with bacterial vaginosis: relation to vaginal and cervical infections. *Sex Transm Infect.* 2004;80:401–405.

Manhart LE, Critchlow CW, Holmes KK, et al. Mucopurrulent cervicitis and *Mycoplasma genitalium. J Infect Dis.* 2003;187:650–657.

Marrazzo JM, Handsfield HH, Whittington WL. Predicting chlamydial and gonococcal cervical infection: implications for management of cervicitis. *Obstet Gynecol.* 2002;100:579–584.

Marrazzo JM, Johnson RE, Green TA, et al. Impact of patient characteristics on performance of nucleic acid amplification tests and DNA probe for detection of *Chlamydia trachomatis* in women with genital infections. *J Clin Microbiol.* 2005;43:577–584.

Marrazzo JM, Martin DH. Management of women with cervicitis. *Clin Infect Dis.* 2007;44(suppl 3):S102–S110.

Marrazzo JM, Wiesenfeld HC, Murray PJ, et al. Risk factors for cervicitis among women with bacterial vaginosis. *J Infect Dis.* 2006;193:617–24.

McClelland RS, Wang CC, Mandaliya K, et al. Treatment of cervicitis is associated with decreased cervical shedding of HIV-1. *Aids.* 2001;15:105–110.

Morrison CS, Bright P, Wong EL, et al. Hormonal contraceptive use, cervical ectopy, and the acquisition of cervical infections. *Sex Transm Dis.* 2004;31:561–567.

Nugent RP, Hillier SL. Mucopurulent cervicitis as a predictor of chlamydial infection and adverse pregnancy outcome. The Investigators of the Johns Hopkins Study of Cervicitis and Adverse Pregnancy Outcome. *Sex Transm Dis.* 1992;19:198–202.

Nyirjesy P. Nongonococcal and nonchlamydial cervicitis. *Curr Infect Dis Rep.* 2001;3:540–545.

Peipert JF, Ness RB, Soper DE, Bass D. Association of lower genital tract inflammation with objective evidence of endometritis. *Infect Dis Obstet Gynecol.* 2000;8:83–87.

Schwebke JR, Schulien MB, and Zajackowski M. Pilot study to evaluate the appropriate management of patients with coexistent bacterial vaginosis and cervicitis. *Infect Dis Obstet Gynecol.* 1995;3:119–122.

16

Acute Pelvic Pain

Mark H. Yudin and Harold C. Wiesenfeld

INTRODUCTION

The accurate clinical diagnosis of a reproductive age woman presenting with acute pelvic or abdominal pain is a challenge. Pelvic pain is a common presenting symptom of many gynecologic disorders. However, it also may be seen with disorders of the gastrointestinal, urinary, and musculoskeletal systems. To determine the etiology of the pain, the clinician must use the history, physical examination, and diagnostic tests as tools. In this chapter, we will present a framework to assist in classifying and diagnosing acute pelvic pain. We will then outline the role of the history, physical examination, and laboratory tests and conclude with a brief discussion of selected specific disorders.

DIFFERENTIAL DIAGNOSIS OF ACUTE PELVIC PAIN

Numerous studies have confirmed that it is often difficult to arrive at a definitive diagnosis in women of reproductive age with acute pelvic pain. A comprehensive evaluation leading to a timely diagnosis will reduce the morbidity associated with delayed diagnosis.

To assist with diagnosing acute pelvic pain, it is convenient to divide the causes into pregnancy related, gynecologic, and nongynecologic. The gynecologic causes can be further subdivided into infectious and noninfectious. This classification is presented in Table 16-1.

HISTORY

The first step in evaluating the patient with acute pelvic pain is to obtain a careful history, which can be the source of important diagnostic clues. The essential features of the history are presented in Table 16-2.

AGE

Infectious causes of pain such as pelvic inflammatory disease (PID) and appendicitis are more common in younger women (adolescents and women younger than 30 years), while disorders such as diverticulitis are more commonly seen in women older than 40 years. The differential diagnosis of pain grouped by patient age is presented in Table 16-3.

PAIN CHARACTERISTICS

Pain of sudden onset suggests an acute event, while pain that is more gradual may be seen with subacute or progressive conditions. The differential diagnosis of pain grouped by time of onset is presented in Table 16-4. The location of the pain may also be helpful, although different etiologies can lead to pain in the same region. The uterus, cervix, and adnexae share visceral innervation with the lower ileum, the sigmoid, and rectum (T10 to L1), and pain from any of these structures may be felt in the same place. Diffuse and generalized pain should alert the clinician to the possibility of peritonitis.

Although pain quality and severity are nonspecific, they may provide some clue about the etiology. Abrupt and severe pain is typically associated with perforation (ectopic pregnancy), strangulation (ovarian torsion), or hemorrhage (ovarian cysts). Crampy pain is often seen with dysmenorrhea or spontaneous abortion. Colicky

TABLE 16-1   The Differential Diagnosis of Acute Pelvic Pain

1. **Pregnancy related**
   Spontaneous abortion
   Threatened
   Complete
   Incomplete
   Septic
   Ectopic pregnancy

2. **Gynecologic: infectious**
   Endometritis
   PID/salpingitis
   TOA

3. **Gynecologic: noninfectious**
   Dysmenorrhea
   Uterine fibroids
   Endometriosis
   Mittelschmerz (midcycle ovulatory pain)
   Ovarian cysts
   Rupture
   Hemorrhage
   Torsion
   Ovarian cancer/tumor
   Ovarian hyperstimulation syndrome

4. **Nongynecologic**
   Gastrointestinal
      Appendicitis
      Gastroenteritis
      Diverticulitis
      Inflammatory bowel disease
      Irritable bowel syndrome
      Bowel obstruction
      Mesenteric lymphadenitis
      Constipation
      Abdominopelvic adhesions
   Urinary tract
      Lower urinary tract infection/cystitis
      Interstitial cystitis
      Pyelonephritis
      Nephrolithiasis
   Musculoskeletal
      Strained tendons/muscles
      Joint infection/inflammation
      Hernia
   Other
      Aortic aneurysm
      Aortic dissection
      Porphyria

PID = pelvic inflammatory disease; TOA = tubo-ovarian abscess.

TABLE 16-2   Historic Data Useful in the Differential Diagnosis of Acute Pelvic Pain

1. **Patient Age**

2. **Pain Characteristics**
   Onset
   Position
   Quality
   Radiation
   Severity
   Aggravating/alleviating factors
   Associated symptoms
   Urinary symptoms
   Gastrointestinal symptoms
   Fever/chills
   Vaginal bleeding
   Vaginal discharge
   Treatment tried

3. **Obstetrical and Gynecologic History**
   LMP
   STIs/PID
   Ectopic pregnancy
   Uterine fibroids/ovarian cysts
   Menstrual history
   Contraceptive history
   Sexual history

4. **Medical/Surgical History**

5. **Social History**
   Marital status

LMP = last menstrual period; STI = sexually transmitted infection; PID = pelvic inflammatory disease

TABLE 16-3 Differential Diagnoses: Grouped by Age

1. **Menarche to Age 21 Years**
   Dysmenorrhea
   PID
   Ovarian cysts
   Rupture
   Hemorrhage
   Torsion
   Pregnancy
   Spontaneous abortion
   Ectopic pregnancy
   Appendicitis
   Inflammatory bowel disease

2. **Aged 21 to 35 Years**
   Ovarian cysts
   Endometriosis
   Pregnancy

   Spontaneous abortion
   Ectopic pregnancy
   PID
   Irritable bowel syndrome

3. **Age 35 to Menopause**
   Uterine fibroids
   Endometriosis
   Ovarian cancer/tumor
   Pregnancy
   Abortion
   Ectopic pregnancy
   Nephrolithiasis
   Irritable bowel syndrome
   Diverticulitis
   Hernias
   PID

PID = pelvic inflammatory disease

Note: There is considerable overlap between age groups, and disorders are not listed in order of frequency.

TABLE 16-4 Differential Diagnoses Grouped by Time of Onset

1. **Acute Onset (seconds–minutes)**
   Ovarian cysts
   Rupture
   Hemorrhage
   Torsion
   Rupture
   TOA
   Abdominal aortic aneurysm
   Ectopic pregnancy
   Aortic dissection
   Nephrolithiasis

2. **Gradual Onset (hours–days)**
   Appendicitis
   Diverticulitis
   Herpes zoster
   Gastroenteritis
   Mittelschmerz
   Primary dysmenorrhea
   Abortion

3. **Slow Onset (days–weeks)**
   Neoplasms
   Cystitis
   Pyelonephritis
   Ectopic pregnancy
   PID
   Diverticulitis
   Abortion
   Abdominal aortic aneurysm

4. **Chronic Onset (weeks–months)**
   Neoplasms
   Endometriosis
   Uterine fibroids
   Chronic pelvic pain
   Domestic violence/sexual abuse
   Diverticular disease
   Irritable bowel syndrome
   Inflammatory bowel disease

TOA = tubo-ovarian abscess; PID = pelvic inflammatory disease.

pain typifies ovarian torsion or nephrolithiasis. Burning or aching pain often occurs with inflammatory processes, such as appendicitis or PID.

ASSOCIATED SYMPTOMS

Associated symptoms are often helpful when trying to narrow in on a diagnosis. Pain with fever suggests an infectious or inflammatory etiology, such as appendicitis, PID, or a tubo-ovarian abscess (TOA). Nausea, vomiting, and anorexia are nonspecific symptoms of peritoneal irritation that can be seen with inflammatory conditions and hemoperitoneum. Vaginal discharge can be seen with infectious conditions of the female genital tract, such as cervicitis or PID. Vaginal bleeding may be associated with pregnancy-related disorders, abnormalities of the menstrual cycle, PID, or pathology of the uterus or cervix.

AGGRAVATING AND ALLEVIATING FACTORS

Changes in pain may occur in relation to menses, coitus, activity, diet, bowel movements, or voiding. These pain characteristics may help in narrowing the differential diagnosis.

OBSTETRIC AND GYNECOLOGIC HISTORY

A complete obstetric and gynecologic history, including menstrual, contraceptive, and sexual histories, is essential. The patient's gravidity, parity, and past obstetric history should be established. The past gynecologic history, including previous episodes of sexually transmitted infections (STIs), PID, and ectopic pregnancy, is important.

A menstrual history, including last normal menstrual period, can be helpful. The results of some studies have suggested that PID is more likely to occur in the first half of the menstrual cycle, while appendicitis is randomly distributed. A contraceptive history is also of diagnostic value. Women not using reliable contraception are at risk for pregnancy. Women not using barrier methods of contraception are at increased risk for STIs and PID, while those using barrier methods or combined oral contraceptives have a reduction in the risk of PID of approximately 50%. The presence of an intrauterine contraceptive device (IUD) increases the risk for developing acute PID, particularly around the time of insertion, but does not increase the absolute risk for developing an ectopic pregnancy. However, an IUD is more effective at preventing

intrauterine versus extrauterine gestation, so a pregnancy that occurs with an IUD in place has a 10-fold increased risk of being ectopic.

Finally, a sexual history is important (see Chapter 2). Information about sexual habits and risky behavior, current partners, new sexual partners in the past 3–6 months, and number of lifetime partners helps the clinician to estimate the patient's risk of STIs and PID.

MEDICAL AND SURGICAL HISTORY

A history of urinary or gastrointestinal tract disorders may be a clue to the current problem. Surgical history may help to rule out certain disorders, such as appendicitis, or heighten awareness of the possibility of other problems, such as ectopic pregnancy in a patient with previous pelvic or tubal surgery.

PHYSICAL EXAMINATION

Observation is an important first step and often helps to assess the severity of the patient's condition. Vital signs, especially temperature, must be obtained. Fever can help to identify an inflammatory process but may not help to specify which one. If hemorrhage is suspected, such as in ruptured ectopic pregnancy or hemorrhagic ovarian cysts, orthostatic pulse and blood pressure should be measured to evaluate for hypovolemia.

The important components of the abdominal examination include inspection, auscultation, percussion, and palpation. Percussion and palpation can help to identify masses and peritoneal irritation. Peritoneal irritation is confirmed by the presence of rebound tenderness, involuntary guarding, and increased pain with motion or cough.

The next step in the physical examination is the pelvic examination. This is most easily organized from external to internal structures. The external genitalia should be carefully inspected for lesions (see discussion in Chapter 4 about examining the female patient). The presence of inguinal adenopathy suggests a local infectious process. On speculum examination, the vagina and cervix should be visualized. Lesions, blood, or discharge should be noted. The presence of cervical discharge, erythema, or friability should alert the clinician to the possibility of cervicitis or PID. Grossly purulent cervical discharge (mucopus) reflects a high concentration of polymorphonuclear leukocytes in the mucus, but the presence of mucopus has not been shown to accurately predict PID. On internal pelvic examination, the first step should be an assessment for cervical motion tenderness (CMT) or "excitation." Its presence is nonspecific and may indicate PID, ectopic pregnancy, endometriosis, ovarian cysts, or appendicitis. Next, a bimanual examination should be performed, with assessment of the uterus and adnexae. Pain on bimanual examination may occur with endometritis, degenerating uterine fibroids, endometriosis, PID, ovarian cysts or torsion, ectopic pregnancy, or appendicitis. Finally, digital rectal and rectovaginal examinations should be considered, especially if the diagnosis is unclear.

When interpreting the pelvic examination, remember that movement of the pelvic organs will be painful if peritoneal irritation is present, regardless of the cause. Therefore, CMT and adnexal tenderness may be found with a variety of disorders. In one study that compared findings in patients with PID and appendicitis, CMT was found significantly more often in patients with PID but was still found in 28% of patients with appendicitis. Adnexal tenderness was found with equal frequency in both groups but was usually limited to the right side in patients with appendicitis and was usually, but not always, bilateral in patients with PID.

■ DIAGNOSTIC TESTS AND IMAGING

Laboratory and diagnostic imaging tests may be helpful with the differential diagnosis of acute pelvic pain but should be interpreted cautiously. Baseline tests should include at least a complete blood count (CBC) and highly sensitive urine pregnancy test. A serum beta human chorionic gonadotropin (β-hCG) pregnancy test may also be considered, although urine tests are highly accurate. In one study, the peripheral white blood cell (WBC) count was significantly higher in those with appendicitis than in those with PID (15.3 vs. 12.7, p < 0.01). However, note that the CBC has a low sensitivity and specificity. The hematocrit is low in roughly one-third of patients with ectopic pregnancy but normal in another third. In studies, a normal WBC count has been found in more than half of patients with PID and in one-third of patients with acute appendicitis, while an elevated WBC count is commonly seen in patients with ectopic pregnancies and bleeding corpus luteum cysts. The erythrocyte sedimentation rate (ESR) is another nonspecific sign of inflammation. It is classically elevated in PID but can be normal in up to 25% of patients.

A urinalysis should be performed on every patient with acute pelvic pain to rule out the presence of a urinary tract infection or stone. Care must be taken with specimen collection to avoid contamination by vaginal or cervical discharge. Cervical, urine, or vaginal swab specimens should be obtained to test for *Neisseria gonorrhoeae* and *Chlamydia trachomatis* (see Chapter 5). Vaginal fluid should be collected for pH measurement, saline wet mount, and potassium hydroxide (KOH) preparation to diagnose bacterial vaginosis, *Trichomonas vaginalis*, and yeast infection (see Chapter 7). The majority of women with PID will have leukocytes present on wet mount.

Imaging studies, especially ultrasound, may be useful in making the diagnosis. Ultrasound is invaluable in evaluating the gynecologic organs and may help to identify ovarian cysts, pelvic masses, and uterine lesions, such as fibroids. Transvaginal ultrasound may offer more information than abdominal or pelvic ultrasound. The utility of ultrasound in the work-up for PID and TOA is discussed elsewhere in Chapter 8. Computed tomography (CT) and magnetic resonance imaging (MRI) scanning may also be useful to evaluate women presenting with pelvic pain, especially if a nongynecologic cause is part of the differential diagnosis.

In difficult cases, diagnostic laparoscopy is perhaps the most definitive way to arrive at a diagnosis in a patient with acute pelvic pain. It is the best and most reliable method to achieve a complete evaluation of the pelvic structures and allows direct visual access to the peritoneal cavity. Although laparoscopy is minimally invasive, it does carry some risks with it. Vascular injuries, injuries to the gastrointestinal tract, and urinary tract have been reported with a risk estimated at 2/1000 to 3/1000.

■ INTERPRETATION OF PATIENT WORK-UP

To establish a working diagnosis in the woman of reproductive age with acute pelvic pain, the clinician must use all of the tools previously discussed. Clinical history, physical examination, laboratory tests, and imaging procedures are useful in providing diagnostic clues, but they may lack adequate sensitivity or specificity to make a final diagnosis. Despite a comprehensive history and physical examination, a significant proportion of patients with acute pelvic pain will continue to have an unclear diagnosis.

■ PREGNANCY-RELATED CAUSES OF ACUTE PELVIC PAIN

The most common pregnancy-related causes of acute pelvic pain are abortion (threatened, incomplete, and septic) and ectopic pregnancy.

Spontaneous Abortion

Spontaneous abortion is defined as a pregnancy that ends spontaneously before 20 weeks of gestation and is estimated to occur in 15–20% of all pregnancies. Classic symptoms are amenorrhea followed by abdominal pain and vaginal bleeding. The pain is typically midline and crampy. The differential diagnosis includes an ectopic gestation until the pregnancy is proved to be intrauterine.

Ectopic Pregnancy

Ectopic pregnancy should be considered as a diagnosis in any sexually active woman who presents with acute pelvic pain. It occurs when a fertilized ovum implants at any site outside of the endometrial cavity. In most cases, implantation occurs in the fallopian tube, but ectopic pregnancies have been reported in the ovary, cervix, and peritoneal cavity. The most important risk factor is a history of salpingitis. Other risk factors include prior tubal surgery or ligation, current IUD use, and prior ectopic pregnancy. After one ectopic pregnancy, there is a 10–20% chance that the next pregnancy will be ectopic.

Pelvic pain is the most common single symptom in patients with ectopic pregnancy. The nature of the pain is variable and may be well localized or more generalized if intraperitoneal bleeding has occurred. A history of abnormal bleeding is also often present. The physical examination of patients with ectopic pregnancy can also be variable and can range from subtle findings to shock if a rupture occurs. An adnexal mass is only palpable in roughly one-third of patients.

The mainstays of diagnosis with ectopic pregnancy are urine or serum β-hCG and ultrasound. Currently available highly sensitive urine tests can detect hCG levels as low as 25 mIU/mL. Current serum assays for β-hCG are also sensitive, and a negative result rules out pregnancy. A single level has limited utility, but serial measurements are useful. The β-hCG should rise by 65% or greater in a 48-hour period in a normal intrauterine gestation. A slow rise or a plateau in the level should alert the clinician to the presence of an abnormal pregnancy. Ultrasound can also be of great value in diagnosing ectopic pregnancy. A viable intrauterine pregnancy should be seen on transabdominal ultrasound at an β-hCG level of 6500 mIU/mL and on transvaginal ultrasound at a level of 1000–2000 mIU/mL. If an intrauterine gestation is seen, an ectopic pregnancy can be essentially ruled out as the likelihood of coexisting gestations is exceptionally rare in spontaneous conception.

■ INFECTIOUS GYNECOLOGIC CAUSES OF ACUTE PELVIC PAIN

Infectious gynecologic causes of acute pelvic pain include endometritis, PID, and tubo-ovarian abscess.

Endometritis

Endometritis is defined as an infection of the lining of the uterus. It may occur postpartum (following vaginal delivery or cesarean section) or as part of the progression of ascending infection from the cervix to the fallopian tubes. It may also be found following instrumentation of the endometrial cavity, such as with elective abortion, hysteroscopy, or dilatation and curettage.

Endometritis is a polymicrobial infection. Organisms include aerobic and anaerobic bacteria, *Mycoplasma hominis, Ureaplasma urealyticum, N. gonorrhoeae, C. trachomatis,* and perhaps *Mycoplasma genitalium.* Patients typically present with fever, abdominal pain, and vaginal discharge. Uterine tenderness is usually found on examination. Patients often have an elevated WBC count. Endometritis can progress to myometritis, parametritis, or peritonitis. Some authors advocate the use of endometrial culture using a sampling device to make the diagnosis. Because of its polymicrobial nature, treatment should be with an antibiotic regimen covering a broad spectrum of bacteria. Dilatation and curettage is necessary in the setting of retained products of conception.

Pelvic Inflammatory Disease (PID) and Tubo-Ovarian Abscess (TOA)

Pelvic inflammatory disease (PID) is discussed in detail in Chapter 8. The clinical diagnosis of PID is often difficult to make. There is no single historical, physical, or laboratory finding that is both sensitive and specific for the diagnosis of PID. The most common nongynecologic disorder to be confused with PID is appendicitis.

Lower abdominal pain is the most consistent symptom in patients with confirmed PID. In most cases, the pain has been present for less than 3 weeks, and often for less than 1 week. Pain lasting longer than 3 weeks is unlikely to be caused by PID. Patients may also complain of other nonspecific symptoms, including vaginal discharge or bleeding, nausea, vomiting, a change in bowel habits, and urinary symptoms. The specificity of any single symptom is low.

On physical examination, fever is sometimes seen but is not always present. On abdominal and pelvic examination, it is common to find bilateral lower abdominal, uterine, adnexal, and cervical motion tenderness (or CMT, known also as cervical excitation). The Centers for Disease Control and Prevention (CDC) in its 2010 guidelines, list lower abdominal pain, and uterine/adnexal or CMT as the minimum criteria for diagnosing PID. Treatment for PID is outlined in Chapter 8 and in the CDC Treatment Guidelines (CDC 2010).

TOAs occur in 15–34% of women with acute PID. The proximity of the ovary to the fallopian tube places it at risk for infection, and the abscess may spread to involve other contiguous structures, such as bowel, bladder, or the opposite adnexa. The diagnosis of TOA is most accurately made with ultrasound, typically appearing as a complex or cystic adnexal mass with multiple internal echoes.

■ NONINFECTIOUS GYNECOLOGIC CAUSES OF ACUTE PELVIC PAIN

Noninfectious gynecologic cause of acute pelvic pain include dysmenorrhea, uterine fibroids, endometriosis, Mittelschmerz, ovarian cysts, adnexal torsion, ovarian cancer or tumors, ovarian hyperstimulation syndrome (OHSS), and pain following sexual assault.

Dysmenorrhea

Dysmenorrhea usually appears within 1 to 2 years of menarche, when ovulatory cycles are established. It is more commonly a cause of chronic than acute pain. It is caused by an increased production of, or response to, endometrial prostaglandins. It typically presents as recurrent and crampy suprapubic pain occurring in the first few days of the menstrual cycle. The treatment is with prostaglandin synthase inhibitors, such as nonsteroidal anti-inflammatory drugs (NSAIDs), or combined oral contraceptives.

Uterine Fibroids

Uterine fibroids are benign estrogen-responsive growths arising from the myometrium. They are the most common neoplasm of the female pelvis and occur in 20–25% of women of reproductive age. The most common age for presentation with pain is older than 35 years. Patients often present with a sensation of pressure in the pelvis, and acute pain is uncommon unless there is fibroid degeneration or torsion. Physical examination may reveal an irregularly enlarged and firm uterus that is often nontender. Diagnostic evaluation is best accomplished with ultrasound. Management is either medical with NSAIDs, hormonal suppression with GnRH agonists, or surgical with myomectomy or hysterectomy.

Endometriosis

Endometriosis is defined as the presence of endometrial tissue (glands and stroma) outside of the uterus. It is most commonly found in the pelvis, on the pelvic organs and peritoneum. The prevalence varies widely in studies but is probably between 5% and 20% of reproductive-aged women. Roughly, one-third of women with endometriosis are asymptomatic. Of those with symptoms, chronic pelvic pain is common, although acute pain may also be seen. Dysmenorrhea that begins after years of pain-free menses suggests endometriosis. Other symptoms that may occur include dyspareunia (painful intercourse) and pain with urination or bowel movements. Classic physical examination findings include a fixed and retroverted uterus, tenderness and nodularity in the cul-de-sac and on the uterosacral ligaments, and ovarian enlargement. Treatment is either medical or surgical. Medical therapy includes oral contraceptives, progestins, Danazol, or GnRH agonists. The objective of surgical therapy is to restore normal anatomy and to remove or ablate as much disease as possible, and this can be accomplished with laparoscopy or laparotomy.

Ovarian Cysts

Physiological cysts of the ovary, such as follicular and corpus luteum cysts, should not cause pain unless they lead to rupture, hemorrhage, or torsion. In the absence of complications, these cysts are best managed expectantly, as they usually resolve spontaneously within 4 to 8 weeks.

Rupture of a follicular cyst leads to release of fluid, which may irritate the peritoneum and cause pain. This pain is typically sudden in onset and may be severe but resolves without treatment. Corpus luteum cysts are vascular, and rupture can lead to severe hemorrhage and pain that can be indistinguishable from the pain of a ruptured ectopic pregnancy. Serum β-hCG and ultrasound are helpful in making a diagnosis. If the diagnosis of a ruptured corpus luteum cyst is confirmed and the patient is stable, expectant management may be appropriate. If significant hemorrhage is suspected or the patient is unstable, surgery is required.

Adnexal Torsion

Adnexal torsion occurs when the adnexa twists on its connection to the uterus, the utero-ovarian ligament. Torsion most commonly involves the ovary but may involve the fallopian tube as well. Torsion is usually preceded by enlargement of the ovary with an ovarian cyst or neoplasm; torsion of the normal ovary and adnexa is uncommon. Adnexal torsion is an acute surgical emergency. With torsion, the blood supply to the adnexa is interrupted, and this can lead to necrosis and infarction.

Adnexal torsion usually occurs in women of reproductive age. Patients typically present with sudden and severe unilateral, colicky, lower abdominal pain. In two-thirds of cases, there is associated nausea and vomiting. Physical examination reveals an enlarged, tender adnexal mass in up to 90% of patients. There may also be abdominal tenderness and guarding. Patients are usually afebrile, but an elevation in the WBC count may be seen. The management is surgical and is typically done with laparoscopy. The current surgical approach involves untwisting the adnexa and assessing its viability. If it is gangrenous, it must be removed. If an ovarian cyst is present, a cystectomy should be done to obtain a histological diagnosis.

Domestic Violence and Sexual Assault

Of particular importance is the patient who presents with pelvic pain following an episode of domestic violence or sexual assault. It is estimated that up to 44% of all women have been the victims of an actual or attempted assault at some time in their lives. Women who have suffered abuse may account for 22–35% of women seeking care for any reason in an emergency department. Finally, it has been estimated that 2 million cases of domestic violence occur each year in the United States. The patient may present with vague symptoms and pain that is not well localized and may not volunteer that she has been the victim of assault. These patients need to be evaluated by clinicians familiar with the appropriate counseling and specimen collection techniques. Most hospitals will have an assault or crisis team with a protocol for evaluating and managing these patients. Physical examination is tailored to a systematic search for injuries and to the collection of samples. Appropriate work-up includes screening for sexually transmitted disease, hepatitis B and C, and pregnancy and human immunodeficiency virus (HIV) testing. Consideration must also be given to emergency contraception and prophylaxis for STDs and HIV. (See Chapter 33.)

■ NONGYNECOLOGIC CAUSES OF ACUTE PELVIC PAIN

Nongynecologic causes of acute pelvic pain include disorders of the gastrointestinal, urinary, and musculoskeletal systems.

Gastrointestinal

Disorders of the gastrointestinal tract that lead to acute pelvic pain include appendicitis, gastroenteritis, diverticulitis, inflammatory bowel disease (IBD), irritable bowel syndrome (IBS), bowel obstruction, mesenteric lymphadenitis, and constipation.

In women of reproductive age, acute appendicitis is the most common nongynecologic disorder for which PID is mistaken. There is often a prodromal period of vague abdominal discomfort followed by periumbilical pain that ultimately shifts to the right lower quadrant. Associated symptoms include nausea, vomiting, and anorexia. Initial physical examination findings are right lower quadrant tenderness and low-grade fever. With progression of the condition, local inflammation of the parietal peritoneum produces peritoneal signs on examination. Diagnostic studies that may be helpful include CBC (which often shows an elevated WBC count) and abdominal imaging. Abdominal ultrasound and CT may demonstrate edema of the appendiceal wall or an abscess. The treatment of acute appendicitis is surgical.

The diagnosis of acute appendicitis in young women is especially difficult because of the significant overlap with gynecologic disorders in symptoms and signs. The most common gynecologic disorder to be confused with appendicitis is PID. Both of these disorders can present with acute pelvic pain, fever, CMT, and adnexal tenderness on physical examination. When peritoneal irritation is present, movement of the pelvic organs (and especially the cervix) during bimanual examination will be painful. Therefore, a finding of CMT does not rule out appendicitis. In one study that compared findings among patients with acute appendicitis and PID, some distinguishing features were identified. Nausea and vomiting were usually present in patients with appendicitis but only in roughly half of those with PID. On physical examination, findings were usually localized to the right lower quadrant in patients with appendicitis, while they tended to be bilateral in patients with PID. Finally, the total WBC count was higher in patients with appendicitis than in those with PID.

Gastroenteritis and diverticulitis may also present with acute pain and fever. Gastroenteritis can occur at any age and is often accompanied by nausea, vomiting, and diarrhea. Diverticulitis is typically seen in women older than 40 years. The presentation is often similar to appendicitis except that the pain is usually on the left side. IBD, IBS, bowel obstruction, mesenteric lymphadenitis, and constipation can all present with acute pelvic pain and should be considered in the differential diagnosis.

Urinary Tract Disorders

Disorders of the urinary tract that lead to acute pelvic pain include lower urinary tract infection, pyelonephritis, and nephrolithiasis (see also Chapter 24). With lower urinary tract infection, typical symptoms and signs include dysuria, urgency, frequency, and suprapubic tenderness. Systemic symptoms are absent. Treatment can usually be accomplished with oral antibiotics. With pyelonephritis, patients are often unwell and typically present with dysuria, urgency, frequency, fever, and chills. Tenderness is localized to the costovertebral angle and flank. Urinalysis is positive for bacteria and white blood cells, and there is usually an elevated WBC count.

Nephrolithiasis leads to pain due to the distention and muscular contraction of the urinary tract against obstruction. Patients present with severe and colicky pain that may radiate down the flank and into the pelvis. There may be associated nausea and vomiting, but no fever. Urinalysis is positive for blood, and imaging studies reveal the stone and a dilated ureter or kidney. Management is usually expectant and involves analgesia and hydration.

Musculoskeletal

Disorders of the musculoskeletal system that lead to acute pelvic pain include muscle or tendon strains, and joint infections or inflammation. Musculoskeletal pain is most commonly confused with pain originating from the urinary tract. The diagnosis can usually be made with history and physical examination alone. On examination, tenderness tends to be superficial. Most pain experienced principally in the lower back rather than in the pelvis is musculoskeletal in origin. Management is usually medical, with muscle relaxants or NSAIDs.

■ CONCLUSION

The woman of reproductive age presenting with acute pelvic or abdominal pain remains one of the great diagnostic dilemmas of clinical medicine. Pelvic pain is a common presenting symptom of many gynecologic disorders. The differential diagnosis also includes various disorders of the gastrointestinal, urinary, and musculoskeletal systems. To assist with the diagnosis, it is convenient to divide the causes into pregnancy related, gynecologic, and nongynecologic. The gynecologic

causes can be further subdivided into infectious and noninfectious. The history, physical examination, and diagnostic tests should then be used to determine the etiology of the pain. By using a methodical and systematic approach, the clinician will increase his or her chance of arriving at the correct diagnosis.

■ KEY POINTS

- It is often difficult to arrive at a definitive diagnosis in women of reproductive age with acute pelvic pain. To determine the etiology of the pain, the clinician must use the history, physical examination, and diagnostic tests as tools.

- The uterus, cervix, and adnexae share visceral innervation with the lower ileum, the sigmoid, and rectum (T10 to L1), and pain from any of these structures may be felt in the same place.

- A menstrual history is essential in evaluating the woman of reproductive age with acute pelvic pain. A pregnancy test must be done to rule out pregnancy. If the test is positive, an ectopic pregnancy must be considered in the differential diagnosis.

- A careful abdominal and pelvic examination is useful. When interpreting the pelvic examination, remember that movement of the pelvic organs will be painful if peritoneal irritation is present, regardless of the cause.

- Transvaginal ultrasound may be useful as a diagnostic tool in women with pelvic pain, as it usually allows good visualization of the gynecologic organs.

- No single historical, physical, or laboratory finding is both sensitive and specific for diagnosing pelvic inflammatory disease (PID). Women present with a wide variety of symptoms and signs that often overlap with other disorders, so the clinician must have a high index of suspicion for this possible diagnosis.

- One-third of women with endometriosis are asymptomatic. Of those with symptoms, the most common are pelvic pain, dysmenorrhea, and dyspareunia. Pain from endometriosis is more often chronic rather than acute.

- Adnexal torsion is an acute surgical emergency.

- The possibility of domestic assault must always be considered when women present with acute pelvic pain.

REFERENCES

Bongard F, Landers DV, Lewis F. Differential diagnosis of appendicitis and pelvic inflammatory disease. *Am J Surg.* 1985;150:90–96.

Brenner PF, Roy S, Mishell DR Jr. Ectopic pregnancy—a study of 300 consecutive surgically treated cases. *JAMA.* 1980;243:673–676.

British Association of Sexual Health and HIV (BASHH). Clinical guidelines. http://www.bashh.org/guidelines.htm.

Centers for Disease Control and Prevention. Sexually Transmitted Diseases Treatment Guidelines 2010. *Morb Mortal Wkly Rep.* 2010;59(RR-12):1–110.

Faro S, Maccato M. Pelvic pain and infections. *Obstet Gynecol Clin North Am.* 1990;17:441–455.

Hewitt GD, Brown RT. Acute and chronic pelvic pain in female adolescents. *Med Clin North Am.* 2000;84:1009–1025.

Quan M. Diagnosis of acute pelvic pain. *J Fam Pract.* 1992;35: 422–432.

Robertson C. Differential diagnosis of lower abdominal pain in women of childbearing age. *Lippincotts Prim Care Pract.* 1998;2:210–229.

Tarraza HM, Moore RD. Gynecologic causes of the acute abdomen and the acute abdomen in pregnancy. *Surg Clin North Am.* 1997;77:1371–1394.

17

Genital Ulcer Disease

Michael Augenbraun

■ INTRODUCTION

In the "real world" of most medical practice, patients only rarely present to the clinician with "neatly" diagnosed conditions. Most often, the clinician is confronted with the task of evaluating a problem or a constellation of problems that present as a disruption of function or anatomy. The test of the clinician's skill is whether he or she can link the complaint and a cause, counsel appropriately, and then institute management strategies.

The patient with a sexually transmitted infection usually presents for the care of a perceived problem, which is usually (but not always) limited to the genitourinary tract. One of the most common of these problems is a noticeable disruption of genital epithelium. Diseases that cause this problem are collectively termed genital ulcer disease (GUD). Disruption of epithelium may occur on either keratinized or nonkeratinized tissue. Lesions can be linear, serpiginous or circular, indurated or nonindurated. They may occur singly or in groups. They can be tender or nontender. They may resolve with or without therapy. Because the long-term sequelae, specific interventions, and response to treatment of GUD may differ depending on the pathogen involved, the clinician needs to know the salient characteristics of each.

Genital ulcer disease can arise from either infectious or noninfectious causes (see Table 17-1). Infectious causes are further divided into sexually transmitted or nonsexually transmitted etiologies. The major sexually transmitted entities include syphilis, herpes simplex virus, chancroid, lymphogranuloma venereum (LGV), and granuloma inguinale. Nonsexually transmit-

ted infectious etiologies are uncommon. They include endemic forms of treponematosis, amebiasis, varicella-zoster, and ectoparasitic infestations (e.g., scabies). Noninfectious causes of GUD are also uncommon but should be considered in the differential diagnosis, particularly when diagnostic or treatment strategies aimed at venereal etiologies do not result in clinical improvement. Nonvenereal dermatoses are reviewed in Chapter 11.

TABLE 17-1 Differential Diagnosis of Genital Ulcer Disease

Sexually Transmitted Diseases
Herpes
Syphilis

Chancroid
Human immunodeficiency virus (primary ulcerations)
Uncommon in United States:
    Lymphogranuloma venereum
    Granuloma inguinale (Donovanosis)
Chronic:
    Epidermal carcinomas

Other Etiologies
Varicella zoster
Cytomegalovirus
Behcet's syndrome
Trauma

SEXUALLY TRANSMITTED GUD

Sexually transmitted GUD is more common in the developing world than in the developed world. The prevalence of specific etiologies differs depending on location, socioeconomic factors and temporal trends. An accurate assessment of the prevalence and incidence of any of these etiologies is hampered by a shortage of accurate diagnostic tests at most sites where clinical care is often rendered. Although each infectious process is associated with certain key clinical characteristics, purely clinical judgment as to the etiology of GUD is notoriously inaccurate. Perhaps 50–70% of cases can be diagnosed in the absence of appropriate laboratory tests. Even with access to laboratory facilities 25–50% of cases will remain undiagnosed.

Lesions of GUD may develop anywhere in the genital, perineal, or perianal region of both men and women. As a result of anatomic differences, females may be less likely than males to notice genital ulcers. In men, they may develop on the scrotum or on the base of the shaft, particularly if condoms are used, illustrating that, although condoms are highly efficient at protecting against the acquisition of infections of mucosal surfaces such as gonorrhea and chlamydia, they are less efficient at protecting against acquisition of GUD. In women, labial, vaginal, or cervical lesions can occur. Therefore, it is imperative that the clinician perform a careful and complete examination. For example, in women, careful examination of the introitus, cervix, and all of the labial folds as well as the external genitalia, perineal, and perirectal region is necessary. Similarly, in men, careful examination of the penile shaft, including retraction of the foreskin in uncircumcised men, and scrotum is required.

EPIDEMIOLOGY AND CLINICAL PRESENTATION OF SPECIFIC PATHOGENS

Syphilis

GUD caused by the spirochete *Treponema pallidum* is common in both the developed and developing world. The incidence of syphilis decreased dramatically in the United States during the 1990s after reaching historically high rates at the end of the preceding decade. In the last several years, case rates have risen again particularly in populations of men who have sex with men (see Chapter 9).

Syphilis is contracted through exposure to an infected lesion, which may often be asymptomatic. Within a mean of 2 to 4 weeks after exposure, patients develop a papule or macule that rapidly erodes to form the classic syphilitic chancre of primary syphilis (see Figure 17-1),

but in rare cases, the latency period may be as long as 3 months. The term *chancre* is a French derivation of the Latin term for *cancer*. Typically, the chancre is a single lesion with well-demarcated borders. It reveals significant subcutaneous induration and is not usually tender. Unless superinfected, the base of the ulcer exudes a serous material. Lesions that develop on surfaces that regularly approximate other epithelial surfaces, such as inner aspects of the labia majora, may result in autoinoculation (kissing lesions). Bilateral nontender inguinal lymphadenopathy is common. Left untreated, primary syphilis lesions resolve, usually within 3 weeks.

The secondary stage of syphilis will develop in untreated patients, usually a mean of 8 weeks after the initial exposure. In some cases, this can occur coincident with healing of the primary chancre of primary disease. During secondary syphilis, spirochetemia develops and is associated with systemic symptoms, such as headache, fever, generalized lymphadenopathy, and rash. In some patients, raised moist lesions develop at a variety of sites, most often in the anogenital region. These are referred to as condylomata lata or mucous patches and are highly infectious (see Figure 17-2). These lesions may occasionally become superinfected or confused with other entities, such as genital warts. The key differential point is that they develop rapidly, usually over the course of a few days, and respond dramatically to therapy. Other lesions associated with secondary syphilis, such as papulosquamous eruptions, may occur in the genital area. However, these lesions are usually generalized and typically involve the trunk and extremities.

Herpes Simplex Virus

Cross-sectional seroprevalence studies in the United States and Western Europe demonstrate rates of HSV-2 antibody

FIGURE 17-1 Primary Syphilitic Chancre

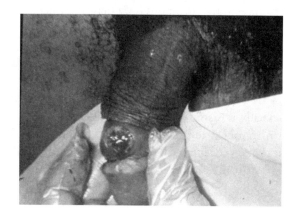

FIGURE 17-2 Condyloma Lata in Secondary Syphilis

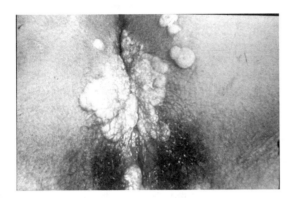

FIGURE 17-3 Penile Genital Herpes, Grouped Vesicular Lesions

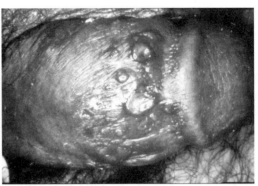

seropositivity between 15% and 25%, and as high as 80% in some urban. Only a minority of these groups will recall suffering anything suggestive of HSV, implying that infection is usually asymptomatic (see Chapter 18).

Genital herpes can be caused by either HSV-1 or HSV-2, two distinct but related viruses. Most recurrent genital disease is caused by HSV-2 and most orolabial disease is caused by HSV-1. Because of changes in the epidemiology of these infections, the rate of HSV-1 genital disease has been increasing in many developed countries. In particular, HSV-1 is now a common cause of primary HSV infection in the United States and Western Europe but tends to recur much less frequently. The clinical course of HSV-1 and HSV-2 genital infection is indistinguishable. Like all herpes viruses (e.g., varicella-zoster, Epstein-Barr, cytomegalovirus), infection is lifelong. Infection can be transmitted through contact with an individual who sheds virus symptomatically or asymptomatically (see also Chapter 18).

Prodromal dysesthesias may precede symptomatic disease. Grouped vesicles can appear anywhere in the genital region. These eventually rupture to leave shallow, nonindurated tender ulcers on an erythematous base (see Figure 17-3). With time, these ulcers may coalesce, dry, scab over, and then heal. Although characteristic, this course can vary considerably from individual to individual. As described in Chapter 18, the first symptomatic outbreak for an individual patient is classified as either a primary outbreak, of the first clinical episode of recurrent infection. These can be differentiated by antibody testing (Chapter 18). Primary outbreaks of genital herpes infection are usually longer and more severe than recurrences of established infection (see Figure 17-4). Lesions of primary disease may persist for 3 to 4 weeks before resolving and are associated sometimes with severe local

and systemic symptoms. Patients may complain of fever, malaise, sore throat, and headache. Recurrences generally last for 1 to 2 weeks. Occasionally, prodromal symptoms without a break in the mucous membrane troubles the patient. Tender bilateral inguinal adenopathy is common in either primary disease or recurrences. Urinary tract symptoms such as dysuria often occurs.

A key point is that lesions resolve whether therapy is provided. In cases in which the ulcers are atypical or asymptomatic, primary syphilis would need to be considered in the differential diagnosis, as both entities spontaneously resolve within 2 to 3 weeks of onset. The frequency of recurrence is variable and the factors that precipitate it are diverse. Stress, sun exposure, menses intercurrent illness, and immunosuppression have all been

FIGURE 17-4 Labial HSV, Vesicular and Ulcerative Lesions

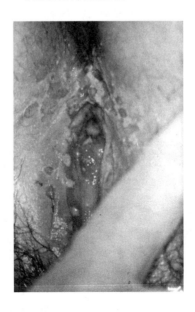

implicated. Although not entirely protective, preexistent HSV-1 orolabial infection appears to reduce the severity and frequency of HSV-2 genital disease.

Chancroid

Genital ulcer disease, caused by the gram-negative, facultative anaerobic bacillus *Hemophilus ducreyi*, is known as chancroid for its clinical similarity to the chancre of syphilis. It has historically occurred in isolated epidemic outbreaks in urban centers in the United States and for a long time was a common cause of GUD in the developing world. Currently global rates of chancroid have declined for reasons that are not entirely clear. Chancroid almost exclusively occurs in persons who have had recent travel and sexual exposure to endemic areas.

Within 3 to 10 days after exposure, an infected individual develops a pustule that rapidly erodes and leaves an irregularly shaped tender ulcer with ragged, undermined edges (see Figure 17-5). The lesions are typically exquisitely painful. In some respects, the lesion of chancroid possesses characteristics of both herpes and syphilis. Single or multiple lesions may occur. Bilateral or unilateral tender inguinal adenopathy, which are often fluctuant and spontaneously drain (i.e., buboe), are common and may be confused with lymphogranuloma venereum. Anatomic variation in the lymphatic drainage patterns between men and women may affect the disease course. Without therapy, chancroid lesions heal only after a long and protracted course and produce scarring. Diagnosis is difficult because it requires cultures that are available only in highly specialized settings. If chancroid is suspected based on presentation and history, and referral services are not available, then empiric treatment may be reasonable. Recommended therapies in 2010 include

FIGURE 17-5 Chancroidal Ulcer

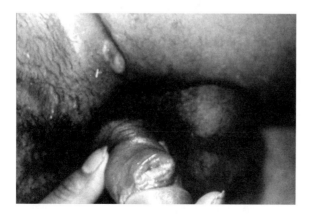

ceftriaxone 250 mg IM, azithromycin 1 g, or ciprofloxacin 500 mg as a single oral dose.

Lymphogranuloma Venereum

Lymphogranuloma venereum (LGV) is caused by *Chlamydia trachomatis* serovars L1, L2, and L3 and can be easily differentiated from other chlamydial causes of genital disease. LGV is much more common in tropical and subtropical countries than in temperate zones. Since 2000, multiple outbreaks of LGV have been reported in US cities and Western Europe, almost exclusively associated with homosexual men. LGV should be suspected in men who have sex with men (MSM) who develop a genital ulcer, fluctuant large inguinal lymphadenopathy, or rectal symptoms, including ulcer, rectal pain, or hematochezia. Although it is not uniformly associated with the development of a genital ulcer, primary disease stages 3 days to 3 weeks after exposure may be associated with a small papule, which can ulcerate and cause a small nontender and nonindurated lesion spontaneously resolves. Less than 30% of patients with LGV recall an ulcer. Concurrently, or sometime thereafter, the untreated patient develops large, unilateral inguinal lymph nodes draining the infected area. In men with genital ulcers, the inguinal nodes are involved and can become highly tender and may become debilitating, impairing ambulation. Adjacent lymph nodes may coalesce. Eventually, fluctuance develops with darkening of the overlying skin. The buboe may spontaneously rupture and discharge pus, which actually provides symptomatic relief. With this development the patient feels greatly relieved. If lymph nodes above and below Poupart's ligament are involved, the disease is noted to demonstrate the classic "groove sign" of LGV (see Figure 17-6).

In men with rectal disease or women with LGV, inguinal lymph nodes are less likely involved because drainage from the upper female genital tract and rectum is to the pelvic lymph nodes and retroperitoneal chain. These patients may come to medical attention complaining of deep pelvic or rectal pain. Chronic untreated LGV may resolve or cause disfiguring or destructive lesions of the genital anatomy.

Granuloma Inguinale (Donovanosis)

Granuloma inguinale is exceedingly rare in developing countries but is endemic in tropical regions of the world, primarily in the South Pacific. Disease is caused by *Klebsiella* (formerly *Calymmatobacterium*) *granulomatis*, a gram-negative bacillus difficult to grow in culture. Although

FIGURE 17-6 "Groove Sign" in Lymphogranuloma Venereum

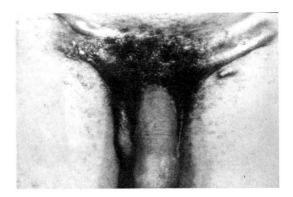

venereal transmission appears to occur, its role in the spread of this disease is poorly defined. After exposure, incubation may last a week to several months. Multiple subcutaneous nodules develop which erode through the skin to form large, painless, heaped-up granulomatous lesions (see Figure 17-7). These can become secondarily infected and may also cause lymphatic obstruction.

DIAGNOSIS

Syphilis

The spirochete, which causes syphilis, cannot ordinarily be cultured. When moist lesions of primary stage disease or condylomata lata are present dark-field microscopy should be performed. This requires an ordinary light microscope fitted with polarizing lenses in the objective and stage. Spirochetes appear white against a dark background and assume a helical shape (see Chapter 20). Although a positive dark-field examination is considered diagnostic,

FIGURE 17-7 Granuloma Inguinale

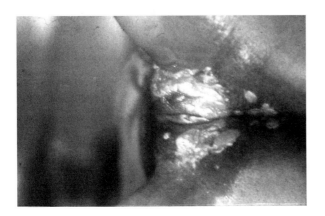

serologic tests are usually performed for confirmation. Serologic tests may be diagnostic when microscopy is unavailable or negative. They also provide a measure with which to follow the success or failure of therapy, rising or falling depending on the activity of disease. Serologic tests are performed in two steps: (1) screening tests like the RPR (rapid plasma reagin) or VDRL (venereal disease research laboratory) are nonspecific, sensitive, relatively inexpensive, and easy to perform. They may be nonreactive shortly after the appearance of the genital ulcer but become reactive soon thereafter. The height of the titer usually, but not always, corresponds to the activity of disease with the highest values recorded during secondary stage disease and dropping with latency or effective therapy. These tests use nontreponemal material to serve as a substrate for the detection of antibodies in patient serum. Reactive nontreponemal tests are confirmed with more specific tests that use *T. pallidum* antigens. These tests include the FTA-ABS (fluorescent treponemal antibody-adsorbed), and the *Treponema pallidum* particle agglutination (TPPA). They are usually reported qualitatively and once reactive are expected, with exceptions, to remain so for the life of the patient. Many clinics now use the *T. pallidum*–specific enzyme-linked immunosorbent (ELISA) test as a screening test. Because syphilis serological testing may be complex, we have included a detailed chapter (see Chapter 20) on this topic.

Herpes Simplex Virus

Unless the clinician has ready access to a virology lab, most cases of HSV GUD will be made on clinical grounds. In terms of clinical diagnosis, patients with herpes will often describe previous episodes of similar outbreaks. Although there is always some similarity in the clinical characteristics of all the etiologies of GUD, HSV lesions are characteristically shallow, tender, and can usually be differentiated from the other causes of GUD. Care should be made to differentiate from syphilitic chancre, which also spontaneously resolves but is usually painless and has a sharply indurated border. Furthermore, because herpes is much more prevalent, simply on epidemiologic grounds alone, the likelihood that a patient in a developed nation presenting with GUD has HSV-2 is high.

Serologic tests for HSV can reliably distinguish between antibodies directed against HSV-1 and HSV-2 (see also Chapter 18). Clinicians should ensure that the tests are type-specific antibody tests. Seroconversion and development of antibodies occurs 4–6 weeks after infection. These tests are useful in defining whether a patient has had previous infection. In the case of a first clinical presentation with a positive lesion culture, if serological assessment is negative, then the diagnosis or primary herpes can be made; if serology is positive, then the diagnosis would be the first clinical episode of recurrent disease.

Given the prevalence of HSV infection, their role in the evaluation of acute GUD is unclear. Tzanck smears, which rely on the identification of multinucleated giant cells in scrapings from the base of an ulcer, are both insensitive and nonspecific and have fallen out of favor. Where possible, culture provides a reliable diagnostic tool for HSV. Provided the genital lesion ascribed to HSV is either in the vesicular or pustular stages, a cotton-tipped swab applied to cellular material at the lesion base and inoculated onto the appropriate cell culture will be positive in 90–100% of cases. This sensitivity drops off significantly with progressive ulceration and healing. Even when culture is available, sensitivity of testing lesions once crusting begins drops to 20–30%. When off-site commercial labs are used, there are typical delays introduced by transport that can be as long as 24 hours, which in turn reduces the sensitivity. Therefore, a negative culture will not rule out herpes if there are delays in the culture processing.

Direct tests on clinical specimens using immunologic techniques, DNA hybridization, and nucleic acid amplification have been used in research and are finding some application in clinical practice.

Chancroid

Chancroid is caused by *Hemophilus ducreyii*, a gram-negative bacillus that requires hemin for growth and an incubation temperature of 35°C. The organism can be isolated from either an ulcer or bubo by inoculation of infectious material onto an agar medium supplemented with hemoglobin and serum. Culture is relatively complex and is performed only in specialized centers or research laboratories. Even with the proper media, rates of isolation are low. Gram's stain of clinical material from ulcers or buboes may be examined for gram-negative coccobacilli in parallel or in clusters, the classic "school of fish" or "railroad track," characteristic of *H. ducreyii*. Although specific, it is insensitive.

Lymphogranuloma Venereum

The diagnosis of LGV is usually clinical and is suspected when a patient presents with a bubo in the inguinal area and no other genital lesions. *Chlamydia trachomatis* isolation in appropriate cell culture using aspirate from a bubo obviously confirms the diagnosis. While very spe-

cific, this test is only 30–50% sensitive. Serologic testing can also be used in the appropriate clinical setting. Microimmunofluorescence testing for antibodies to *C. trachomatis* in the appropriate clinical setting can be suggestive of LGV. Commercially available nucleic acid amplification tests on appropriate clinical specimens can identify *C. trachomatis* species. Further identification of L1, L2, and L3 serovars may require use of noncommercially approved NAAT tests.

Granuloma Inguinale

This infection should be considered in persons with non-healing ulcers and sexual exposure in the South Pacific region. *Klebsiella* (formerly *Calymmatobacterium*) *granulomatis* cannot be cultured by routine methods. Diagnosis is based on the clinical appearance of the lesion in conjunction with the demonstration of Donovan bodies from tissue scrapings or a biopsy using Giemsa or Wright's stain.

Tests are currently under development using nucleic acid amplification (e.g., polymerase chain reaction) technology to detect multiple GUD pathogens from a single clinical specimen. These are available to clinicians in the UK via the Health Protection Agency (HPA) and will be available more widely in the future.

■ HIV INFECTION AND GENITAL ULCER DISEASE

There seems little doubt that a bidirectional effect between genital ulcer diseases and HIV exists (see Chapter 10). A number of studies strongly support the notion that the breakdown of epithelium associated with genital ulcer disease can serve as either a portal of entry or a point of transmission for HIV. There is also considerable evidence that underlying HIV infection and its attendant immunosuppression modify the clinical presentation and response to therapy of the various genital ulcer disease etiologies. Aggressive forms of syphilis (both primary and secondary disease), herpes simplex virus infection, and chancroid have all been described in HIV-infected patients. Genital herpes in advanced immunosuppression may lead to large, severely painful atypical ulcerations. Lesion recurrences may be frequent. Unlike in the immunocompetent patient, these lesions may not spontaneously heal after a month. This should alert the clinician to the underlying immunodeficiency. Syphilis lesions may also persist beyond the expected time course in the setting of HIV infection. The rash of secondary syphilis may more commonly be seen before the primary chancre resolves and signs of neurosyphilis can occur quite early after infection despite appropriate treatment. Failure of therapy for chancroid has been seen where there is underlying HIV infection.

A Suggested Approach to the Patient Presenting with a Genital Ulcer

There is an old maxim in infectious disease that neither the patients nor the microorganisms "read the textbook" and are thus unsure as to how they should present to the examining clinician. This is particularly true with regard to genital ulcer disease. Although there are certain key distinguishing characteristics between the specific etiologic agents, there is also enough overlap to make diagnosis difficult.

A detailed history is critical. Epidemiologic factors might warrant primary initial consideration in the evaluation of a patient with a genital ulcer. If the clinical encounter occurs in a developed country, the patient most likely has HSV. While chancroid typically occurs more commonly in the tropics, even there, the incidence of herpes is on the rise. Although occasionally suspect, the report from a patient that no recent sexual contact has occurred makes nearly all the venereal causes of genital ulcer unlikely except for HSV. If the patient reports that the current problem has occurred and resolved on previous occasions in the past, then HSV again becomes likely.

Besides a detailed history, a thorough examination is always warranted, including a speculum exam of the female patient. An examination of nongenital skin and mucosal surfaces should also be performed for findings consistent with secondary syphilis. Inguinal lymph nodes, although often present in venereal-genital ulcer disease is fluctuant only in LGV and chancroid. Tender shallow ulcers are characteristic of HSV while nontender deeply indurated lesions are more common in syphilis. Chancroid lesions tend to possess findings similar to both, that is, tender, deeply indurated, heaped-up lesions. A suggested algorithm is presented in Figure 17-8, which incorporates evaluation for all of the common causes of GUD.

When possible, certain tests should be done in all cases of genital ulcer disease if only because the presence of one etiologic agent does not necessarily exclude the presence of another. Dark-field microscopy of the lesion's exudate and serologic tests for syphilis should be performed. If access to a virology laboratory exists, a culture (or PCR) of lesions scrapings for HSV should be sent. Most labs in developed countries see too little chancroid for staff to be proficient in identifying the characteristic Gram's stain appearance of *H. ducreyii*, and maintaining a ready supply of *H. ducreyii* culture media in these circumstances is not considered cost effective.

FIGURE 17-8 Practical Scheme for Differential Diagnosis of Genital Ulcers in Developed Country Setting

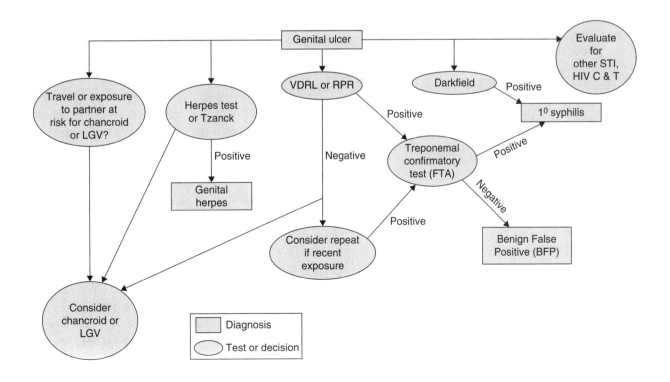

Tests for LGV and Donovanosis should only be conducted when clinical suspicion for these problems is high. HIV counseling and testing should be performed for all patients with genital ulcer disease (see Chapter 29). Nonvenereal causes of genital ulcer disease should be considered when venereal causes have been eliminated. Aphthous ulcers sometimes occur as a result of HIV or other immunomodulatory conditions, such as Behçet's disease. Candida infection occasionally results in macerated tissue with painful linear fissures. Carcinoma of the penis can cause fungating masses with overlying ulcers. Other conditions such as scabies, fixed drug eruption, and trauma warrant consideration although they rarely cause distinct genital ulcers that appear like venereal disease.

■ THERAPY

Therapy for each of the venereal etiologies of genital ulcer disease is summarized below (CDC: 2010 Guidelines for Treatment of Sexually Transmitted Diseases; BASHH guidelines www.bashh.org). Before selecting any therapy, the possibility of pregnancy in the sexually active female patient should be assessed:

Primary syphilis and secondary syphilis
Recommended: Benzathine penicillin G 2.4 million units IM once
Alternative: Doxycycline 100 mg orally twice daily for 2 weeks
OR Tetracycline 500 mg orally four times daily for 2 weeks

Herpes simplex virus
First Episode: Acyclovir 400 mg orally three times daily for 7–10 days
OR Acyclovir 200 mg orally five times daily for 7–10 days
OR Famciclovir 250 mg orally three times daily for 7–10 days
OR Valacyclovir 1 g orally twice daily for 7–10 days

Recurrent episode
Acyclovir 400 mg orally three times daily for 5 days
OR Acyclovir 800 mg orally twice daily for 5 days
OR Famciclovir 125 mg orally twice daily for 5 days
OR Famciclovir 1000 mg orally twice daily for 1 day

OR Valacyclovir 500 mg orally twice daily for 3 days
OR Valacyclovir 1 g orally once a day for 5 days

Chancroid
Recommended: Azithromycin 1 g orally once
OR Ceftriaxone 250 mg IM once
OR Ciprofloxacin 500 mg orally twice daily for 3 days
OR Erythromycin base 500 mg orally 3 times daily for 7 days

LGV
Recommended- Doxycycline 100 mg twice daily for 21 days
Alternative: Erythromycin base 500 mg orally 4 times daily for 21 days

Granuloma inguinale
Recommended: Doxycycline 100 mg orally twice daily for a minimum of 3 weeks
Alternative: Azithromycin 1 g orally per week for a minimum of three weeks and until all lesions have completely healed
OR Ciprofloxacin 750 mg orally twice daily for a minimum of 3 weeks
OR Erythromycin base 500 mg orally 4 times daily for a minimum of 3 weeks
OR Trimethoprim-sulfamethoxazole one double strength table twice daily for a minimum of 3 weeks

In many, if not most instances, therapy for genital ulcer disease will be initiated at the time of the clinical encounter and before the receipt of complete laboratory data that can assist in the diagnosis. Decisions about therapy should be guided by clinical judgment. In many circumstances, empiric therapy for syphilis and chancroid would be appropriate considering the efficacy of therapy and the potential for serious long-term consequences if left untreated (see also Chapter 41).

The sexual partners of any patient with venereal or suspected venereal GUD should be counseled and examined. Partners to index cases with syphilis should usually be treated whether or not they have clinical disease. The course of therapy (i.e., penicillin once versus three weekly injections) may depend on serologic results. Individuals who have had sexual contact with index cases of chancroid, LGV, and Donovanosis within proscribed periods (10 days, 30 days, 60 days, respectively) should be treated as noted previously even in the absence of overt disease. Individuals exposed to index cases of HSV do not warrant therapy unless they demonstrate findings of active disease.

KEY POINTS

- In most developed country settings, the primary differential diagnosis of genital ulcer disease is syphilis and genital herpes. GUD caused by both of these infections will spontaneously heal without specific treatment.

- Lymphogranuloma venereum causes a fleeting genital ulcer and local adenopathym and is seen primarily in homosexual men. Diagnosis is made primarily by serology.

- Chancroid is caused by Hemphilus ducreyi and is seen in hyperendemic settings, almost exclusively heterosexual.

- Diagnostic testing is warranted to establish the correct treatment course, and also to provide partner notification services, especially if syphilis, LGV, or chancroid are diagnosed.

- Clinical differentiation of primary versus recurrent HSV ulcerations is difficult and should not be done without serology.

- GUD in women may be subtle and missed, especially if the lesions are interior.

- GUD is more common in uncircumcised men. During the examination, the foreskin should be fully retracted to effect a complete examination.

- HIV acquisition and transmission are associated with GUD disease. All persons with GUD should receive HIV counseling and testing.

REFERENCES

Centers for Disease Control and prevention. 2010 guidelines for treatment of sexually transmitted diseases. *Morb Mortal Wkly Rep*. 2010;59(RR-12):1–110.

Chapel T, Brown J, Jeffries C, et al. How reliable is the morphological diagnosis of penile ulcerations? *Sex Transm Dis*. 1977;4:150–152.

Dillon S, Cummings M, Rajagopalan S, et al. Prospective analysis of genital ulcer disease in Brooklyn, New York. *Clin Infect Dis*. 1997;24:945–50.

Fast M, D'Costa L, Nsanze H, et al. The clinical diagnosis of genital ulcer disease in men in the Tropics. *Sex Transm Dis*. 1984;11:72–76.

Greenblatt R, Lukehart S, Plummer F, et al. Genital ulceration as a risk factor for human immunodeficiency virus infection. *AIDS*. 1988;2:47–50.

Johnson R, Nahmias A, Magder L, et al. A seroepidemiologic survey of the prevalence of herpes simplex virus type 2 infection in the United States. *N Engl J Med*. 1989;321:7–12.

Lafferty W, Coombs R, Benedetti J, et al. Recurrences after oral and genital herpes simplex virus infection: influence of site of infection and viral type. *N Engl J Med*. 1987;316:1444–1449.

Mertz G, Trees D, Levine W, et al. Etiology of genital ulcers and prevalence of human immunodeficiency virus coinfection in 10 US cities. *J Infect Dis*. 1998;178:1795–1799.

Nsanze H, Fast M, D'Costa L, et al. Genital ulcers in Kenya: clinical and laboratory study. *Br J Vener Dis*. 1981;57: 378–381.

Rolfs R, Joesoef R, Hendershot E, et al. A randomized trial of enhanced therapy for early syphilis with and without human immunodeficiency virus infection. *N Engl J Med*. 1997;337:307–14.

Schmid G, Sanders L, Blount J, et al. Chancroid in the United States: reestablishment of an old disease. *JAMA*. 1987;258:3265–3268.

18

Genital Herpes Infections

Raj Patel and Anne Rompalo

INTRODUCTION

In both the developed and developing world, most genital ulcers are caused by herpes simplex virus (HSV). Most cases are latent. Because most genital ulcer diseases are caused by herpes simplex virus infections, what is the best method of diagnosis? Given the high prevalence of HSV-2, should all patients be offered serologic screening, and if serologically positive, should all HSV-2-infected persons be offered suppressive therapy to decrease possible transmission to others? Because HSV-2-infected individuals are at a two- to threefold increased risk for HIV acquisition and because HSV/HIV coinfected persons are more likely to transmit either or both infections, should the diagnosis, treatment, and suppression of HSV-2 be a priority?

In this chapter, we will review clinical presentations, currently available diagnostic and screening tests, and current treatment options for genital herpes and discuss practical approaches to address difficult questions in the management of this sexually transmitted infection.

EPIDEMIOLOGY

The two types of herpes simplex viruses are HSV-1 and HSV-2. They share 83% sequence homology of their protein-coding regions but can be distinguished serologically. Clinically, the lesions they cause are indistinguishable. Most recurrent episodes of genital herpes are caused by HSV-2, but HSV-1, which is usually associated with orolabial infection acquired during childhood ("fever blisters" or "cold sores"), has been increasingly reported as causing most first-episode genital herpes in the young, where it is thought to be principally associated with oral sex.

At least 50 million persons in the United States have genital HSV-2 infection for a prevalence of approximately 17%. Other country-specific prevalence estimates vary from 10% to 60%, and even higher rates are observed in parts of sub-Saharan Africa. As with any sexually transmitted infection (STI), the risk of acquiring genital HSV-2 increases with increased numbers of lifetime sexual partners, previous history of STIs, and early age of first sexual intercourse.

NATURAL HISTORY AND CLINICAL FEATURES

Herpes simplex causes a chronic infection of the sensory nerve roots and dorsal root ganglia. The initial infection occurs through inoculation of the virus into abraded keratinized epithelium or directly onto mucous membranes. Local viral replication within epithelial cells occurs in parallel with infection of the dendritic processes of sensory neurons.

It is currently believed that most primary genital HSV-1 infections are acquired through oral sex, and most primary genital HSV-2 infections is acquired through genital-to-genital exposure. The incubation period can be as fast as 24 hours but is usually within a week after inoculation. Clinical symptoms may range from none to severe, bilateral, painful ulcerations accompanied by bilateral, often painful, regional lymphadenopathy and nearly 40% of men and 70% of women report fever, headache, malaise, and myalgias. Lesions develop through a number of phases: papules form on erythematous bases, rapidly evolve to become fragile vesicles that form ulcers on minimal abrasion. The ulcers are superficial and frequently coalesce to acquire serpiginous edges. Ulcers are painful and if abraded usually exude blood. Ulcers may be present on any of the primary contact areas—typically the penis, external female genitalia, and rectum, depending on type of sexual exposure. Without antiviral therapy, signs and symptoms of primary genital herpes may persist in the range of 3 weeks. Healing with the formation of scabs occurs on keratinized epithelium, while on mucous membranes, soft exudates and crusts form over reepithelializing ulcers. Both local and distant complications are described (see Table 18-1). Viral shedding may occur until the lesions are fully crusted over, however.

In primary infection, symptoms begin to appear 3–5 days after infection, and persist for up to 10 days afterward (see Figure 18-1). Signs and symptoms of HSV-1 and HSV-2 are similar.

There is a wide range of clinical presentations. Genital HSV may present as classic grouped vesicular lesions, which may be present on the penis, vulva, or rectum (Figures 18-2, 18-3, and 18-4). There is a prodrome that presents with burning, neuropathic pain, low-grade fevers, arthralgias, and myalgias. Following this prodrome, blister- or vesicular-type lesions will develop, which are typically painful, pruritis, or both. On the mucosal surfaces, these lesions will often present as shallow ulcers,

TABLE 18-1 Complications of Genital Herpes

Local
- Superinfection (principally candidal species and streptococci)
- Adhesion formation
- Urinary retention

Neurological
- Autonomic neuropathy
- Encephalitis
- Meningitis
- Radiculitis
- Transverse myelitis

Dissemination (neonates, immunocompromised, and rarely in pregnancy)
- Autoinoculation
- Corneal involvement
- Herpetic whitlow

Psychosexual pathology

Erythema multiforme

FIGURE 18-1 Natural History of Genital Herpes

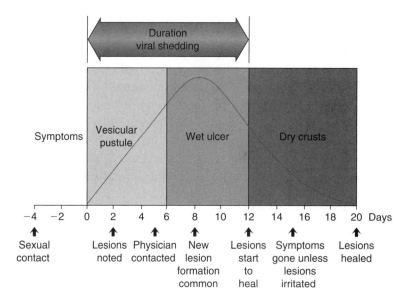

FIGURE 18-2 Penile HSV

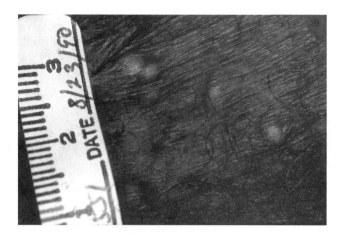

FIGURE 18-4 Vulval and Labial HSV

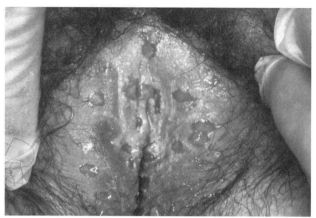

and in women, vulvar lesions can be mistaken for shallow mucosal tears. After 3 to 5 days, these lesions will crust over and heal spontaneously. In cases of true primary herpes, the signs and symptoms may be severe, with often more aggressive clinical presentations, such as bullous herpes disease (see Figure 18-5). In up to two-thirds of the cases of primary HSV, there may be associated urethritis (Figure 18-6), manifesting as pyuria/dysuria syndrome in women (Chapter 24), or nongonococcal urethritis (Chapter 14) in men

It is currently believed that many HSV-2-infected individuals have atypical or unrecognized signs and symptoms, which may include burning, itching, fissures, linear ulcerations, or patchy erythema. Many are unaware of their infection. For example, depending on the serologic study, only 10–25% of people with HSV-2 antibodies are aware that they have genital infection. Despite their lack of symptoms, they shed virus and can infect any susceptible sex partners.

ESTABLISHING LATENCY

Various virological mechanisms exist to limit and delay the development of a full local immune response; however, virus will be cleared from the epithelium in time. The virus, however, maintains a latent state in the dorsal root ganglia, which is a sequestered site, and infection is lifelong. Clearance does not occur within neuronis and virus persists as extrachromosomal DNA (viral episomes), which may intermittently reactivate, migrate to the neuronal dermal junction, and cause productive infection in adjacent epithelium. When this migration/reactivation phenomena occurs, nerve root irritation is manifest as the pain and tingling sensation reported by many patients. Recovery from infection requires a functioning cell-mediated immune response and may explain the protracted nature of acquisition disease in the immunocompromised. Women appear to be more susceptible to HSV-2 infections than men and tend to have a much

FIGURE 18-3 Perirectal HSV

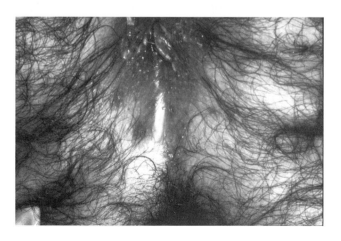

FIGURE 18-5 Bullous HSV in Primary Herpes

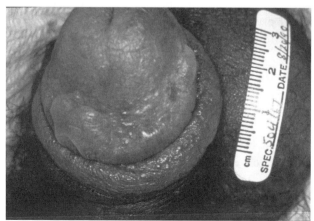

FIGURE 18-6 HSV with Urethritis

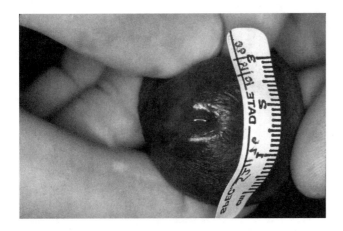

more extensive and protracted initial illness. However, once infected, both women and men will shed virus both symptomatically and asymptomatically.

Any individual who presents for care and is found on examination to have a genital ulcer should have a diagnostic test for herpes. However, not all HSV-infected persons present with ulcers and the clinical diagnosis of genital herpes is typically unreliable. Furthermore, tests for HSV can be falsely negative, especially if there presentation is late in the course of the disease or if there are specimen transport issues. As described in Chapter 17, both primary syphilis and herpes have a similar natural history even with no specific therapy—both are genital ulcer diseases, and both resolve spontaneously without treatment, although the course of HSV healing is more rapid.

■ DIAGNOSIS

The diagnosis of genital herpes, therefore, is not simple. Clinicians and patients often expect to see classically described herpetic lesions. If an individual who has not been previously infected with HSV-1 or HSV-2 in the orolabial or genital area and has no serologic evidence of any prior infection becomes inoculated in the genital area with either HSV-1 or HSV-2 through close contact with an infected person who is shedding virus from skin or genital secretions, the susceptible person may become primarily infected.

Serological evaluation can confirm the differentiation between primary and nonprimary (recurrent) infection. First clinical episodes may represent either primary infection or recurrent infection with a previously unrecognized latent primary episode.

Nonprimary first-episode genital herpes are usually newly acquired HSV-2 genital infection in someone with previous HSV-1 orolabial disease. The clinical presentation may be modified and milder, but the previous HSV-1 infection is not protective against infection with HSV-2. For counseling purposes, the first clinical presentation of genital herpes may not mean recent infection, because almost 25% of people presenting with these initial complaints have serological evidence of past HSV-2 infection, suggesting that their initial infection was asymptomatic. Such a view is supported by data from prospective studies in serodiscordant couples, indicating that more than one-third of acquisitions are asymptomatic and that many are atypical or associated with minimal symptoms.

Recurrences after primary infection are variable. Individuals with symptomatic primary or first episode genital herpes due to HSV-1 or HSV-2 can expect to have symptomatic recurrences during the next year. Of those with HSV-2, 70–90% recur, and of those with HSV-1, 20–50% recur. After their first episode, HSV-2-infected individuals have on average 4 recurrences a year, 40% have at least 6, and 20% have more than 10. Recurrent lesions tend to be less severe, fewer in number, and the duration of lesions without antiviral treatment is usually 5 to 10 days. Over time, symptomatic recurrences may lessen in frequency, and one prospective study reported a median reduction of two recurrences per year between years 1 and 5. Recurrent disease may rarely be associated with complications such as recurrent meningitis or erythema multiforme (see Chapter 11). It is frequently associated with psychological morbidity.

Many genital herpes lesions are atypical. Genital HSV may be misdiagnosed as fissures, furuncles, excoriations, urinary tract infections, yeast vaginitis, patchy erythema, or trauma from intercourse. Clinicians should be aware of these atypical presentations and consider serologic testing when applicable.

Whether an individual has typical or atypical herpetic lesions, subclinical or asymptomatic shedding may occur intermittently. The greatest frequency of shedding is within the first year of acquisition and then gradually declines to lower stable levels over a 2- to 3-year period. The rate of subclinical or asymptomatic shedding is individual for each infected person but usually mirrors the levels of symptomatic disease. The majority of episodes of shedding are short-lived, last for less then 1 day, and can involve more than one anatomic site such as the cervix, anus, or urethra. Infected individual are infectious to their sex partners during these episodes of shedding and should be counseled in this regard (see Chapter 31).

CLINICAL PRESENTATIONS IN HIV-INFECTED INDIVIDUALS

Limited data are available on HSV-2 seroprevalence in HIV-positive patients in the United States, but it is estimated that 60–70% of patients who were infected with HIV are also coinfected with HSV-2.

In patients with severe immunosuppression, symptomatic genital lesions may be extensive and difficult to treat. Chronic persistent genital ulcers caused by HSV were among the opportunistic infections included in the early definitions of AIDS. In the pre-HAART era, painful and sometimes extensive lesions could persist for months in HIV-infected patients with very low CD4 counts, but effective antiretroviral therapy can improve HSV clinical manifestations and ameliorate the ulcers. Individuals coinfected with HSV-2 also shed HSV-2 more frequently than do HIV-uninfected persons, and the frequency of shedding is inversely correlated with the degree of immunosuppression. HIV-infected persons with lower CD4+ cell counts shed HSV-2 in higher quantity, at multiple anatomic sites, and more frequently. Highly active antiretroviral therapy reduces the frequency of genital lesions, but subclinical reactivation is still frequently detected.

DIAGNOSING GENITAL HERPES: WHAT TO EXPECT

Available Diagnostics

Genital Ulcers

The prevalence and etiology of genital ulcers is different in geographical regions and populations. In developed countries, the most common cause of genital ulcers among individuals in both urban and nonurban settings is HSV-2. In developing countries, especially in Africa, the etiology of genital lesions has been changing over the past two decades from bacterial causes, such as syphilis or chancroid, to mainly HSV-2. Therefore, ideally, anyone who presents for evaluation of a genital ulcer should be tested for herpes.

For decades, viral isolation in cell culture was considered the gold standard with a specificity of 100%. The amount of viral shedding, the specimen quality, and the time and condition of specimen transport affect the sensitivity of culture. Culture performs best for diagnosis of primary HSV lesions, preferably vesicular lesions, when the amount of virus present should be plentiful (sensitivity about 80%). Performance declines with time since lesion onset with sensitivities of 52–93% for vesicles, 41–72% for ulcers, and 19–27% for crusted lesions.

Polymerase chain reaction (PCR) is currently considered the gold standard for diagnosing genital HSV lesions but is not widely available. It is up to four times more sensitive than culture, does not depend heavily on collection and transport conditions, and provides faster results than the 4 to 5 days usually required for viral culture. The rapid turnaround of negative samples is a distinct advantage. PCR is, however, expensive to initiate and requires trained technicians, sophisticated machinery, and reliable power sources. Once PCR facilities are established, they can be cost saving and are increasingly recommended as the diagnostic method of choice.

Other direct lesion testing methods are available, which include detection of viral antigen by direct immunofluorescence assay using fluorescein-labeled monoclonal antibodies on smears (sensitivity of 74% and specificity of 85%) and enzyme immunoassay on swabs (62–100% sensitivity and >95% specificity compared with culture).

Serologic Tests

Current Centers for Disease Control and Prevention Sexually Transmitted Diseases Treatment Guidelines recommend serologic tests to confirm a clinical diagnosis of genital herpes in patients with recurrent genital symptoms, atypical lesions, or with healing lesions and negative HSV cultures. Serology may also be used to manage sex partners of people with known HSV infection or to diagnose and counsel individuals with atypical or unrecognized lesions. Currently, serologic testing is not recommended for screening of general populations, but some argue that it may be beneficial to screen people with HIV to offer suppressive therapy, people with other STIs or who have multiple sexual partners, and men who have sex with men. A major issue in providing screening services is also providing accurate and relevant counseling (see Chapter 31).

When choosing serologic tests for HSV antibody detection, clinicians must be aware that no good IgM test is currently available. In addition, IgM is often produced to respond to recurrent episodes. IgG tests that have the best sensitivity and specificity are type-specific glycoprotein G-based tests, which detect antibody to HSV-specific glycoprotein G2 (HSV-2) and glycoprotein G1 (HSV-1). Since IgG antibodies may take 2 weeks to 3 months to develop, patients with newly acquired HSV infection may initial test negative and then test positive after 12 weeks.

When compared with the labor-intensive and costly Western blot analysis, which is considered the gold standard serologic test for herpes, type-specific IgG2 herpes tests have reported sensitivity of 97–100% and specificity of 94–98% among U.S. populations. False positives may occur and in low prevalence settings, and a poor positive predictive value has dampened its generalized use. Take care to interpret HSV-1 results because some commercially available tests are significantly poorer at detecting these infections. Nonetheless, serologic testing for HSV should be offered or available for all who request it.

■ ISSUES RELATED TO SEROLOGICAL TESTING

Latency and Seroconversion

Serologic tests (both Western blot and type-specific gG-based) are frequently negative during the early stages of infection and may take a variable time to become positive as the humoral response matures.

Sensitivity and Specificity

Serological assays have sensitivity and specificity of approximately 92-97% each for HSV-1 and HSV-2. Therefore, if prevalence is low in the tested population, the positive predictive value is low. Therefore, wide population-based screening in asymptomatic populations is not recommended.

Temporality

Antibody tests do not determine the timing of infection but can only determine whether the individual has become infected within the past 3–6 months.

■ CLINICAL UTILITY OF TESTING

Serologic tests can be used diagnostically in symptomatic patients, as an aid to counseling, for assessing the partners of those who have infection, and for screening patients who are at high risk for HSV. Screening low-risk patients is not recommended. Screening for pregnant women is a controversial area.

Symptomatic Patients

HSV serology in first-episode disease can help stage (primary or initial) the diagnosis when lesion antigen direct tests or cultures failed or were inconclusive. Testing potentially can confuse; anecdotal cases are reported in which the attribution of recurrent genital symptoms to HSV-2 infection (following sero-identification) has delayed a more appropriate and accurate dermatologic diagnosis. Serology was found to be rarely helpful with atypical, nonulcerative symptoms.

Partner Evaluation and Counseling

Serologic testing can help with counseling couples in which one partner has diagnosed HSV infection. Where seroconcordance is found, it may be appropriate to retest the previously undiagnosed partner if they are asymptomatic. Following education and counseling, most such partners will recognize some HSV-related symptoms and signs even if asymptomatic at diagnosis. Usefulness is diminished when a partner's HSV type is unknown. Serodiscordant couples need careful counseling regarding the risks for transmission and possible interventions, as discussed later. More detailed recommendations for counseling are provided in Chapter 31.

High-Risk Patients

High rates of HSV-2 infection are reported among STI clinic attendees, and there is some debate about whether it is appropriate to offer high-risk groups serologic testing for HSV in the context of an evaluation for STI. Proponents of testing develop four arguments.

1. Patients want HSV testing. Surveys of patient views on testing show that most patients would want type-specific HSV testing if it were available to them. However, when serologic identification is made available with counseling (STI clinic patients), fewer patients choose to be tested, suggesting that informed take-up may be far from universal even among higher-risk groups.

2. Testing will provide for better symptomatic control for patients. Most of the new infections identified serologically will prove to be symptomatic. Most HSV disease is likely to be atypical. Serologic identification will provide for easier and earlier symptom recognition. However, detractors from a screening strategy would argue that much of the disease detected is likely to be mild or trivial in nature.

3. Testing will reduce the risk for onward HSV transmission to sexual partners through education and behavioral change or antiviral therapy. For this group, benefit remains highly theoretic and assumes that behavioral change can be realized through education and counseling.

■ THERAPEUTIC INTERVENTIONS

Three commonly used antiviral drugs are effective for treating and suppressing genital herpes: acyclovir, valacyclovir, and famciclovir. Treatment for initial episode, recurrences, and suppression listed in Table 18-2.

Valacyclovir is the prodrug of acyclovir, famciclovir is the prodrug of penciclovir, and both drugs have higher oral bioavailability and less frequent dosing than acyclovir. These drugs are nucleoside analogs that are substrates for HSV-specific thymidine kinase (TK). They are phosphorylated by TK only within actively infected cells, incorporated into the growing HSV DNA chain and cause chain termination. No antiviral therapy cures herpes, but they do offer clinical benefits that include faster healing and decreased shedding. All drugs are comparable, but ease of administration and cost may be important considerations for the patient. Because these drugs interfere with viral replication, antiviral treatment should be initiated as soon as possible and not delayed by waiting for laboratory confirmation of the diagnosis. Recommended regimens for first clinical episode of genital herpes are shown in Table 18-2.

Because most individuals with symptomatic, first-episode genital herpes infection will experience recurrent episodes as well as asymptomatic shedding, options for future treatment should be discussed. Options include episodic therapy for recurrent recognized lesions to ameliorate or shorten the duration of recurrence or suppressive therapy to reduce the frequency of prodromal symptoms, recurrences, and viral shedding.

Episodic therapeutic options are listed in Table 18-2. Patients should be counseled to identify their prodromal symptoms and initiate therapy as soon as possible, preferably within 1 day of symptoms or lesion onset. Patients, therefore, should have a supply of antiviral drugs available for immediate access. Extending episodic therapy beyond a few days has little benefit, and a traditional 5-day course can no longer be seen as ideal.

Suppressive Therapy

Suppressive therapy is often the best option for those with severe, complicated disease and for those with psychosexual morbidity. The typical settings in which suppressive therapy is given include

- Frequent recurrences, typically >5 per year
- Severe lifestyle impact of symptomatic HSV disease
- Persons with previously controlled disease who are immunosuppressed
- Managing dichotomous couples to prevent transmission to uninfected partner

TABLE 18-2 Treatment Strategies for Herpes (2010 CDC STD Treatment Guidelines)

Treatment for First Clinical Episode
Acyclovir 400 mg orally three times a day for 7–10 days
OR
Acyclovir 200 mg orally five times a day for 7–10 days
OR
Famciclovir 250 mg orally three times a day for 7–10 days
OR
Valacyclovir 1 g orally twice a day for 7–10 days

Treatment for Symptomatic Recurrent Disease Recommended Regimens
Acyclovir 400 mg orally three times a day for 5 days
OR
Acyclovir 800 mg orally twice a day for 5 days
OR
Acyclovir 800 mg orally three times a day for 2 days
OR
Famciclovir 125 mg orally twice daily for 5 days
OR
Famciclovir 1000 mg orally twice daily for 1 day
OR
Famciclovir 500 mg once, followed by 250 mg twice daily for 2 days
OR
Valacyclovir 500 mg orally twice a day for 3 days
OR
Valacyclovir 1.0 g orally once a day for 5 days

Suppression to Prevent Recurrences
Acyclovir 400 mg orally twice a day
OR
Famciclovir 250 mg orally twice a day
OR
Valacyclovir 500 mg orally to 1 gram orally once a day

Source: BASHH Genital Herpes Treatment Guideline at www.bashh.org; CDC Treatment Guidelines 2010, at www.cdc.gov/STD/treatment

Therapeutic doses of antivirals may need to be adjusted in line with levels of disease control. It is often difficult to render patients completely disease free. However, a reduction of 70–80% in frequency (and a significant reduction in severity) should be anticipated. Suppressive therapy has been shown to reduce the frequency of asymptomatic shedding of virus by 85%. The acyclovir class of drugs used to treat HSV have a favorable side effect profile and can be taken for long periods.

Treatment to Prevent Transmission

Daily treatment with valacyclovir 500 mg orally has been shown to decrease the rate of HSV-2 transmission in discordant, heterosexual couples in whom the source partner had a history of genital HSV-2 infection. Counseling of partners with herpes (see Chapter 31) should emphasize the following issues:

- Herpes may be transmitted between partners even when asymptomatic.

- The average transmission rate between discordant partners 5–8% per year.

- Decisions whether to institute suppressive therapy should also include a frank discussion of the potential disease severity or lack thereof. In many couples, a joint decision is made not to use treatment.

- Couples should be counseled that condoms are highly effective in preventing transmission when used consistently.

- Couples should be counseled that the vast majority of women with HSV-2 can become pregnant and deliver vaginally. However, if a discordant (seropositive male and seronegative female) couple plans pregnancy, then they should be counseled about potential risks to the fetus if primary infection occurs during pregnancy.

- Treatment to prevent transmission primarily prevents *symptomatic* transmission.

- Treatment to prevent transmission does not relieve the infected person from informing his or her sexual partner of infection status.

Acyclovir Resistance

In vitro resistance to acyclovir (ACV) can result from thymidine-kinase (TK) deficient, TK-altered, or DNA-polymerase-resistant strains of HSV. These mutant viruses are generally less virulent, have not increased in number or isolation in immunocompetent individuals for the past 30 years, and most likely represent a random mutation rapidly cleared by the immune system in the healthy host. In immunocompromised individuals who undergo multiple courses of acyclovir-based drugs, acyclovir-resistant mutants can occur. In one study in HIV-positive patients, ACV-resistance risk was increased with low CD4 count and use of topical ACV therapy. Because resistance is rare, routine HSV cultures for ACV-resistance testing are not indicated. However, in patients with persistent HSV infections that are unresponsive to ACV-based drugs, especially those patients with advanced HIV disease, testing for ACV resistance should be performed.

Therapy for ACV-Resistant HSV

Foscarnet, a viral DNA polymerase inhibitor similar in structure to phosphonoacetic acid, has potent antiviral activity but is intravenously or topically administered only. It has systemic toxicity, including renal insufficiency and metabolic disturbances, especially hypophosphatemia.

Cidofovir is another nucleotide analog with good antiherpetic activity, which does not require TK for phosphorylation. A randomized, double-blind, placebo-controlled trial of topical cidofovir gel 0.3% or 1.0% in 30 patients with AIDS who did not respond to ACV therapy showed that 10 of 20 cidofovir recipients healed by at least 50% compared with none of the placebo recipients. Cidofovir has been administered intravenously, but it causes significant renal toxicity and, therefore, is not used.

Resiquimod and imiquimod have been evaluated in clinical trials for genital herpes. Both work in animal models and are applied topically during a recurrence to stimulate local immune response in which the antigen is present. Imiquimod is not effective in delaying the time of the next genital HSV recurrence, and resiquimod results have been inconsistent. Therefore, further commercial development of this compound for HSV therapy has ceased.

■ RARE COMPLICATIONS

Spread and Dissemination

Unlike the six other members of the herpes family, viremic spread of HSV is extremely rare. Although systemic symptoms are often present in primary infection, these are not related to any widespread dissemination, and whole virus cannot be identified in blood at any disease stage. Disseminated infection occurs in three situations:

- Severely immunocompromised, such as systemic chemotherapy/radiation associated with hematological malignancies or organ transplantation

- Neonates associated with vertical transmission

- Sporadic primary infection in pregnancy

Dissemination is a serious complication that may rapidly progress to and organ failure. Prompt initiation of intravenous acyclovir is required.

Autoinoculation

Initial infection results in the development of a cell-mediated and antibody response. Until these develop, it is fairly easy to inoculate virus into other parts of the body, and up to 10% of patients demonstrate such contemporaneous inoculations with the establishment of infection. Animal experiments suggest that autoinoculation outside of the initial exposure are extremely rare and difficult to achieve in those with a functioning and intact immune system. Late autoinoculation most commonly occurs into the cornea. It is often seen in those with eczema. HSV can be easily inoculated into areas of eczematous activity where high doses of antivirals in conjunction with expert dermatological care will be required to control the disease

Distant Complications

HSV is the most common cause of recurrent erythema multiforme (see Chapter 11). Whole virus cannot be isolated from the target lesions. Lesions often occur within a few days of an HSV episode. Most affected individuals will respond favorably to suppressive antiviral therapy.

Managing Herpes in Pregnancy

The frequency of neonatal herpes varies from 1:3000 to 1:60000 live births, with the highest rates reported in North America. This risk is maximal for those women who acquire disease in late pregnancy, although an excess of risk does remain for those who acquire disease before the third trimester. Arguments for screening women and their partners during pregnancy are based on developing strategies that would diminish third-trimester acquisitions of new disease and extend ideal medical management to those already infected to limit either neonatal transmission (e.g., antivirals, selective cesarean section) or early identification of active neonatal infection.

New infections during pregnancy carry the highest risks. Infections in the first and second trimester can result in fetal loss. Infections in late pregnancy can precipitate premature delivery. Late acquisitions will result in a limited immune response and high levels of viral shedding at term. If vaginal delivery proceeds and shedding is present, a risk of 50% transmission of HSV to the neonate has been described.

Most clinicians advocate the judicious use of ACV in acquisition episodes despite its not being licensed in pregnancy. All guidelines agree that cesarean section is mandatory for primary herpes acquired in the third trimester. The management of women with established infection before the third trimester is more controversial and subject to local practice and custom. Routine cesarean section is not recommended in these cases, and a more conservative approach is increasingly applied. Cesarean section is still conducted in many centers when recurrent lesions are seen at term. The instigation of continuous acyclovir (400 mg two or three times daily) from 36 weeks onward may be an effective strategy to avoid cesarean section in these otherwise lower-risk pregnancies.

Although a wide serologic testing strategy involving pregnant women and their partners is, superficially, extremely attractive, cost–benefit analysis in many countries suggests that, unless the local rate of neonatal disease is high, any screening policy is unlikely to be valuable. Although screening may not be practical or currently advised, many potentially serodiscordant couples will self-identify to the clinician. Management should aim at keeping these pregnant women disease free during the third trimester. Despite the absence of data supporting interventions for this group, many clinicians would advocate either abstinence or condoms and continuous suppressive therapy with valacyclovir.

Managing HSV in Those with HIV

STD guidelines usually acknowledge that short-course treatment doses for initial and recurrent HSV in those with HIV cannot be based on trial data (BASHH Genital Herpes Treatment Guideline, www.bashh.org; CDC Treatment Guidelines, www.cdc.gov/STD/treatment/). Evidence is extremely limited, and most authorities recommend that, in those with CD4 <500/ml that twice the standard doses of antivirals be used and that they are continued until healing occurs.

Suppressive therapy with twice-daily doses of antivirals is most effective, but here again treatment may need to be adjusted in line with the clinical response. Every effort should be made to boost the patient's background immune status, because if deteriorates, the development of resistant disease becomes much more likely.

In the current STD treatment guidelines, the CDC recommends considering suppressive therapy with an oral antiviral agent to decrease the clinical signs and symptoms of genital herpes among patients with HIV infection. Therefore, some specialists suggest that HSV type-specific serology should be offered to HIV-positive patients during their initial evaluation and that suppressive antiviral therapy be considered in HIV-positive patients who have HSV-2 infection. Perhaps the strongest argument to test HIV-infected individuals for HSV during their initial HIV evaluation visit comes from studies that look at the effect of suppressive therapy for HSV on HIV viral loads and CD4 cell decline. Numerous small studies have shown an impact of valacyclovir not only on genital HSV shedding but also on HIV plasma viral loads for those not on effective antiretrovirals. A large placebo-controlled study in 3381 heterosexual participants in Africa dually infected with HIV and HSV-2 has recently demonstrated that ACV therapy 400 mg twice daily over a 2-year period reduced the proportions reaching CD4 counts of <350 cells/ml by 19% (Celum 2008). The implications of these studies are that HSV suppression may provide clinical benefits to persons not receiving highly active ART.

Treatment of HSV-2 to Prevent HIV

Multiple studies have shown that the risk of HIV acquisition is significantly increased with HSV-2 seropositivity. It is theorized that mucosal barrier breakage and open lesions may increase susceptibility to the HIV virus. In addition, infection with HSV-2 has been shown to result in an influx of CD4+ T cells and macrophages to the genital region. Other studies have confirmed that HSV-2 reactivation or shedding increase HIV viral replication, further evidence for the increase in HIV acquisition with HSV-2 disease. On the basis of these data, a proof-of-concept, randomized, placebo-controlled trial (HPTN 039) was designed to assess whether HSV-2 suppression with twice-daily antiherpetic therapy (acyclovir 400 mg) reduces the risk of HIV acquisition among 1380 women in Africa and 1871 men who have sex with men (MSM) in the Americas (Celum 2008). Despite excellent adherence to the study drug, HIV incidence rates in the treatment and placebo arms of the study were identical among all the studied groups. A large study to evaluate the effect of HSV-2 suppression in HIV-infected individuals on HIV transmission to their HIV-uninfected partners has been recently reported. These too indicate that, despite the strong epidemiological links between HSV and HIV transmission, continuous suppression with currently available antivirals does not impact HIV transmission.

PREVENTION OF HERPES INFECTION

Transmission of HSV remains a major concern for patients and their partners. Various strategies are effective but rely on the disclosure of the index case's diagnosis. Chemical barriers, such as topical microbicides, that inactivate the virus directly and block viral binding and entry are currently under investigation. Vaccines that have been tested have had marginal success. Two studies tested an HSV-2 recombinant glycoprotein-D vaccine and showed efficacy of 39–46% for prevention of HSV-2 infection and a greater significant impact on disease (Stanberry et al. 2002). However, efficacy was only seen in the subgroup of women who were seronegative for both HSV-1 and HSV-2. Concern remains regarding the ability of this vaccine to limit infection and its impact on asymptomatic disease and viral shedding. Another larger vaccine trial among HSV-1 and HSV-2 seronegative women is under way. Other vaccines under development include live, attenuated vaccines, replication-defective viral mutant vaccines, recombinant-vector-based vaccines, and DNA vaccines. No phase III studies of these other candidates are currently under way.

Strategies to prevent HSV transmission to sexual partners include abstention from sexual activity if lesions or prodrome are present (although cognizant that asymptomatic shedding may occur), consistent and correct condom use, and daily suppressive therapy. Daily suppression with valacyclovir 500 mg daily was given in an international, randomized, placebo-controlled trial in heterosexual couples in which one partner had genital HSV-2 and the other was susceptible. Valacyclovir lowered HSV-2 transmission to the susceptible partner by 48% compared with placebo over the 9-month study period.

Symptom Recognition

Patients can be taught to recognize some of their symptomatic and clinical disease episodes and may be able to reduce risk through selective abstinence during these times and immediately afterward. The levels and extent of exposure to their partner will be reduced, but this will not reduce risk in relation to asymptomatic shedding; that risk will still remain in these instances. Some weak natural history data suggest that patients are able to use disease recognition to modify the timing of sex and that, for couples aware of their discordance, sexual behavior can be timed to avoid episodes of overt clinical disease.

Condom Use

Despite the virtual impermeability that latex presents to herpes viruses, condoms can fail to protect against herpes viral transmission. Three factors are thought to contribute to this: (1) HSV is frequently shed from multiple sites, some of which are not amenable to protection by male condom use; (2) many couples engage in considerable unprotected genital contact before using condoms for penetrative sexual intercourse; and (3) condoms may fail during penetrative sex because of breakage or slippage. Studies of the effectiveness of condom use for preventing HSV transmission are difficult to perform ethically and practically. Indirect evidence for condom effectiveness comes from well-documented natural history studies of transmission in serodiscordant couples where diaries of sexual activity, symptomatology, and condom use were kept. These show that the male condom, when used consistently, will protect men and women from genital HSV acquisition but also that consistent condom use is difficult to achieve. Estimates of the prevention impact of consistently reported condom use are 50–60%.

Summary

Herpes simplex virus genital infections are common STIs that are lifelong, incurable, and recurrent. Most infections go undiagnosed or unrecognized in HSV-infected individuals. Any patient who presents with genital ulceration should have a diagnostic evaluation for genital herpes with either culture, direct antigen test for HSV from the lesion, or PCR, which is the most sensitive test. Antiherpetic viral therapy should be initiated presumptively and immediately before test results are available to stop disease progression, increase healing time, and decrease viral shedding. In persons newly diagnosed with HSV, therapeutic options of episodic therapy or suppressive therapy should be discussed. For recurrent disease, therapy should be tailored to patients' needs. Antivirals can be used to manage many of the complications of infection, including psychosexual problems and

transmission anxiety. In those with early HIV infection, antivirals have been shown to delay progression.

Type-specific HSV serologic assays may be useful in the diagnostic workup of patients with recurrent genital symptoms or atypical symptoms with negative HSV cultures and when a clinical diagnosis of genital herpes is suspected without laboratory confirmation. It may also help in counseling a partner. If serology is ordered, the serologic type-specific glycoprotein G (gG)-based assays should be requested because nontype-specific antibodies are not accurate, and results are impossible to interpret meaningfully. Some experts believe that HSV serologic testing should be included in a comprehensive evaluation for STIs, among persons with multiple sex partners, HIV infection, and among MSM at increased risk for HIV acquisition. Currently, however, screening the general population for HSV-1 or HSV-2 is not recommended.

Getting the Best from Antiviral Therapy

1. Be realistic with your patient about what impact therapy will have on his or her disease symptoms:

   Episodic therapy: Up to 30% of episodes will be aborted at an early stage if patients take their therapy early in a lesional episode. Other episodes will be shortened. There is limited or no impact on prodromal symptoms.

   Suppressive therapy: Most patients will experience a dramatic reduction in disease frequency. However, even on full doses of suppressive therapy, most patients will continue to have occasional recurrences. Frequent disease should lead a review of therapy and the diagnosis.

2. Timing of Treatment

   Episodic therapy: For therapy to be effective, it must be taken at the earliest stages of lesion development. Ideally, therapy should be instigated during the prodromal (warning) phases or early on before papules have become blisters. There is some evidence that treatment taken after 24–48 hours does not affect healing at all in HSV lesions. Because treatment must be started early, a supply of medication should be made available to the patient at home, ready for the next recurrence. Patients should be encouraged to carry one day's therapy at all times.

   Suppressive therapy: Studies have shown that infrequent medication leads to poor control of disease. Acyclvoir therapy is particularly sensitive to drug timing and where possible treatment should be taken at equal intervals throughout the day.

3. Review Effectiveness

Episodic therapy: Many patients find only a limited impact of episodic therapy. If disease is frequent, prodromes absent or false prodromes present (prodromal-like symptoms in the absence of other features of disease), episodic therapy is usually inappropriate and better control can be provided by suppressive therapy.

Suppressive therapy: After starting therapy, patients may need to have their dose adjusted if the disease does not adequately respond (two recurrences within a 3-month period should trigger a such review for most patients). Compliance with therapy, dosage, and dose timing, as well as the possibility of misdiagnosis should all be considered. If the patient has normal liver and renal function blood tests are not required.

4. Review Patient Needs

Disease patterns and the patient's needs from therapy change with time. Transmission concerns may no longer exist within mature relationships, or frequent disease may make episodic therapy less attractive. Clinicians should ensure that patients are aware that current therapeutic recommendations may need review.

■ KEY POINTS

- Herpes simplex virus infections are the most common cause of genital ulcers worldwide. Herpes is highly prevalent, with rates as high as 50–60% in some populations.

- Most prevalent HSV infections are asymptomatic. Because primary infections may be asymptomatic, in cases of first clinical presentation, clinical differentiation of *primary* from *recurrent* herpes is not possible without serological testing.

- Herpes simplex virus type 2 (HSV-2) is the cause of most genital herpes and is usually sexually transmitted.

- Herpes simplex virus type 1 (HSV-1) is usually transmitted during childhood through nonsexual contact, but it has become an important cause of genital herpes in some developed countries.

- Among individuals infected with genital herpes, an estimated 20% have classically described painful genital ulcers, 20% are completely asymptomatic, and 60% have atypical or unrecognized signs and symptoms.

- The clinical features of genital HSV and its complications are amenable to medical intervention.

- All infected individuals, whether symptomatic or asymptomatic, will shed herpes simplex virus and can transmit the virus to uninfected sexual partners. Partner transmission occurs most frequently via asymptomatic shedding.

- The highest risk in pregnancy for vertical transmission is when primary infection occurs during the last trimester.

- Infection with HSV-2 may at least double the risk for acquisition of HIV and may accelerate HIV progression and increase the infectiousness of HIV. HSV is associated with HIV transmission even when genital ulcers are not present.

REFERENCES

BASHH (British Association for Sexual Health and HIV). Genital herpes treatment guideline. www.bashh.org.

Benedetti JK, Corey L, Ashley R. Recurrence rates in genital herpes after symptomatic fist-episode infection. *Ann Intern Med.* 1994;121:847–854.

CDC treatment guidelines (2010). www.cdc.gov/STD/treatment/.

Celum C, Wald A, Hughes J, et al. Effect of acyclovir on HIV-1 acquisition in herpes simplex virus 2 seropositive women and men who have sex with men: a randomised, double-blind, placebo-controlled trial. *Lancet.* 2008;371(9630): 2109–2119.

Celum C, Wald A, Lingappa, et al. Acyclovir and transmission of HIV-1 from persons infected with HIV-1 and HSV-2. *N Engl J Med.* 2010;362(5):427–439.

Corey L, Wald A, Patel R et al Reduction in the Transmission of Genital Herpes with suppressive valacycloviracyclovir. *N Engl J Med.* 2004;350(1):11–20.

Fleming D, McQuillan G, Johnson R, et al. Herpes simplex virus type 2 in the United States, 1976–1994. *N Eng J Med.* 1997;337:1105–1111.

Gupta R, Warren T, Wald A. Genital herpes. *Lancet.* 2007;370: 2127–2137.

Lingappa JR, Baeten JM, Wald A, et al. Daily acyclovir for HIV-1 disease progression in people dually infected with HIV-1 and herpes simplex virus type 2: a randomised placebo-controlled trial. *Lancet.* 2010;375:824–833.

Stanberry LR, Spruance EK, Cunningham AL, et al. Glycoprotein-D-adjuvant vaccine to prevent genital herpes. *N Engl J Med.* 2002;347:1652–1661.

19

Laboratory Interventions

Charlotte A. Gaydos

A common dilemma for practicing clinicians who treat patients with sexually transmitted infections (STIs) is how to most accurately and specifically diagnose an STIs so that proper therapy can be administered. With the advent of new molecular-based tests, the choice of available diagnostic tests has increased significantly, as well as the availability of specimen choices, such as urine. The ability to amplify the nucleic acids, DNA, and RNA from agents that cause STIs has resulted in a revolution of new knowledge about STIs.

Another consideration for clinicians is who to test or screen, especially in the absence of symptoms. It has become increasingly apparent that many, if not most, patients who have an STI are asymptomatic. Therefore, which patients to test is an important decision. In addition to more accurate molecular-based tests, rapid, but less sensitive point-of-care tests have become available for clinicians who have access to an office-based or easily accessed, licensed laboratory. This chapter will focus on chlamydia and gonorrhea, two highly prevalent STIs, for which commercial molecular assays are available. It will consider both the older assays, the new molecular tests, and point-of-care tests. The chapter will discuss which patients to screen and which specific tests should be used, when and how to use them, which specimen type to use, and how to interpret the results with regard to sensitivity and specificity.

▮ CHLAMYDIA TRACHOMATIS

Taxonomy

Chlamydia trachomatis is an obligate intracellular bacteria and one of several species that also includes *C. pneumoniae*

and *C. psittaci*, which cause many types of diseases. There are 18 serovars of *C. trachomatis*, which are divided into the trachoma serotypes A–C, the occulogenital serovars, D–K, and the lymphogranuloma venereum (LGV) serovars L_1–L_3. Serovars can be distinguished by serological typing using monoclonal antibodies or by molecular methods but are not clinically important, since the antibiotic susceptibility pattern is the same. Serovar is important only if LGV is suspected, because the length of time for treatment needs to be longer. LGV is quite rare in the United States and Europe and is the cause of a distinct systemic clinical syndrome quite different from genital chlamydia infections commonly encountered clinically (Janda and Gaydos 2007). LGV infections are characterized by acute lymphadenitis with bubo formation or acute hemorrhagic proctitis. Recently, however, there has been a resurgence of LGV in rectal specimens from men who have sex with men (MSM). Serovar typing can be useful for epidemiological studies, which focus on transmission and geographical differences. In the developed world, the occulogenital strains are predominantly the strains that are routinely prevalent, while trachoma is a sequelae of ocular disease in developing countries and continues to be a leading cause of preventable blindness.

Epidemiology and Clinical Syndromes

C. trachomatis is the etiologic agent of urogenital, ocular, and pneumonic infections. The urogenital infections are sexually transmitted and may be transmitted to infants born to infected women. *C. trachomatis* infections are among the most common sexually transmitted diseases, especially among young adults and adolescents. More than 50 million cases occur worldwide and approximately 3 million to 4 million cases occur in the United States annually.

Clinically, chlamydia occulogenital infections are associated with many syndromes, ranging from cervicitis, salpingitis, acute urethral syndrome, endometritis, ectopic pregnancy, infertility, and pelvic inflammatory disease (PID) in the female; conjunctivitis and pneumonia in infants born to infected mothers; and urethritis, proctitis, and epididymitis in the male. Women bear the burden of morbidity due to chlamydia infections because of the seriousness of the sequelae of infections. Untreated chlamydia infections lead to PID, and multiple episodes of PID can lead to tubal factor infertility. Unfortunately, symptoms of genital infection are often completely absent or very mild among infected patients, especially women, creating a large reservoir of infected persons who continue transmission to new sexual partners. Studies estimate that up to 80–90% of women and more than 50% of men with chlamydial infections lack symptoms.

Chlamydial infections occur primarily among young sexually active persons. Prevalence rates encompass all socioeconomic groups and geographical areas and may range from 5 to 20% in various groups of young adults. Because symptoms are absent in most infected individuals, the prevalence in population groups may be severely underestimated. Thus, widespread screening of individuals at greatest risk, for example, those individuals who are young, sexually active, and have new or multiple partners, has been recommended.

◼ OLDER DIAGNOSTIC TOOLS FOR DETECTION OF CHLAMYDIA INFECTIONS

Previously, detection of chlamydia has been accomplished either (1) staining of chlamydial inclusions grown in tissue culture cells, (2) direct examination of patient clinical specimens to detect elementary bodies using monoclonal antibodies or direct fluorescent antibody (DFA) staining, (3) antigen detection in enzyme immunoassay (EIA) or (4) nucleic acid probe hybridization (see Table 19-1).

TABLE 19-1   Diagnostic Tests to Detect *Chlamydia Trachomatis**

Diagnostic Method	Chlamydia trachomatis	
	Sensitivity	Specificity
Tissue Culture	70–85%	100%
Direct Fluorescent Antibody	80–85%	>99%
Enzyme Immunoassay	53–76%	95%
Hybridization (Pace 2)	65–83%	99%
Polymerase Chain Reaction (COBAS)		
Cervical	89.7%	99.4%
Female Urine	89.2%	99.0%
Male Urine	90.3%	98.4%
Strand Displacement Amplification		
Cervical	92.8%	98.1%
Female Urine	80.5%	98.4%
Male Urine	94.5%	91.4%
Male Urethral	94.6%	94.2%
Transcriptional Mediated Amplification		
Cervical	94.2%	97.6%
Female Urine	94.7%	98.9%
Male Urine	97.0%	99.1%
Male Urethral	95.2%	98.2%

*Compared to infected patient status; package inserts, clinical trials.

Culture

Until about 10 years ago, isolation of *C. trachomatis* in cultured cells was felt to be the gold standard for detecting chlamydia in clinical specimens; however, the sensitivity may vary from 70% to 85% (see Table 19-1). Culture is no longer recommended for routine diagnosis by the Centers for Disease Control and Prevention (CDC) because of its lack of sensitivity and its technical complexity. However, *C. trachomatis* culture is still recommended for medicolegal cases for detecting chlamydia in investigations of sexual abuse, because of its near perfect specificity, but this is changing to increased use of molecular tests. The use of nucleic acid amplification test (NAATs) for medicolegal investigations has received some attention and the demonstrated accuracy may enable the legal system to accept these tests in the future.

Direct Fluorescent Antibody

In the early 1980s, monoclonal antibodies directed against the major outer membrane protein of *C. trachomatis* permitted the implementation of a specific Direct Fluorescent Antibody (DFA) test. As with other tests, the performance of the DFA to detect *C. trachomatis* from invasive urogenital specimens (female cervical and male urethral swabs) varied with respect to the reference gold-standard test. Multisite studies that used culture as a reference demonstrated a sensitivity and specificity of 92% and 98%, respectively (Microtrak package insert). However, when DFA is compared with NAATs, it had an approximate sensitivity and specificity of 80–85% and greater than 99%. The DFA is cleared by the Food and Drug Administration (FDA) for female cervical specimens and male urethral specimens. In addition, since the DFA test is FDA cleared to detect *C. trachomatis* infections in the pharynx and rectum, it can be used to test these samples from MSM. Persons who have receptive anal intercourse are at risk of rectal *C. trachomatis* infections and the CDC has recommended annual screening for such individuals (Gaydos and Rompalo 2002).

Enzyme Immunoassay

In the 1980s, the development of enzyme immunoassay (EIA) tests for direct detection of chlamydial antigen in patient samples provided a cheaper alternative to tissue culture. The sensitivity of the EIA had been comparable to culture, and this technology increased laboratory throughput. However, EIA tests are no longer recommended by CDC to detect chlamydia

(http://www.aphl.org/aphlprograms/infectious/std/Documents/CTGCLabGuidelinesMeetingReport.pdf).

Leucocyte Esterase Test

The Leucocyte Esterase Test (LET) is a rapid dipstick test to use with urine specimens to detect urinary infections. It determines the presence of the esterase enzyme produced by polymorphonuclear (PMN) white cells, which accumulate in urine during any bacterial infection. It is a nonspecific test for diagnosing urethritis because it is only detects PMNs and not the etiologic agent. It has never been recommended for women, and the CDC does not recommend its use for detecting chlamydia in men. Large studies in asymptomatic men have indicated a sensitivity of 57.9% with a specificity of 78.3%; sensitivity of 58.9%, specificity of 94.9%; and sensitivity of 45.8%, specificity of 97.4%. Positive predictive values ranged from 13.8% to 38.4%. Thus, LET is not recommended as a screening test for *C. trachomatis* infection.

Rapid Point-of-Care Tests

Although there are a number of rapid, point-of-care (POC) antigen tests on the market that are FDA-c-cleared for use for cervical samples, none can be recommended for screening for chlamydia, especially in asymptomatic men and women. There is some use of these rapid assays for diagnostic testing of symptomatic patients (as opposed to "screening" of asymptomatic persons). These "point-of-care tests" were designed to be performed while the patient waits for results. One study reported sensitivities for Testpack, Surecell, and Clearview of 70%, 67.3%, and 67.7%, respectively. However, Testpack and Surecell are no longer commercially available, but the Clearview (Unipath, Mountain View, CA), assay is still manufactured. It is FDA cleared for use with male urethral swabs and female cervical swabs but not urine. It is a moderate complexity test and is not a waived test for laboratories approved by the Clinical Laboratory Improvement Act (CLIA). In addition, the QuickVue Chlamydia Test (Quidel Corporation, San Diego, CA) is another marketed rapid test, but it is only intended for females (endocervical swabs or cytobrushes). The Chlamydia Optical Immunoassay (OIA; Thermo Scientific, Waltham, MA, previously called Biostar) is another example of a rapid test and has been shown to be useful, when patients are not likely to return for test results. It is only FDA cleared to use with female endocervical specimens and is not approved for males. A modeling study favored the use of a lower-sensitivity rapid test if treatment can be given before infected persons infect their partners. In general, the rapid tests have very low sensitivities (i.e., 50–70%), compared with NAAT assays and cannot be used with noninvasive specimen types. Most rapid test kit evaluations that received FDA clearance were compared with culture, which being approximately 65–85% sensitive, made the package insert report artificially higher sensitivity than if they were compared with the more sensitive NAAT tests.

Probe Hybridization

The first molecular FDA-approved DNA test for *C. trachomatis* was the nonamplified direct probe test (Pace 2, GenProbe, San Diego, CA). It is only cleared for use with cervical and urethral samples and cannot be used for urine samples or vaginal swabs. When compared with assays employing amplified technology, its sensitivity is much lower. While the probe hybridization assay increased laboratory throughput above culture or DFA, the sensitivity is only comparable to EIA.

■ NEW MOLECULAR DIAGNOSTIC TESTS TO DETECT CHLAMYDIA INFECTIONS

New molecular technologies are now available that amplify nucleic acids of chlamydia in clinical specimens. These assays or NAAT, which are available commercially, include polymerase chain reaction (PCR; Roche Molecular Diagnostics, Branchburg, NJ); transcription-mediated amplication (TMA; GenProbe, San Diego, CA); and strand displacement amplification (SDA; Becton Dickinson, Sparks, MD). These methods offer greatly expanded sensitivities of detection, usually well above 90%, while maintaining very high specificity. These assays are cleared by the FDA for use with chlamydia and are commercially available for use with cervical swabs, male urethral swabs, or urine specimens. These assays have specificity in the range of 98–99%; confirmatory assays had been previously recommended by the CDC if the positive predictive value is less than 95% (low prevalence settings) but is no longer recommended.

Polymerase Chain Reaction

For polymerase chain reason (PCR; Roche), in addition to the microwell format, there is an automated method

(COBAS), which also detects gonorrhea, as well as chlamydia. In the clinical trial for chlamydia, the sensitivity was 89.7% for endocervical samples, 89.2% for female urine specimens, 88.6% for male urethral swabs, and 90.3% for male urines.

Strand Displacement Amplification

For strand displacement amplification (SDA; Becton Dickinson), which also detects gonorrhea, the sensitivity for chlamydia was 92.8% for cervical swabs, 80.5% for female urine, 92.5% for male urethral swabs, and 93.1% for male urine.

Transcription-Mediated Amplification

For transcription-mediated amplification (GenProbe), there is a Combo2 test that tests for both chlamydia and gonorrhea, as well as individual tests ("stand-alone" ACT and AGC) for each organism. The sensitivity for chlamydia in the original clinical trial was 94.2% for cervical swabs, 94.7% for female urine, 97.0% for male urine, and 95.2% for male urethral samples. This assay is also the only FDA cleared for use with clinician and self-administered vaginal swabs.

Choice of assay depends on cost and preference of the laboratory, as all of these NAATs are comparable in sensitivity and specificity, with the TMA assay being slightly more sensitive. Whereas culture was once thought to be the gold standard for detecting chlamydia in clinical specimens, it is now known, because of the extremely high sensitivity of DNA-amplified technology, that culture may have a sensitivity ranging from only 50% to 85%, depending on the specimen type and laboratory performing the culture.

Because older nonculture tests, such as DFA and EIA, were traditionally compared to culture as a gold standard, the sensitivities reported in the older literature can no longer be viewed as accurate. A meta-analysis that adjusted the sensitivities of such assays based on a sensitivity of culture of 85% has been reported. Table 19-1 shows a comparison of the sensitivities and specificities of diagnostic assays available for the detection of *C. trachomatis* in clinical specimens.

One other molecular hybridization test for chlamydia is available, the Digene hybrid capture II CT-ID test (Digene, Silver Spring, MD). It does not amplify the nucleic acid but rather the detection signal is amplified. It has had limited evaluation. It is not FDA cleared for urine specimens.

The ensuing revolution in diagnostic testing that took place after the introduction of NAAT has resulted in a dramatic increase in estimates of the population prevalence of this infection. The number of infections detected by NAAT may be up to 80% higher than those found with older technology. Therefore, widespread screening programs of sexually active individuals using NAAT are in use and are recommended by public health officials. In the United Kingdom, a national program to screen all women aged 15–25 years is currently underway.

If the sensitivity of POC tests can be improved, they will be able to be used in settings in which it is doubtful that the patient will return for test results, such as in homeless shelters, detention centers, and some clinic sites. If such a test had a high enough specificity to warrant its use in such settings, it may be important to accept a less sensitive test for use, rather than treat no one at all because of the inability to locate such infected patients after results from routine tests are available. If the POC test result is negative and the test has a high specificity, a testing algorithm could be set up to continue on to a more sensitive assay as a next step.

■ NEW SPECIMEN TYPES AVAILABLE TO DETECT *C. TRACHOMATIS*

NAAT is so powerful that theoretically even one organism can serve as a target for amplification in clinical specimens. Because of this improved sensitivity of detection, alternative specimen types have been found to be useful for chlamydia diagnosis. First-void urine from both men and women can be used with DNA amplification tests with great accuracy. Because urines are easily obtained, noninvasive specimens, they offer a great advantage for large public health screening programs, where there is no opportunity to obtain a cervical or urethral specimen. In addition, urine specimens are highly acceptable to individuals who may be asymptomatic and who are unwilling to submit to a medical examination. Because a clinician is not required for urine collection, cost savings are also generated when screening large numbers of individuals.

Another type of specimen that has been shown to be both sensitive and specific for detecting chlamydia when amplified tests are used and which has high acceptability by the female patient is a vaginal or vulvar swab. Many studies have reported the successful use of vaginal swabs, which can be self-administered.

Although sexually transmitted infection clinics and family planning clinics have been the source of specimens for chlamydia screening programs, usefulness of alternative specimens types have made alternative sites for screening programs attractive to public health officials. Some of these include schools, prisons, military reception stations, health vans, shopping malls, street outreach sites, and teen centers, as well as the Internet.

■ CHOICE OF DIAGNOSTIC TEST, WHO AND HOW OFTEN TO SCREEN, AND SPECIMEN FOR SCREENING

Even though molecular amplification assays are generally more expensive than older nonculture tests, cost-effectiveness assays, which are done from a societal perspective, have shown NAAT to be more cost-effective in preventing the sequelae associated with chlamydia infections, even when screening is performed in men to reduce sequelae in women. If a female patient has urogenital symptoms or if a pelvic examination is being performed on a patient, clinicians should obtain a cervical swab for a NAAT, because cervical swabs have a higher sensitivity than urine specimens. If an individual is not receiving a pelvic examination, such as in a screening program or because an examination is not indicated, clinicians should take advantage of the ease of obtaining a urine specimen or even a self-administered vaginal swab for amplification testing. The CDC now recommends the vaginal swab as the specimen of choice for screening.

For male patients, the urine specimen is usually always the choice of specimen for testing for chlamydia with an amplification assay. Although, in general, there have been no large ongoing national screening programs for men, several studies have indicated that they also demonstrate high prevalences of chlamydia, ranging from 3% to 8%. Male military recruits presenting for basic training from diverse geographical areas of the United States have a prevalence of approximately 5% and a national household survey sample demonstrated a prevalence of 2.8%.

Age has been determined to be an excellent predictor of risk for chlamydia infections. Those 25 years or younger and those younger than 30 years have been found to be useful in large screening programs. Studies have also shown that individuals who practice high-risk sexual behaviors, such as new or multiple sex partners or who do not use condoms, are at greater risk for chlamydia infections.

Caution should be exercised in using DNA amplification tests for cure assays. Residual DNA from cells rendered noninfective by antibiotics may give a positive test until 3 weeks after therapy, when the patient is actually cured. Studies that examined incidence rates have shown that adolescents may get reinfected with chlamydia frequently. Therefore, sexually active asymptomatic women 25 years or younger should be screened at least once a year with the NAAT. Those patients who have had a chlamydia infection should be screened again at 3 months after treatment.

In summary, clinicians who serve individuals at risk for chlamydia infections now have a new type of test for detecting chlamydial infections, which is a new gold standard that is more sensitive than culture and other nonculture tests. The NAATs, which amplify chlamydial DNA or RNA in a clinical specimen, are so powerful that they can be also used with urine specimens and even self-administered vaginal swabs. Such tests offer clinicians a cost-effective way to diagnose a highly prevalent disease, to prevent serious sequelae and morbidity, and to address the control of a significant public health problem.

■ NEISSERIA GONORRHOEAE

Neisseria gonorrhoeae, first described by Neisser in 1879, is a gram-negative, nonmotile, non-spore-forming diplococcus, belonging to the family Neisseriaceae, which is the etiologic agent of gonorrhea. The other pathogenic species is *N. meningitidis,* to which *N. gonorrhoeae* is genetically closely related. Although *N. meningitidis* is not usually considered to be a sexually transmitted infection, it may infect the mucous membranes of the anogenital area of homosexual men. The other members of the genus, including *N. lactamica, N. polysaccharea, N. cinerea,* and *N. flavescens,* which are related to *N. gonorrhoeae,* and saccharolytic strains, such as *N. subflava, N. sicca,* and *N. mucosa,* which are less genetically related, are considered to be nonpathogenic and are normal flora of the nasopharyngeal mucous membranes.

Gonococcal infection may be either symptomatic or asymptomatic and can cause urethritis, cervicitis, proctitis, Bartholinitis, or conjunctivitis. Gonorrhea is the second most frequently reported bacterial infection in the United States. In males, complications may include epididymitis, prostatitis, and seminal vesiculitis. In MSM, rectal infection and pharyngitis can occur. In females, most cases are asymptomatic, and infections of the urethra and rectum often coexist. Complications can include pelvic inflammatory disease, pelvic pain, ectopic pregnancy, infertility, chorioamnionitis, spontaneous abortion, premature labor, and infections of the neonate, such as conjunctivitis. Other serious sequelae, such as disseminated gonococcal infection (DGI), occur rarely and can result in septicemia, septic arthritis, endocarditis, meningitis, and hemorrhagic skin lesions.

■ OLDER DIAGNOSTIC TOOLS FOR DETECTION OF GONOCOCCAL INFECTIONS

Direct Smear Examination

A direct Gram's stain may be performed as soon as the specimen is collected on site, or a smear may be prepared and transported to the laboratory. Urethral smears from males with symptomatic gonorrhea usually contain intracellular gram-negative diplococci in polymorphonuclear leukocytes (PMNs). Extracellular organisms may be seen also, but a presumptive diagnosis of gonorrhea requires the presence of intracellular diplococci. The sensitivity of such smears in males is 90–95.0%. However, endocervical smears from females and rectal specimens require diligent interpretation, because of colonization of these mucous membranes with other gram-negative coccobacillary organisms. In females, the sensitivity of an endocervical Gram stain is estimated to be 50–70.0% (see Table 19-2).

Antigen Detection

Gonococcal antigen may be detected by an enzyme immunoassay (Abbott Laboratories, Abbott Park, IL) for a presumptive diagnosis. This EIA is about as sensitive and specific as a Gram stain in males but is less sensitive for use with endocervical specimens.

Culture

The isolation and identification of *N. gonorrhoeae* is the currently accepted gold standard to diagnosis gonococcal infections (see Table 19-2). Specimens should be inoculated onto nonselective media (chocolate agar), upon which all *Neisseria* spp. will grow, or selective media, such as modified Thayer-Martin (MTM), Martin-Lewis (ML), or New York City (NYC). Selective media contain antimicrobial agents to inhibit commensal bacteria, nonpathogenic *Neisseria* sp., and fungi. Because pathogenic *Neisseria* are nutritionally and environmentally fastidious, the ideal method for transporting organisms for culture is to plate the specimens directly onto the culture medium and immediately incubate the plates in an increased humidity atmosphere of 3–5% CO_2, at 35–37°C. The CO_2-enriched atmosphere is very important, and with the advent of commercial zip-locked bags with CO_2-generating tablets, specimens should no longer be transported in Stuart's or Amies medium.

TABLE 19-2. Diagnostic Tests to Detect *Neisseria Gonorrhoeae**

Diagnostic Method	Neisseria Gonorrhoeae	
	Sensitivity	**Specificity**
Culture	80–95%	100%
Gram Stain		
Males—symptomatic	90–95%	95–100%
Males—asymptomatic	50–70%	95–100%
Females	50–70%	95–100%
Hybridization (Pace2)	92.1–96.4%	98.8–99.1%
Polymerase Chain Reaction (COBAS)		
Cervical	92.4%	99.5%
Female Urine	64.8%	99.8%
Male Urine	94.1%	99.9%
Strand Displacement Amplification		
Cervical	96.6%	98.9–99.8%
Female Urine	84.9%	98.8–99.8%
Male Urine	98.1%	96.8–98.7%
Male Urethral	98.1%	96.8–98.7%
Transcriptional Mediated Amplification		
Cervical	99.2%	98.7%
Female Urine	91.3%	99.3%
Male Urine	97.1%	99.2%
Male Urethral	98.8%	98.2%

*Compared with infected patient status; package inserts, clinical trials.

Identification

Two levels of identification of isolated organisms may be used: presumptive and confirmatory. An isolate may be presumptively identified as *N. gonorrhoeae* when a gram-negative, oxidase positive diplococcus has been isolated. Confirmatory identification requires that biochemical, fluorescent antibody, chromogenic enzyme substrate, serological, or coagglutination tests be performed to distinguish the isolate from *N. meningitidis*, and *Branhamella catarrhalis*, *Kingella denitrificans*, as well as non-pathogenic *Neisseria* spp. Many of these methods are commercially available, none are perfect, and most require an isolated subculture or colony. Some of these rapid methods include QuadFERM+ (bioMerieux Vitek, Hazelwood, MO); Gonochek II (bioMerieux Vitek); Identicult-Neisseria, IDN (Adams Scientific, West Warwick, RI); Polyvalent Fluorescent-Antibody Test (Difco Laboratories, Detroit, MI); *Neisseria gonorrhoeae* Culture Confirmation Test (a monoclonal fluorescent-antibody test, Syva Co, San Jose, CA); Phadebact GC OMNI (Karo Bio Diagnostics AB, Huddinge, Sweden); Gonogen I and Gonogen II (New Horizons Diagnostics, Columbia, MD); the Meritec GC (Meridian Diagnostics, Cincinnati, OH); and the GC Monoclonal Antibody Test (Boule Diagnostics International AB, Stockholm, Sweden). A DNA probe test (Accuprobe, GenProbe, San Diego, CA) for culture confirmation was a test similar to PACE (GenProbe), which is used for the direct detection of gonococci in clinical specimens, but it has now been replaced by PACE 2, which can be used for either direct detection or culture confirmation.

■ MOLECULAR DIAGNOSTIC TESTS FOR DETECTION OF GONORRHEA INFECTIONS

Molecular techniques for identifying, sequencing, and amplifying genes from *N. gonorrhoeae* have obviated the requirement for viable organisms for diagnosing infections and for epidemiological typing studies. In particular, the technology to amplify nucleic acids from clinical specimens is so powerful that theoretically one gene copy in a sample can be detected. The power of the amplification methods have also lead to the use of nonconventional specimens types that are unsuitable for culture, such as urine, vaginal swabs, and tissue from the upper reproductive tract.

There are now several FDA-approved nucleic acid tests for *N. gonorrhoeae*: the unamplified probe test (Pace 2, GeneProbe, San Diego, CA) and the amplified DNA or RNA tests, the PCR test for the co-amplification of both *N. gonorrhoeae* and *C. trachomatis* (Roche Molecular Systems, Branchburg, NJ), transcription-mediated amplification TMA; GenProbe, San Diego, CA), and strand displacement amplification (SDA; Becton Dickinson, Sparks, MD) (see Table 19-2).

Pace 2 Assay

Although this is not an amplified test, sensitivity and specificity both appear to be very good for this assay. Sensitivity, as compared with culture, ranges from 90.8% to 96.3% for women and for men, 99.1% to 99.6% (package insert). Specificity is uniformly high, ranging from 97.5% to 100% for men and women (package insert). An advantage of this method is that there are no stringent transport conditions required, which makes it attractive for use with specimens that must be transported to an off-site laboratory. Clinical evaluations of the assay have supported the reported high sensitivity and specificity of the assay. Of published reports, the sensitivity ranged from 96.3% to 100% and specificity from 98.8% to 99.6%.

Ligase Chain Reaction

Multicenter trials and other studies demonstrated that the overall sensitivity and specificity of LCR (Abbott) for *N. gonorrhoeae* were 97.3% and 99.8%, respectively, from 1539 female endocervical specimens; and for 1639 males a sensitivity and specificity of 98.5% and 99.8% for 808 urethral swabs and 99.1% and 99.7% for urine, respectively. Although this assay is no longer available commercially, it represents the power of NAAT assays compared with culture.

Other NAATs

Other NAATs are similarly sensitive and specific for detecting gonorrhea in clinical genital samples with the

exception that although the PCR test (Roche Amplicor) is not FDA cleared to use for gonorrhea with urine from females, it has been used successfully in research studies. In addition, there have been problems with specificity for gonorrhea with this assay, as it occasionally identified nonpathogenic *Neisseria* sp. as gonorrhea. For PCR (Roche), there is an automated method (COBAS), which detects both gonorrhea as well as chlamydia. For gonorrhea, the sensitivity was 92.4% for endocervical samples but 64.8% for female urine specimens; 94.1% for symptomatic male urines; and 42.4% for urines from asymptomatic men. For SDA (Becton Dickinson), which also detects both chlamydia and gonorrhea, the sensitivity for gonorrhea was 96.6% for cervical swabs, 84.9% for female urine, 98.5% for male urethral swabs, and 97.9% for male urine. For the APTIMA Combo2 (GenProbe) assay, sensitivity for gonorrhea in cervical samples was 99.2%, 91.3% for female urine, 97.1% for male urine, and 98.8% for male urethral specimens. There is also an individual APTIMA assay for gonorrhea (AGC).

■ THE CHANGING EPIDEMIOLOGY OF CHLAMYDIA AND GONORRHEA

A main advantage of using amplified tests to detect STIs is the ability to use the same sample type, whether it is urine or a self-administered vaginal swab, to detect both chlamydia and gonorrhea. While most outreach screening studies have used NAATs primarily for chlamydia testing, also screening for gonorrhea has distinct advantages, especially in populations and regions that have demonstrated high prevalences for gonorrhea. Other alternative sites for screening programs have been attractive to public health officials, including schools, prisons, military personnel, health vans, shopping malls, household surveys, street outreach sites, and teen centers. Such studies give public health officials the ability to direct future control efforts toward populations where high prevalences of disease exist in asymptomatic and untreated persons not ordinarily seeking health care.

Hospital emergency departments have also been sites for screening programs in young adults presenting for reasons other than reproductive health care and have demonstrated high prevalences using urine screening. Therefore, widespread screening programs of sexually active individuals using NAAT are justified and are supported by recommendations of public health officials. Finally, the effectiveness of expanded screening programs in reducing chlamydia prevalence has been shown in areas where the screening programs have been in existence for an extended time.

■ General Diagnostic Issues

Because NAATs measure DNA or RNA rather than live organisms, care should be used in using NAATs for test-of-cure assays. Residual nucleic acid from cells rendered noninfective by antibiotics may still give a positive amplified test up to 3 weeks after therapy, when the patient is actually cured of viable organisms. Therefore, clinicians should not use NAATs for test-of-cure until after 3 weeks.

Even though molecular amplification assays are more expensive than older nonculture tests, cost-effectiveness assays, have shown NAAT to be more cost-effective in preventing the sequelae associated with chlamydia infections. In general, if a female patient has urogenital symptoms or if a pelvic examination is performed on a patient for reasons other than screening, clinicians should obtain a cervical swab for a NAAT, because cervical swabs usually have a higher sensitivity than urine specimens. However, if an individual is not receiving a pelvic examination, clinicians should take advantage of the ease of obtaining a urine or vaginal specimen for amplification testing for chlamydia and gonorrhea. Screening of males for chlamydia can also be recommended as cost-effective in preventing sequelae in women due to chlamydia.

■ Positive Predictive Values and Testing

One of the major issues in diagnostic testing is the concept of positive predictive value (PPV)—the probability that a positive test is truly positive. The major determinants of PPV are the underlying prevalence in a given population and the specificity of the test. The specificity is, indirectly, a measure of the number of false-positives. With newer generation NAAT tests, specificity is routinely >98%, and often above 99%, and therefore is highly optimized. However, the major challenge, even with highly specific tests, is in dealing with low prevalence populations. The PPV conundrum is that as the prevalence drops, the proportion of false positive tests rises. With STIs, this may present a number of difficulties.

In STI practice, therefore, the clinician should be particularly careful to offer testing in settings where the likelihood of false positives is lower. This in practice may be difficult, since there is an imperative to screen and identify asymptomatic and subsymptomatic infections.

■ Summary

In conclusion, the availability of amplification assays and the ability to obtain noninvasive urine and vaginal specimens to diagnose chlamydia and gonorrhea infections in both symptomatic and asymptomatic patients have led to a revolution in how detection of infected individuals can be accomplished. Because of their increased detection capability, the ease of sample collection, and the high prevalences of both chlamydia and gonorrhea in non-healthcare-seeking persons, clinicians, and public health officials alike should be encouraged to use these amplified tests in their practices and screening programs for STIs. Only by increased surveillance, detection, and treatment of infected patients and their partners can the epidemic of STIs in this country be halted.

References

Association of Public Health Laboratories. Guidelines for the laboratory testing of STDs. http://www.aphl.org/aphlprograms/infectious/std/Pages/stdtestingguidelines/aspx. 2009. Accessed March 30, 2010.

CDC. STD treatment guidelines 2010. *Morb Mortal Week Rep.* 2010;59(RR-12):1–110.

Finelli L, Schillinger JA, Wasserheit JN. Are emergency departments the next frontier for sexually transmitted disease screening? *Sex Trans Dis.* 2001;28:40–42.

Gaydos CA. Nucleic acid amplification tests for gonorrhea and chlamydia: practice and applications. In: Zenilman JJ, Moellering RC Jr, eds. *Infectious Disease Clinics of North America, Sexually Transmitted Infections.* Vol. 19, no. 2. Philadelphia; 2005;367–386.

Gaydos CA. Chlamydiae. In: Spector S, Hodinka RL, Young SA, Wiedbrauk DL, eds. *Clinical Virology Manual.* 4th ed. Washington, DC: ASM Press; 2009:630–640.

Gaydos CA, Ferrero DV, Papp J. Laboratory aspects of screening males for *Chlamydia trachomatis* in the new millennium. *Sex Transm. Dis.* 2005;35(suppl):S44–S50.

Gaydos CA, Rompalo AM. The use of urine and self-obtained vaginal swabs for the diagnosis of sexually transmitted diseases. *Curr Infect Dis Rep.* 2002;4:148–157.

Howell MR, Quinn TC, Brathwaite W, Gaydos CA. Screening women for *Chlamydia trachomatis* in family planning clinics: the cost-effectiveness of DNA amplification assays. *Sex Transm. Dis.* 1998;25:108–117.

Janda WM, Gaydos CA. *Neisseria.* In: Murray PR, Baron EJ, Jorgensen JH, Landry MR, Pfaller MA, eds. *Manual of Clinical Microbiology.* Washington, DC: American Society for Microbiology; 2007:601–620.

Kuypers J, Gaydos CA, Peeling RW. Principles of laboratory diagnosis of STIs. In: Holmes KK, Sparling PF, Stamm WE, et al, eds. *Sexually Transmitted Diseases*. 4th ed. New York: McGraw Hill; 2008;937–957.

Mehta SD, Rothman RE, Kelen GD, Quinn TC, Zenilman J.M. Clinical aspects of diagnosis of gonorrhea and *Chlamydia* infection in an acute care setting. *Clin Infect Dis.* 2001;32:655–659.

Mertz KJ, Levine WC, Mosure DJ, Berman SM, Dorian KJ. Trends in the prevalence of chlamydia infections: the impact of community-wide testing. *Sex Transm Dis.* 1997;24:169–175.

Rompalo AM, Gaydos CA, Shah N, et al. Evaluation of use of a single intravaginal swab to detect multiple sexually transmitted infections in active-duty military women. *Clin Infect Dis.* 2001;33:1455–1461.

Schachter J, Stephens RS. Biology of *Chlamydia trachomatis*. In: Holmes KK, Sparling PF, Stamm WE, et al, eds. *Sexually Transmitted Diseases*. 4th ed. New York: McGraw-Hill Companies, Inc; 2008:555–574.

US Preventive Services Task Force. Screening for chlamydial infection: recommendations and rationale. *Am J Prev Med.* 2001;20(suppl):90–94.

Wiesenfeld HC, Lowry DLB, Heine RP, et al. Self-collection of vaginal swabs for the detection of Chlamydia, gonorrhea, and trichomonas. *Sex Transm Dis.* 2001;28:321–325.

20

Syphilis Serology

Klaus-Peter Hunfeld and Hans-Jochen Hagedorn

Syphilis is caused by *Treponema pallidum* subsp. *pallidum*, a member of the family of Spirochaetaceae. The variety of clinical symptoms (see Chapters 9 and 17), and the frequent latency of infection, presents a challenge to clinical diagnosticians. Therefore, serological laboratory testing is an important part of diagnosing the presence or absence of syphilis.

SAMPLE COLLECTION AND TRANSPORT

T. pallidum cannot be grown in in vitro culture. The most frequently used direct clinical specimens for direct diagnosis are fresh preparations from genital ulcers viewed by dark-field microscopy. Because of the difficulty in diagnosis, serological testing is most frequently used with whole blood, serum, or plasma. Serological testing can also be performed on cerebrospinal fluid (CSF) in cases where neurosyphilis is suspected. Serum is the preferred material and is stable at room temperature, but CSF specimens that are shipped should be refrigerated. All materials should be accompanied by a short report containing the essential clinical information required for accurate interpretation of and clinical comment on the laboratory test results.

METHODS FOR THE LABORATORY DIAGNOSIS OF SYPHILIS

The diagnosis of syphilis depends on the synopsis of clinical findings, direct examination of lesion material for treponemes, or serological testing (see also Chapter 9).

The full complement of laboratory diagnostic tests is described in Table 20-1.

DIRECT DETECTION BY MICROSCOPY

Spirochetes were first demonstrated in syphilitic lesions by Schaudin and Hoffman in 1905. Dark-field or India ink microscopy (see Figure 20-1) is the diagnostic method of choice for diagnosing *T. pallidum* from cutaneous lesions and lymph nodes in early primary syphilis.

Diagnostic Value

Except for cutaneous ulcers, the number of organisms in clinical specimens is low, which directly impacts sensitivity. The detection cutoff is 100 treponemes/μl. Sensitivity is also affected by prior antibiotic therapy (even if ineffective) or the use of ointments, which patients often place directly on the lesions. Moreover, direct microscopy cannot reliably distinguish *T. pallidum* from the other *Treponema* species. This is especially important in oral lesions, where the presence of *T. denticola* and other commensals impact test specificity.

DIRECT DETECTION OF *T. PALLIDUM* BY POLYMERASE CHAIN REACTION

Because of the low sensitivity of direct detection techniques, DNA amplification techniques, such as polymerase chain reaction (PCR), hold promise for etiological diagnosis of genital ulcers, and specific PCR tests

TABLE 20-1 Direct and Indirect Detection Methods for the Laboratory Diagnosis of Syphilis

Direct Detection Methods	Indirect Detection Methods
Dark-field or India ink microscopy[1]	*T. pallidum* particle agglutination (TPPA)[1]
Direct fluorescent-antibody testing[2]	*T. pallidum* hemagglutination (TPHA)[1]
Animal inoculation[2]	Fluorescent treponemal antibody absorption (FTA-ABS) test (polyvalent)[1]
	Enzyme immunoassay (EIA), polyvalent[1]
Polymerase chain reaction (PCR)[2]	Immunoblot[2]
	Venereal disease research laboratory (VDRL) test[1]
	Cardiolipin complement fixation test (CFT)[1]
	Rapid plasma reagin (RPR) test[1]
	Class-specific EIA (IgG, IgM[2])[2]
	IgM-FTA-ABS[1]
	IgM-immunoblot[2]

Laboratory diagnosis of syphilis: (1) standard assays; (2) supplementary or research procedures.

have been developed to target specific sequences of the organism. However, these are available only in the research environment.

INDIRECT DETECTION OF THE PATHOGEN (SEROLOGICAL APPROACHES)

Wasserman developed the first serological tests in 1906. Diagnosis based on testing for specific anti–*T. pallidum* antibodies has since been widely used. Serological tests are divided into nontreponemal and treponemal tests that are best employed in a combined stepwise diagnostic approach. Whenever possible, antibody testing should be performed in a semiquantitative manner because the relative amount of specific antibodies as

measured in titers or units per milliliter (U/mL) can be correlated to the clinical course and disease activity and is useful in monitoring treatment success.

Diagnostic Value

The capabilities and limitations of some frequently used serological tests are described in Table 20-2.

NONTREPONEMAL (REAGINIC) TESTS

Nontreponemal tests (see Table 20-2), such as the rapid plasma reagin (RPR), the venereal disease research laboratory (VDRL) test, and the cardiolipin complement

FIGURE 20-1 *T. Pallidum*, Dark-Field Microscopy, Magnification 1000×

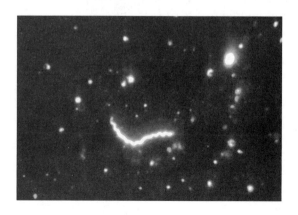

BOX 20-1 How to Do a Dark Field

- Clean the suspicious lesion with sterile saline
- Abrade the base of the lesion with gauze and squeeze gently
- Apply a coverslip to the exuding serous fluid and then place slip without bubbles on a clean glass slide
- Inspect immediately by use of a special microscope with a dark-field condenser (magnification 400×)
- Look for spiral-shaped bacterial organisms (see Figure 20-1) and their characteristic motility

TABLE 20-2   Diagnostic Properties of Common Reaginic and Treponeme-Specific Tests

Assay	Reaginic Tests		Treponeme-Specific Tests		
	Rapid Plasma Reagin (RPR) Test	**Venereal Disease Research Laboratory (VDRL) test**	**Treponema pallidum Hemagglutination Assay (TPHA)**	**Fluorescent Treponemal Antibody Absorption (FTA-ABS) Test**	**Immunoblot**
Test Principle	Charcoal flocculation	Microflocculation	Hemagglutination	Immunofluorescence	Enzyme-linked antibody detection
Positive After	2 weeks postexposure	2 weeks postexposure	2 weeks postexposure	2 weeks postexposure	10–14 days postexposure
Remains Positive					
Treated	3 mos. to >1 yr.	3 mos. to >1 yr.	Lifelong	Lifelong	Lifelong
Untreated	Decades	Decades	Lifelong	Lifelong	Lifelong
Sensitivity					
Primary Syphilis	86% (77–100%)	78% (74–87%)	76% (69–90%)	84% (70–100%)	>95% (80–100%)
Secondary Syphilis	98% (95–100%)	95% (88–100%)	100%	100%	100%
Latent/Late Syphilis	73%	71% (37–94)	100%	100%	100%
Specificity					
	93–99%	96–99%	98–100%	94–100%	98–99%

Adapted from Orton et al. (2001).

fixation test (CFT) are reagin-based assays that use precipitation, flocculation, or complement fixation to qualitatively or quantitatively measure antilipoid IgM- and IgG-antibodies. These antibodies are directed against a lipid hapten called cardiolipin, which can be found in a variety of tissues as well as within the spirochete. The relative amount of reagin titers correlates well with disease activity and is used to define treatment success. In primary syphilis, however, reaginic tests can be negative in up to 20-50% of cases, especially early in the course of disease. This occurs because antibodies develop after the onset of lesions. Nonspecific test titers against cardiolipin tend to decline in later disease stages or during latency and may be undetectable in treated and untreated individuals alike. The cardiolipin antigen is found in a number of tissues, and antibodies may be detected in a number of other situations, such as collagen-vascular disease (especially systemic lupus), intravenous drug users, and in a number of adverse drug reactions.

Diagnostic Value

Reaginic tests should be used to monitor disease activity and the success of antibiotic treatment in syphilis patients. CFT is laborious but slightly more sensitive than the widely used RPR and VDRL tests. Because of the cross reactivity, these tests should not be used as single screening procedures. All positive tests should be confirmed by a specific treponemal assay.

■ TREPONEMAL (SPECIFIC) TESTS

Treponemal tests (see Table 20-2) detect treponeme-specific cellular antigens and are largely used for confirmation of non-treponemal tests. Conventional polyvalent treponemal tests for the simultaneous detection of specific IgG and IgM include the *T. pallidum* hemagglutination assay (TPHA), the *T. pallidum* particle agglutination assay (TP-PA), and the polyvalent fluorescent treponemal antibody absorption test (FTA-ABS). Agglutination assays, such as TPHA and TPPA (overall sensitivity: 69–100%, specificity: 98–100%), apply ultra sonicated or SDS-treated *T. pallidum* antigens and are widely used as screening tests. Both TPHA and TPPA can be adapted to automated test performance. Polyvalent FTA-ABS uses whole cell *T. pallidum*-antigen (Nichols strain) fixed onto glass slides and serves mainly as a confirmatory assay.

In primary syphilis, treponemal tests become positive slightly earlier than with reagin-based assays, usually within 2–4 weeks after infection. The overall sensitivity

and specificity of FTA-ABS is reported to be 70–100% and 94–100% respectively, and false-positive results are unusual (~1–2%). Accurate reading of test results in these manual assays, however, correlates strongly with the expertise of the laboratorian and this is a clear disadvantage compared to the enzyme immunosorbent assays (EIA) format.

Diagnostic Value

Treponemal tests are more sensitive and specific than nontreponemal tests, and false-positive reactions are less likely to occur (see Table 20-2). TPHA, TPPA, and FTA-ABS tests are still regarded as the serologic gold standards in laboratory screening for and confirmation of specific anti–*T. pallidum* antibodies. Although promising, recent diagnostic approaches, such as EIA and immunoblot, have been less well assessed. Moreover, the quality of the commercially available EIA and immunoblot assays can differ substantially.

■ DETECTION OF SPECIFIC IgM-ANTIBODIES

When testing is available, a qualitative or quantitative test for specific anti–*T. pallidum* IgM-antibodies can be helpful in assessing the stage of infection and the need for antibiotic therapy. Such tests, however, are not readily available in most routine or field laboratories but require the capabilities of expert or specialist laboratories. At present, IgM-FTA-ABS test, IgM-EIA, and IgM-immunoblot are available to test for specific IgM in syphilis infections, mostly in Europe. The classical IgM-FTA-ABS test is still regarded as the gold standard (see Table 20-3). After absorption of cross-reacting group-specific antibodies and following separation of the IgM and IgG fractions by gel filtration or immune absorption with anti-IgG serum (rheuma factor absorbent or protein G), detection of specific anti–*T. pallidum*–IgM by use of a fluorochrome-marked μ-chain-specific antihuman antibody takes place. The assay can be evaluated in a qualitative or quantitative manner. Titration of immune absorbed sera is usually begun at a serum dilution of 1:5 or 1:10, depending on the methodological details and the antigen preparation used. The strength of fluorescence is graded as + (borderline reactive) up to ++++ (strongly reactive). A result of ++ in the screening dilution is generally regarded as specific.

Commercially available IgM-EIAs lack sensitivity in reinfected patients as well as in latent and late syphilis. Moreover, the quality of such commercially available IgM-EIA and IgM-immunoblot assays, however, can

TABLE 20-3   Diagnostic Properties of Common Treponeme-Specific IgM-tests

	Treponeme-Specific IgM-Tests		
Assay	IgM-Enzyme Immunoassay (EIA)	IgM-FTA-ABS	IgM-Immunoblot
Test Principle	Enzyme-linked antibody detection	Immunofluorescence	Enzyme-linked antibody detection
Positive After	10–14 days postexposure	10–14 days postexposure	10–14 days postexposure
Remains Positive			
Treated	6–12 mos.	6–18 mos.	6–12 mos.
Untreated	Mos. to yrs.	Mos. to yrs.	Mos. to yrs.
	Sensitivity		
Primary Syphilis	69–100%	97%	90–100%
Secondary Syphilis	100%	100%	~100%
Latent/Late Syphilis	Variable	Variable	Variable
	Specificity		
	90–99%	98–100%	98–99%

Under conditions of a field laboratory, IgM-assays are regarded as supplementary procedures.

differ substantially from one manufacturer to another. Thus, to date, they cannot be regarded as a viable alternative to classical IgM-FTA-ABS testing.

Diagnostic Value

Together with treponemal and reaginic tests specific anti–*T. pallidum* IgM-testing is helpful in assessing the stage of infection and provides a baseline for monitoring the effects of treatment. Nevertheless, the specific IgM-test result always should be interpreted in the context of other treponemal and reaginic assay results and against the backdrop of additional clinical information. In critical cases, the IgM-FTA-ABS test remains the gold standard for specific anti–*T. pallidum* IgM-antibody detection, especially in the very early and in the latent stage of infection.

■ STAGE-DEPENDENT ANTIBODY KINETICS IN NATURAL SYPHILIS INFECTION

The natural course of syphilis is extremely variable (see Figure 20-2). The immune response to *T. pallidum* involves the production of antibodies to a broad range of antigens, only few of which are regarded as highly specific. The production of specific anti–*T. pallidum* IgM-antibodies commences approximately 2 weeks after infection and is followed by specific IgG at about 4 weeks. By the time that clinical symptoms actually occur, most patients show a detectable specific anti–*T. pallidum* IgM- and IgG-response. Antibody levels rise as the disease progresses, and, in late syphilis, TPHA/TPPA titers (predominantly IgG) into the millions can be found in some

FIGURE 20-2 Possible Courses of the Natural Immune Response, As Detected by Different Assays in Patients with Syphilis

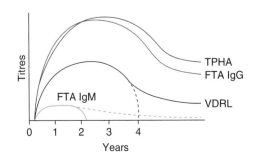

individuals. The specific IgM-response, however, can decline during latency or in late syphilis and may become nonreactive in some persons during the natural course of the infection. The reactivity of nontreponemal tests varies with the level of anticardiolipin IgG- and IgM-antibodies, which do occur slightly later than the specific anti–*T. pallidum* IgM-response. Early on in the disease, when the sensitivity of nontreponemal tests is only 62–76%, reaginic test results may be nonreactive. Reaginic test titers commonly peak during secondary syphilis, when the sensitivity of such tests approximates 100% but tend to decline afterward and can revert to nonreactive in 25% of untreated patients. This explains why sensitivities of reaginic tests average only 70% in late syphilis.

The natural course of the immune response can be influenced by treatment, by immunocompromising diseases, such as HIV, and by previous syphilis infection. HIV can eventually reduce or delay the specific immune response, but usually the response is normal or even exaggerated.

Exact diagnosis of secondary infection or relapse clearly requires knowledge of quantitative test results in the previous medical history. A sharp rise in the specific IgG response paralleled by a boost in reaginic test titers can be observed. In such cases, however, the specific IgM-response can vary considerably, ranging from highly positive to nonreactive.

▪ STANDARD SERODIAGNOSIS OF SYPHILIS

In clinical practice, serological tests for syphilis are used for screening asymptomatic individuals, such as blood donors, organ tissue donors, and pregnant women. Serology is also applied in patients with a recent risk of acquiring a sexually transmitted disease, and for testing patients with a history or symptoms consistent with syphilis. The testing strategy varies depending on the patient population and whether a specialized laboratory needs to detect all stages of syphilis and to monitor and comment on the effects of treatment. Smaller laboratories or blood banks might wish to screen their patients solely with the intention of sending all screening test-positive samples to a specialized laboratory for further confirmation and commentary. A stepwise diagnostic approach (see Figure 20-3),

FIGURE 20-3 Rational Stepwise Algorithm for Serological Diagnosis of Syphilis.

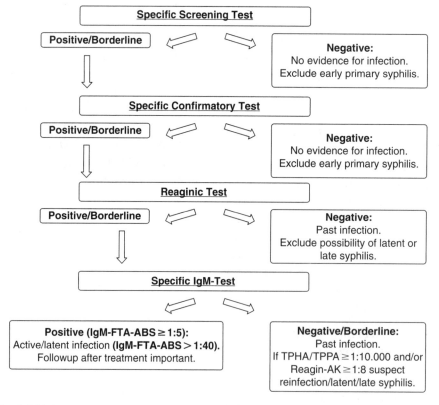

Under conditions of a field laboratory, IgM-assays are regarded as supplementary procedures.

including a treponemal screening test, a confirmatory assay, a reagin test, TPHA, TPPA, and polyvalent EIA are the best single screening tests within the routine clinical laboratory setting.

In the event of a positive screening test, the result should be *confirmed* by another treponemal test, that is, EIA or FTA-ABS, if TPPA is used for screening, or TPPA or FTA-ABS, when EIA is employed for screening. Reaginic assays (RPR or VDRL) are the tests of choice for determining the serological *activity* of syphilis and for monitoring the effect of treatment. Follow-ups are best performed in parallel with the initial serum at the same laboratory that performed the original testing.

■ RATIONAL INTERPRETATION OF SEROLOGIC FINDINGS

If the serological screening in patients with potential primary or secondary syphilis but without typical clinical symptoms yields a negative result, no further diagnostic testing should be performed. If, however, clinical suspicion persists because of typical symptoms or potential exposure of the patient, serologic screening with a treponemal test should be repeated at weekly intervals to confirm or exclude early primary syphilis. In such cases, a parallel examination of suspicious lesions by direct microscopy can be helpful in ruling out early manifestations before the onset of a specific immune response. A positive reaginic test result together with a negative treponemal test points to a nonspecific reaction and excludes early syphilis. These are classified as biological false positives (BFP) and are seen often in patients with leprosy, patients chronic inflammatory disorders, intravenous drug users, patients with rheumatological diseases, patients with drug reaction, and patients who are pregnant. BFP titers are rarely greater than 1:16. In cases showing a positive screening test together with a positive confirmatory assay, the disease activity should be determined by performing a reagin-based assay.

In asymptomatic patients, a highly positive screening test, that is, TPPA/TPHA titers of greater than 5000, and a positive confirmatory test provide evidence for persistent (latent) infection. In such cases, the results of reaginic tests can vary from strongly reactive to negative. All patients without evidence for any specific therapy in their medical history should be treated to avoid possible late-stage manifestations. Some examples for classical constellations of serologic test results are shown in Table 20-4.

■ LABORATORY DIAGNOSIS IN NEUROSYPHILIS

After local infection, *T. pallidum* disseminates systemically, including the CNS. Neurosyphilis can present as part of the secondary syphilis syndrome or as late syphilis. In suspected neurosyphilis, a negative treponeme-specific blood test clearly excludes *T. pallidum* infection of the CNS. In patients with serologically *confirmed* syphilis and suspicion of neurosyphilis, a lumbar puncture is indicated. In the CSF, total protein, albumin, immunoglobulin levels, and the total number and kind of inflammatory cells should be determined together with a search for reagin- and treponeme-specific antibodies. The CSF-VDRL is most widely used. Even in research settings, PCR has proved to be of minimum value in detecting *T. pallidum* in the CSF of patients with syphilis.

Under the conditions of a field laboratory, the serological examination of the CSF alone cannot provide sufficient diagnostic evidence to confirm or exclude neurosyphilis. Instead, paired serum and cerebrospinal fluid (CSF) samples obtained on the same day should be analyzed. Independent of a possible *T. pallidum* infection, the immunoglobulin content and, consequently, the concentration of treponemal and nontreponemal antibodies in the CSF is significantly influenced by three major factors:

- *The concentration of immunoglobulins in serum*: An increase in the concentration of immunoglobulins or a rise in specific antibody titers in serum can lead to a subsequent increase in the corresponding CSF concentrations.

- *A possible dysfunction of the blood-CSF barrier*: Increased permeability of the blood-CSF barrier results in a greater influx of serum proteins and in rising concentrations of these proteins in the CSF.

- *Ongoing local immunoglobulin synthesis within the CNS*: Autochthonous antibody production can result in a relative increase of specific antibody concentrations within the CSF, independent of the blood-CSF barrier function.

Under the conditions of a specialist laboratory, a more precise assessment of whether *T. pallidum*–specific antibodies detected in the CSF originate from peripheral blood or whether they have been synthesized within the CNS (autochthonous antibody production) can be made by simultaneous examination of the total IgG- or IgM (Ig) concentration (mg/L) and the pathogen-specific IgG- and/or IgM-antibodies (as determined in

TABLE 20-4   Typical Constellations of Test Results in Patients with Active or Past Syphilis Infection

Material	TPHA/TPPA/EIA	FTA-ABS	Reaginic Test	IgM-FTA-ABS Test*	Comment
Serum	Negative	—	—	—	No evidence for infection, follow-up if early primary infection is suspected
Serum	1:80	Negative	Negative	—	False-positive reaction, follow-up if early primary infection is suspected
Serum	1:1280	1:640	1:2 to 1:4	Negative	Past infection
Serum	1:5120	1:5120	1:8 to >1:16	Positive (1:40 to >1:160)	Active infection
Serum	≥1:10.000	≥1:10.000	≥1:8	Negative/ borderline	Active infection or reinfection, endogenous blocking of IgM-response
Serum CSF	1:1280 1:16	1:640 1:8	1:16 1:4	Positive (1:80) positive (1:8)	Active infection with probable CNS-involvement, AI determination necessary for confirmation!
Serum CSF	1:1280 Negative	1:640 Negative	1:16 Negative	Positive (1:80) Negative	Active syphilis infection CNS-involvement not likely (if cell count in CSF is negative)
Serum CSF	1:20,000 1:640	1:10,000 1:320	1:8 1:4	Negative or positive Negative or positive	Active (re-?)infection with possible CNS-involvement, AI determination necessary for confirmation!
Serum CSF	1:80 Negative	Negative Negative	1:4 1:4	Negative Negative	Past infection or false positive reaction CNS-involvement not likely

*Commonly done in specialist laboratories only.

titers or EIA absorption), as determined in serum and CSF obtained on the same day. In mathematical terms, so-called antibody-specific indices (AI) are calculated by means of the following formulas:

$$AI = \frac{Tp - specific\ Ig\ CSF \times Total\ Ig\ serum\ (mg/L)}{Tp - specific\ Ig\ serum \times Total\ Ig\ CSF\ (mg/L)}$$

When using polyvalent TPHA, TPPA, or FTA-ABS for specific antibody determination, an AI of less than 2 gives no evidence for specific intrathecal antibody production. An AI of 2–3 is regarded as *elevated* and compatible with neurosyphilis, whereas an index of greater than 3 definitely indicates a specific local antibody production in the CNS and *demonstrates* recent or past treponemal CNS infection. The determination of specific intrathecal IgG- or IgM-antibody synthesis is also possible using this formula if assays with adequate sensitivity are selected for both the measurement of total IgM and the determination of *T. pallidum*–specific IgM in the CSF. Today, the corresponding protein analysis can be performed using automated laboratory analyzers, which, at the same time, permit software-assisted calculation and evaluation of the findings. In our experience, the determination of the specific intrathecal antibody response as outlined earlier is also reliable in most HIV patients with neurosyphilis.

RATIONAL INTERPRETATION OF LABORATORY FINDINGS IN THE CSF

The detection of a specific intrathecal antibody synthesis indicates a recent or past infection of the CNS but does not necessarily imply the diagnosis of active neurosyphilis. That is because persistence of a specific antibody response for years in the CSF has been reported even in patients with neurosyphilis who had received adequate treatment. For the assessment of disease activity, nonspecific parameters, such as mononuclear pleocytosis, increased total CSF protein, and function of the blood-CSF barrier, must be taken into consideration.

- A positive TPHA/TPPA or FTA-ABS test together with an increased number of mononuclear cells and an elevated total autochthonous IgG- and or IgM-response in the CSF provide circumstantial evidence for neurosyphilis (Table 20-4).

- A positive VDRL- or specific IgM-test is seen as a more direct index for active neurosyphilis because in primary, secondary, and latent syphilis without CNS involvement the VDRL- and specific IgM-antibody titers in serum usually are too low to induce positive reactivity in the CSF.

- A positive treponeme-specific or reaginic test alone in the CSF does not definitely confirm the diagnosis of neurosyphilis but requires the immediate calculation of the AI.

- A negative VDRL- or IgM-test result in the CSF as well as a normal cell count do not necessarily rule out active neurosyphilis, because in cases with early neurosyphilis, specific antibodies in the CSF may be absent. Alternatively, intrathecal antibody synthesis in the CNS may not yet be detectable. In such cases, the findings should be reconfirmed by a follow-up examination in 3–4 weeks. Similarly, reaginic assays can be negative in neurosyphilis and the number of mononuclear cells normal in the CSF of patients with late parenchymatous neurosyphilis.

- Clearly, a positive TPPA/TPHA-AI together with elevated mononuclear cell counts or a positive re-

aginic test in the CSF provides definitive evidence of neurosyphilis.

- On rare occasions, an isolated positive treponeme-specific IgM- or reagin-test result in the CSF of TPPA/TPHA- and FTA-ABS-positive but reaginic test-negative patients with late neurosyphilis can be observed, which underlines the necessity of lumbar puncture to exclude or confirm suspected cases of neurosyphilis in seropositive patients.

As a rule, however, all serological findings in the CSF of suspected cases of neurosyphilis should be diagnostically evaluated in conjunction with the results of classical cytological and biochemical testing.

SYPHILIS SCREENING IN BLOOD AND ORGAN DONORS

Screening of blood donations and organ donors for syphilis is mandatory in many countries. Despite the high specificity of the currently applied test systems, the routine use of screening tests in a low-risk setting (blood and organ donors) will result in a high proportion of false-positive test results and a low positive predictive value. All persons tested in these settings require confirmatory testing.

LABORATORY DIAGNOSIS IN PREGNANCY AND IN THE NEWBORN

In many countries, all expectant mothers are routinely screened for syphilis early in pregnancy and testing should be repeated during the third trimester in areas of high-prevalence and in high-risk groups. If a treponemal or nontreponemal screening test is positive, further assessment of the stage of infection by FTA-ABS, EIA, or immunoblot, and the additional determination of specific IgM, is required since both treponeme-specific and reaginic tests are known to yield false-positive results during pregnancy. Moreover, titers of nontreponemal tests may increase nonspecifically, and this increase is easily confused with reinfection or relapse. Clinical and serological examination of all infants born to mothers with positive serologic tests for syphilis should be performed within the first month of life. Serum is the preferred material inasmuch as cord blood may show false-positive results. Sera of suspicious neonates must be continuously monitored in monthly intervals by quantitative treponeme-specific and reaginic assays, and, additionally, should be screened for *T. pallidum*–specific

IgM to detect or exclude active neonatal infection and to assess the need for treatment. CSF analysis (see earlier) of the newborn should be performed in cases with abnormal physical examination or serologic test results that are consistent with an active infection.

The diagnosis of neonatal syphilis is complicated by potential passive transfer of maternal treponeme-specific and reaginic IgG-antibodies to the infant through the placenta. These antibodies, however, are metabolized during the first 6–12 months of life, leading to a continuous decline of titers in noninfected infants. A neonatal syphilis infection is ruled out if TPHA/TPPA and reaginic tests show a significant fourfold decline of titers at serologic follow-up within 3–4 months. A significant increase of treponeme-specific and reaginic test titers or the presence of a specific IgM-response, however, strongly suggest syphilis infection in the newborn. Initial investigations of maternal and neonatal antibody titers should be carried out in parallel and are best performed at identical IgG concentrations to adjust for titer differences resulting from postpartum disturbances of fluid metabolism in mother and child. Serologic test results should always be interpreted within the context of additional clinical findings and, more important, after reviewing the maternal test results and medical history recorded during pregnancy. In cases in which maternal records of adequate treatment of active or recent syphilis are inconclusive, however, the initiation of treatment in the newborn is mandatory regardless of the actual serologic test results.

■ MONITORING THE EFFECTS OF TREATMENT

The effect of antibiotic treatment in patients with syphilis is monitored at 1, 3, 6, and 12 months after treatment by use of a quantitative reaginic assay. In HIV-patients, follow-up should be more frequent, that is, at 1, 3, 6, 12, 18, and 24 months. Treatment success is indicated by a significant decline, that is, a fourfold decrease of titers at parallel examination of sera obtained before and after chemotherapy. The earlier treatment is initiated following the onset of the infection, the more rapid titers will decline. In cases showing no continuous decrease of titers or even a rise of the antibody response after the conclusion of antibiotic therapy, a possible relapse or reinfection should be suspected.

■ PITFALLS IN THE SERODIAGNOSIS OF SYPHILIS

False-positive and false-negative test results can be observed both in reaginic and treponemal tests.

False-positive reaginic tests

- In reaginic tests, false-positive reactions may be seen during pregnancy, after recent myocardial infarction, after recent immunization, and in many acute febrile illnesses.

- In addition, autoimmune diseases, leprosy, chronic liver disease, intravenous drug abuse, pregnancy, and old age are associated, in part, with chronic false positive anti-lipoid test results.

False-positive treponemal tests

- False-positive screening test results in treponemal assays (TPHA, TPPA, FTA-ABS) occasionally can be observed in HIV infection, during pregnancy, and in autoimmune disorders but can be excluded by the additional use of a specific EIA or immunoblot.

- Extensive cross reactivity of *T. pallidum* with other spirochetes, such as *Leptospira*, *Borrelia*, *Cristispira*, as well as with nonpathogenic and pathogenic treponemes does exist.

- Antibodies directed against *T. pallidum* subsp. *endemicum* (endemic syphilis), *T. pallidum* subsp. *pertenue* (yaws, frambesia), and *T. carateum* (pinta), the causative agents of endemic treponematoses, are known to cross-react in treponemal and nontreponemal tests. Antibodies to these endemic treponemes cannot be distinguished from *T. pallidum* subsp. *pallidum*–specific antibodies by using conventional serologic tests. The most important aspect of ascertainment is from the history. Individuals from areas with endemic treponematoses should be screened and, in the event of a suspicious test constellation, should be treated as for syphilis.

- In addition, false-positive reactions can be seen in Lyme borreliosis patients and result from the close antigenic relationship between *Borrelia burgdorferi* and *T. pallidum*. Such false-positive reactions mainly occur in the FTA-ABS test. This phenomenon can be avoided by routine preabsorption of sera with *T. phagedenis* sonicate antigens.

False-negative reaginic tests

- Early on in the disease, reaginic test results may be negative and can revert to nonreactive in patients with latent or late syphilis.

False-negative treponemal tests

- False-negative test results occur early on in cases with primary syphilis and in rare instances have been observed in immunocompromised individuals (e.g., HIV).

CRITICAL ASSESSMENT OF TEST QUALITY AND STANDARDIZATION IN THE CLINICAL LABORATORY

It is critical that the laboratory and the clinician pay careful attention to quality control issues. The accuracy of diagnostic tests is critical for successful control measures of epidemic syphilis outbreaks, including case finding, prompt therapy of infected individuals, and mandatory testing of potential transmitters.

Promotion of quality control and standardization of diagnostic procedures remain relevant public health issues. The ongoing participation of laboratories in proficiency testing and the production and use of standard preparations are important interventions to achieve in more reliable test systems and in a high quality of syphilis serology outside the specialized laboratory.

KEY POINTS

- Despite some limitations, serologic testing remains the mainstay in the laboratory diagnosis of syphilis.

- Direct detection methods are used in early localized infection or for special indications only.

- In case of neurosyphilis or syphilis in pregnant women and the newborn, the correct interpretation of test results requires special laboratory expertise.

- For laboratory testing, several types of assays are commercially available but can vary concerning their sensitivities, specificities, and test quality.

- Internal and external quality control measures are key to guarantee diagnostic accuracy and safety.

REFERENCES

CDC. STD treatment guidelines 2010. *Morb Mortal Week Rep.* 2010;59(RR-12):1–110.

DGHM-Verfahrensrichtlinie 3.1. (1981). Serodiagnostik der Syphilis (Lues). In: *DGHM-Verfahrensrichtlinie.* Stuttgartt: Gustav Fischer Verlag; 1981:1–6.

Eggelstone SI, Turner AJL. Serological diagnosis of syphilis. *Commun Dis Public Health.* 2000;3:158–163.

Goh BT, van Voorst Vader PC. European guideline for the management of syphilis. *Int J STD AIDS.* 2001;12(suppl 3):14–26.

Golden RM, Marra CM, Holmes KK. Update on syphilis: resurgence of an old problem. *JAMA.* 2003;17:1510–1514.

Goldmeier D, Guallar C. Syphilis: an update. *Clin Med.* 2003; 3:209–211.

Hagedorn H-J. Syphilis. In: Mauch H, Lütticken R, eds. *Qualitätsstandards in der mikrobiologische-infektiologischen Diagnostik (MIQ).* No. 16. München: Urban & Fischer Verlag; 2001.

Hagedorn H-J, Müller F. Syphilis. In: Thomas L., ed. *Labor und Diagnose.* Frankfurt: Thomas Books; 2005:1629–1638.

Hunfeld K-P, Oschmann P, Kaiser R, Schulze J, Brade V. Diagnostics. In: Oschmann P, Kraiczy P, Halperin J, Brade, V., eds. *Lyme-Borreliosis and Tick-Borne Encephalitis.* 1st rev English ed. Bremen: Unimed Verlag AG, International Medical Publishers; 1999: 80–108.

Larsen SA, Steiner BM, Rudolph AH. Laboratory diagnosis and interpretation of tests for syphilis. *Clin Microbiol Rev.* 1995;8:1–21.

Muller I, Brade V, Hagedorn HJ, et al. Is serological testing a reliable tool in laboratory diagnosis of syphilis? meta-analysis of eight external quality control surveys performed by the German infection serology proficiency testing program. *J Clin Microbiol* 2006;44:1335–1341.

Orton S. Syphilis and blood donors: what we know, what we do not know, and what we need to know. *Transf Med Rev.* 2001;15:282–292.

Singh AE, Romanowski B. Syphilis: review with emphasis on clinical, epidemiologic, and some biologic features. *Clin Microbiol Rev.* 1999;12:187–209.

Wheeler HL, Agarwal S, Goh BT. Dark ground microscopy and treponemal serological tests in the diagnosis of early syphilis. *Sex Transm Infect.* 2004;80:411–414.

World Health Organization. Sexually transmitted infections: management's guidelines. Geneva: WHO. http//:www.who.int./HIV_AIDS. Accessed December 12, 2005.

21

Epididymitis

Janet D. Wilson

▓ BACKGROUND

Definition

Acute epididymitis is a clinical syndrome consisting of pain, swelling, and inflammation of the epididymis. The most common route of infection is local extension and is mainly due to infection that has spread from the urethra (sexually transmitted pathogens) or the bladder (urinary pathogens).

Anatomy

The epididymis is a markedly coiled duct that is continuous with the vas deferens at its lower pole. Several efferent ducts from the testis unite the upper pole of the epididymis to the upper pole of the testis. It lays posterolateral to the testis, on the right side of the right testis and the left side of the left testis. It is nearest to the testis at the upper pole with the lower pole connected to the testis by fibrous tissue. The vas deferens lays posteromedial to the epididymis.

There are two testicular appendages: the appendix testis and appendix epididymis. The appendix testis is present in 92% of testes and is usually located at the superior pole of the testis in the groove between the testis and epididymis. The appendix epididymis is present in 23% of testes and may be of variable location.

Incidence

It is difficult to know the exact incidence of epididymitis as it is a syndrome rather than due to a specific infection. Figures collected from sexually transmitted infection (STI) clinics in the United Kingdom show an increasing rate of epididymitis due to STIs from 1996 to 2008 (see Figure 21-2). Data from Hospital Episode Statistics in England suggest that 0.06% (7397) of all hospital

FIGURE 21-1 Epididymitis in the United Kingdom

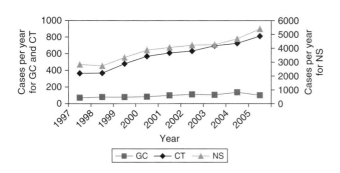

FIGURE 21-2 Number of Cases of Epididymitis Due to STIs Reported from Sexually Transmitted Disease Clinics in the United Kingdom

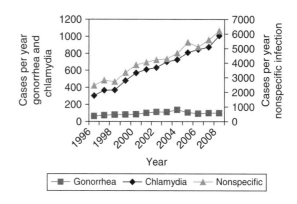

consultant episodes were for epididymitis and orchitis during 2002 to 2003; 87% of these episodes required emergency hospital admission, occupying 0.027% (14,009) of hospital bed days. It is estimated that epididymitis accounts for about 600,000 office visits per year in the United States and 0.9% of male outpatient visits to urologists in Canada.

Etiology

Most cases of epididymitis are caused by infection spreading from the urethra or bladder, down the vas deferens, and into the epididymis. Infections resulting in acute epididymitis can be divided into two main causes.

In men younger than 35 years of age, epididymitis is mainly caused by sexually transmitted pathogens, such as *Chlamydia trachomatis* and *Neisseria gonorrhoeae* (see Chapter 5). Approximately two-thirds of such cases will be due to *C. trachomatis* and between 4% and 25% due to *N. gonorrhoeae*. Any role of *Mycoplasma genitalium* in acute epididymitis has yet to be established. *Ureaplasma urealyticum* is often found in men with epididymitis, frequently in association with *N. gonorrhoeae* or *C. trachomatis* infection. However, evidence supporting it as a cause of epididymitis is lacking. Studies suggest that no microbiological cause will be found in up to 30% of cases; however, there is usually a clinical response to antimicrobial therapy that covers nongonococcal urethritis.

In men older than 35 years of age, epididymitis is mainly caused by nonsexually transmitted gram-negative enteric organisms causing urinary tract infections. There can be crossover between these groups and complete sexual history taking is imperative. Epididymitis caused by sexually transmitted enteric organisms also occurs in men who engage in insertive anal intercourse.

Gram-negative enteric organisms are more commonly the cause of epididymitis if recent instrumentation or catheterization has occurred. Anatomical abnormalities of the urinary tract are common in the group infected with gram-negative enteric organisms and further investigation of the urinary tract should be considered in all such patients.

Between 20% and 40% of postpubertal males with mumps will develop epididymo-orchitis. This is mainly unilateral but may be bilateral. Characteristic bilateral parotid swelling is usually present, but scrotal involvement can occur without other symptoms.

Occasionally, epididymitis is a complication of systemic infections, such as *Mycobacterium tuberculosis*, brucella species, and various fungi. Such infections are more likely to cause bilateral epididymitis than STIs or urinary pathogens and are often associated with immunosuppression. The incidence of tuberculomatous epididymitis may be increasing due to the increase of tuberculosis and its association with HIV infection.

Epididymitis can also be due to systemic, noninfectious disorders and has been described in 12–19% of men with Behçet's disease. This is noninfective and thought to be part of the disease process. Epididymitis has also been reported as an adverse effect of amiodarone treatment due to lymphocytic infiltration and fibrosis.

■ CLINICAL PRESENTATION

Symptoms

The first presentation of epididymitis is usually onset of unilateral scrotal pain. This occurs over several hours in most cases, although a significant number describe it as sudden onset. The pain may radiate along the spermatic cord into the groin where pain may first be felt in the early stages of epididymitis due to inflammation of the vas deferens. If the causative agent is a sexually transmitted organism, then there may be symptoms of urethritis, such as urethral discharge and dysuria; however, the urethritis is often asymptomatic. If the causative organism is a urinary tract pathogen, then urinary frequency, urgency, and dysuria may be present, but in studies of men with epididymitis due to such pathogens, urinary symptoms are frequently absent. There may also be symptoms of urinary tract outflow obstruction, such as urinary hesitancy or slow stream. (See Table 21-1.)

Signs

A visible urethral discharge may be present even in those who deny any urethral symptoms, but asymptomatic urethral infection without discharge is common. There may also be pyrexia.

There may be tenderness in the groin over the spermatic cord with thickening of the cord by edema. The scrotum on the affected side is usually enlarged, and the overlying skin may be erythematous and edematous with visible swelling of the scrotal contents (Figure 21-3). The position and lie of the testicle within the scrotum will be in the normal position. The epididymis will be tender to palpation on the affected side with palpable swelling. The process of epididymitis starts at the tail, which connects to the vas deferens, so the initial swelling will be in the lower part adjacent to the lower pole of the testis. However, with time, the swelling spreads to the head of the epididymis so

TABLE 21-1   Common Symptoms and Signs with Epididymitis

Symptoms	Signs
Gradual onset of unilateral pain	Enlarged scrotum ± erythema and edema of overlying skin
Pain radiating to groin	Tenderness in groin over spermatic cord
Possible symptoms of urethritis (urethral discharge and dysuria)	Tender swollen epididymis starting at lower pole of testis
Possible symptoms of urinary tract infection (frequency, dysuria, urgency, nocturia)	Late presentation—infection may have spread to testis, resulting in one mass involving epididymis and testis
Possible symptoms of urinary tract outflow obstruction (urinary hesitancy or slow stream)	Urethral discharge may be present

the palpable swelling extends to the upper pole. Early in the course of acute epididymitis, the enlarged indurated tender epididymis may be distinguished from the testis. Eventually, the inflammatory process spreads to involve the testis, resulting in one mass where it becomes impossible to distinguish the epididymis from the testis. In severe cases, the inflamed epididymis and testis become adherent to the scrotum. Palpation may be hampered by the presence of a secondary hydrocele, which can be present in most conditions that cause acute scrotal pain.

With mumps, there is usually bilateral parotiditis and no urethral abnormalities. The tender scrotal swelling is mainly testicular and unilateral but occasionally may be just in the epididymis.

Chronic painless induration can be due to granulomatous infections, such as tuberculosis or endemic fungal disease. Pain and significant fever are rarely present. The epididymis is usually distinguishable from the testis on palpation; the spermatic cord is often thickened and "beading" of the vas deferens may be felt. Chronic painless swelling is also the main presentation of testicular cancer, which is the most common cancer in young men. With this, a firm or hard mass can be palpated within, or attached to, the testicle.

■ DIFFERENTIAL DIAGNOSIS

Torsion of the spermatic cord, causing testicular ischemia, is the main differential diagnosis. Unless treated within 3 to 4 hours, testicular infarction and atrophy can occur; hence, this is a surgical emergency so should be considered in all patients and should first be excluded as testicular salvage becomes decreasingly likely with time. Torsion is more common in men who are younger than 20 years of age (the peak incidence is in adolescents) but can occur at any age. Previous episodes of scrotal pain are more common with torsion than epididymitis, presumably due to previous episodes of intermittent torsion. Torsion is more likely if the onset of pain is sudden and the pain is severe. There are often systemic symptoms, such as nausea and vomiting. With vascular occlusion, there is edema of the testis and cord up to the point of occlusion. Examination of torsion usually reveals a swollen tender testicle that is retracted upward because of shortening of the cord by twisting and loss of the cremasteric reflex. Testes apt to undergo torsion lie horizontally when the patient is standing. In the early stages of torsion, if the epididymis can be felt in an abnormal position (i.e., anterior) and if it is not as tender as the testis, this indicates the diagnosis. However, unless the examination is performed early the signs in epididymitis and torsion are similar, as after a few

FIGURE 21-3   Bilateral Epididymitis

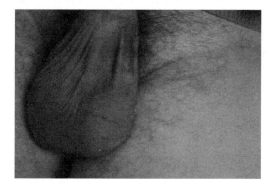

Prominent clinical features are the bilateral swelling and erythema, which is accompanied by testicular and epididymal tenderness.

hours, the area becomes so swollen that the epididymis cannot be distinguished from the testis by palpation. Torsion is more likely if investigations show no evidence of urethritis or probable urinary tract infection. Torsion can usually be differentiated from epididymitis by color Doppler sonography. Absence of arterial flow is typical of torsion; hypervascularity suggests inflammation. Radionuclide imaging can also be used to differentiate testicular torsion from inflammatory lesions.

Torsion of the appendix of the testis also presents as scrotal pain, but systemic symptoms are usually absent. The pain and any tenderness are usually localized to the superior pole of the testis. There may be a paratesticular nodule palpable at the superior aspect of the testis and a "blue-dot" appearance on the scrotal skin. The necrotic tissue of the appendix is reabsorbed without any sequelae in most cases, and pain usually resolves within 1 week.

Parotiditis usually accompanies mumps orchitis, and there are no urethral or urinary abnormalities.

Uninfected hydroceles and spermatoceles do not commonly cause pain and can be diagnosed by transillumination. A varicocoele may cause a dull ache in the testicle that increases with heavy exercise. Varicoceles are found in about 10% of young men and consist of dilatation of the pampiniform plexus above the testis, with the left side most commonly affected. If the man is examined upright, a mass of dilated tortuous veins lying posterior to, and above, the testis can be palpated. They are often tender. The degree of dilatation can be increased by the Valsalva maneuver, and in the supine position, the venous distension abates.

The first symptom of an early indirect inguinal hernia may be referred testicular pain, but this will usually be reducible and have a cough impulse. Pain from a stone in the upper ureter may be referred to the testicle.

About 25% of men with testicular tumors experience some scrotal discomfort. The peak age for tumors and epididymitis is similar, and the signs can be similar if epididymitis has spread to involve the testis or if the tumor has invaded the epididymis. Reactive hydroceles can be present with both. Failure of improvement of testicular swelling during treatment for epididymitis should raise suspicion of a tumor and an urgent ultrasound scan should be performed.

DIAGNOSIS

The following investigations should be performed:

- Urethral smear stained by Gram's method and examined microscopically for the diagnosis of ure-

thritis, (≥5 polymorphonuclear leucocytes per high power field 1000×) and presumptive diagnosis of gonorrhea.

- Urethral culture for *N. gonorrhoeae* or a nucleic acid amplification test (NAAT) for *N. gonorrhoeae* of urethral swab or first-void urine.

- A NAAT for *C. trachomatis* of first void urine or urethral swab.

- If the Gram-stained urethral smear is negative, a Gram-stained preparation from a centrifuged first void urine sample should be examined microscopically for the diagnosis of urethritis (≥10 polymorphonuclear leucocytes per high power field 1000×).

- Microscopy and culture of midstream urine for pyuria and bacteria.

If there is any doubt about the diagnosis, either color Doppler ultrasound, radionuclide imaging, or urological consultation for surgical exploration of the scrotum should be performed without delay to differentiate between epididymitis and torsion. This is especially important in adolescents or young men, as the incidence of torsion is higher in these age groups.

As there is no evidence to support *U. urealyticum* as a cause of epididymitis routine investigation for it is not recommended. The role of *M. genitalium* in epididymitis has not yet been established, so the value of a NAAT test for *M. genitalium* is currently unknown. A clinical diagnosis of mumps can be confirmed with IgM serology.

There is no role for epididymal aspiration in routine clinical practice. However, it may be useful in infections that fail to respond to initial therapy or in recurrent infections in which the organism has not yet been identified, or if tuberculosis is suspected. When tuberculosis is suspected, or within the differential diagnosis, three early morning urine samples should be obtained for mycobacterial culture, and a purified protein derivative (PPD) skin test should be performed.

All patients with sexually transmitted epididymitis should be screened for other sexually transmitted infections.

MANAGEMENT

Treatment

Most patients can be treated as outpatients, but hospitalization should be considered when the patient is febrile and systemically unwell. Empirical therapy should be

TABLE 21-2 Main Differential Diagnoses of Scrotal Pain with Associated Symptoms, Signs, and Investigations

Diagnosis	Epididymitis	Testicular Torsion	Testicular Tumor
Onset and Type of Testicular Pain	Gradual onset of pain	Sudden and severe	Gradual onset of discomfort
Associated Symptoms	Urethral discharge Urinary symptoms Pain radiating to groin	Nausea, vomiting	Heavy feeling in scrotum Dull aching in lower abdomen
Signs	Tender swollen epididymis starting at tail Normal position and lie of testicle Hydrocele may be present Fever Urethral discharge	Swollen, tender testicle retracted upward Loss of cremasteric reflex Hydrocele may be present	Firm/hard mass within or attached to testicle Normal position and lie of testicle Hydrocele may be present
Microbiological Investigations	Evidence of urethritis or UTI	No evidence of urethritis or UTI	No evidence of urethritis or UTI
Ultrasound Scan Findings	Enlargement of the epididymis with hypervascularity	Absence of arterial flow with color Doppler sonography	Focal intratesticular lesion

started in all patients with acute epididymitis once microbiological testing has been performed but before culture results are available. The antibiotic regimen chosen should be determined in light of the immediate tests as well as age, sexual history, any recent instrumentation or catheterization and any known urinary tract abnormalities in the patient. Antibiotics used for sexually transmitted epididymitis may need to be varied according to local knowledge of antibiotic sensitivities for gonorrhea. The therapy may need to be modified once the cultures and sensitivity profiles are available.

Recommended Regimes

For epididymitis most probably due to gonococcal infection:

- Ceftriaxone 250 mg intramuscularly single dose, plus

- Doxycycline 100 mg orally twice daily for 10–14 days

For epididymitis most probably due to chlamydia infection or other nongonococcal, nonenteric organisms:

- Doxycycline 100 mg orally twice daily for 10–14 days

For epididymitis most probably due to enteric organisms:

- Ofloxacin 200–300 mg orally twice daily for 10–14 days, or

- Ciprofloxacin 500 mg orally twice daily for 10 days, or

- Levofloxacin 500 mg orally once daily for 10 days

For epididymitis where likely cause cannot be determined at initial assessment:

- Ceftriaxone 250 mg intramuscularly single dose, plus

- Ofloxacin 200–300 mg orally twice daily for 10-14 days

Allergy

For epididymitis of all causes where the patient is allergic to cephalosporins or tetracyclines:

- Ofloxacin 200–300 mg by orally twice daily for 10–14 days.

In these cases, careful follow-up should be ensured because of the concern of quinolone-resistant gonorrhea,

General Advice

Scrotal elevation and support and nonsteroidal anti-inflammatory drugs are recommended. Corticosteroids have been shown not to be beneficial in treating acute epididymitis.

Partner Notification

If the epididymitis is caused by, or likely to be caused by, a sexually transmitted pathogen, recent sexual contacts must be evaluated. It is unclear what duration of "look-back" should be used, but up to 6 months has been suggested. All partners should be treated epidemiologically. This will prevent illness and complications in the contact and will prevent reinfection of the index patient. Patients should be advised to avoid unprotected sexual intercourse until they and their partner(s) have completed treatment and follow-up.

Follow-Up

Most patients show improvement within 48 to 72 hours of starting treatment. If there is no improvement in the patient's condition after 3 days, then the diagnosis should be reassessed and therapy reevaluated. Reassessment is required if symptoms persist after antimicrobial therapy is completed or if there has been little resolution of the swelling and tenderness. Surgical assessment may be appropriate in these cases. The differential diagnoses to consider include testicular ischemia/infarction, abscess formation, testicular or epididymal tumor, mumps epididymitis, chronic epididymitis due to tuberculosis, or fungal infections.

   If the epididymitis is due to a urinary pathogen, investigation of the urinary tract for structural abnormalities and outflow obstruction should be considered.

■ PROGNOSIS AND COMPLICATIONS

Abscess formation and infarction of the testis can occur with epididymitis. Infarction probably results from spermatic vessel thrombosis secondary to inflammation. However, with early diagnosis and appropriate treatment, both of these are rare complications. Older studies reported high (15%) levels of chronic epididymitis; however, recent clinical audits suggest high rates of complete resolution.

   Bilateral occlusion of the vas deferens can occur after bilateral epididymitis leading to azoospermia. The development of sperm during passage through the epididymis is essential for their full function of motility and the ability to fertilize an ovum. It is not clear what long-term effect, if any, epididymitis has on this process and hence on fertility.

■ KEY POINTS

- Acute epididymitis in men younger than 35 years is mainly caused by sexually transmitted pathogens such as *Chlamydia trachomatis* and *Neisseria gonorrhoeae*. In men older than 35 years, it is mainly caused by gram-negative enteric organisms that cause urinary tract infections.

- The first presentation of epididymitis is usually the gradual onset of unilateral scrotal pain, and the scrotum on the affected side is usually tender and enlarged and the overlying skin, erythematous and edematous.

- Torsion of the spermatic cord, causing testicular ischemia, is the main differential diagnosis.

- Investigations for nongonococcal urethritis, *N. gonorrhoeae*, *C. trachomatis*, and a urinary tract infection should be performed. Empirical therapy should be started once microbiological testing has been performed and the regimen chosen in view of the likely cause.

- If the epididymitis is likely to be caused by a sexually transmitted pathogen, recent sexual contacts must be evaluated and treated epidemiologically, and patients should be advised to avoid sex until they and their partner(s) have completed treatment and follow-up.

- If the epididymitis is due to a urinary pathogen, further investigation of the urinary tract should be considered.

REFERENCES

Berger RE. Acute epididymitis: etiology and therapy. *Semin Urol.* 1991;9:28–31.

CDC. STD treatment guidelines 2010. *Morb Mortal Week Rep.* 2010;59(RR-12):1–110.

Ciftci AO, Senocak ME, Tanyel FC, et al. Clinical predictors for differential diagnosis of acute scrotum. *Eur J Pediatr Surg.* 2004;14:333–338.

Clinical Effectiveness Group. National guideline for the management of epididymo-orchitis. *Sex Transm Infect* 1999;75(suppl 1):551–553. Updated 2009 on http://www.bashh.org.

Eickhoff JH, Frimodt-Moller N, Walters S, et al. A double-blind randomised, controlled multicentre study to compare the efficacy of ciprofloxacin with pivampicillin as oral therapy for epididymitis in men over 40 years of age. *BJU Int.* 1999;84:827–834.

Hagley M. Epididymo-orchitis and epididymitis: a review of causes and management of unusual forms. *Int J STD AIDS.* 2003;14:372–378.

Hoosen AA, O'Farrell N, Van den Ende J. Microbiology of acute epididymitis in a developing country. *Genitourin Med.* 1993;69:361–363.

Luzzi GA, O'Brien TS. Acute epididymitis. *BJU Int.* 2001;87: 747–755.

Stehr M, Boehm R. Critical validation of colour Doppler ultrasound in diagnosis of acute scrotum in children. *Eur J Pediatr Surg.* 2003;13:386–392.

22

Genital Warts

Hiok-Hee Tan and Roy Chan

INTRODUCTION

Anogenital warts are caused by infection with the human papillomavirus (HPV). Infection occurs via close mucosal contact, typically sexual contact.

Papillomaviruses are a group of small DNA viruses that have been detected in a large number of vertebrates; they induce epithelial cell proliferation and highly species-specific infections. Utilizing nucleic acid hybridization studies, more than a hundred HPV types are known, of which more than 30 infect the genital tract. HPV is one of the most common sexually transmitted infections and causes cutaneous disease, precancer lesions, and anogenital malignancies. The most common subtypes that cause HPV are types 6 and 11, which are generally not premalignant.

EPIDEMIOLOGY

The true prevalence of HPV anogenital infection is difficult to determine, as the majority of infections are asymptomatic and subclinical infections are common (also see Chapter 6). Epidemiological investigations are made more difficult by the lack of tests that can detect the time of infection.

Surveillance data are based on passive surveys, since the disease is not reportable. In the United States, 500,000 to 1,000,000 new cases annually are reported as new patients presented to physicians' offices, which is thought to be a profound underestimate of the true figure. The highest rates of genital warts are found in adults aged 18–28 years, and it is estimated that viral warts are present in approximately 1% of sexually active adults in the United States and at least 15% have subclinical infection, as detected by HPV DNA assays.

Similar trends exist in the United Kingdom. A retrospective analysis showed that the rate of attendance for genital warts increased by 390% and 594% for men and women, respectively, between 1971 and 1994, with rates of attendance for first attack in men highest in the 20- to 24-year age group, whereas for women, it peaked in those aged 16–24 years.

The most common HPV types to infect the genital tract are HPV-6 and HPV-11 (which cause classic condyloma acuminata), and HPV-16 and HPV-18 (which cause less common flat warts). Types 6 and 11 are considered low risk, as they are not associated with cervical cancer. Types 16 and 18 are classified as high-risk types. For a discussion on high-risk HPV epidemiology and cervical cancer screening, please refer to Chapter 6.

Table 22-1 lists the association between HPV types and clinical lesions found in the anogenital region (this list is not meant to be exhaustive).

CLINICAL FEATURES

Anogenital Warts

Anogenital warts, occurring as single or multiple lesions, appear as epidermal and dermal papules or nodules on the perineum, genitalia, crural folds, and anus. They vary in size and can form large, exophytic masses, especially in the moist environment of the perineum. They are largely asymptomatic and painless. Warts tend to occur over areas that are subject to trauma during sexual intercourse. The clinical presentation of genital warts

TABLE 22-1 HPV Types and Associations

Lesion	Associated HPV types
Condylomata acuminata	6, 11 (most common)
Giant condylomata of Buschke and Lowenstein and other verrucous carcinoma	6, 11, 57, 72, and 73
Bowenoid papulosis	16, 34, 39, 40, 42, and 45
Vulvar intraepithelial neoplasia	56, 59–64, 67, and 71
Cervical squamous intraepithelial lesions (SIL)	
Low-grade squamous intraepithelial lesions (LSIL)	6, 11, 16, 18, 26, 27, 30, 31, 33–35, 40, 42–45, 51–58, 61, 62
High-grade squamous intraepithelial lesions (HSIL)	6, 11, 16, 18, 31, 33, 35, 39, 42, 44, 45, 51, 52, 56, 58, 59, 61, 64, 66, 68, and 82
Penile intraepithelial neoplasia (PIN) Perianal intraepithelial neoplasia (PAIN) Anal intraepithelial neoplasia (AIN)	6, 11, 16, 18, 30, 31, 33, 34, 35, 39, 40, 42–45, 51, 52, 56–59, 61, 62, 64, 66, 67, and 69
Cervical cancer	16, 18, 31, 33, 35, 39, 45, 51, 52, 54, 56, 58, 59, 62, 66, and 68

Sources: De Villiers (1997), Oriel (1971), Chuang et al. (1984), Chao and Gibbs (2005), and Chen and Cheung (2003).

were described in detail in a series of prospective case series conducted by Oriel (1971) and Chuang et al. (1984). In sum, the lesions are distributed throughout the genital tract, highlighting the importance of a careful and thorough physical examination.

In Oriel's (1971) study of 191 mostly uncircumcised men, the glans, frenum, and corona were affected in 52% of cases, with the prepuce being the next most commonly affected site (33%), followed by the urethra (23%), the penile shaft (18%), the perianal region (8%), and the scrotum (2%) (Maiti and Hay 1985). This contrasts with a study by Chuang et al. (1984), on 246 mostly circumcised men, where the penile shaft was affected in 51% of cases, with the perianal region being the next most commonly affected site (34%), followed by the glans, the frenum and corona (10%), the urethra (10%), the prepuce (8%), the perineum (3%), and the scrotum (1%).

The same authors also studied the distribution of anogenital warts in women. In Oriel's (1971) study on 141 women, warts were found on the introitus in 73%

of cases. The next most common site was the labia majora and minora, where 63% of warts were located, followed by the perineum (23%), the anus (18%), the vagina (15%), urethra (8%), and the cervix (6%).

Chuang and colleagues' study (1984) of 500 women with warts showed that the most common location was the labia majora and minora (66%), followed by the introitus (37%), the perineum (29%), the anus (23%), cervix (8%), and the urethra (4%).

The clinical lesions of anogenital warts appear as condylomata acuminata, papular, keratotic, and flat warts. Subclinical lesions are often only visible after application of acetic acid and latent infections are diagnosed when HPV DNA can be demonstrated in the absence of clinical or histological evidence of infection.

Condylomata acuminata are fleshy, sessile, or pedunculated exophytic lesions. On keratinized skin, they appear as whitish gray protuberances with an acuminate or pointed structure of the top of the lesion. On mucosal surfaces, it appears as a red papilliferous structure, often with visible capillaries.

FIGURE 22-1 Fleshy Hyperplastic Warts Presenting as a Moist-Looking Exophytic Mass on the Prepuce and Glans Penis

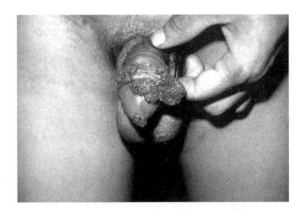

Differential diagnoses of condylomata acuminata include pearly penile papules, vestibular papillae, skin tags, sebaceous and Tyson's glands, molluscum contagiosum, and condylomata lata (see Chapter 11). Pearly papules tend to be distributed around the corona and have a fairly similar appearance. Moluscum contagiosum are pearly pink, often with a central dimple. Condylomata lata are usually moist, fleshy lesions, which appear with relative rapidity and have a positive syphilis serology test.

Buschke-Lowenstein tumors, or giant condylomas, are variants characterized by large cauliflower-like lesions on the penis or perianal area. Despite its histologically benign appearance, it behaves in a malignant fashion, destroying adjacent tissues, and is regarded as an entity intermediate between an ordinary condylomata acuminatum and squamous cell carcinoma.

Papular warts are flesh-colored, dome-shaped papules, usually 1–4 mm in diameter; they may resemble lesions of psoriasis, lichen planus, pearly penile papules, and melanocytic naevi. A variant known as bowenoid papulosis, caused mainly by HPV-16, presents as asymptomatic hyperpigmented papules with a flat and sometimes verrucous surface. Keratotic warts have a thick, crustlike layer and may resemble common skin warts or seborrheic keratoses. Flat warts appear as slightly raised lesions, and differential diagnoses include psoriasis, seborrheic dermatitis, and lichen planus (see also Chapter 11).

Squamous intraepithelial lesions

Squamous intraepithelial lesions (SIL) of the cervix caused by HPV are seldom visible to the naked eye, and diagnostic tools currently in use include cytology as a screening method, followed by colposcopic localization of areas with cellular atypia, and a histologic diagnosis through a colposcopic-directed biopsy. Vulval SILs are usually detected when the patient complains of symptoms related to vulval dystrophy, such as itch

FIGURE 22-2 Keratinised Warts Presenting as Greyish-White Lesions Clustered Together Forming a Cauliflower-Like Growth

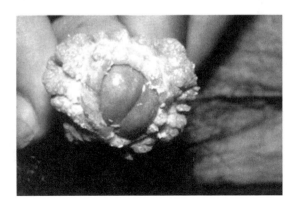

FIGURE 22-3 Bowenoid Papulosis

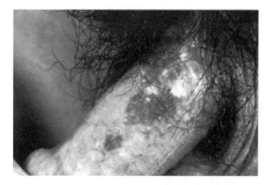

This often presents as pigmented popular lesions that can resemble warts. It has a distinctive histology of Bowenoid dysplasia and a few case reports have associated this condition with malignant transformation.

and soreness. Examination may reveal a white patch, which could indicate SIL or early cancer (Sauder et al. 2003). Differentials include lichen sclerous et atrophicus, postinflammatory hypopigmentation, vitiligo, or leukoplakia. If SIL is clinically suspected, Pap smear testing with reflex HPV testing, if available, should be performed and arrangements made for prompt follow-up and specialist referral, if indicated. SILs of the penis and anal canal are often subclinical infections and can be identified with a colposcope or operating microscope after the application of acetic acid.

FIGURE 22-4 Pearly Penile Papules

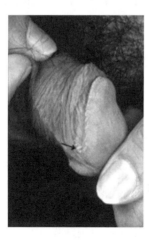

These present as rows of small white papules along the coronal sulcus, consisting of hypertrophic papillae. It is important to reassure patients that these are not warts.

FIGURE 22-5 Florid Meatal Warts Extending into the Urethra

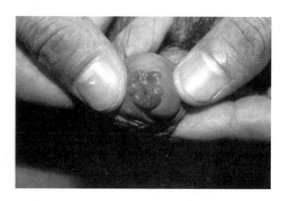

■ DIAGNOSIS

Anogenital warts on the external genitalia can generally be diagnosed based solely on clinical features. Clinical inspection of the entire anogenital region should be carried out with the aid of a clear and powerful light and with a magnifying lens. A careful clinical inspection of the external genitalia will detect most abnormalities except for subclinical infections.

For inspection of urethral warts, the meatal lips should be parted using the fingers so that the entrance to the urethral canal can be examined. This method generally allows the observer to inspect up to 5 mm within the canal. In the presence of meatal warts, efforts should be made to detect how deep the lesion extends.

Clinical pearl: A nasal speculum may be introduced to allow a deeper inspection of the urethral canal. The

FIGURE 22-6 Urethral Wart

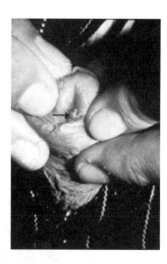

This is a single papular lesion.

FIGURE 22-7 Anal Warts

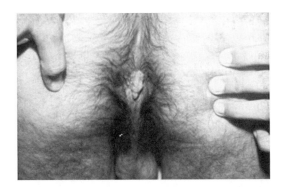

authors have found the otoscope is useful in visualizing the deeper parts of the urethral canal as well. A meatal spreader is an instrument that can be introduced into the meatus, with the advantage that once opened, it does not have to kept in the operator's hand.

Anoscopy or proctoscopy should be performed in all patients presenting with warts in the perianal region.

Cervical lesions, however, are seldom detected by the naked eye. Most lesions are identified only by colposcopy, in women in whom a Pap smear suggested the presence of an abnormality. The appearance of these lesions is variable, and a detailed description is beyond the scope of this chapter.

Acetic Acid Application

The use of 3% or 5% acetic acid onto HPV-associated lesions produces a whitening effect. This can be applied onto discrete as well as suspected subclinical lesions; the mechanism for this acetowhitening effect is not clear. One hypothesis is that acetic acid causes a reversible coagulation of some epithelial and stromal proteins.

Acetic acid is applied to the area and left for at least 3 minutes before observing the effect. This whitening

FIGURE 22-8 Prostoscopy Should Be Performed in Patients with Anal Warts

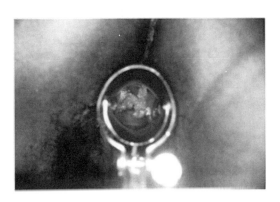

FIGURE 22-9 Extensive Keratinised Warts on the Scrotum

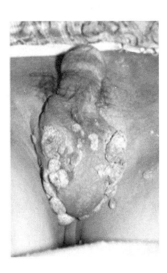

effect may also occur in areas of abrasions or nonspecific inflammation and may also be seen in other infections, such as candidiasis, and thus is not specific for HPV infection. However, the acetowhite obtained from HPV infection tends to have a sharper and more defined border than that seen with inflammation.

Biopsy

Biopsies can be done to confirm the diagnosis of a clinical lesion, although this is seldom necessary. They are more likely to be performed to exclude malignancy. A biopsy should be considered if there is a doubt to the diagnosis, of the patient is immunocompromised,

FIGURE 22-10 Warts Affecting the Labia Majora and Minora

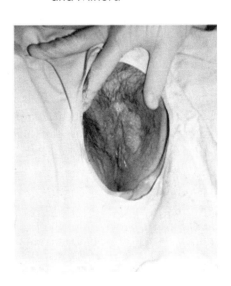

or if the lesion is worsening despite treatment. On the external genitalia, punch or forceps biopsies can be performed under local anesthesia.

Cytology—Anal Lesions

Cytological examination at annual intervals can be performed and is recommended for homosexual and bisexual men, particularly those that are immunocompromised. The procedure is somewhat similar to that of a cervical Pap smear. A cytobrush is inserted into the anal canal and rotated several times, and a smear is prepared and immediately fixed. A major challenge is laboratories proficient in reading anal smears.

Molecular Detection

As far as clinical utility is concerned, clinical examination and colposcopy remain the best tools for diagnosing HPV infection of the external genitalia and the cervix. With the development of polymerase chain reaction (PCR) technology based on HPV DNA and mRNA for various HPV genotypes, there is potential for its use in distinguishing high-risk HPV types from the low-risk genotypes.

■ TREATMENT OF ANOGENITAL WARTS

General Considerations

Patients should be given a detailed explanation of their condition. They should appreciate the long-term implications for their health and of their partners. Condom usage with regular sex partners has not been shown to affect the treatment outcome in HPV-related disease, such as CIN 1, but many patients and their partners feel more comfortable using condoms when the warts are visible. Condom usage should be encouraged to prevent possible transmission to new sexual partners. Some patients may be psychologically disturbed by the diagnosis, and should be referred for counseling, if needed.

The choice of treatment depends on the type, distribution and number of warts, as well as patient preference. Treatments can either be patient applied or provider administered. They consist of either chemical applications or various forms of physical ablation.

Chemical Methods

Podophyllin

Podophyllin resin is a cytotoxic plant compound. It is applied to warts as a 10% to 25% solution in tincture

of benzoin and allowed to dry. This procedure is done in the clinic once or twice a week. Care should be taken to avoid splashing the surrounding skin during application. The unaffected surrounding skin should be covered with a layer of white soft paraffin as protection before the resin is applied. Patients must wash off the chemical after 4 hours.

Comparable results with this treatment have been achieved using 0.5%-2% ethanol solution applied by the patient at home.

There are concerns with the use of podophyllin. It is semiquantitatively produced, and is a nonstandardized compound composed of numerous chemical substances and varying amounts of cytotoxic compounds known as lignans. The ingredients may thus vary considerably between batches, and the stability of the compound may not be reliable. The biologically active lignans can be broken down into inactive isomers such as quercetin and kaempherol, which are potentially mutagenic. For these reasons, there are some authors who are against using this compound to treat warts.

Patients must be strongly advised against excessive use of the treatment, as severe adverse local and systemic side effects can occur.

Podophyllin can cause local side effects, such as itching, swelling, pain, ulceration, and severe genital burns. Increased absorption is likely if it is used internally, and applications should be limited to 10 cm² or 0.5 ml for external warts, and less than 2 cm² for vaginal warts. As it is potentially oncogenic, it should not be used on the cervix or in the anal canal and is contraindicated in pregnancy.

Podophyllotoxin

Podophyllotoxin is a purified extract of podophyllin and is available as a 0.5% alcoholic solution or 0.15% cream. This is a patient-applied formulation, suitable for home use. However, it is recommended that the physician or nurse should apply the first treatment to demonstrate the proper method of application and to identify which warts should be treated. Treatment cycles consist of twice daily application for 3 days, followed by 4 days' rest. If the warts persist, treatment can be repeated at weekly intervals for four cycles. Patients may find the cream easier to apply, especially in the perianal area.

Side effects from podophyllotoxin include mild tenderness, pain, burning, and redness, swelling and minor erosions. The precautions on its use are similar to podophyllin's: avoid if pregnant and not exceed a total treatment area of 10 cm² or a volume of 0.5 ml of the solution per session.

Compared with podophyllin, podophyllotoxin solution and cream are associated with increased short-term effectiveness and increased odds of remission of all warts. However, long-term recurrence rates (measured at 12 weeks) are similar.

Imiquimod

Imiquimod is an TLR7 agonist and immune-response modifier that induces a cytokine response, including the production of interferon alfa, tumor necrosis factor-alpha, as well as interleukins 1, 6, and 8, when applied to skin infected with HPV.

Imiquimod 5% cream has been found to be an effective treatment for external genital and perianal warts, providing a significant benefit in comparison with vehicle cream, independent of gender, initial wart size, duration of current outbreak of warts, previous wart treatment, or tobacco use. Clinical trials have shown response rates comparable to that of other chemical agents but an encouragingly low relapse rate. Clearance rates of warts in patients treated with imiquimod have been reported as high as 75%, although 50% would be a reasonable expectation. Recurrence rates are lower than with chemical methods. Clearance rates are also reported to be higher in women compared with men.

It is suitable for use on all external genital warts but is not approved for use in pregnancy or internally. The cream is applied to the lesions three times weekly and washed off 6-10 hours later for up to 16 weeks.

The most common side effect with the use of imiquimod is the development of erythema, which occurs in most individuals. Excoriation and erosions are seen in roughly half of patients. Less commonly encountered adverse events include induration, scabbing, and ulceration.

The efficacy of imiquimod in HIV-infected patients or others with immune deficiency is not known and may be an issue because of the drug's unique mechanism of action. Therefore, imiquimod is not recommended in these patient populations.

Trichloroacetic Acid (TCA) or Bichloroacetic Acid (BCA)

TCA and BCA are caustic agents that are applied directly to the warts in the physician's office. Most physicians use 25–70% TCA (higher concentrations are available) or 80–90% BCA. This treatment can be repeated weekly, if necessary.

A small amount of the chemical is applied to the warts, taking care to avoid contact with clinically normal skin. As the product is allowed to dry, a white "frosting" develops. The application of TCA or BCA usually causes several minutes of mild to moderate discomfort at the site. The main complication is the development of local skin irritation, including burns and ulcers, if excessive amounts are applied. If an excess amount is applied, liquid soap should be used to remove any unreacted acid. The acid can also be prevented from causing further damage if the entire treated area is quickly dusted with talc or sodium bicarbonate.

As local side effects can be severe, it is usually not recommended for use on very large areas of warts. TCA and BCA, however, are not associated with significant systemic absorption. Overall success rates of between 63–70% have been reported with its use.

5-Fluorouracil (5-FU)

5-FU interferes with DNA synthesis by blocking the methylation of deoxyuridylic acid and inhibits thymidylate synthetase, which subsequently reduces cell proliferation. It is not commonly used in treating warts and is recommended mainly for use on warts resistant to other forms of treatment.

5-FU has not been approved by the FDA to treat warts, and its use in this situation is off-label. It can be used to treat urethral and vaginal warts and can be used at home by the patient after he has been taught how to apply the medication by a healthcare professional. 5-FU can also be used as an adjunct to laser therapy, where it may reduce recurrence rates.

It is applied as 5% cream or 1% in ethanol one to three times per week for several weeks as needed to clear the warts. To reduce skin sensitivity, the cream should be washed off 3 to 10 hours after application. The surrounding normal tissue can be protected with petroleum jelly to prevent irritation. For men, the skin at the tip of the penis should be protected with an ointment. Patients should be advised against wearing tight-fitting underwear because it might smear the medication to other areas. A skin reaction may not occur until 3 or 4 days after application. It may cause dysuria if used to treat urethral warts, and severe local irritation, burns, and ulcers can occur. 5-FU is contraindicated in pregnancy.

Interferons

Interferons have direct and indirect activity against viruses and therefore are a theoretically attractive treatment option. Various regimens have been described, using interferons alfa, beta, and gamma as creams or gels and as intralesional or systemic injections. Topical, systemic, and intralesional interferon regimens have been evaluated. However, because of the toxicity and high costs, interferons are not used in routine practice.

Physical Methods
Cryotherapy

In cryotherapy, a cryogen is applied to a lesion to produce local destruction. The basic cryotherapy principle is to freeze the lesion with subzero temperature and allow a later sloughing of the damaged tissue. The depth of damage depends on the technique and the freezing time.

Liquid nitrogen is the most commonly used cryogen. It is a liquefied gas with a temperature of −196°C. Skin freezes at a temperature range of 0 to −2°C, and for tissue destruction to occur, tissue must be cooled to between −18 to −30°C. The major challenge to using cryotherapy is having the appropriate instruments available, as well as a reliable supplier for liquid nitrogen. Busy clinics usually manage with a weekly resupply. There are several ways to apply liquid nitrogen to warts.

Dipstick Method

A cotton wool-tipped applicator is immersed in a vacuum flask of liquid nitrogen and then applied to the wart. When this is applied four times within 60 seconds, the temperature of the skin is lowered to −18°C up to a depth of 2 mm. The degree of injury is roughly proportional to the intensity of freezing. The intensity and extent of freezing are determined by the duration of freezing, the size of the area in contact with the freezing agent, and the pressure applied.

The rate of freezing is also important, as repeated freezing and thawing is more destructive than a single freeze. A new dipstick is to be used for every application.

The Spray Method

In this method, a hand-held insulated and pressurized flask filled with liquid nitrogen is used. The spray applicator should be about 1 to 2 cm away from the lesion. A rubber cone can be used to limit the area sprayed. An intermittent spray is more efficacious than a continuous spray, as conversion of the liquid nitrogen to the gaseous phase will not be interrupted. Care should be taken to avoid spraying surrounding skin.

Cryoprobe Contact Method

Here a precooled metal accessory is applied directly on the lesion. The preferred time interval between treatment for warts is 1 to 2 weeks. The efficacy of cryotherapy for external warts in clinical trials ranges from 27% to 88%.

Complications of Cryotherapy

Freezing warts produces a stinging, burning pain. Take care to avoid excessive freezing, as the blisters that form may be large or hemorrhagic. If blisters form, they should not be unroofed, but instead decompressed with a sterile needle if necessary. Secondary infection and ulceration can also develop as complications.

Electrosurgery

In electrosurgery, heat is produced in tissue at the point of entry of high-frequency currents. There are basically three modalities: (1) electrodessication/electrofulguration, (2) electrocoagulation, and (3) electrosection (cutting). Electrosurgery requires trained operators and the necessary equipment, which can be costly. Surgical options may be particularly attractive in treating larger lesions.

Factors that influence tissue damage will include the surface area of the electrode, the duration of contact, the power setting, and the type of current selected. The longer the electrode is kept in contact with the lesion, the greater the amount of tissue destruction, keeping the electrode moving reduces the amount of tissue damage. There are no randomized trials of surgery compared with chemical methods. Reported clearance and remission rates are 57–94%. However, these data may be biased by preferences for surgery among specific groups of patients.

Scabs will form posttreatment, and saline washes and an antibiotic ointment can be applied to the area postsurgery. For larger lesions, nonstick gauze can be used.

Scissors Excision

Among the various treatment modalities for condyloma acuminatum, excisional cold-blade surgery appears excellent but it has been little studied and little used, particularly for lesions not located in the perianal area.

After infiltration of local anesthetic, warts are removed with fine-pointed curved scissors by cutting at the base of the wart. Clinical trials are small but show results in a similar range as electrosurgery.

Laser Therapy

The carbon dioxide laser can be used to treat warts and can be used at difficult anatomical sites, such as the urethral meatus, cervical, and intra-anal region. It can also be used to treat large volume warts, but this often requires general anesthesia and is not routinely done as an outpatient procedure. Laser therapy is expensive and is no more effective than cryotherapy, podophillotoxin, and trichloroacetic acid.

Choosing a Treatment and Follow-Up

Patients with external anogenital warts can be offered either home-based or clinic-based therapies. The choice of treatment would depend on the patient's preference, and type and number of warts.

First-line therapies would include cryotherapy or podophyllotoxin [or podophyllin]. Imiquimod, a more costly option, can also be considered. Recurrent warts are common, and repeated treatment cycles are often needed. Patients should be made aware of this. Warts that are heavily keratinized should be initially treated with cryotherapy, as self-applied preparations are less likely to penetrate the thickened epithelial surface.

Patients should be reviewed to monitor their response to therapy and assess need for changes in treatment. If the patient is responding well, and the original lesions have cleared or improved significantly but new lesions are evolving, then the current therapy can be extended. The treating physician should consider changing therapy if the patient has less than 50% response to a current treatment after 2 to 3 months or sooner if the patient cannot tolerate or is not able to comply with the current treatment.

For intravaginal warts, cryotherapy and trichloroacetic acid are recommended. If podophyllin is used, be careful not to exceed a total area of 2 cm² weekly. When cervical warts are detected, colposcopy and biopsy should be performed before any treatment decisions are made. If CIN is not detected, then cryotherapy or trichloroacetic acid can be used. If CIN is detected, a referral to the gynecologist is needed—a large loop excision of the transformation zone can be performed.

When warts are detected at the urethral meatus, standard therapies can be used if the base of the warts can be seen. If the wart extends far into the urethra and the base cannot be seen, referral to the urologist should be made. The use of 5-FU cream for urethral warts has been recommended by some—applied two to three times per week after micturition for up to 6 weeks. This can result in severe inflammation and dysuria, and patients should be warned about this side effects and told to discontinue treatment if they occur.

Intra-anal warts can be treated with any of the standard first-line therapies. However, in view of the mitogenicity of podophylline, it is probably unwise to use in the anal canal or on the cervix.

Anal intraepithelial neoplasia can be problematic to manage. These patients should be referred.

■ TREATMENT OF ANOGENITAL WARTS IN IMMUNOCOMPROMISED INDIVIDUALS

In immunocompromised patients, the clinical spectrum of HPV disease is similar to that in nonimmunocompromised patients, but HIV-associated disease may be more extensive and more severe.

In particular, HIV-positive men and women have a high burden of HPV-associated anogenital disease, and disease manifestations range from condylomata acuminata to lesions with malignant potential such as high-grade AIN, CIN, and VIN. A high incidence of cervical cancer in HIV-positive women has resulted in a recommendation of more frequent interval cervical Pap screening, and anal Pap screening has been recommended for HIV-positive individuals, but more clinicians need to be trained to identify and treat AIN.

The treatment options are the same as for immunocompetent patients, but all things being equal, treatment of HPV infection is less effective in immunosuppressed patients than in immunocompetent patients. Combined medical and surgical procedures may have to be considered to achieve the best outcome.

■ TREATMENT OF ANOGENITAL WARTS IN PREGNANCY

Imiquimod, podophyllin, podophyllotoxin, and 5-FU should not be used during pregnancy. Genital warts can proliferate and become friable during pregnancy, and many specialists advocate their removal during pregnancy.

Cryotherapy, trichloroacetic acid, and surgical methods can be used. Although HPV can cause respiratory papillomatosis in infants and children, the preventive value of cesarean section is unknown and should not be performed solely to prevent transmission of HPV infection to the newborn.

TREATMENT OF ANOGENITAL WARTS IN CHILDREN

Genital warts in children have serious medical, social, and legal implications. Although the warts on the anogenital area may have arisen from autoinoculation of common warts, the question of sexual abuse inevitably arises, and there are concerns about vertical transmission from the mother as well as the potential for development of malignancies in the future that must be addressed.

Any child with genital warts requires a complete medical examination, including a careful examination of the anus and genitalia for possible signs of sexual abuse. An oral examination for warts should also be conducted. If sexual abuse is suspected, a screen for other infections is warranted. Parental history of genital warts or other sexually transmitted infections should be obtained, and the mother's Pap smear results should be reviewed. Other aspects of management include a complete psychosocial assessment, and where abuse is suspected, notifying the relevant authorities.

KEY POINTS

- Genital warts are caused by a number of human papillomavirus types, predominantly types 6 and 11.

- In most cases, these are not premalignant lesions.

- There is a long (at least several month) latency period for genital wart disease.

- There are multiple clinical presentations. Genital warts can occur at any external mucosal site, as well as intrameatus, on the cervix, and in the rectum.

- Clinical treatment is based on either tissue-destructive therapies or immune modulation. Recurrence is common.

- HPV is latent in normal appearing areas adjacent to the clinical lesion.

- Genital wart disease is more severe and prone to higher rates of recurrence in immunocompromised persons.

REFERENCES

Beutner KR, Wiley DJ. Recurrent external genital warts: a literature review. *Papillomavirus Rep.* 1997;8:69–74.

Challenor R, Alexander I. A five-year audit of the treatment of extensive anogenital warts by day case electrosurgery under general anesthesia. *Int J STD & AIDS.* 2002;13:786–789.

Chan YC, Ng KY, Chan RK. The epidemiology and treatment of anogenital warts in Singapore: a retrospective evaluation. *Ann Acad Med Singapore.* 2002;31(4):502–508.

Chao MW, Gibbs P. Squamous cell carcinoma arising in a giant condyloma acuminatum (Buschke-Lowenstein tumour). *Asian J Surg.* 2005;28(3):238–240.

Chen CW, Cheung KB. Clinical significance and management of cervical atypical glandular cells of undetermined significance. *Hong Kong Med J.* 2003;9(5):346–351.

Chuang TY, Perry HO, Kurland LT, Ilstrap DM. Condylomata acuminatum in Rochester, Minn., 1950–1978. I. Epidemiology and clinical features. *Arch Dermatol.* 1984;120(4):469–475.

de Villiers EM. Papillomavirus and HPV typing. *Clin Dermatol.* 1997;15(2):199–206.

Eron LJ, Judson F, Tucker S, et al. Interferon therapy for condylomata acuminata. *N Engl J Med.* 1986;315:1059–1064.

Haidopoulos D, Diakomanolis E, Rodolakis A, et al. Safety and efficacy of locally applied Imiquimod cream 5% for the treatment of condylomata acuminata of the vulva. *Arch Gynecol Obstet.* 2004;270(4):240–243.

Hornor G. Anogenital warts in children: sexual abuse or not? *J Pediatr Healthcare.* 2004;18(4):165–170.

Koutsky L. Epidemiology of genital human papillomavirus infection. *Am J Med.* 1997;102(5A):3–8.

Lacey CJ, Goodall RL, Tennwall GR, et al; Perstop Pharma Genital Warts Clinical Trial Group. Randomised controlled trial and economic evaluation of podophyllotoxin solution, podophyllotoxin cream and podophyllin in the treatment of genital warts. *Sex Transm Infect.* 2003;79(4):270–275.

Maiti H, Hay KR. Self treatment of condylomata acuminata with podophyllin resin. *Practitioner.* 1985;229:37–39.

Maw R. National guidelines for the management of anogenital warts. *Sex Transm Inf.* 1999;75(suppl 1):S71–S75.

Oriel JD. Natural history of genital warts. *Br J Vener Dis.* 1971; 47:1–13.

Sauder DW, Skinner RB, Fox TL, Owens ML. Topical Imiquimod 5% cream as an effective treatment for external genital and perianal warts in different patient populations. *Sex Transm Dis.* 2003;30(2):124–128.

Simms I, Fairley CK. Epidemiology of genital warts in England and Wales: 1971 to 1994. *Genitourin Med.* 1997;73(5):365–367.

Skinner RB Jr. Imiquimod. *Dermatol Clin.* 2003;21(2):291–300.

Von Krogh G, Longstaff E. Podophyllin therapy against condylomata should be abandoned. *Sex Transm Infect.* 2001;77(6):409–412.

Wiley DJ, Douglas J, Beutner K, et al. External genital warts: diagnosis, treatment, and prevention. *Clin Infect Dis.* 2002;35(suppl 2):S210–S214.

23

Anorectal Infections

Darren Russell

INTRODUCTION

The anorectal area is rich in nerve endings, second only to the lips in sensitivity. Yet for all this sensitivity, many people have traditionally regarded the anus as a taboo area as far as sensual pleasure is concerned because of its association with excretion. However, anal intercourse is commonly practiced. Even in persons who have had receptive anal intercourse, most anorectal symptoms are not due to sexually transmitted infections though they may, in some part, be due to sexual activity. The feeling of embarrassment and shame that accompanies anal intercourse may lead to people presenting late to their physician. There are a variety of symptoms that may be experienced, including pain, discharge, bleeding, ulceration, and itching.

ANAL INTERCOURSE

Anal intercourse is common. Most men who have sex with men (MSM) have engaged at some time or other in anal sex, in which they have tried both receptive and insertive intercourse. Many of these men, however, do not have regular anal intercourse in their current relationships, despite a widely held community perception that this is the case.

Less is known about the frequency of heterosexual anal intercourse. A California study published in 1995 showed that of 3,545 sexually active adults sampled by telephone interview, 7% (8% of males and 6% of females) of respondents reported having anal sex at least

once a month during the year before the survey (Erickson 1995). A more recent survey from the United States showed that of sexually transmitted infection (STI) clinic attendees, 39.3% engaged in heterosexual anal sex in a 12-month period, with most of them not using condoms (Tian 2008). Furthermore, manual anal stimulation is also a widespread practice.

There are few data on prevalence of anal intercourse in developing countries, an issue that is complicated by societal taboo in many countries. Some authorities suggest that previous analyses of HIV risk may have overestimated the risk of penile-vaginal intercourse by not asking about anal intercourse in heterosexual couplings, an issue that would have major implications for education and health-promotion interventions.

Serious complications of anal intercourse are not particularly common except when force, as in sexual assault, is involved. Prolapsed hemorrhoids, anal tears, anal fissures, rectal ulcers, and the presence of foreign bodies have all been reported to occur as a result of anal sex and are not particularly common. There is no good evidence that regular, consensual anal intercourse leads to sphincter laxity or incontinence in later life.

Specific practices such as *fisting* (also known as *handballing*, medically defined as *brachioproctic eroticism*), or the insertion of large sex toys, may lead to rectal perforation or tearing of the internal (deep) anal sphincter. When identified, the health professional should adopt a nonjudgmental approach to dealing with such information and concentrate on the presenting medical issues.

Unprotected anal intercourse may also lead to HIV transmission, and this should be raised with patients when appropriate.

Anatomy

Given the sensitivity of the anus, some conditions are capable of causing exquisite pain. The perianal skin is keratinized, stratified squamous epithelium. The anus proper extends from the anal verge to the dentate line and is only 2–3 cm (about 1 inch) in length. The epithelium changes from stratified squamous to stratified cuboidal epithelium.

The rectum extends from the dentate line to the sigmoid colon and is lined by columnar epithelium, as is the rest of the colon. The rectum is insensitive to pain caused by inflammation or damage to the mucosa and may be biopsied without the need for anesthetic agents. However, the rectum is able to appreciate the sensation of stretch, as with the urge to defecate, or with anorectal intercourse. Inflammation of the rectum is termed *proctitis*.

Enteritis is inflammation of the duodenum, jejunum, or ileum. Sigmoidoscopy performed on a patient with enteritis will show no abnormalities. Infection is usually contracted by the ingestion of infected food or water or by certain sexual practices. Oral–anal contact, known as *anilingus* (referred to colloquially as *rimming*), may transmit enteric pathogens. Another portal of entry for pathogens is direct intrarectal inoculation by the penis.

■ SEVERE PAIN

Severe anal pain is generally due to one of two conditions, perianal herpes simplex infection (usually an initial, as opposed to a recurring, infection) or a perianal abscess. More recently, lymphogranuloma venereum (LGV) has emerged in MSM populations in Western Europe, North America, and Australia, and if left untreated may lead to severe anorectal symptoms, including pain.

It will usually be obvious to the health professional that the patient is in significant pain, and he or she may evince discomfort while walking. The patient will usually prefer to stand during the consultation or to sit gingerly on the corner of the chair and will walk with a wide-based, tentative gait. He or she will often state that the pain is severe and constant or throbbing.

There may be sleep disturbance, fever, and malaise with both initial herpes simplex infections and perianal abscess.

Other conditions to keep in mind with severe pain are prolapsed, strangulated hemorrhoids with spasm of the anal sphincter (an uncommon presentation nowadays) and the possibility of a foreign body in the rectum (usually present for some days if the pain is severe). With the latter condition, patients may be reticent to give a history of insertion of a foreign body, and examination is therefore mandatory in patients with severe pain.

Primary Perianal Herpes Simplex Infection

Perianal herpes simplex (see Figure 23-1) may be acquired through penile–anal intercourse, or through anilingus. As with genital herpes (see Chapter 18) in the developed world, an increasing proportion of anorectal HSV genital infections are now due to herpes simplex type 1 (HSV-1) infection, especially in younger adults. These are less likely to cause symptomatic recurrences though the initial episode is often as severe as that caused by an infection with HSV-2. The incubation period is 2 to 7 days, and there may be a prodrome of malaise and fever before the onset of perianal pain and ulceration (see Figure 23-1). There is frequently tenesmus and constipation. Rectal discharge and slight bleeding is not uncommon, and urinary retention and erectile dysfunction may also occur.

On examination, the patient often has a fever and may look unwell. There is usually typical herpetic ulceration of the perianal region, although occasionally no

FIGURE 23-1 Primary HSV Infection

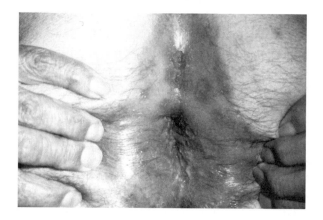

ulceration is seen. Inguinal lymphadenopathy is generally present as the groin nodes drain the perianal region. Anoscopy may not be possible because of severe pain but may reveal internal mucosal ulceration or severe generalized edematous proctitis *without* obvious ulceration. The anal mucosa often bleeds on contact.

Diagnosis is best made with the combination of an ulcer swab for herpes culture or a NAAT (nucleic acid amplification test) for herpes simplex types 1 and 2 (if available), along with type-specific HSV serology (see Chapter 18). A positive culture or NAAT along with negative serology (that subsequently becomes positive some weeks later) is evidence of a true primary herpetic episode, with implications for natural history and viral shedding.

Treatment for anorectal HSV is similar to treatment for genital infections and is based on using the antivirals acyclovir, famciclovir, or valacyclovir in the appropriate doses, as well as analgesia. If no lesions are visible externally and a diagnosis cannot be confirmed, proctoscopy or sigmoidoscopy may be warranted. Recurrent infections are much milder than the primary infection and can be delayed or even averted altogether using suppressive antiviral therapy with antiherpetic medications in the appropriate doses.

Perianal Abscess

Perianal abscess is a common surgical condition that also occurs in persons who have not had receptive anal intercourse. There is no evidence that anal intercourse makes this condition more likely. However, in patients who report anal sex, evaluation for sexually transmitted pathogens (especially *Neisseria gonorrhoeae*, chlamydia, and LGV) should be performed. The usual microbiology, however, is an enteric polymicrobial flora, with *Escherichia coli*, *Enterococcus* spp., and *Bacteroides* spp. as the predominant organisms. Rarely, *Mycobacterium tuberculosis* and endemic fungi can also cause perianal abscesses. Perianal abscesses are most common in those aged 30 to 40 years, and are two to three times more common in males than females. About a third of patients with perianal abscesses give a history of previous abscesses. It is thought that abscesses arise as a result of obstructed anal crypts, with subsequent suppuration and abscess formation in the anal gland.

The patient usually presents with dull anal pain and may have fever, chills, and malaise, especially if the abscess extends more deeply. Sitting and defecation worsen the pain. Examination reveals an erythematous, well-defined, fluctuant, acutely tender mass near the anus. The diagnosis is generally made on clinical grounds. In severe cases, CT or MRI scanning may provide valuable information about the extent of the abscess and any associated fistulas.

Treatment is incision and drainage, either under local or general anesthesia. As mentioned previously, pus should be cultured, and the laboratory should test for gonorrhea and chlamydia in those who give a sexual risk history. Antibiotic therapy is based on treating for enterics, including anaerobes, and regimens such as amoxicillin and clavulanic acid for 5–10 days are often used. In the appropriate patient, where incision and drainage is carried out and laboratory culture is omitted, failure of the abscess to resolve suggests that the etiology may be gonococcal or chlamydial.

■ PAINFUL ULCERS

Painful, though not *severely* painful, ulceration is usually due to recurrent genital herpes, chancroid (in endemic areas), or trauma. Genital herpes has been discussed previously, though it is worth reiterating that the lesions of recurrent genital herpes are commonly misdiagnosed, as the diagnosis is either not considered or the lesions are atypical and testing for HSV is not carried out. We recommend that all perianal ulcerative lesions should be tested for HSV.

Chancroid

Chancroid, caused by the gram-negative bacillus *Haemophilus ducreyi*, is rarely seen in the developed world. It was formerly the most common cause of genital ulceration in Africa, but it has now been overtaken by genital herpes. It is still relatively common in endemic areas, however, and, of course, it is not uncommon to have multiple etiological agents (such as syphilis and chancroid, or HSV and chancroid) in the one lesion. Anal infection occurs in women and in homosexually active men and the resulting nonindurate, often painful, multiple ulcers can be locally destructive. Tenesmus and rectal bleeding are common symptoms.

Diagnosis of chancroid is difficult, because the testing is difficult to do and is not widely available. Culture is difficult for this fastidious organism, though selective, enriched culture media are available. Although polymerase chain reaction (PCR) tests have been developed, they have not been commercialized and are therefore available only in specialized centers. Presumptive treatment for chancroid using an approved regimen, such as azithromycin or quinolones (see CDC 2010 STD Treatment Guidelines), may be a reasonable approach in persons in which the diagnosis is suspected on clinical or epidemiological grounds.

■ PAIN ON DEFECATION

Pain that occurs *only* on defecation is usually due to a perianal fissure (see Figure 23-2). This relatively common condition is a painful linear tear in the distal anal canal. It only involves the epithelium initially but with time may come to involve the full thickness of the anal mucosa. Perianal fissures are said to occur equally in both sexes and are more common in younger persons, particularly those in the 20- to 40-year-old age group. Constipation, with the passage of hard stools, is said to predispose to fissures, although, counterintuitively, fissures can also occur after episodes of diarrhea.

Prior anal surgery predisposes to perianal fissures, but there is no evidence that anal intercourse leads to this condition. Anal intercourse can cause small splits or tears in the anal mucosa, but these do not seem to progress to ulceration and fissures. It is generally accepted that homosexual men are at no greater risk of perianal fissures than are heterosexual men. In fact, the reverse might theoretically be the case as resting anal tone is likely to be less in the man who is experienced in receiving anal intercourse and has learned to relax his sphincter muscles at will.

FIGURE 23-2 Aggressive Perirectal HSV with Fissure Development in an Untreated HIV-infected Patient

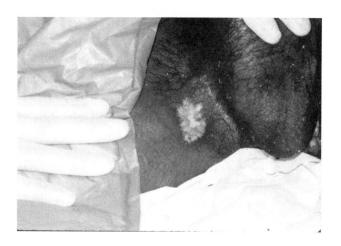

The diagnosis is usually apparent on history alone. The patient complains of severe pain during a bowel movement (as the stool passes over the raw area of the ulcer, with subsequent painful spasm of the internal anal sphincter), with this pain lasting for minutes or up to 1–2 hours. The patient comes to dread the prospect of another bowel action and worsening constipation may ensue. About 70% of patients notice bright red blood in the toilet bowl or on the toilet paper but significant bleeding does not occur.

On examination, the fissure may initially just be a tear in the anal mucosa (see Figure 23-2), but with time, a chronic fissure develops and the fibers of the internal anal sphincter are then present in the base of the fissure. In addition, an enlarged anal skin tag, sometimes referred to as a *sentinel pile*, may be visible distal to the fissure.

The differential diagnosis includes inflammatory bowel disease, local or systemic malignancy, anogenital herpes, syphilitic chancre, early LGV, trauma, and tuberculosis. These diagnoses should particularly be considered when lesions are atypical (multiple, or large and irregular).

Initial treatment for a perianal fissure is conservative, and 80% of fissures will heal without further therapy. Stool-bulking and softening agents are recommended to keep the bowel actions soft and less painful. Analgesic agents may help before a bowel action. Topical application of 0.2% glyceryl trinitrate ointment relaxes the internal anal sphincter and improves blood flow to the mucosa. This assists resolution of the fissure. Unfortunately, the side effects of a throbbing headache and dizziness limit its use. Botox (botulinum toxin A) injected into the internal anal sphincter produces an effect within hours, resulting in much less pain almost immediately. The effect then lasts for approximately three months and causes a chemical sphincterotomy, which allows healing to occur. There is a very low rate of fecal incontinence or relapse after using Botox.

Calcium channel blockers nifedipine and diltiazem in both oral and topical forms have also been tried and seem to have fewer side effects. They may well be the mainstay of future treatment.

If the fissure fails to heal after a few months of medical therapy, then surgical treatment is warranted. A lateral internal sphincterotomy is performed, either in the surgeon's rooms or under general anesthetic as a day procedure with the patient returning home the same day. Analgesics and stool softeners are prescribed postoperatively, and the patient can usually resume usual activities (excluding anal intercourse) within a day or two. There remain some concerns about the long-term consequences to young adults of surgically damaging their anal sphincters, and the risk of incontinence of flatus, and sometimes feces, are low, but real.

■ BLEEDING

Painless bleeding is the hallmark of *hemorrhoids*, or *piles*. The peak age range is 45–65 years, and it is thought that a low fiber diet is largely to blame for the high prevalence of this condition; however, genetics also plays a part. Pregnancy predisposes women to hemorrhoids, though most women become asymptomatic after delivery. Most patients, and many health professionals, attribute *all* perineal symptoms to hemorrhoids.

The patient will usually complain of bright red blood that drips into the toilet bowl with or after a bowel action. Blood may also be evident on the toilet paper. There may also be some mucus production and perianal itching can occur. Pain is most unusual and indicates prolapse of the hemorrhoids with subsequent spasm of the sphincter complex. Strangulation with necrosis may then worsen the pain.

Hemorrhoids are not visible on examination of the perianal area unless they are prolapsed. Neither are they palpable with a digital rectal examination as the soft, vascular hemorrhoids compress readily as the gloved finger slides over them. Anoscopy is the examination of choice and allows the soft hemorrhoids to fill the proximal lumen of the anoscope. In patients older than 40 years, rectal bleeding mandates referral to investigate the rest of the colon to exclude carcinoma.

Treatment should be limited to those with symptoms. Asymptomatic hemorrhoids need no treatment at all (your treatment won't make them feel any better when they have no symptoms to begin with!). Many symptoms resolve with adopting a high fiber diet as the sole intervention. The usual treatment for *symptomatic* hemorrhoids is rubber band ligation. Less frequently used treatments include injection sclerotherapy and cryotherapy. Stapling and surgical resection is reserved for severe prolapsing hemorrhoids and is carried out relatively rarely nowadays.

■ PAINFUL LUMP

A painful perianal lump is nearly always due to a perianal hematoma, sometimes referred to as an external hemorrhoid. Acute thrombosis of an external hemorrhoidal vein leads to acute pain, as the rapid distension of innervated skin by the blood clot occurs. This is often precipitated by an acute event, such as physical exertion (heavy lifting or sometimes receptive anal intercourse), straining with constipation, or a bout of diarrhea. Sometimes, though, the patient presents after becoming aware of the perianal hematoma with no history of a causative event.

On examination, there is a tender hematoma adjacent to the anal verge. This may appear tense and bluish and may become grape sized. The pain can be quite severe initially but tends to settle over one to two weeks. A skin tag may remain after the hematoma has been absorbed.

Treatment is generally best centered on analgesics initially, as the natural history of perianal hematomas is spontaneous resolution. Occasionally, it may be warranted to inject some local anesthetic into the hematoma and then to incise and enucleate the clot. This is only justified the first day or two after the hematoma has occurred, and even then, one is generally better to wait for the condition to become less painful on its own. If the hematomas recur frequently, then definitive surgery with excision of the hematoma and the offending vein at the base of the clot may be required.

■ PAINLESS LUMPS

Painless lumps are usually due to perianal warts caused by infection from the human papillomavirus. They are common in those who practice anal intercourse but also occur in sexually active people who do not practice anal intercourse. Warts may extend into the anal canal though they rarely extend beyond the dentate line. Immunocompromised patients are more likely to have extensive lesions and to suffer frequent recurrences.

Warts are usually noticed as lumps around the anus (see Figure 23-3), though sometimes some bleeding may occur. Itch is uncommon. Diagnosis is clinical, and anoscopy may be required to assess the anal canal. Occasionally, if there is difficulty making the diagnosis, histopathological examination of a biopsied lesion is helpful. With long-standing warts, particularly in the HIV-positive population (both male and female), malignant change can occur. Squamous cell carcinoma (SCC) of the anus is an uncommon condition but is many times more common in those who are HIV-positive. As people with HIV now live much longer because of antiretroviral treatments, there is concern that the incidence of anal SCC will increase. The risk of anal cancer developing is associated with oncogenic strains of HPV, particularly type 16 (and less commonly type 18), and is higher for smokers and for those individuals with a lower CD4+ cell count.

FIGURE 23-3 (a) Perirectal Condyloma Acuminate (Warts); (b) Aggressive Perirectal Warts in an HIV-Infected Patient

(a)

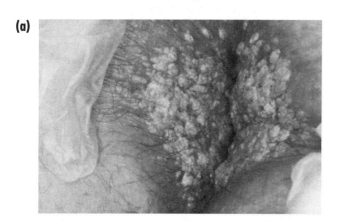

(b)

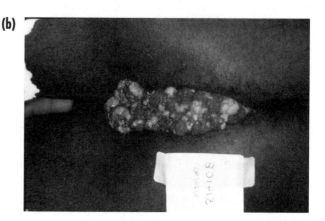

Studies are under way to determine whether there is a place for screening anal cytology (wryly referred to as *chap smears*) in HIV-positive men and women, and in HIV-negative MSM. In the interim, any suspicious perianal lesions deserve biopsy and histopathological assessment.

Treatment of external perianal warts is with ablative therapies such as cryotherapy, surgical excision, or the application of 0.5% podophyllotoxin paint or solution, or 0.15% podophyllotoxin cream. Imiquimod 5% cream (Aldara) is an effective treatment for perianal warts (see Chapter 22). One of the difficulties with the application of topical therapies is that one's own anus can be quite difficult to visualize adequately. This may necessitate the dexterous use of a mirror or sometimes the assistance of a (very) close friend.

With regards to prevention, two prophylactic HPV vaccines have become available. The Merck Gardasil vaccine targets types 6 and 11, which cause genital warts, as well as types 16 and 18, which are the primary causes of cervical and anorectal cancer. The U.S. Food and Drug Administration has approved the 4-type vaccine to prevent genital warts. To maximize effectiveness, these vaccines should be administered before the individual commences sexual activity and will, it is hoped, greatly reduce the incidence of carcinoma of the cervix and of the anus over the coming decades, as well as lead to a dramatic decline in the presentations of people with anogenital warts.

■ PAINLESS ULCER

A painless ulcer may be due to a syphilitic chancre, though other possibilities such as neoplasia, HSV, trauma, and chancroid must be kept in mind. All of these, with the exception of an anal carcinoma, generally cause pain, however. Donovanosis (granuloma inguinale) may cause perianal ulceration and the lesions of this infection are usually not painful.

Syphilis

Epidemics of syphilis have occurred in recent years in homosexual populations in Europe, the United States, and Australia and now account for most cases in these areas. Of particular concern is that in many areas, more than half of the cases involve HIV infection, and there has been a strong association with illicit drug use, especially stimulants such as methamphetamine.

Syphilis is the usual cause of a painless perianal ulcer. There may be one or more chancres present in the perianal region and associated inguinal lymphadenopathy is common. The patient may not notice perianal chancres and chancres within the anal canal, and so these infections will not come to the health professional's attention. *Rectal* chancres are even less commonly seen and may be mistaken for carcinomatous lesions during sigmoidoscopy or colonoscopy. A chancre will heal spontaneously (or after treatment with penicillin or some other antibiotics), whereas carcinomas obviously do not behave in this way.

The diagnosis of an anorectal syphilitic chancre is usually made with the help of serology, though histology may also yield the diagnosis. Histology characteristically reveals a dense plasma infiltrate and numerous blood vessels with prominent endothelial swelling. Silver impregnation techniques may then reveal the presence of treponemes. Indirect immunofluorescence is also employed.

Dark-field microscopy of the transudate of the ulcer is not generally helpful because of the presence of commensal organisms such as intestinal treponemes—these may be mistaken for *Treponema pallidum*. PCR testing has also been used but may not yet be widely available. Many multiplex PCR kits have been developed and include primers for other causes of anogenital ulceration, including HSV-1, HSV-2, CMV, *Klebsiella granulomatis*, *Haemophilus ducreyi*, and LGV.

Condylomata lata—moist, polypoid lesions that teem with spirochetes—in the perianal and perineal regions (see Figure 23-4) are classic signs of secondary syphilis. The other signs of secondary syphilis, such as fever, generalized lymphadenopathy, a generalized maculopapular rash, and mucous patches, will generally accompany the presence of condylomata lata. A primary chancre will often still be present when secondary syphilis develops, especially in HIV-positive individuals. Treatment for anorectal syphilis is similar to treatment for genital syphilis (see Chapter 9).

Donovanosis

Donovanosis is rare in the Western world. Only one case was reported in Australia in 2009, and it is close to being eliminated there. In countries such as South Africa, Zambia, Zimbabwe, southern India, Papua New Guinea, Brazil, and Vietnam still have endemic donovanosis, however. Primary perianal donovanosis has been reported and is said to be more common in homosexual men.

Late presentation with advanced disease still occurs because of the shame associated with this disease, made worse because of the highly offensive odor associated with large, ulcerated lesions. Poor access to medical care in some parts of the world also increases the likelihood of late presentation. The ulcers spread with soft tissue destruction, and the resulting sclerosis can result in anal canal stenosis. Distinguishing chronic lesions in the rectum from malignancy can be difficult, and in endemic areas, a trial of antibiotics should always be given if there is the slightest possibility that the lesions are due to donovanosis.

Various staining techniques to identify the Donovan bodies, along with new PCR techniques, enable the diagnosis to be made. Tissue from biopsy can also be subjected to histological examination.

◼ ANAL DISCHARGE

Both *N. gonorrhoeae* and *Chlamydia trachomatis* can cause a variety of anorectal symptoms. They frequently (perhaps more than 50% of times) cause no symptoms at all and are readily transmitted sexually. When symptoms occur, they may result in an anal discharge, bleeding, discomfort, or itch.

Gonorrhea

In previous studies during the 1970s and 1980s, anorectal gonorrhoea in MSM was more common than was gonorrhea in the urethra or pharynx. Recent studies also support this assertion, and it is likely that asymptomatic, or mildly symptomatic anorectal gonorrhea, is the main reservoir of gonorrhea in gay men. Increased prevalences of anorectal gonorrhea have been reported among MSM in recent years and up to 85% may be asymptomatic.

Anorectal gonorrhea in women has traditionally been attributable to secretions from the vagina running down the perineum to the anus, though it is more likely caused by direct inoculation from penile–anal intercourse (and subsequent nonreporting of this act by the patient, or nonasking by the health professional!). Studies conducted in the 1970s and early 1980s found rates of anorectal gonorrhea in women named as contacts as high as 47%, with the rectum as sole site of infection in 2% of cases. This led to the common practice of performing concurrent rectal cultures. However, with the advent of NAATs, as culture methods became more sensitive, rectal cultures and testing is not as critical except in patients who exclusively report receptive rectal intercourse.

Gonorrhea may be transmitted to the anorectum through the penis, the tongue, or sometimes fingers. Sex toys can also carry the gonococcus. Receptive penile–anal

FIGURE 23-4 Perianal Condylomata Lata

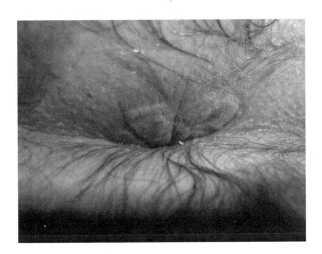

intercourse is not a sine qua non for contracting anorectal gonorrhea. Anoscopy may reveal normal mucosa, mucopus (especially around the anal crypts), or erythema and contact bleeding. Rarely, fistulas, abscesses, strictures, or disseminated gonococcal infection may occur. Diagnosis is with Gram staining and culture of an anal swab. Microscopy has only 30–40% the sensitivity of culture, though it is highly specific. Using a "blind" anorectal swab is almost as sensitive as taking direct vision swabs through an anoscope. Culture is both highly sensitive and specific. NAATs are highly accurate and more sensitive than culture.

Treatment of anorectal gonorrhea is the same as for urethral infections, with single-dose intramuscular ceftriaxone or oral cefixime. Spectinomycin, when available, has been used in persons with penicillin sensitivity; however, it has only a 50% efficacy in treating rectal gonorrhea. Treatment should also be given for *C. trachomatis* as concomitant infection rates are high.

Chlamydia trachomatis

Anorectal infection with *C. trachomatis* is more common than infection with the gonococcus. It occurs predominantly in MSM.

Non-LGV serotypes can cause anorectal pain or a mucoid or mucopurulent discharge, though it is probable that most infections are asymptomatic. Gram staining of an anal swab may show the presence of increased numbers of polymorphs. When performed on anorectal specimens, chlamydial culture or immunofluorescent antibody testing has poor sensitivity (i.e., many false-negative results), and enzyme linked immunosorbent assay (EIA) has poor specificity (i.e., many false-positive results). NAATs have now been validated by many laboratories around the world for anorectal chlamydial infections and should be considered as the diagnostic tool of first choice. Treatment with azithromycin 1 g as a single dose is the preferred treatment, though doxycycline and erythromycin are reasonable alternatives.

Lymphogranuloma Venereum

This condition is caused by *C. trachomatis* serovars L1–L3 and has recently reemerged in homosexual communities in continental Europe, the United Kingdom, the United States, and Australia. The L2b serovar has been responsible for these outbreaks. Unlike other chlamydial infections, which are generally restricted to epithelial surfaces, LGV is invasive and causes severe inflammation, with a preference for lymphatic tissue.

It has especially been associated with HIV-positive men, in those with ulcerative anorectal disease, and in those who undertake more "adventurous" sexual activities, including unprotected receptive anal sex with multiple partners.

LGV infection is characterized by three stages. In the first stage, the primary lesion is usually an asymptomatic small genital ulcer that heals spontaneously. This is followed by a painful inguinal lymphadenopathy associated with systemic features, including malaise and fever. Lymph node inflammation may progress to involve the surrounding subcutaneous tissue, causing an inflammatory mass (bubo) or abscess.

Complications occur in 30% of cases as a result of bubo rupture or sinus tract or fistula formation. Most of the recent cases in MSM have presented with a bloody proctitis, which may mimic inflammatory bowel disease. In anorectal disease, acute hemorrhagic inflammation of the colon and rectum is associated with involvement of perirectal lymphatic tissue. The third stage is characterized by chronic granulomatous inflammation leading to lymphatic obstruction, fibrosis, and stricture formation.

The notable absence of the typical "bubonic" presentation of LGV (classical genital ulcers, the "groove" sign, suppurating lymph nodes, etc.)—usually seen in parts of Africa, Asia, South America, and the Caribbean—has often delayed diagnosis and allowed further transmissions and complications to occur. If left untreated, rectal strictures and fistulas may occur. Recently, however, several cases of the classical "bubonic" presentation have been reported in the United Kingdom in gay men.

Identifying the L-serovars of *C. trachomatis* is important as longer treatment regimens are required for these serovars, especially in invasive disease. Commercially available NAATs for *C. trachomatis* will also detect the LGV-causing serovars but are unable to differentiate them from the B-K serovars that cause the usual oculogenital chlamydial diseases. Specialized PCR tests are now available to detect LGV-causing serovars and are available in some specialized laboratories. Serological testing for LGV (using microimmunofluorescence or complement fixation testing) is available, though the results are not always reliable, especially at low titers. A high index of suspicion for LGV is required when seeing MSM with anogenital symptoms, especially if they are also HIV positive.

Recommended treatment is doxycycline 100 mg twice daily for 21 days, although azithromycin 1 g once weekly for 3 weeks is also likely to be effective. It is quite possible that the early stages of LGV infection are diagnosed and treated as "standard" chlamydia infection of the anorectum and are adequately treated with usual antibiotic treatment courses for this infection.

■ ANORECTAL INFECTIONS IN CONJUNCTION WITH HIV—POINTS TO REMEMBER

- The inflammatory and ulcerative sexually transmitted infections (STIs) facilitate the spread of HIV infection.

- HIV infection may facilitate the spread of some STIs.

- Anorectal infections may have a more aggressive course in HIV-infected persons.

- Increased rates of anorectal intraepithelial neoplasia and squamous cell carcinoma of the anus occur in individuals with HIV infection.

HIV has greatly complicated the clinical presentation and occurrence of many anal conditions. In the HIV-infected person, the clinician may encounter the following:

1. Common conditions found in the general population (e.g., anal fissures, hemorrhoids)

2. Common disorders with altered pathogenesis or treatments (syphilis, HSV, HPV)

3. Conditions unique to, or much more common in, people with HIV/AIDS (aphthous ulcers, CMV, MAC, cryptosporidiosis, and anorectal cancers, such as squamous cell carcinoma, lymphoma, and Kaposi's sarcoma)

Keep these in mind when dealing with those individuals who have HIV infection. Advice from an HIV-experienced colleague should be sought if there are concerns about diagnosis or treatment.

■ KEY POINTS

- Sexually transmitted anorectal infection needs to be considered and assessed in homosexual men and in women reporting receptive rectal intercourse. Persons at risk should be routinely screened for gonorrhea, chlamydia, syphilis, and HIV.

- The major differential diagnosis of rectal discharge is gonococcal or chlamydial infection. Herpes can also cause a painful discharge syndrome.

- The differential diagnosis of anorectal ulcer is herpes, syphilis, and lymphogranuloma venereum. Chancroid is rare.

- Treatment regimens for anorectal infections are the same as for genital infections, with the exception of gonorrhea, where spectinomycin is ineffective.

- In developed countries, HIV coinfection rates in persons with anorectal sexually transmitted diseases, especially homosexual men, are high.

REFERENCES

CDC. STD treatment guidelines 2010. *Morb Mortal Week Rep.* 2010;59(RR-12):1–110.

Erickson PI, Bastani R, Maxwell AE, Marcus AC, Capell FJ, Yan KX. Prevalence of anal sex among heterosexuals in California and its relationship to other AIDS risk behaviours. *AIDS Educ Prev.* 1995;7(6):477–493.

Joesoef MR, Gultom M, Irana ID, et al.. High rates of sexually transmitted diseases among male transvestites in Jakarta, Indonesia. *Int J STD AIDS.* 2003;14(9):609–613.

Kent CK, Chaw JK, Wong W, et al. Prevalence of rectal, urethral, and pharyngeal chlamydia and gonorrhoea in 2 clinical settings among men who have sex with men: San Francisco, California, 2003. *Clin Infect Dis.* 2005;41(1):67–74.

Kinghorn GR, Rashid S. Prevalence of rectal and pharyngeal infection in women with gonorrhoea in Sheffield. *Br J Vener Dis.* 1979;55(6):408–410.

McMillan A, Young H, Moyes A. Rectal gonorrhoea in homosexual men: source of infection. *Int J STD AIDS.* 2000; 11(5):284–287.

Sethi G, Allason-Jones E, Richens J, et al. Lymphogranuloma venereum presenting as genital ulceration and inguinal syndrome in men who have sex with men in London, UK. *Sex Transm Infect.* 2009;85(3):165–170.

Stansfield VA. Diagnosis and management of anorectal gonorrhoea in women. *Br J Vener Dis.* 1980;56(5):319–321.

Tian LH, Peterman TA, Tao G, et al; Respect-2 Study Group. Heterosexual anal sex activity in the year after an STD clinic visit. *Sex Transm Dis.* 2008;35(11):905–909.

Wiley DJ, Harper DM, Elashoff D, et al. How condom use, number of receptive anal intercourse partners and a history of external genital warts predict risk for external anal warts. *Int J STD AIDS.* 2005;16:203–211.

24

Urinary Tract Infections

Michael Dan

INTRODUCTION

Acute urinary tract infection (UTI) is a common clinical problem in women of reproductive age. UTIs typically occur in an anatomically normal urinary tract. The primary risk factors for UTI in these women are sexual intercourse and spermicidal contraceptives, both of which facilitate introduction of intestinal flora into the urinary tract.

Cystitis, the most common UTI, is characterized by dysuria, urgency, and frequency concomitant with pyuria and bacteriuria. Pyelonephritis occurs as result of ascending infection involving the renal parenchyma and pelvicaliceal system. Symptoms include flank pain, chills, and fever, with or without manifestations of cystitis. Recurrent UTI can be either due to relapse (recurrent infection after therapy resulting from persistence of the pretherapy isolate in the urinary tract) or reinfection (recurrent infection with an organism originating from outside of the urinary tract, either a new strain or a strain previously isolated that has persisted in the flora of the gut or vagina). The management of UTI has been made more complicated in recent years by increasing antimicrobial resistance, especially to beta-lactams and trimethoprim-sulfamethoxazole. This chapter will deal with the epidemiology, pathogenesis, diagnosis, and therapy of uncomplicated UTI in sexually active women.

EPIDEMIOLOGY

Urinary tract infections are exceedingly common in female patients: 60% of women report having had a UTI in their lifetime, and about one-third of all women will

have at least one episode of UTI requiring antibiotics by age 24 years. The incidence of acute cystitis in sexually active young women is 0.5% to 0.7% per year. Approximately 30–40% of women with an initial UTI will experience at least one recurrence, and one-third of those recurrences occur within the first 6 months. More than 90% of recurrences in young women are episodes of reinfection, occurring months apart. In approximately 3–5% of women, there are multiple recurrences over many years. Risk factors associated with recurrence include frequent intercourse, a new sexual partner, long-term spermicide use, diaphragm use, young age at first UTI, and a maternal history of UTI. Episodes of recurrent UTI tend to cluster, with the highest risk of recurrence immediately after initial infection. There also seems to be seasonal variation, with more UTI episodes occurring in the summer than in the winter.

Asymptomatic bacteriuria in young women is common, is usually transient, but strongly predicts subsequent symptomatic UTI. Asymptomatic bacteriuria is defined as the presence of at least 10^5 colony-forming units of the same urinary tract pathogen per milliliter in two consecutive voided urine specimens but without the local or systemic genitourinary signs or symptoms. In a prospective evaluation of 796 sexually active, nonpregnant American women 18–40 years of age followed for 6 months, asymptomatic bacteriuria was found in 5%, although persistent bacteriuria with the same *E. coli* strain was rare (Hooton 2000). Symptomatic urinary tract infection developed within 1 week after 8% of episodes of asymptomatic bacteriuria, as compared with 1% of occasions when urine cultures did not detect significant bacteriuria ($P < 0.001$). This association was stronger if pyuria was present. The increased risk of symptomatic infection remained at 1 month after new-onset bacteriuria. No difference was observed in the genotypes of *E. coli* in isolates from symptomatic and asymptomatic episodes. Others have found that *E. coli* strains isolated from women with asymptomatic bacteriuria are characterized by fewer virulence characteristics than are those isolated from women with symptomatic infection. For healthy women, the prevalence of asymptomatic bacteriuria increases with advancing age and can be detected in 11–16% of elderly women in the community. Although patients with asymptomatic bacteriuria are at increased risk for symptomatic episodes, studies have consistently found no short-term or long-term adverse outcomes (such as renal scarring, hypertension, renal failure, genitourinary cancer, or decreased duration of survival) that could be directly attributed to asymptomatic bacteriuria. Treatment is generally not recommended.

UTI in pregnant women and diabetic patients often present difficult management challenges. Diabetic women have symptomatic and asymptomatic bacteriuria twice as often as nondiabetic women, may be caused by more atypical uropathogens, and may lead to severe complications, such as emphysematous cystitis and emphysematous pyelonephritis. Women with diabetes were 6 to 24 times more likely than nondiabetic women to be hospitalized for pyelonephritis.

In pregnancy, lower tract infection more easily leads to complications, both because of the biomechanical and hormonal changes that occur. Pyelonephritis is the most common severe bacterial infection complicating pregnancy and the most common cause of septic shock in pregnancy. Asymptomatic bacteriuria is detected in 4–10% of pregnant women, a prevalence similar to that of nonpregnant women. Acute pyelonephritis affects 1–2% of pregnant women; 80–90% of cases have been reported to occur in the second and third trimesters. Risk factors include young age and nulliparity. Women with prior history of UTI are at increased risk of UTI during pregnancy. Other risk factors for asymptomatic bacteriuria or acute cystitis during pregnancy include lower socioeconomic status, increased parity or older age, a history of childhood UTIs, and minimal medical care throughout the pregnancy. Women with asymptomatic bacteriuria in early pregnancy have a 20- to 30-fold increased risk of developing pyelonephritis during pregnancy, compared with women without bacteriuria. Pyelonephritis has

been associated with prematurity and low birth weight. Therefore, asymptomatic bacteriuria during pregnancy should be treated with the objective of reducing the upper tract complications. Treatment reduces the risk of ascending infection from 20–40% to 1–4%. Prevention of gestational pyelonephritis by early screening for asymptomatic bacteriuria during pregnancy is highly recommended.

The incidence of UTI among HIV-seropositive women seems to be higher than among women who are HIV seronegative, and organisms other than *E. coli* (such as *Enterococcus* species) are isolated more frequently.

■ RISK FACTORS

Susceptibility to UTI is associated with a number of behavioral and genetic determinants. The most important risk in anatomically normal women is sexual intercourse. Specific risks include increased frequency of sexual intercourse among premenopausal women, use of spermicides for contraception, use of a diaphragm, condom use by partner, estrogen deficiency, a prior history of UTI, and nonsecretory status of ABO blood-group antigens. Multiple studies have shown a strong dose-response relationship between the frequency of vaginal intercourse in the preceding 2 weeks and the risk of first-time UTI. Vaginal intercourse with a condom increases the risk of UTI by 43%, compared with vaginal intercourse using oral contraceptives or no birth control, with higher risk among those who used unlubricated condoms.

The strong association between a history of urinary tract infection and current urinary tract infection could reflect a biologic predisposition to urinary tract infection among certain women. Women with frequent episodes of UTI are more likely to have a maternal history of cystitis and to have had cystitis at an early age. Women with recurrent UTIs are three times more likely to be nonsecretors of blood-group antigens than are women who do not have such infections.

Women of all ages are at increased risk of UTI after antimicrobial use. Data from a prospective study correlated antecedent antibiotic use 2 to 4 weeks before the onset of UTI increased the relative risk for that UTI by 2.6 to 5.8. The increased risks were noted both for women whose antimicrobial use was to treat a previous UTI and for women who received antimicrobials for other illnesses. The most frequently associated antibiotics were beta-lactams, especially those with broad spectrum.

BACTERIOLOGY

Uncomplicated UTI in young women is caused by a narrow spectrum of etiologic agents, nearly all of which are enteric flora. *E. coli* is responsible for 70–95% of the cases, *Staphylococcus saprophyticus* is isolated in 5–15%, and occasionally *Klebsiella* species, *Proteus mirabilis*, or other microorganisms (such as *Enterobacter* sp., *Enterococcus* sp., and group B streptococci) are detected. The latter are more often associated with structural abnormalities of the urinary tract, indwelling catheters, and renal calculi.

In as many as 10% of symptomatic patients, no organisms are found on routine urine cultures. False-negative cultures may be the result of using antimicrobial agents, soap from the preparation falling into the urine, total obstruction below the anatomical site of the infection, infection with a fastidious organism, and diuresis. Another consideration in women with negative cultures is the dysuria-pyuria syndrome, which is caused by infection of the urethra by sexually transmitted pathogens such as *Chlamydia trachomatis, Neisseria gonorrhoeae*, and herpes simplex. This syndrome is diagnosed by the presence of pyuria in the first-void specimen, with a normal midstream urinalysis. Because comprehensive etiological evaluation of pyuria-dysuria is often difficult in a primary care setting, syndromic treatment for the STI pathogens may be an option.

Antimicrobial resistance among community-acquired uropathogens has increased during the past decades: in the United States, resistance of cystitis-causing *E. coli* strains to TMP-SMX and, more recently, to quinolones, has dramatically increased. Similar resistance rates (9–15%) were reported from Europe for 1999–2000, except for Spain and Portugal, where the rate was nearly 35%. TMP-SMX resistance has been associated with concurrent resistance to other antibiotics recommended in UTI. *E. coli* strains resistant to TMP-SMX, for example, are 14 times more likely to be resistant to ciprofloxacin than are susceptible strains (9.5% vs. 0.7%), and they are four times more likely to be resistant to nitrofurantoin (1.9% vs. 0.5%). Community-acquired UTI caused by organisms resistant to multiple antibiotics such as the *Klebsiella pneumonia* carbapenemase (KPC) producers have been encountered.

PATHOGENESIS

The normal urinary tract resists bacterial colonization by eliminating microorganisms that gain access to the bladder. The major defenses include unobstructed flow of urine and washout of transient uroepithelial colonizers, the antibacterial effect of urine, glycoproteins that block adherence of bacteria to the vesical and vaginal mucosa, and local immunologic responses. UTI in women is most often caused by perineal and periurethral bacteria of intestinal origin that gain entrance to the bladder.

Host Factors

The female urethra is markedly shorter than males, and women susceptible to UTIs are more likely to have a shorter distance between the anus and the urethra than control subjects. Vaginal intercourse increases the risk of infection because of meatal trauma, urethral massage, and probably, changes in vaginal flora. Intercourse facilitates the transfer of potential uropathogens to the vagina and the entrance of potential uropathogens into the urethral meatus from the vagina. A statistically significant increase in the level of vaginal colonization with *E. coli* has been documented after intercourse. Furthermore, heterosexual couples may be colonized with the same uropathogenic strains. Using a diaphragm with spermicide or a cervical cap during sexual intercourse increases the rate of vaginal colonization by uropathogenic flora and decreases the rate of colonization by lactobacilli.

The increasing prevalence of UTI with advancing age might be due to the hypoestrogenic state, which is responsible for vaginal mucosal atrophy, lactobacillary depletion, and impaired voiding. The higher occurrence of pyelonephritis during gestation is due to pregnancy-induced physiological changes in the urinary system. Dilatation of the ureters and renal calyces occurs as early as 12 weeks gestation and is thought to be caused by progesterone-induced relaxation of their muscular layers. In addition, the enlarging uterus compresses the ureters at the pelvic brim, particularly on the right. Anatomical changes in bladder position occur in late pregnancy. Impaired emptying of the bladder leads to increased bladder residual volume and ureterovesical reflux. Relative stasis of urine in the ureters results in hydronephrosis.

Adherence

In women susceptible to UTI, uropathogens adhere avidly to the vaginal, bladder, and buccal epithelial cells. Epithelial cells receptivity may vary and is genetically determined, as evidenced by higher susceptibility to UTIs among women of some families. Women who are nonsecretors of blood-group antigens have increased presence of specific *E. coli*–binding glycosphingolipids on their uroepithelial cells. The glycosphingolipids are components of the glycocalyx that surrounds epithelial cells. As a result of the enhanced susceptibility of human epithelial cells to bacterial adherence, women with recurrent cystitis have a more frequent and more prolonged colonization of the perineum, including the periurethral region, with coliform bacteria. Vaginal cell receptivity for bacterial attachment varies significantly from day to day in both healthy controls and patients. For instance, when adherence was correlated with the days of a woman's menstrual cycle, increased numbers of bacteria adhered in the early phase, and this number diminished shortly after the time of expected ovulation. This observation suggests that hormonal fluctuations, as seen with estrogen, may modify vaginal cell receptivity and the pathogenesis of UTIs. It is also well established that women experience clustering of UTIs followed by infection-free intervals.

Other behavioral factors, such as using sanitary napkins for menstrual protection, direction of wiping after bowel movements, and douching have not been clearly been linked to recurrent UTIs.

Bacterial Factors

Most of the involved bacterial strains are uropathogenic *E. coli* belonging to a small number of O:K:H serotypic groups. They possess adherence factors and other virulence factors that allow them to initiate and propagate infections in the anatomically normal urinary tract. Bacterial adhesins are filamentous appendages called pili, or fimbriae, that project from the bacterial cells (numerous uropathogenic strains adhere, however, in the absence of pili). The two main pili found in uropathogenic *E. coli* (type 1 and type P) differ in their ability to mediate hemagglutination in the presence of mannose. Type 1 pili, which are mannose sensitive, are associated with persistence of *E. coli* in the urinary tract. Type P pili are mannose resistant and were named so because of their high incidence in pyelonephritis and their association with the P blood group system. About 90% of pyelonephritis-causing *E. coli* possess the P pili that seem to be associated with high virulence. This same category of *E. coli* is also a common cause of urosepsis but is rarely present in healthy patients with cystitis or asymptomatic bacteriuria. Other virulence factors, such as hemolysin and carbohydrate capsules, increase resistance to serum bactericidal activity and resistance to host phagocytic activity. Other Enterobacteriaceae and *S. saprophyticus* adhere to uroepithelial cells through different adhesive mechanisms. Adherence of pathogens to epithelial cells is the first step

in the pathogenesis of UTI. The binding of pathogens to epithelial cells is followed by a complex set of events and interactions between bacterial and host mechanisms, such as influx of neutrophils into the bladder, elaboration of cytokines, replication of bacterial clusters inside superficial cells, exfoliation of superficial epithelial cells, differentiation and proliferation of the underlying transitional cells, and encasement of bacteria in a polysaccharide-rich matrix or biofilm.

■ CLINICAL MANIFESTATIONS

An episode of cystitis in a young female causes an average 6.1 days of symptoms, 2.4 days of restricted activity, 1.2 days of absence from classes or work, and 0.4 days in bed. Symptoms of acute bladder infection are sudden onset and burning or pain during urination (dysuria), frequent voiding of small volumes of urine (frequency), and the urge to void immediately (urgency). Hematuria is noted in approximately 40% of cases. Discomfort in the lower abdominal area can also accompany acute cystitis, and the suprapubic area may be tender on palpation. Approximately one-half of lower UTI episodes clear spontaneously after 2–4 weeks if untreated, although symptoms may persist for up to several months.

Onset of pyelonephritis is usually abrupt, with fever, chills, and aching pain in one or both lumbar regions. Anorexia, nausea, and vomiting are common and can worsen dehydration associated with fever. Symptoms of cystitis may or may not be present. Tenderness can be elicited by percussion in one or both costovertebral angles. The presentation of acute pyelonephritis varies from a mild to moderate illness; rarely, the condition can be life threatening with multiple organ system failure, including a sepsis syndrome with or without shock. Approximately 12% of patients hospitalized for pyelonephritis will have bacteremia; however, there is no evidence that bacteremia is associated with worse prognosis or warrants longer therapy in otherwise healthy individuals with pyelonephritis.

■ DIAGNOSIS

Distinction between uncomplicated and complicated UTIs, and between cystitis and upper UTI is important because of implications regarding pre- and posttreatment evaluation, type and duration of antimicrobial regimens, and extent of investigation of the urinary tract. UTI is considered complicated in the presence of diabetes mellitus, immunocompromised conditions, pregnancy, and urinary tract obstruction (e.g., strictures, neurogenic bladder); some consider older age (>65 years) and prolonged symptoms (>14 days) to be complicating factors. It is generally safe to assume that a premenopausal, sexually active, nonpregnant woman with recent onset of typical symptoms who has not been recently instrumented or treated with antibacterial agents and who has no history of genitourinary tract abnormalities has an uncomplicated UTI.

The traditional approach to UTI diagnosis was based on the presence of typical urinary tract symptoms, demonstration of pyuria on urinalysis, and isolation of a pathogen on urine culture. However, these tests are rarely necessary with uncomplicated cystitis. Cystitis can be established in most patients using history alone: the probability of cystitis in a woman with dysuria, urinary frequency, or gross hematuria is about 50% in primary care settings. Symptoms suggesting vaginitis or cervicitis, such as vaginal irritation or discharge, reduce the likelihood of a diagnosis of cystitis by about 20%. Specific combinations of symptoms (e.g., dysuria and frequency without vaginal discharge or irritation) raise the probability of cystitis to greater than 90%. When a woman with a history of cystitis has symptoms suggesting a recurrence, there is an 84–92% chance that an infection is present. In such circumstances, empiric ther-

apy can be offered without further tests. In contrast, history taking (as well as physical examination and dipstick urinalysis) cannot rule out UTI when a patient presents with one or more symptoms. In patients who present with some symptoms of UTI but with mostly negative history and physical examination findings, a urine culture and pelvic examination should be considered. In conclusion, obtaining a history of the presence of certain symptoms (e.g., dysuria, frequency, hematuria) coupled with the absence of other symptoms (e.g., vaginal irritation or discharge) is a useful method to diagnose cystitis, while significantly decreasing urinalysis, urine culture, and office visits.

Differentiating between UTI, cervical sexually transmitted infections, and vaginal infections may be difficult because symptoms and signs commonly overlap (see Table 24-1).

Because historical information is the basis for diagnosing uncomplicated cystitis, telephone-based management is often done in primary care settings with no excessive adverse outcomes. Moreover, patients managed via telephone are extremely satisfied; in one survey, 98% have stated that they would prefer to receive telephone-based management if symptoms of presumed cystitis recur rather than have an office visit with a healthcare provider. However, the positive predictive value of the

TABLE 24-1   Major Infectious Causes of Acute Dysuria in Women

Condition	Pathogens	Pyuria/Hematuria	Colony count (CFU/mL)	Comment
Cystitis	*E. coli* *Staphylococcus saprophyticus* *Proteus* spp. *Klebsiella* spp.	Usually/sometimes	10^2–10^5	Abrupt onset. "Internal" dysuria, frequency, urgency, suprapubic pain
Urethritis	*Chlamydia trachomatis* *Neisseria gonorrhoeae* Herpes simplex virus	Usually/rarely	$10^2>$	Gradual onset Mild symptoms, possible discharge (due to cervicitis). Risk factors for STI
Vaginitis	*Candida* spp. Trichomonas vaginalis	Rarely/Rarely	$10^2>$	Gradual onset. "External" dysuria, discharge, vulvar irritation/burning, pruritus, dyspareunia

Adapted from Stamm WE, Hooton TM. Management of urinary tract infections in adults. *N Engl J Med.* 1993;329:1328–1334. CFU, colony-forming units.

telephone-based guidelines remains uncertain, leading to concerns that these guidelines may result in overdiagnosis of cystitis and unnecessary antimicrobial therapy in some patients. Published protocols have included only women at low risk who have not recently had another UTI, who do not have symptoms suggesting vaginitis or cervicitis, and, in some institutions, who are younger than 55 years old. Women who do not meet these criteria should usually be seen and examined. Despite this limitation, telephone-based treatment appears to be cost effective and safe for carefully selected patients.

The physical examination has a limited role in diagnosing cystitis. A pelvic examination is recommended in all women reporting vaginal discharge; the presence of vaginal discharge on examination suggests vaginal infection. The physical examination may also be useful to distinguish between lower urinary tract (cystitis) and upper urinary tract (pyelonephritis) disease: the presence of fever or costovertebral angle tenderness in a woman with dysuria indicates infection of the upper urinary tract rather than cystitis. However, normal temperature in the presence of UTI symptoms does not exclude the possibility of an upper urinary tract infection, especially in diabetics. It has been suggested that most cystitis cases that fail to respond to short-course antimicrobial therapy are misdiagnosed upper urinary tract infections that should have been treated with a longer course of antibiotics.

In contrast to lower tract disease, laboratory workup, including urinalysis, urine culture, and antimicrobial susceptibility testing of isolates, is required when pyelonephritis is suspected.

Specimen Collection for Urine Culture and Urinalysis

The midstream clean-catch technique has long been considered the standard method for collecting urine cultures from women. The patient must first wipe her introitus from front to back with a gauze pad moistened with tap water or saline, spread her labia, discard the initial urine sample, and then collect a midstream sample in a sterile container (use of a disinfectant may alter the colony count). This requires a fair amount of manual dexterity and coordination. A recent randomized trial of consecutive women presenting with symptoms of cystitis found that a non-midstream urine specimen provided in a clean container without performing any cleansing had a contamination rate similar to a specimen obtained by the midstream clean-catch technique. Because enteric bacteria may proliferate quickly at room temperature, thereby

leading to false-positive results of quantitative bacterial evaluation, the urine specimen should reach the microbiology laboratory within a few hours of its collection to avoid inaccurate results. Alternatively, the urine specimen can be stored overnight in a refrigerator until processed.

Urinalysis is used to demonstrate the presence of bacteriuria and pyuria. The most accurate method to detect pyuria is examining an unspun urine sample with a hemocytometer; the finding of ≥ 10 leukocytes per mm^3 is considered abnormal. Pyuria on urinalysis has high sensitivity (95%) but a relatively low specificity (71 percent) for infection and is thus present in almost all women with acute symptomatic UTI; its absence strongly suggests a different diagnosis. Gram staining of an uncentrifuged specimen is an easy, rapid, and relatively reliable way to detect significant numbers of organisms. The presence of ≥ 1 bacterium per oil immersion field in a midstream, clean-catch, Gram stained, uncentrifuged urine correlates with $\geq 10^5$ bacteria/mL of urine. The absence of bacteria in several fields in a stained sedimented specimen indicates the probability of $<10^4$ bacteria/mL. Although microscopic evaluation of the urine for bacteriuria cannot detect low numbers of bacteria ($\leq 10^4$ CFU/mL), the test is quite specific for UTI (85–95%) if a predominance of bacteria with the same morphology is seen. The leukocyte esterase test and the nitrite test (urinary "dipstick" evaluation) is a useful indicator of the presence of bacteriuria or pyuria. Dipstick testing of urine has largely replaced microscopy and urine-culture analysis, because the dipstick method is cheaper, faster, and more convenient. The nitrite test is used to detect gram-negative bacteria capable of converting urine nitrates to nitrites. It will not detect gram-positive organisms, such as *S. saprophyticus*, and other bacteria that do not produce nitrite (such as *Pseudomonas aeruginosa*). Although highly specific ($\geq 90\%$), the nitrite test lacks adequate sensitivity when used alone (60–85%). In research conditions, the leukocyte esterase test has a good sensitivity (75–96%) and specificity (94–98%) in detecting significant leukocyturia, although it may not perform as well in daily practice. A negative result on a dipstick test cannot, however, reliably rule out an infection in symptomatic women: for patients with a negative leukocyte esterase dipstick test who have urinary symptoms, microscopical evaluation for pyuria or a culture should be performed.

The gold standard for diagnosis is quantitative urine culture. The most commonly used technique for obtaining an adequate specimen is the midstream clean catch. Among asymptomatic patients, bacteriuria is designated as significant when there are bacteria $\geq 10^5$ CFU/mL of voided urine. The term *significant bacteriuria* indicates that the number of bacteria in the voided urine exceeds the number that can be expected from contamination from the anterior urethra (these criteria apply only to the Enterobacteriaceae). Applying the same criteria in women with clinical symptoms suggesting uncomplicated cystitis was found to be of low sensitivity; it is now accepted that using a definition of $\geq 10^2$ CFU/mL has the best combination of sensitivity (95%) and specificity (85%). It has been postulated that low-count bacteriuria may represent an early phase of urinary infection. In pyelonephritis the bacterial counts are usually higher than those in acute cystitis, and 80–95% of episodes of pyelonephritis are associated with $\geq 10^5$ CFU/mL uropathogens. Because the causative organisms and their antimicrobial susceptibility are so predictable in women with uncomplicated cystitis and culture results are available only after the patient's symptoms have resolved, culturing urine in these patients is not recommended. Urine cultures should be reserved only for women with atypical symptoms of UTI, if clinical improvement does not occur within 48 hours of empiric treatment or in the case of recurrence and should also be performed routinely in women with pyelonephritis. Blood cultures are not routinely recommended; they are advocated in cases that are complicated by sepsis, temperature of at least 39°C, or respiratory distress syndrome. Renal ultrasound evaluation should be reserved for women who are unresponsive to initial treatment. An intravenous pyelography also may be useful to evaluate renal collecting system obstruction. Contrast-enhanced computed tomography or magnetic resonance imaging is indicated to rule out a perinephric abscess or phlegmon. The use of a postvoid residual volume measure, urodynamic testing, cystourethroscopy, or radiologic imaging is not cost effective in premenopausal women with no evidence of relapsing UTI.

Therapy

Treatment of lower tract UTI is generally empirical. Unfortunately, drug resistance among uropathogens has increased steadily during the past several decades, resulting in more complex treatment choices. If available, local surveillance data should be reviewed to guide empirical therapy for UTIs. These data should be periodically updated as susceptibility patterns change over time. Resistance rates higher than 20% necessitate a change in antibiotic class.

Therapy should be based on two sets of considerations: (1) the choice of the appropriate drug and (2) the determination of the duration of its administration. Choice of drug depends on the antimicrobial spectrum of the agent, the prevalence of resistance among local uropathogens, the duration of adequate urinary or renal tissue concentrations achieved, the effect of the antimicrobial agent on the vaginal flora, the potential adverse effects, and cost. Considering these factors altogether, three drugs (1) trimethoprim-sulfamethoxazole (TMP-SMX), (2) trimethoprim, and (3) ciprofloxacin (as representative of fluoroquinolones) have been most successfully used. Beta-lactams, such as first-generation cephalosporins and amoxicillin, are less effective in treating uncomplicated acute cystitis than the agents mentioned earlier. This is because of increasing resistance among the common uropathogens, rapid excretion from the urinary tract, and the inability to completely clear gram-negative rods from the vagina, increasing the risk for recurrence.

TMP-SMX and trimethoprim have long been considered the drugs of choice for treating uncomplicated cystitis. They are highly effective for treating this condition, well tolerated, and inexpensive. In its guidelines published in 1999, the Infectious Diseases Society of America (IDSA) recommended TMP-SMX (FDA Pregnancy Category C) as first-line treatment for acute cystitis. The efficacy of trimethoprim (FDA Pregnancy Category C) is similar to that of TMP-SMX, and it can be prescribed to patients who are allergic to sulfa although trimethoprim can also cause hypersensitivity and rashes. The efficacy of fluoroquinolones (FDA Pregnancy Category C) equals or exceeds that of TMP-SMX. In addition to their activity against most typical gram-negative uropathogens, fluoroquinolones are also active against *S. saprophyticus* but against only 60–70% of enterococci. Despite their excellent efficacy and safety profile, fluoroquinolones have not been regarded as a first-line agents because of their much higher cost and because of concern about promoting bacterial resistance. However, faced with the increasing resistance among uropathogens to TMP-SMX experts were compelled to reexamine the recommendations for empirical therapy for cystitis. In Israel and in the western United States, where in vitro resistance of *E. coli* to TMP-SMX approaches 30%, the rate of clinical failure with this agent was 23% overall and 46% among patients with pathogens that were resistant to TMP-SMX. Some authorities now advocate using TMP-SMX only if the patient has no known allergy, if she has not recently received antibiotics, and if the local prevalence of resistance in urinary isolates is below 20% (see Table 24-2). Fluoroquinolones are now recommended as first-line therapy for uncomplicated UTI in areas where resistance to TMP-SMX is ≥20%. However, at least 50% of women infected with a resistant organism are successfully treated with TMP-SMX, and overall microbiologic and clinical cure rates of 80–85% can still be expected, even when the prevalence of resistance approaches 30%. This probably occurs because of the extraordinarily high concentration of antibiotics achieved in urine. Reported risk factors for infection with a TMP-SMX-resistant strain include recent hospitalization, diabetes, antibiotics, and TMP-SMX within the previous 3–6 months. Clinicians should include such information in their patient assessments to help determine when TMP-SMX is to be avoided. However, increasing fluoroquinolone resistance is a serious public health threat; it is essential that the indiscriminate use of these agents for treating mild-to-moderate acute uncomplicated cystitis is avoided to preserve their efficacy.

To minimize exposure of uropathogens to fluoroquinolones, nitrofurantoin (FDA Pregnancy Category B) is increasingly used. However, nitrofurantoin, unlike fluoroquinolones, does not eliminate effectively *E. coli* from the vagina, and it is associated with less satisfactory results using a 3-day course even with susceptible microorganisms (85% vs. 95%). Nitrofurantoin is inactive against most *Proteus* species, and some *Klebsiella* and *Enterobacter* strains, but it is active against enterococci. Side effects are more common, although the frequency of major adverse reactions, such as acute and chronic pulmonary syndromes, has been remarkably low. The monohydrate macrocrystal formulation, which is given twice daily, is more convenient to use and associated with less side effects. Nitrofurantoin should be avoided in patients with glucose-6-phosphate dehydrogenase deficiency because it can rarely induce hemolytic anemia in these patients.

Cefixime (FDA Pregnancy Category B) seems to be effective for treating uncomplicated UTI, although published data are scant and it might not be effective against *S. saprophyticus*. Other beta-lactams (e.g., amoxicillin and cephalexin) should be avoided because of frequent bacterial resistance to these agents and low cure rates.

For treating *acute uncomplicated cystitis*, a 3-day regimen of TMP-SMX, trimethoprim, or a fluoroquinolone appear adequate, with efficacy comparable to a 7-day regimen (approximately 95% cure rate), but with fewer side effects (18% vs. 30%) and lower cost. Seven-day regimens should be reserved for patients with risk factors, including pregnancy, that may result in lower cure

TABLE 24-2   Empiric Treatment for Acute Uncomplicated Cystitis

TMP-SMX	Nitrofurantoin	Fosfomycin	Fluoroquinolone
Patient has no history of allergy to the drug AND has had no antibiotic treatment (especially TMP-SMX) in the previous 3 months AND has had no recent hospitalization AND lives in a community in which *E. coli* resistance to TMP-SMX is not known to be ≥20% in women with acute uncomplicated cystitis.	Patient has allergy to TMP-SMX, OR antibiotic treatment in previous 3 months (except for nitrofurantoin) OR lives in a community in which *E. coli* resistance to TMP-SMX is known to be ≥20% in women with acute uncomplicated cystitis.	Patient has allergy to TMP-SMX, OR antibiotic treatment in the previous 3 months (except for fosfomycin) OR lives in a community in which the *E. coli* resistance to TMP-SMX is known to be ≥20% in women with acute uncomplicated cystitis.	Patient has allergy to TMP-SMX OR antibiotic treatment in previous 3 months (except for fluoroquinolone) OR live in a community in which *E. coli* resistance to TMP-SMX is known to be ≥20% in women with acute uncomplicated cystitis.

Adapted from Hooton TM, Besser R, Foxman B, Fritsche TR, Nicolle LE. Acute uncomplicated cystitis in an era of increasing antibiotic resistance: a proposed approach to empirical therapy. Clin Infect Dis. 2004;39:75–80.

rates with shorter regimens or when beta-lactams or nitrofurantoin are used.

Recurrent cystitis should be documented by culture at least once and then managed as a sporadic cystitis, although some experts would recommend a longer regimen of 7 days for frequently recurring episodes. A urine culture test of cure 1–2 weeks later to confirm clearance is suggested by some experts. Management of recurrent UTIs should include a search for known risk factors associated with recurrence. Behavioral changes, such as using a different form of contraception instead of spermicide, should be advised. Prophylaxis should not be initiated until the eradication of active infection is confirmed by a negative urine culture at least 1 to 2 weeks after treatment is discontinued. One of three prophylactic strategies can be offered: (1) continuous prophylaxis, (2) postcoital prophylaxis, or (3) therapy initiated by the patient. Patient-initiated therapy undertaken when symptoms arise provides a convenient, safe, inexpensive, and effective management.

In postmenopausal women, *Staphylococcus saprophyticus* is rarely isolated; however, gram-negative bacteria and enterococci are common, with *E. coli* remaining the most common causative organism. More attention should be paid to potential drug interactions. Antibiotic treatment of 3–6 days appears to be equivalent to longer courses of treatment (7–14 days), with fewer adverse events. A randomized, controlled trial assessing the optimal duration of antibiotic therapy for uncomplicated UTIs in women aged 65 years or older concluded that

the 3-day regimen was equally effective but better tolerated than a 7-day course.

Except for pregnant women, treatment of *asymptomatic bacteriuria* neither decreases the frequency of symptomatic infection nor prevents further episodes of asymptomatic bacteriuria. Screening for and treating asymptomatic bacteriuria in premenopausal, nonpregnant women is therefore not indicated. Similarly, screening for or treating asymptomatic bacteriuria in women with diabetes mellitus is not recommended because it does not reduce the rate of pyelonephritis or hospitalization for pyelonephritis. Treatment is also not recommended for older patients, whether they live in a community setting or institution; for patients with spinal cord injuries; or for patients with indwelling catheters. Treatment is indicated, however, in women undergoing a urologic procedure in which mucosal bleeding is anticipated and in women in whom catheter-acquired bacteriuria persists 48 hours after catheter removal.

Pyelonephritis can safely be treated orally in an outpatient setting if the infection is mild and if the patient is able to take medication orally, is trustworthy, can be easily reached by telephone for early follow-up, and is likely to return to the clinic promptly if symptoms do not resolve rapidly. Oral regimens for uncomplicated pyelonephritis are displayed in Table 24-3. Hospitalization for initial parenteral therapy is indicated for patients with nausea, vomiting, other conditions that precludes oral hydration and medication, uncertain social situation or concern about compliance, uncertainty

TABLE 24-3 Oral Antimicrobial Agents for Uncomplicated UTI

Antimicrobial Agent	Dosage in Cystitis	Dosage in Pyelonephritis
TMP-SMX	1 DS tab. twice daily	1 DS tab. twice daily
Trimethoprim	100 mg twice daily	NR**
Norfloxacin	400 mg twice daily	400 mg twice daily
Ofloxacin	200 mg twice daily	200-300 mg twice daily
Ciprofloxacin	250 mg twice daily	500 mg twice daily
Levofloxacin	250 mg once daily	500 mg once daily
Nitrofurantoin*	100 mg 4× a day	NR
Nitrofurantoin* Monohydrate	100 mg twice daily	NR
Fosfomycin	3 g single dose	NR
Cefixime	400 mg once daily	400 mg once daily

*Macrocrystals.

**NR, not recommended.

about the diagnosis, pregnancy, and moderate-to-severe illness. The optimal empiric regimens should be based on the local antimicrobial susceptibility profile of uropathogens. The recommended empiric parenteral regimens for pyelonephritis include a cephalosporin, an aminoglycoside, a fluoroquinolone, or a combination of ampicillin and gentamicin (see Table 24-4). TMP-SMX can be used empirically only in areas where there is no problem of resistance of uropathogens to this agent. In selected patients, parenterally administered ceftriaxone can be used as outpatient therapy. Treatment should be administered for no longer than 10–14 days, even in patients with positive blood cultures. Shorter regimens of 7 days are often satisfactory in patients treated with a non-beta-lactam agent who defervesce rapidly, although well-controlled trials are lacking. If fever and flank pain persist after 72 hours of therapy, cultures should be repeated and ultrasonography or computed tomography should be considered to rule out perinephric or intrarenal abscesses, unrecognized urologic abnormalities, or obstruction.

Urinary analgesics, such as phenazopyridine 200 mg three times daily, for 1 to 2 days, can be offered to patients with severe dysuria. This compound, now available over the counter, is not free of adverse effects, including gastrointestinal upset, headaches, rash, hemolytic reactions (in patients with glucose-6-phosphate dehydrogenase deficiency), and (rarely) nephrotoxicity. Increased fluid intake is usually advocated for women with UTI to hasten the removal of uropathogens by increased micturition; however, the increased hydration may be detrimental to the patient because the urinary concentration of antimicrobials is decreased by diluting the urine. Urinary acidification is frequently difficult to achieve and is rarely if ever necessary.

■ CLINICAL GUIDELINES FOR THE MANAGEMENT OF ACUTE UNCOMPLICATED CYSTITIS

Because the causative organisms and their susceptibility to antimicrobial agents are so predictable in women with acute cystitis, several authors have advocated a shortened laboratory workup followed by empirical therapy. In patients with typical symptoms, the diagnosis can be presumed if pyuria is present on microscopy or leukocyte esterase testing. No urine culture is performed, and a short course of empirical antimicrobial therapy is administered. No follow-up visit or culture after therapy is necessary unless symptoms persist or recur. If pyuria is absent, or there are atypical clinical features or factors that suggest a complicated infection, a culture should be performed before therapy is started. This approach was found to be efficacious, safe, and cost effective.

■ PREVENTION

Women with recurrent infection and who use spermicides, condoms, or diaphragms should consider alternative methods of contraception and STI prevention. Those with frequently recurring UTIs (≥ 3 episodes annually) can benefit from antimicrobial prophylaxis. Three different strategies can be offered to highly motivated and trustworthy patients. Continuous antimicrobial prophylaxis consists of daily administration of low-dose antibiotic (trimethoprim, TMP-SMX, or nitrofurantoin) at bedtime (see Table 24-5). Continuous prophylaxis diminishes recurrences by 95% and may prevent pyelonephritis. Prophylaxis is usually continued for 6 months but has been safely and effectively used for 2 to 5 years without the emergence of resistant organisms.

TABLE 24-4   Parenteral Treatment Regimens for Uncomplicated Pyelonephritis

Antimicrobial Agent	Dosage
Cefazolin	1000–2000 mg q 8 h
Cefuroxime	750–1500 mg q 8 h
Ceftriaxone	1000–2000 mg q 24 h
Ciprofloxacin	500 mg q 12 h
Ofloxacin	400 mg q 12 h
Levofloxacin	500 mg q 24 h
TMP-SMX	960 mg q 12 h (800 mg TMP + 160 mg SMX)
Gentamicin	3–5 mg/kg q24 h, or 1 mg/kg q 8 h
Ampicillin (with gentamicin)	1 g q 6 h

TABLE 24-5   Prophylactic Regimens for Uncomplicated UTI

Antimicrobial Agent	Dosage
TMP-SMX	1 single-strength tab. (80/400) every night or postcoitus
Trimethoprim	100 mg every night or postcoitus
Nitrofurantoin macrocrystals*	50 or 100 mg every night or postcoitus
Norfloxacin	200 mg every night or postcoitus
Ciprofloxacin	250 mg every night or postcoitus
Cephalexin*	250 mg every night or postcoitus
Cefuroxime axetil*	250 mg every night or postcoitus
Cefixime*	200 mg every night or postcoitus

* Can be used during pregnancy.

The most common adverse effects are gastrointestinal symptoms, rash, and yeast vaginitis. Postcoital antibiotic administration is intended for women with temporal association of UTI recurrence and intercourse. Postcoital prophylaxis is as effective as daily prophylaxis although it uses only one-third of the amount of drug used in the daily prophylaxis. Single-dose fluoroquinolone, nitrofurantoin, or TMP-SMX are the drugs of choice for this strategy (see Table 24-5). Patient-initiated intermittent self-treatment is recommended to educated women with lower recurrence rates. Women are given a prescription for one of the 3-day dosage regimens and are instructed to start therapy when symptoms develop. If symptoms do not improve in 48 hours, clinical evaluation should be performed.

Preventing or reducing the recurrence of UTI episodes with means other than antibiotics appeals to many. Cranberries are a longtime traditional prophylactic and therapeutic agent for UTI, either in juice or tablet form. Cranberries contain proanthocyanidins, which prevent the adherence of bacterial pathogens to uroepithelium, and thereby prevent UTIs, although data to show effectiveness are minimal. The use of topical estrogen creams in postmenopausal women with a history of recurrent UTIs decreased the number of episodes of UTI by 10-fold from 5.9 episodes to 0.5 episodes per year. Revitalization of the mucosa by local estrogen reinstitution of a more acidic environment created a favorable environment for the premenopausal lactobacillary flora and reduced the density of Enterobacteriaceae in the periurethral area. The benefit of vaginal lactobacilli application remains unproven.

No convincing data exist to corroborate the protective role of postcoital voiding. There is also no evidence that poor urinary hygiene is associated with recurrent infections, and there is no rationale for giving women instructions regarding the frequency of urination, timing of voiding, wiping patterns, douching, using hot tubs, or the wearing of pantyhose. There is not enough evidence to support the use of methenamine salts (methenamine hippurate and methenamine mandelate) for urinary prophylaxis.

■ KEY POINTS

• Screening for and treatment of asymptomatic bacteriuria is not recommended in nonpregnant women.

• A history of urinary symptoms (i.e., dysuria, frequency, hematuria) coupled with the absence of vulvovaginal symptoms (e.g., vaginal irritation, itching, discharge) is a useful method to diagnose cystitis.

• A 3-day antimicrobial regimen is the preferred treatment duration for uncomplicated acute bacterial cystitis in women.

• Trimethoprim-sulfamethoxazole and fluoroquinolones are the preferred agents for the treatment of acute uncomplicated cystitis. Nitrofurantoin is an acceptable alternative.

• Resistance rates higher than 15–20% necessitate a change in antibiotic class.

• In acute pyelonephritis, 10–14 days of total antimicrobial therapy should be completed.

REFERENCES

American College of Obstetricians and Gynecologists. ACOG Practice Bulletin No. 91: treatment of urinary tract infections in nonpregnant women. *Obstet Gynecol.* 2008;111:785–794.

Bent S, Nallamothu BK, Simel DL, Fihn SD, Saint S. Does this woman have an acute uncomplicated urinary tract infection? *JAMA.* 2002;287:2701–2710.

Fihn SD. Acute uncomplicated urinary tract infection in women. *N Engl J Med.* 2003;349:259–266.

Harding GKM, Shanel GG, Nicolle LE, Cheang M. Antimicrobial treatment in diabetic women with asymptomatic bacteriuria. *New Engl J Med.* 2002;347:1576–1583.

Hooton TM, Besser R, Foxman B, Fritsche TR, Nicolle LE. Acute uncomplicated cystitis in an era of increasing antibiotic resistance: a proposed approach to empirical therapy. *Clin Infect Dis.* 2004;39:75–80.

Hooton TM, Scholes D, Gupta K, Stapleton AE, Roberts PL, Stamm WE. Amoxicillin–clavulanate vs ciprofloxacin for the treatment of uncomplicated cystitis in women: a randomized trial. *JAMA.* 2005;293:949–955.

Hooton TM, Scholes D, Stapleton AE, et al. A prospective study of asymptomatic bacteriuria in sexually active young women. *N Engl J Med.* 2000;343:992–997.

Nicolle LE, Bradley S, Colgan R, C. Rice JC, Schaeffer A, Hooton TM. Infectious Diseases Society of America guidelines for the diagnosis and treatment of asymptomatic Bacteriuria in Adults. *Clin Infect Dis.* 2005;40:643–654.

McLaughlin SP, Carson CC. Urinary tract infections in women. *Med Clin N Am.* 2004;88:417–429.

Raz R, Chazan B, Dan M. Cranberry juice and urinary tract infection. *Clin Infect Dis.* 2004;38:1413–1419.

Raz R, Chazan B, Kennes Y, et al. Empiric use of trimethoprim-sulfamethoxazole (TMP-SMX) in the treatment of women with uncomplicated urinary tract infections in a geographical area with a high prevalence of TMP-SMX resistant uropathogens. *Clin Infect Dis.* 2002;34:1165–1169.

Sheffield JS, Cunningham FG. Urinary tract infection in women. *Obstet Gynecol.* 2005;106:1085–1092.

Warren JW, Abrutyn E, Hebel JR, Johnson JR, Schaeffer AJ, Stamm WE. Guidelines for antimicrobial treatment of uncomplicated acute bacterial cystitis and acute pyelonephritis in women. Infectious Diseases Society of America (IDSA). *Clin Infect Dis.* 1999;29:745–758.

25
Viral Hepatitis: Screening and Vaccination Strategies

M. Gary Brook and David Mutimer

■ INTRODUCTION

Viral hepatitides A–D are extremely important in practicing sexual and reproductive health, not only because each, in varying degrees, is transmitted sexually but also because each causes significant morbidity and mortality in infected people. They are largely preventable and therefore knowing patients' immune or infection status is important.

Viral hepatitis as a sexually transmitted infection (STI) first came to prominence in the 1970s when hepatitis B was found to be especially common in MSM, sex workers, and others. Subsequently types A, C, and D have also been shown to transmit readily through various forms of sexual contact. Since the early 1990s, numerous outbreaks of hepatitis A have been reported in MSM, and recently, acute hepatitis C in MSM, especially in those who are HIV positive. The consequences of these infections, both in health and in economic terms, are substantial, and therefore all healthcare workers should treat them extremely seriously.

■ HEPATITIS A VIRUS

Clinical and Epidemiological Features

This picornavirus is endemic worldwide and the major route of transmission is feco-oral, through food, water, and close personal contact. Parenteral spread has been reported in injecting drug users (IDUs), men with hemophilia using contaminated factor VIII, and other recipients of blood products. These high-risk groups for parenteral exposure have in common a significant prevalence of chronic hepatitis B virus (HBV) and hepatitis C virus (HCV) infection. In patients with chronic hepatitis B or C or any other chronic liver disease, acute HAV infection can cause severe hepatitis leading to fulminant hepatic failure.

The incubation period of hepatitis A virus (HAV) is 2 to 6 weeks. Disease usually starts with a flu-like prodromal illness lasting for up to 2 weeks and then icteric hepatitis, which lasts for a few weeks and rarely longer than 3 months. The disease severity and likelihood of symptoms is very much age related. For instance, only 5–20% of children younger than 5 years old will develop jaundice during acute infection, and HAV-related mortality is rarely seen in this age group. In highly endemic countries, infection typically occurs at a young age and therefore is usually without symptoms. Conversely, adult-acquired infection is much more frequently associated with symptoms that include jaundice (possibly 75–90% of cases), though mortality remains generally low at around 0.3%. Thus, HAV infection is associated with significant morbidity and greater risk of mortality when it occurs in older patients and in those with underlying chronic liver disease.

The World Health Organization recognizes three levels of hepatitis A virus (HAV) prevalence.

High endemicity: developing countries with poor sanitary/hygienic conditions—parts of Africa, Asia, and Central and South America. Infection is mostly in children and therefore usually mild or asymptomatic. Disease incidence may reach 150/100,000 population per year with approximately 1 million cases per year in these areas.

Intermediate endemicity: countries where sanitary conditions are variable—south and east Europe, parts of the Middle East. Many children escape infection; therefore, clinical disease incidence may be high as infection occurs more frequently in adults.

Low endemicity: countries with good sanitary and hygienic conditions—northern and western Europe, Japan, Australia, New Zealand, United States, and Canada. Infection rates are low and disease tends to occur among specific risk groups. Disease incidence of 5–10/100,000/year.

Improved sanitation in many countries has led to a fall in childhood HAV infection with a concomitant rise in adults susceptible to symptomatic disease and outbreaks.

Sexual Transmission

Men who have sex with men are the group for whom there is the best evidence of sexual transmission of HAV, with numerous outbreaks reported. In MSM, risk factors for HAV infection include visits to saunas and "darkrooms," sex with anonymous partners, group sex, oroanal and digital-rectal intercourse, and number of partners. The actual mechanism of sexual transmission remains uncertain but is presumably feco-oral and related to oral, penile, or digital contamination during sex. Reported outbreaks have been in large cities, including Melbourne, New York, London, Amsterdam, and Tokyo. However, most MSM do not acquire HAV infection this way, and there are several studies showing a prevalence of HAV-IgG (an indicator of past infection with hepatitis A) that is no higher in MSM than in heterosexual men attending STI clinics. For these routes of

transmission, condoms are unlikely to prevent infection. There is no evidence for heterosexual spread of HAV. As HAV is largely a childhood infection in many countries, unsurprisingly there is also no evidence for sexual transmission as a significant route of infection in adults in resource-poor countries.

Screening

Two situations in the STI clinic in which screening should be considered are: (1) investigating someone with symptoms suggesting acute hepatitis and (2) testing at-risk asymptomatic patients with a view to recommending vaccination.

Investigation of symptoms: Appropriate biochemical tests for suspected acute viral hepatitis are listed in Table 25-1. Two serological tests for HAV are HAV-IgM and HAV total antibody. In acute infection, the serum IgM anti-HAV antibody becomes positive during the prodromal illness and persists for up to 6 months. Thus, positivity indicates recent infection. The total HAV antibody test becomes positive also within the prodromal illness but persists for many years, and therefore a positive test does not distinguish between acute and past infection. Contacts of known cases (sexual, household, or other close contact) should also be tested. A positive total HAV-antibody test signifies that the person is immune to hepatitis A.

Screening of asymptomatic people: Regarding the STI clinic, screening identifies those at risk by their sexual behavior in order that they may be offered vaccination if

TABLE 25-1 Biochemical Features of Acute Viral Hepatitis

Test	Notes
Serum Amino-transferases (ALT, AST)	Will usually peak at 500–10,000 IU/L within the first 2 weeks. Takes up to 6 months to become normal, except for when chronic hepatitis ensues (for HBV, HDV, or HCV) and the abnormality may persist.
Serum Bilirubin	Can be raised to >100 mcmol/L. The bilirubin is both conjugated and unconjugated with bilirubinuria detectable. Prolonged jaundice with high bilirubin may be seen in patients with the cholestatic variant of hepatitis. Jaundice may persist after transaminases settle.
Serum Alkaline Phosphatase	Usually normal or only mildly raised (<300 IU/L) except in the uncommon cholestatic variant of acute viral hepatitis.
Prothrombin Time	May be slightly prolonged by 1–5 seconds. Prolongation >5 seconds (INR > 1.5) reflects more severe liver damage and identifies patients who may be at risk for developing hepatic failure. These cases should be discussed with a hepatologist.

nonimmune. The 2010 CDC STD Guidelines suggest screening may be cost effective only in populations in which past exposure to HAV (with naturally acquired immunity) is highly prevalent.

Some clinics may choose to screen all MSM men. Others may choose to screen those MSM men at highest risk; that is, those living in areas where HAV in MSM is prevalent and if one or more of the following criteria are met:

- More than two partners within 3 months
- Anonymous partners
- Sex in public venues, such as saunas or "dark rooms"
- Group sex
- Oroanal or digitorectal sex

Given that injecting drug users are also at risk and may attend STI clinics as their only contact with health services, they also should be screened and vaccinated.

The screening test for asymptomatic patients is for serum total HAV antibodies, and a positive result indicates natural immunity with no need for vaccination. If nonimmune patients are vaccinated, then there is no need for subsequent screening. However, if vaccination is contraindicated or may not have worked (for instance, in someone with HIV infection), then those with continuing risk should be asked to return for repeat tests should symptoms suggest acute hepatitis in the future.

Vaccination

Preexposure vaccination: Vaccination is recommended in all nonimmune (total HAV-antibody-negative) persons at risk, which, within the STI clinic setting, would include injecting drug users, at-risk MSM (all MSM in the 2010 CDC STD Guidelines), or those with concurrent chronic liver disease. Others requiring vaccination, but not necessarily in the STI clinic, include people intending to travel to intermediate/high-endemic areas. Some countries have a universal hepatitis A vaccination policy for all citizens. The CDC Advisory Committee on Immunization Practices (ACIP 2006) recommends vaccination for all infants 12–23 months, older children in selected areas, MSM, IDUs, and travelers.

The vaccine is formaldehyde-inactivated hepatitis A virus grown in human diploid cells and is available as a single formulation or combined hepatitis A and B and hepatitis A and typhoid vaccines. All formulations seem to be equally efficacious. They are given intramuscu-

larly into the deltoid (not buttock) or subcutaneously if there is a bleeding disorder. In HIV-negative recipients, 95–100% will respond to a course of vaccine for disease prevention. The commercially available test for serum total HAV antibodies is not sensitive enough to detect vaccine-induced immunity, so vaccine response cannot be confirmed in clinical practice. Successful immunization (as outlined in the schedules that follow) in an adult prevents disease for at least 10 years and current opinion suggests that immunity may be lifelong. Response rates to vaccination in HIV-positive people is reduced and this correlates with the CD4 count, with best response at CD4 counts >500 cells/μL. There is a low rate of mild injection-site reaction and rare transient systemic illness following vaccination and those with allergy to the vaccine or its components should not be vaccinated.

Administration intervals: The initial course is of two doses at 0 and 6–12 months for the monodose vaccine. The combined A plus B vaccine is given at 0, 1, and 6 months or 0, 1, 3 weeks, and 12 months. Manufacturers recommend booster doses after 5 years although it is now widely held that in immune-competent patients boosters are not required.

Practical issues: Given the unreliable attendance by many people using STI clinics, it is best to give the first dose of vaccine at the initial clinic attendance to all those at risk of infection, especially if there is no history of prior vaccination or disease. The serum total HAV antibody test should be measured at the same time, and the vaccination schedule can be continued or not, depending on whether this test subsequently shows the recipient to have been previously infected. Many patients at risk for HAV are also at risk for hepatitis B and so the combined A plus B vaccine would be an appropriate choice. However, if it is felt that the patient may not return for further doses, then monodose HAV and monodose HBV vaccines should be administered, as they contain more antigen and are therefore more likely to be effective after a single dose.

Postexposure prophylaxis: If a nonimmune patient presents within 2 weeks of exposure to a known case of hepatitis A, then disease may be prevented by administering human normal immunoglobulin with known anti-HAV activity (HNIG, 500 mg IM or 0.02 mL/kg in the United States). Commercially available HNIG may no longer be reliably effective against hepatitis A, and advice and supplies should be sought from public health bodies. HNIG use is therefore now usually restricted to those at highest risk of HAV complications such as people who are immunocompromised or pregnant. The hepatitis A vaccine course is normally started at the same time as HNIG or given without HNIG and in its own right offers significant protection. It is unlikely that HNIG or vaccine will offer any immediate protection if given more than 2 weeks after exposure to infection.

■ HEPATITIS B VIRUS

Clinical and Epidemiological Features

Hepatitis B virus (HBV) is an extremely common hepadnavirus worldwide with chronic carriage rates as high as 40% in parts of China. Although vertical (mother-to-infant), child-to-child, and sexual transmission account for most cases (see Table 25-2), other nonsexual routes of spread include horizontal transmission in institutionalized populations, and parenteral exposure such as occurs among injecting drug users.

As with HAV, acute infection of children with HBV is typically asymptomatic. Adult-acquired infection may also be asymptomatic, especially if the person is immunocompromised, such as with HIV infection. Between 50% and 90% of adult-acquired infections present with acute icteric hepatitis, which tends to be more severe than that due to HAV. The incubation period is usually 6 to 12 weeks but can be as long as 6 months. Acute HBV infection also causes fulminant hepatitis and can be followed by chronic hepatitis, liver cirrhosis, and liver cancer. Approximately 1% of those with acute symptomatic infection will develop fulminant liver failure, which has a mortality of at least 50%. More important than the morbidity and mortality associated with HBV in the acute phase is chronic infection that can lead to cirrhosis and liver cancer. Ninety percent of infants, 50% of preschool children, and 5–10% of adults with HBV will become chronically infected following acute infection. For adults with HIV who have primary HBV infection, chronic HBV results in 20–25% of cases. Frequently, chronic infection will persist lifelong. Most chronically infected people acquired infection as infants or in early childhood. For infection acquired at that age, the predicted lifetime mortality attributed to HBV infection is as high as 25%. Typically, death is due to liver failure or liver cancer during the fifth and subsequent decades of life. Approximately 1 million people worldwide die of HBV annually. Liver cancer complicating chronic HBV infection is one of the world's 10 most common cancers.

Sexual transmission: In developed countries, most cases of HBV are transmitted sexually. HBV is efficiently transmitted during heterosexual and male homosexual contact. For instance, the transmission rate from patients with acute or chronic HBV to nonimmune heterosexual

TABLE 25-2 Hepatitis B, C, and D Carriage Worldwide

Hepatitis Type	Prevalence Worldwide	High Prevalence Areas	Major Routes of Transmission
B	2 billion have been infected at some time in their life. 350 million chronic carriers	Africa, Asia, and South America 5–10%. China and Taiwan 10–20% Albania and eastern Europe up to 5%	Mother to infant (vertical) Child to child Sexual
C	170 million carriers	2–5% of the population in many developing countries. 10% in northern China and parts of Africa (highly prevalent in Egypt)	Parenteral: reusable medical equipment, tattooing, traditional scarification and circumcision practices, blood products, injecting drug use
D	10 million carriers	Mediterranean basin, Middle East, Central Asia, West Africa, Amazon basin, and some Pacific Islands. Also now identified in China, Japan, northern India, and Albania	Parenteral: injecting drug users Horizontal, nonsexual, intrafamilial spread (exact mechanism unknown)

partners may be as high as 40%. This is assumed to be via vaginal sex, though oral sex is also a possible route. Studies of selected groups of MSM in the United States and Europe have found evidence of past infection in 50% or more and HBsAg-positivity rates of up to 6%. Transmission of HBV in MSM correlates with duration of sexual activity, number of partners, and oroanal and genitoanal sexual contact. Despite the availability of an effective vaccine, HBV continues to be a significant problem in MSM in developed countries.

Screening

Investigation of symptoms: Appropriate biochemical tests for someone suspected of having acute viral hepatitis are listed in Table 25-1. Serological tests for HBV include IgM anticore antibody (IgM anti-HBc), IgG anticore antibody (anti-HBc), antihepatitis B surface antibody (anti-HBs), hepatitis B surface antigen (HBsAg), hepatitis B "e" antigen (HBeAg), antihepatitis B: "e" antibody (anti-HBe), and serum HBV DNA (a direct measure of serum HBV titer). Various patterns of these tests will be found at different stages of infection (see Table 25-3). Chronic carriers who are HBeAg positive or have and HBV-DNA >10^5 copies/mL are most infectious and most at risk of disease progression to cirrhosis.

Screening of asymptomatic people: The World Health Organization recommends universal vaccination against hepatitis B, but some countries, including the United Kingdom, do not do so. The United States began universal childhood immunization in the mid-1980s, so persons born before that time are susceptible unless they were subsequently vaccinated. In countries without universal vaccination, screening is used to find those who are at risk so that they may be vaccinated if they are nonimmune. In addition to the nonimmune susceptible person, screening can also identify chronic HBV carriers so that they may be investigated for evidence of chronic liver disease that may require antiviral treatment. Also, their contacts can be screened. Depending on local HBV prevalence and policies, some clinics screen all STI clinic attendees. Hepatitis B testing should be especially considered for MSM, sex workers (of either sex), injecting drug users, HIV-positive patients, sexual assault victims, people from countries where hepatitis B is common (i.e., outside of northern Europe, North America, and Australasia), needle-stick victims, and sexual partners of positive or high-risk patients. The 2006 American STD Guidelines also include all patients with more than one sex partner in the last 6 months. The most suitable initial test to identify people who have not had exposure to HBV is the serum anti-HBc antibody (see Figure 25-1), though a positive result does not distinguish natural immunity from the chronic HBV carrier. When the anti-HBc antibody is present, serum HBsAg should be sought (see Figure 25-2). If there is a clear history of previous hepatitis B vaccination, evidence for this can be obtained by testing for anti-HBs antibody. If someone is HBV nonimmune and has not responded to the vaccine, then periodic screening for HBV is recommended if that person is at continuing risk. The frequency of screening depends on the degree of infection risk and may vary from 3 to 12 months.

TABLE 25-3   Hepatitis B Serology

Stage of Infection	Surface Antigen (HBsAg)	"e" Antigen (HBeAg)	IgM Anticore Antibody	IgG Anticore Antibody	Hepatitis B Virus DNA	Anti-HBe	Anti-HBs
Acute (Early)	+	+	+*	+	high	–	–
Acute (Resolving)	+	–	+	+	Low	±	–
Chronic (High Activity)	+	±	–	+	high	±	–
Chronic (Low Activity)	+	–	–	+	Low	+	–
Resolved (immune)	–	–	–	+	–	±	±
Successful Vaccination	–	–	–	–	–	–	+

* In very early infection, the IgM anticore can be negative and so can the IgG.

FIGURE 25-1 Flow Chart for Hepatitis B Screening Using Serum Anti-HBc Antibodies

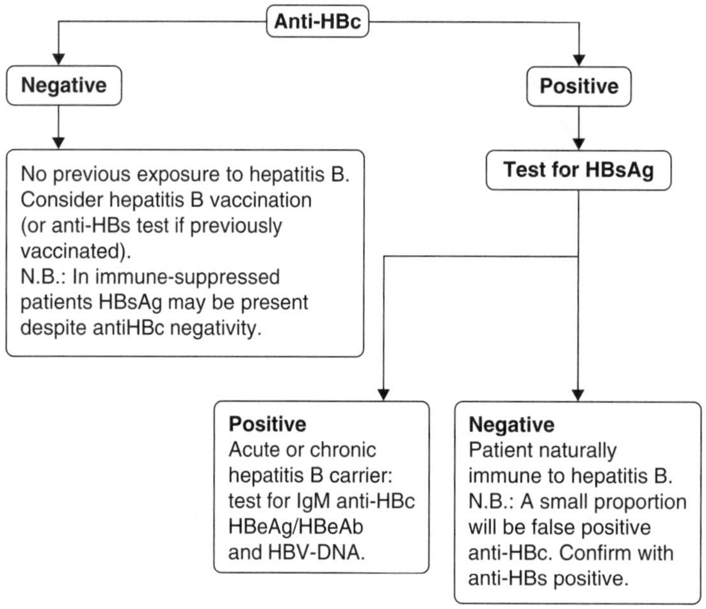

Vaccination

Preexposure vaccination: Vaccination is recommended in all nonimmune (anti-HBc and anti-HBs antibody-negative) persons at risk, (see "Screening of asymptomatic people"). Others requiring vaccination, but not necessarily in the STI clinic, include healthcare workers and people with chronic liver disease. The vaccine is biosynthetic HBV surface antigen made using recombinant technology. There is also a combined hepatitis A and B vaccine. It is administered intramuscularly (IM) into the deltoid (not buttock) or subcutaneously if there is a bleeding disorder. In immune-competent recipients, approximately 90% will respond to a course of vaccine to achieve serum anti-HBs levels >10 IU/L. This rate can be improved by revaccination of nonresponders with up to three more doses and possibly by using a double dose. New vaccines that include additional HBV protein epitopes or novel adjuvants may provide hope for previous vaccine nonresponders. Successful immunization of an adult prevents disease for more than 10 years, and current opinion suggests that immunity may be lifelong. Some people will become infected during this time, but this is mostly transient and subclinical. Response rate to vaccination in HIV-positive people is reduced and this correlates strongly with the CD4 count. Rates of achieving anti-HBs levels >10 IU/L after standard vaccination are about 80% at CD4 count >500 cells/μL and only 25% with counts <200 cells/μL .

There is a low rate of mild injection-site reaction to the vaccine and the main contraindication is known allergy.

Schedule of administration: Initial courses of 0, 1, 6 months or 0, 1, 3 weeks, 12 months show similar efficacy for both the single hepatitis B and combined A and B vaccines and the 0, 1, 2, 12 months schedule for single hepatitis B vaccine. In the United States, 0-, 1-, 4-month and 0-, 2-, 4-month schedules are also licensed. The ultrarapid 0-, 1- ,3-week, 12-month course leads to earlier immunity. Manufacturers recommend booster doses after 5 years although it is now widely held that in immune-competent patients who have responded to the vaccine, boosters are not required.

Practical issues: If the patient's HBV status is unknown, it is safe and practical to start vaccination at the first patient visit, testing HBV serology at the same time. The ultrarapid 0-, 1-, 3-week, 12-month vaccination course is recommended, as adhering to this regimen is likely to be higher. However, even if three doses are spread out over 4 or more years, vaccination is frequently effective. Therefore, if someone fails to return for scheduled doses, the course can be continued years later without the need to administer all three doses again. Serum anti-HBs may be measured 4 to 6 weeks after the third vaccine dose and should be at levels >10 IU/L. After the ultrarapid course, anti-HB antibodies may take longer to develop and so a further test may be taken up to 11 months later or a fourth dose can be

FIGURE 25-2 Flow Chart for Hepatitis B Screening Using Serum HBsAg

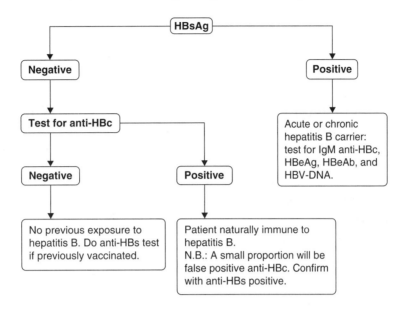

administered immediately if anti-HBs is undetectable. Ten percent of people remain anti-HB negative and should be offered a repeat three doses of vaccine. About 5% will not respond, even to two courses, and should be considered at continuing risk of infection. In the 2010 CDC STD Guidelines, postvaccination serology is only recommended in HIV-positive and other immunocompromised patients or those people who share needles or sex partners who are hepatitis B infected.

Treatment: Chronic hepatitis B is susceptible to treatment either with interferons or with a variety of antiviral agents. Patients considered for treatment include those who are HBeAg+, or have serum HBV-DNA > 10^4 copies/mL if HBeAg. "Cure" in terms of loss of HBeAg can be achieved in up to 30%, and the rest can usually achieve a state of full viral suppression and normalization of liver function if placed on long-term antivirals. Such people should be treated in specialized centers as this is a rapidly evolving field requiring specific management expertise. A benefit of antiviral therapy for patients with acute hepatitis B has not been shown, although it may be considered in severe acute hepatitis B and in cases of acute hepatitis B that are slow to resolve.

■ HEPATITIS D VIRUS

Clinical and Epidemiological Features

Hepatitis D virus (HDV, Delta) is an incomplete RNA virus that requires the hepatitis B virus outer coat. Three main types of epidemiological pattern are (1) endemic

carriage (e.g., Mediterranean basin, indigenous people in parts of South America), (2) areas of mainly parenteral spread (e.g., western Europe, North America), and (3) areas with sudden epidemics (e.g., the Amazon basin or Africa) (Table 25-2). Rarely, vertical (mother-to-infant) spread may also occur.

HDV is only found in patients with hepatitis B and, in many parts of the world is largely an infection of injecting drug users (IDUs) and their sexual partners. It also seen in female sex workers and sporadically in other groups, such as tattoo recipients and prisoners. Acute hepatitis due to HDV, due to concurrent HBV infection, or due to superinfection of a chronically HBV-infected person is associated with a significant risk for fulminant liver failure (which can be as high as to 10%). As well as causing severe acute infection, the liver disease of chronic HBV/HDV coinfection can be rapidly progressive (leading to cirrhosis in as many as 40% within 10 years), and liver cancer develops in cirrhotics at a rate of 10% within 5 years.

Sexual transmission: Several studies have described sexual transmission of HDV in both heterosexual couples and homosexual men. This route appears significant in endemic areas and in relation to sexual partners of IDUs in low-prevalence countries.

Screening

Screening of asymptomatic and symptomatic people: Screening finds those who are infected with HBV and who might also have HDV infection so that they may be investigated with a view to therapy, disease monitoring, and screening of their contacts. Patients to be particularly considered for screening include anyone with parenterally acquired HBV and those with severe acute or chronic HBV-related liver disease. Though HBV infection is a prerequisite for HDV coinfection, HDV appears to suppress HBV replication. Thus, HDV infection should be considered when a patient has severe hepatitis despite low levels of serum HBV-DNA. Diagnosis is confirmed by a positive serum anti-HDV antibody, serum HDV antigen, or HDV-RNA (PCR) test.

Vaccination: There is no HDV vaccine, and therefore, any vaccination strategy is based on the prevention of HBV infection. Since HDV cannot occur without presence of HBV, HBV vaccination is highly effective.

■ HEPATITIS C VIRUS

Clinical and Epidemiological Features

Hepatitis C virus (HCV) is an RNA virus in the flaviviridae (genus *Hepacivirus*) family. It is endemic worldwide with high prevalence rates in Egypt, South and East Asia, and eastern Europe (see Table 25-2).

Parenteral spread accounts for most cases through shared needles/syringes in IDUs, transfusion of blood or blood products (pre-1990s), renal dialysis, needlestick injury, or sharing a razor with an infected individual. Higher rates of infection are also detected in former prisoners, tattoo recipients, and alcoholics. Vertical (mother-to-infant) spread also occurs at a low rate (5% or less in most studies), but higher rates (up to 8%) are seen if the woman is both HIV and HCV positive. Among HCV-positive blood donors, 50% do not admit to an identifiable recognized risk factor.

Jaundice is seldom seen during the acute phase of HCV infection. The incubation period is 4 to 20 weeks. About 80% of acute infections are asymptomatic, and cases of acute icteric hepatitis are clinically indistinguishable from acute hepatitis A or B infections. Fulminant hepatitic failure during the acute phase of HCV infection is rare (<1% of all hepatitis C infections). Fulminant failure may be observed during HAV or HBV infection of an HCV carrier. Following acute HCV infection, 15–25% of patients eradicate infection, and 75–85% of infected patients become chronic carriers. They are normally asymptomatic but may have nonspecific symptoms. Once established, the chronic carrier state rarely resolves without treatment. A proportion of carriers will progress to cirrhosis. HCV-infected people may die of liver failure or liver cancer after decades of infection. More rapid progression to cirrhosis is observed for males, for those who are infected at an older age, and for those with aggravating factors such as alcoholism, chronic HBV infection, or immune deficiency. HIV coinfection is associated with a more rapid progression to cirrhosis.

Sexual transmission: This occurs at a low rate of approximately 0.2–2% per year of a relationship, or 1–11% of spouses in long-term relationships. These rates are increased if the index patient is also HIV infected. There is also an increased rate of carriage (2%) in MSM attending STI clinics, but this is again largely linked to HIV coinfection. In recent years, there have been increasing reports of acute HCV in HIV-positive MSM in developed countries. The exact route of transmission remains to be elucidated but is linked to traumatic anal sex, concurrent ulcerative STIs of the penis or anus, such as syphilis and lymphogranuloma venerum (LGV), and may also include noninjecting recreational drug use, such as cocaine snorting through a shared straw. Increased rates of HCV infection have been reported in female sex workers, and the relative importance of parenteral versus sexual transmission is also unclear.

Screening

Investigation of symptoms: Appropriate biochemical tests for someone suspected to have acute viral hepatitis are listed in Table 25-1. The screening test for hepatitis C is an enzyme-linked immunosorbant assay (ELISA) (see Figure 25-3). Serum HCV RNA detection confirms a positive ELISA result. The antibody test may take 3 or more months to become positive after someone is exposed to HCV, and therefore, in early infection, it may be necessary to check for HCV RNA to refute recently acquired infection.

Screening of asymptomatic people: Screening is performed to identify those patients who are chronically infected so that they may be treated and their partners counseled. The screening algorithm is described in Figure 25-3. The main targets for HCV screening would be injecting drug users and their sexual partners, recipients of potentially untested blood or blood products, needle-stick victims, men who have sex with men, sex workers, ex-prisoners, HIV-positive people, tattoo recipients, partners of known HCV-positive people, and anyone with unexplained abnormal liver function tests. If negative, and if the patient has ongoing risk for HCV exposure, the HCV screening test should be repeated at intervals (according to risk which may be every 3 to 12 months).

FIGURE 25-3 Flow Chart for Hepatitis C Testing Using an Antibody Assay

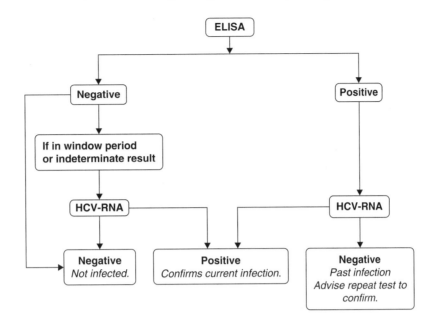

Vaccination and Postexposure Prophylaxis

There is no vaccine against HCV nor is there any suitable antibody preparation for postexposure. All HCV-infected people should be vaccinated against HAV and HBV if they are nonimmune, as acute superinfection may be clinically severe for those with chronic HCV.

Treatment: In the minority of patients who are identified during acute hepatitis C, the majority can be cured with pegylated interferon treatment, with the addition of ribavirin if they are also HIV+. Additional therapies are becoming available and are beyond the scope of this chapter. Cure of chronic hepatitis C (loss of HCV-RNA) is also achievable with pegylated interferon/ribavirin given for 6–12 months. Success can be as high as 90% in HIV-negative people with low HCV viral load and particular viral genotypes (2 or 3). Sustained virological response will be lower if the HCV viral load is high, if the genotype is 1 or 4 or if the patient is HIV positive. Such people should be treated in specialized centers as this is a rapidly evolving field requiring specific management expertise.

▪ KEY POINTS

- Hepatitis B is the most readily sexually transmitted viral hepatitis in both heterosexual men and women and men who have sex with men (MSM).

- Hepatitis C can be sexually transmitted in both heterosexual men and women and MSM but spread is inefficient and uncommon except in HIV-positive people.

- Hepatitis A is sexually transmitted only between MSM.

- Hepatitis A and B are vaccine-preventable infections, and these vaccines should be offered to all nonimmune patients at risk.

- Hepatitis C is not vaccine preventable. Prevention strategies include condom use and safe injecting practices.

- Hepatitis A and B vaccines are protective after a single course of injections in more than 90% of immunocompetent vaccinees. Protection lasts at least 10 years and may be lifelong.

- HIV-positive people are more susceptible to acquisition and chronic carriage of viral hepatitis and respond to vaccine less well.

- Screening for evidence of previous exposure to hepatitis B should be considered in all sexually transmitted infection clinic attenders, and groups to be screened for hepatitis A and C should include MSM and injecting drug users.

REFERENCES

Brook MG. Sexually transmitted hepatitis. *Sex Transm Infect.* 2002;4:235–40.

Brook MG, Nelson M, Bhagani S. On behalf of the Clinical Effectiveness Group (British Association of Sexual Health and HIV). Management of viral hepatitides A, B and C, 2008. http://www.bashh.org/guidelines/ceguidelines.htm.

Centers for Disease Control and Prevention. Recommendations and guidelines. Advisory Committee on Immunization Practices (ACIP). http://www.cdc.gov/vaccines/recs/acip/.

Centers for Disease Control and Prevention. Sexually transmitted diseases treatment guidelines, 2010. *MMWR.* 2010;59(RR-12):78–86.

Department of Health. Immunisation against infectious disease—"The Green Book," 2006. http://www.dh.gov.uk/en/Policyandguidance/Healthandsocialcaretopics/Greenbook/DH_4097254.

Fiore AE, Wasley A, Bell BP, Centers for Disease Control and Prevention. Prevention of hepatitis A through active or passive immunization. Recommendations of the Advisory Committee on Immunization Practices (ACIP). http://www.cdc.gov/mmwr/preview/mmwrhtml/rr5507a1.htm. *MMWR.* 2006;55(RR07):1–23.

26

Vulvar Pain and Vulvodynia

Sarah Edwards

INTRODUCTION

Vulvar pain is a common presentation both in the community and in sexual health settings and can be attributed to a variety of conditions (see Table 26-1). Although sexually transmitted infections (STIs) are clearly in the differential diagnosis, many cases are caused by noninfectious etiologies. Vulvar pain causes significant psychosexual problems and poor sexual function. Because of the associated stigma, most authorities believe that the syndrome is substantially underreported and diagnosed. For example, a study of female attendees at a sexual health clinic showed an incidence of vulvar pain of 13.3%, where symptoms were predominantly caused by infective conditions (mainly candidiasis and genital herpes) (Denbow and Byrne 1998). However, many women have significant symptoms in the absence of either infection or a dermatosis, and these have been categorized as vulvodynia.

The International Society for the Study of Vulvovaginal Disease divides vulvar pain into cases related to a specific disorder and vulvodynia. Vulvodynia has been defined as vulvar discomfort in the absence of gross anatomic or neurologic findings and is subdivided dependent on whether it is generalized or localized and whether it is provoked, unprovoked, or mixed.

VULVODYNIA

Vulvodynia has been described for more than a century but continues to cause significant morbidity among women of reproductive age and beyond. It was originally thought that the problem was more common in Caucasian women, but a recent study in the United States found that, in a survey of 4915 women, 7% had chronic unexplained vulvar pain, and that there was no difference in prevalence between white and African American women (Harlow and Stewart 2003). Similar rates of symptoms have been found in both English and Scandinavian studies. About 40% of women with such symptoms seek medical advice, and many see several clinicians before receiving a formal diagnosis.

The International Society for the Study of Vulval Disease has classified the conditions based on the history and findings on clinical examination (Moyal-Barracco and Lynch 2004). Two conditions of importance are provoked vestibulodynia (previously known as vulval vestibulitis) and generalized vulvodynia. Despite an agreed classification, little systematic research has been conducted. The effectiveness of most treatment modalities have been reported only in small and uncontrolled case series.

PROVOKED VESTIBULODYNIA

Although Skene described the symptom complex we now know as vestibulodynia in 1888, the syndrome was further described and named by Friedrich in 1987 (Friedrich 1987).

The triad of cardinal features are as follows:

1. Severe pain on vulvar vestibular touch or at penetration during intercourse

2. Vestibular erythema

3. Associated point tenderness in the absence of an underlying dermatosis

TABLE 26-1   Causes of Vulvar Pain

Infective	Inflammatory	Other	Vulvodynia
Candidiasis	Lichen planus	Neoplastic (e.g., Paget's disease, Squamous cell carcinoma)	Generalized
Genital herpes	Lichen sclerosus	Neurologic (e.g., Herpes neuralgia)	Localized: Vestibulodynia
Chancroid	Pemphigus		
Trichomoniasis	Pemphigoid		
Group A streptococcus	Infected eczema		
Vulval herpes zoster	Psoriasis		
	Behçet's syndrome		
	Stevens–Johnson syndrome		
	Major aphthous disease		
	Crohn's disease		
	Acrodermatitis enteropathica		
	Vulval fragility		

This condition is predominantly found in women of reproductive age and peaks in the 20- to 30-year age group. It accounted for 1.3% of unselected female genitourinary clinic attendees in one study and accounts for up to 10% of patients with vulval pain. It can be split into primary and secondary, depending on whether the pain was present from first attempted vaginal penetration or whether sexual intercourse had previously been achieved without discomfort. Severity also varies and may be sufficient to prevent any sexual intercourse. Evidence from small trials of treatment suggests that symptoms may resolve spontaneously, although this appears less likely in primary cases, but long-term prospective studies are lacking.

The etiology is unknown and is likely to be multifactorial. Many patients give a previous history of vulvovaginal candidiasis but may also wrongly attribute the symptoms of vestibulitis to ongoing infection. A variety of other infections, including *Neisseria gonorrhoeae*, *Gardnerella vaginalis*, herpes simplex, and cytomegalovirus, have been postulated as triggers, but no association has been found. Human papillomavirus (HPV) has been extensively investigated as a possible cause with some conflicting results, but no causal link has been proven. A history of sensitivity to topical preparations, such as anticandidal creams, soaps, and other hygiene products, is quite frequent, although studies have failed to show true contact sensitivity and may reflect a low-grade irritant reaction. Other associations include early use of the contraceptive pill, early coitarche (15 years or younger), and the development of vestibulitis following laser or 5 fluorouracil treatment for vulval warts.

Biopsy-based histological studies are generally not helpful and tend to show a nonspecific inflammatory infiltrate, which has also been demonstrated in normal controls. No fungal or viral elements are identified in these cases. More recent studies suggest some nerve fiber proliferation and a close association with serotonin-producing neuroendocrine cells. Pain perception has been shown to be increased both locally and distally in women with vulval vestibulitis.

Psychological studies show significant sexual dysfunction but disagree on whether this is an underlying phenomenon or a reaction to the chronic pain syndrome.

Diagnosis

Diagnosis is made on clinical grounds based on the patient's history and associated examination findings. There should be a history of severe pain on vulvar vestibular touch or at penetration during intercourse, vestibular erythema, and associated point tenderness in the absence of an underlying dermatosis. On clinical examination, the vulvar erythema and point tenderness is usually located at 5 o'clock and 7 o'clock on the vestibule toward the hymenal ring, where it can be easily overlooked by clinicians who are unaware of the disorder (see Figure 26-1).

FIGURE 26-1 Clinical Findings in Vestibulitis

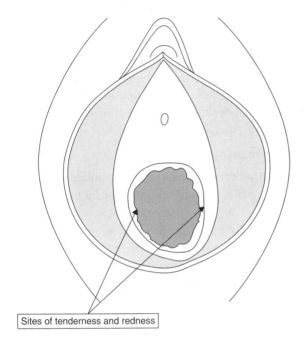

Sites of tenderness and redness

Management

At the initial evaluation, screening for genital infection should be undertaken, as a firm diagnosis is difficult in the presence of coexistent conditions. Screening should include testing for *Neisseria gonorrhoeae, Chlamydia trachomatis,* herpes simplex, trichomonas, and vulvovaginal cultures for candida and bacterial pathogens. Empirically, treatment of infections such as candidiasis, bacterial vaginosis, or streptococcal infection may improve symptoms.

Initial management should include a clear explanation of the condition and reassurance, particularly as many women will have seen several physicians before a formal diagnosis is reached. The discussion should cover the natural history of the condition, that vestibulodynia is well recognized and common (patients can also feel isolated as they are unaware that others have similar problems), and an overview of treatment options.

In mild cases, a thorough explanation may enable the individual to cope with the symptoms, but symptomatic, medical, and surgical treatments can be offered.

Symptomatic Management

General skin care advice, including avoiding irritants and using aqueous cream for genital washing, may be soothing, especially in patients who give a history of sensitivity to topical applications (although many will already have adopted these strategies). Using lubricants

during sexual intercourse will alleviate discomfort in milder cases. In addition, topical local anesthetic agents (e.g., lidocaine gel) can be used for symptomatic relief—these need to be applied 30 minutes before intercourse to take effect and can be applied digitally or by on a tampon. Some women may find regular use of topical local anesthetic agents may reduce sensitivity, but there is a small risk of sensitization to the active component.

Medical Management

There is a paucity of trials for any treatment modality. Treatment agents can be split into local and systemic therapy.

Local application of steroids either alone or in combination with other agents (antifungals or antimicrobials) have been reported to be helpful in small series, but this may reflect treatment of an additional inflammatory component. Intralesional injections of steroids have also shown some improvement. The application of local anesthetic (lidocaine 5%) has been used both regularly and for symptomatic relief with intercourse. More recently, injecting botulinum toxin has shown some promise, as vulvar pain may be associated with pelvic floor hypertonicity.

The current systemic pharmacotherapeutic approaches are similar to those used for peripheral neuropathy. First-line drugs include the tricyclic antidepressants and gabapentin. Tricyclic antidepressant, usually amitriptyline, can be initiated in low doses for its effect on pain. The starting dose of 10 mg each night may be increased gradually, depending on response and side effects. The optimum rate of increase and maximum dose have not been identified because of the lack of formal trials, but dose increments should be implemented at least 1 week apart. Some improvement will be seen in most cases, but the dose may be limited by side effects, especially drowsiness and mucosal membrane dryness. Given the increase in pain perception found in some studies, patients intolerant of amitriptyline have also tried other medications for neuralgic pain (e.g., carbamazepine, gabapentin). The only reported study of carbamazepine showed little benefit, and there is little published evidence relating to gabapentin. Gabapentin (and pregabalin) have become widely used in recent years, and the former has been used at escalating doses starting at 100 mg three times daily, up to 600 mg three times per day.

Surgical Management

Perineoplasty, vestibulectomy, and local excision have all been tried, with some effect. Of these options, vestibulectomy (or modified perienoplasty) appears to be the most effective, but a substantial proportion of patients (up to 50%) continue to have symptoms after the procedure, and therefore it should be avoided in most cases. Local ablative therapy (e.g., laser treatment) have also been tried with some response. These approaches should be reserved for the most severe cases and administered in consultation with a gynecological expert who has particular experience and expertise in this area.

Physical and Behavioral

Some women will benefit from psychosexual counseling and behavioral techniques, while good results were obtained in a study of pelvic floor electromyographic biofeedback. Repeated contraction/relaxation of the pelvic floor muscles is used with the aim of decreasing hypertonicity. Cognitive behavioral therapy has also shown improvements in pain scores, and although pain reduction with these therapies may not be as great as for some surgical interventions, there may be more lasting improvements in psychosexual function.

Other

Acupuncture and hypnotherapy also have been tried with success in small trials (Landry et al. 2008; Rogstad 2000; Neill and Ridley 1999).

■ GENERALIZED VULVODYNIA

Generalized vulvodynia (previously known as dysesthetic vulvodynia) differs from vestibulodynia in that the pain is usually unprovoked, although it may be exacerbated by touch. The pain is dull and burning sometimes with exacerbations of sharp pain. An older patient population (often postmenopausal) tend to be affected and is less likely to complain of an initiating event than patients with vestibulodynia, although the condition may develop following an inflammatory condition (Neill and Ridley 1999). Vestibulodynia patients can develop an element of unprovoked discomfort and a mixed picture of provoked and constant pain is common (Edwards 2004).

Diagnosis

The diagnosis is made on clinical grounds and depends on a characteristic history with normal vulval examination. Candidiasis and other bacterial infections should be excluded, although screening for other sexually transmitted infections may not be required, depending on the patient's risk status. Patients should usually indicate

areas of burning discomfort over the introital and labial area, with the absence of any skin lesions. There may or may not be associated allodynia (provoked pain on light touch). In patients developing constant burning pain who have coexisting inflammatory skin conditions, generalized vulvodynia may be suspected if any discomfort changes or fails to be controlled, despite clinical improvement of the underlying dermatosis.

Management

There are no specific investigations required (and screening for sexually transmitted infections is only indicated if the history suggests risk behavior, given that the condition is usually found in the older age group) although it may be advisable to take a vulval swab to rule out candidal infection. An association with sacral meningeal cysts was found in one small observational study, and although these data have not been reproduced by others, an MRI may be appropriate (particularly if the patient complains of low back pain).

Although patients with vulvodynia are less likely to complain of sensitivity to topical preparations, general skin care advice and soothing agents, such as emollients, are appropriate. Some patients may gain relief from topical local anesthetic agents, such as lidocaine; however, benefit is less marked than in patients with vestibulodynia, and as the pain is constant rather than situational (e.g., with sexual intercourse), results tend to be poorer. Unlike vestibulodynia, there is no role for surgical intervention.

Medical Management

The mainstay of management is the same as for other chronic pain syndromes. Low-dose tricyclic antidepressants, such as amitriptyline tend to be effective if the patient can tolerate side effects (McKay 1993). The regimen is the same as for vestibulodynia (10 mg each night, increasing gradually, depending on response and side effects) but usually has greater efficacy. The optimum dose is uncertain because of the lack of controlled trials, but a maximum of 50 mg seems to be effective. Other tricyclic antidepressants such as nortryptiline may be used if sedation is a problem. Carbamazepine and other anticonvulsants have been used in other pain syndromes, but there is little literature to support their use in vulvodynia. Gabapentin (and pregabalin) have become widely used in recent years although current evidence only extends to a small number of case reports supporting its efficacy, and the former has been used at escalating doses, starting at 100 mg three times daily up, to 600 mg three times per day.

Other Therapies

There is little published evidence on the treatment of vulvodynia. Biofeedback (electromyography) can be useful ion this condition, and if there is increased muscle tone or instability of pelvic floor muscles, specific exercises may be valuable. Other modalities that have been tried include acupuncture, regional nerve blocks, topical capsaicin, transdermal electrical nerve stimulation (TENS), and laser. Other work has looked at the psychological aspects of the condition and has found that women with vulvodynia have more psychiatric morbidity than controls, but this may be due to the effects of the condition on sexual functioning and the presence of chronic pain. Awareness of the psychological aspects of the condition and appropriate support may enable women to mange symptoms and improve functioning (Haefner et al. 2005; Neill and Ridley 1999).

▮ SUMMARY

Vulvodynia is a common and often underrecognized condition. Although there are few randomized controlled trials, significant improvement can be achieved using pain modifiers (such as amitriptyline), local anesthetic agents, and physical and behavioral therapies. Improvements in psychosexual function can occur even with incomplete resolution of the vulvar pain.

REFERENCES

Denbow MC, Byrne MA. Prevalence, causes, and outcome of vulval pain in a genitourinary medicine clinic population. *Int J STD AIDS*. 1998;9:88–91.

Edwards L. Subsets of vulvodynia: overlapping characteristics. *J Reprod Med*. 2004;49(11):883–837.

Friedrich EG. Vulvar vestibulitis syndrome. *J Reprod Med*. 1987; 32:110–114.

Haefner HK, Collins ME, Davis GD, et al. The vulvodynia guideline. *J Low Genit Tract Dis*. 2005;9(1):40–51.

Harlow BL, Stewart EG. A population-based assessment of chronic unexplained vulvar pain: have we underestimated the prevalence of vulvodynia? *J Am Med Womens Assoc*. 2003;58(2):82–88.

Landry T, Bergeron S, Binik YM, et al. The treatment of provoked vestobulodynia: a critical review. *Clin J Pain*. 2008; 24(2):27–42, 155–171.

McKay M. Dysesthetic ("essential") vulvodynia: treatment with amitriptyline. *J Reprod Med*. 1993;38:9–13.

Moyal-Barracco M, Lynch PJ. 2003 ISSVD terminology and classification of vulvodynia: a historical perspective. *J Reprod Med*. 2004;49(10):772–777.

Neill SM, Ridley CM, eds. Vulvodynia. *The Vulva*. 2nd ed. London: Blackwell Science; 1999.

Rogstad KE. Vulvar vestibulitis: aetiology, diagnosis and treatment. *Int J STD AIDS*. 2000;11:557–562.

27

Prostatitis and Chronic Pelvic Pain

Graz Luzzi and Lamont Law

◼ INTRODUCTION

Infections of the prostate gland were described more than a century ago. Later, in the first half of the twentieth century, clinicians recognized prostatitis as a disease entity distinct from other conditions affecting the prostate, and techniques to confirm prostatic infection by localization studies were developed. Whereas acute infections of the prostate, including prostatic abscess, were uncontroversial entities, whether a true state of chronic bacterial infection of the prostate existed was debated into the 1950s. In the 1960s and 1970s, the advent of the localization technique pioneered by Meares and Stamey (the four-glass test) and their subsequent proposed classification of prostatitis, stimulated three decades of clinical and research interest in a new era for prostatitis syndromes. Critical appraisal of the four-glass test in the context of evidence-based medicine and the development of modern imaging techniques and molecular diagnostics have essentially confined this diagnostic approach to history. An international consensus in 1995, leading to new nomenclature and definitions for the prostatitis syndromes, formed the basis for a renewed understanding of this group of conditions in the modern era.

◼ NOMENCLATURE AND CLASSIFICATION

The broad term *prostatitis* historically has been loosely applied to encompass a collection of clinical syndromes, including acute and chronic infections of the prostate and much more common problem of chronic genital and pelvic pain in adult males. The 1978 classification included acute and chronic bacterial prostatitis, chronic nonbacterial prostatitis (inflammation of the prostate without evidence of infection), and prostatodynia (no evidence of inflammation or infection). The three chronic categories were based on the results of the Meares-Stamey four-glass test.

This classification was revised and updated in 1995 (see Table 27-1). The terms *chronic nonbacterial prostatitis* and *prostatodynia* were replaced by one category, *chronic pelvic pain syndrome* (CPPS), and a new diagnostic category of asymptomatic inflammatory prostatitis was introduced.

Although the new classification identifies inflammatory and noninflammatory subcategories of CPPS, based on the four-glass test or other evidence of inflammation (such as leucocytes in semen), this distinction does not seem to have any clinical value. The symptomatology of each subcategory is identical, and evidence now suggests that they reflect a single condition with the same pathophysiological basis.

◼ DEFINITIONS

In the past, the potential for confusion arose because of (1) lack of agreed definitions for the prostatitis syndromes, (2) research papers that often did not include even an attempt at defining chronic prostatitis, and (3) reliance on the poorly validated four-glass test in diagnosing chronic bacterial prostatitis (leading to the diagnosis of CBP [chronic bacterial prostatis] in men who in fact had CPPS, because bacteria, of unlikely significance, were identified in the expressed prostatic secretions).

TABLE 27-1   NIH Classification of Prostatitis Syndromes[a]

Category

I   Acute bacterial prostatitis

II   Chronic bacterial prostatitis

III   Chronic pelvic pain syndrome

    IIIA   Inflammatory[b] (formerly chronic nonbacterial prostatitis)

    IIIB   Noninflammatory[c] (formerly prostatodynia)

IV   Asymptomatic inflammatory prostatitis[b]

[a]US National Institutes of Health 1995.

[b]Leucocytes detected in expressed prostatic secretions (EPS), or urine after prostatic massage urine, or semen.

[c]Leucocytes not found in EPS, or urine after prostatic massage urine, or semen.

The major categories form distinctive syndromes.

I. *Acute prostatitis* denotes acute infection of the prostate (usually bacterial).

II. *Chronic bacterial prostatitis* denotes persistent bacterial infection of the prostatic parenchyma, causing recurrent urinary tract infection (UTI).

III. *Chronic pelvic pain syndrome* causes genital or pelvic pain in adult males, lasting more than 3 months and is diagnosed when other conditions, in particular infections and neoplasms of the urogenital tract, have been excluded.

ACUTE PROSTATITIS

The incidence of acute prostatitis is unknown; however, it is a rare but well recognized complication of UTI and occasionally follows invasive procedures. The cause is usually bacterial, and the range of organisms is similar to UTI, that is, predominantly (85% or so) uropathogens of the genus *Enterobacteriaceae*, and mostly *E. coli*. However, a broad range of bacteria have been implicated, including gram-positive cocci such as *Staphylococcus aureus*. In immunosuppressed men, invasive fungal pathogens may cause acute prostatitis. The range of organisms that can cause acute prostatitis is given in Table 27-2.

Among sexually transmitted infections (STIs), prostatitis caused by *Neisseria gonorrhoeae* has a particular significance, especially in younger men. However, it is now rarely seen in developed countries.

The pathogenesis of acute prostatitis is that of acute bacterial infection of the prostatic parenchyma usually from infected urine (i.e., UTI) via the prostatic ducts. This may arise following urinary tract instrumentation,

especially when UTI is present. Infection may be introduced during invasive procedures such as prostatic biopsy. Rarely, prostatic infection may arise from blood-borne infection during a bacteremic illness.

Acute prostatitis causes a distinctive clinical syndrome of abrupt onset. Typically, the history is a few days in duration; the patient develops symptoms suggesting severe UTI (frequency, urgency, dysuria) with systemic disturbance (fever, rigors, prostration) and, in addition, symptoms suggesting prostatic involvement (perineal pain and obstructive urinary symptoms). A gentle rectal examination usually reveals a tender, swollen prostate. The responsible organism is generally cultured from urine without difficulty if urine samples are obtained before starting antibiotics, and blood cultures may be positive. Following recovery, the urinary tract should be investigated by imaging as is usual following UTI in adult males.

Patients with acute prostatitis may be sufficiently ill to require hospital admission for intravenous antibiotic therapy. Until the sensitivities of the relevant organism are known, treatment should be with broad-spectrum antibiotics appropriate to cover complicated UTI. After a few days, a switch to oral antibiotics is based on antimicrobial sensitivities. In particular, in areas where quinolone resistance is commonly seen in uropathogens, we would recommend that careful susceptibility testing be done (see Chapter 24). Treatment is conventionally prolonged to complete at least 3 weeks of therapy, but this is not based on controlled trials.

Acute urinary obstruction is a recognized complication of acute prostatitis that requires urinary catheterization by the suprapubic route to avoid damage to the swollen prostate by attempted urethral catheterization. *Prostatic abscess* may arise as a complication of acute prostatitis and

TABLE 27-2   Infections of the Prostate

Syndrome	Organisms
Acute Bacterial Prostatitis	*E. coli* (60–65%)
	Pseudomonas aeruginosa
	Proteus spp.
	Klebsiella spp.
	Enterobacter spp.
	Serratia spp.
	Enterococci; other streptococci
	Staphylococcus aureus
	Neisseria gonorrhoeae
	Anaerobes, e.g., *Bacteroides*
	Other (very rare)[a]
Chronic Bacterial Prostatitis[a]	See text
Fungal Prostatitis[b]	*Candida* spp.
	Cryptococcus neoformans
	Aspergillus
	Coccidioidomycosis
Granulomatous Prostatitis[c]	*Mycobacterium tuberculosis* (TB)
	Intravesical BCG therapy[d]
Other[e]	Trichomonas vaginalis

[a]Isolated case reports (prostatic abscess): *Brucella, Rhodococcus equi*; chronic infection: *Burkholderia pseudomallei.*
[b]Usually immunosuppressed patients.
[c]TB, BCG, and fungal infections are among the causes of granulomatous prostatitis, which is frequently an idiopathic condition.
[d]Bacillus Calmette-Guerin.
[e]Causal relationship not certain.

may be a presenting feature. CT scan and MRI are suitable imaging modalities for suspected abscess. Drainage of confirmed abscess by the transurethral route is generally recommended. Although granulomatous prostatitis and chronic bacterial prostatitis are described in the literature as occasional complications of acute prostatitis, the incidence of these complications is unknown.

▆ CHRONIC BACTERIAL PROSTATITIS

The medical literature on chronic bacterial prostatitis is confusing because of unclear and varying definitions. It is best regarded as a condition typified by recurrent UTI caused by the same organism, related to persistent prostatic infection. In between UTIs, patients are usu-

ally symptomless. However, many authors have defined CBP on the basis of the four-glass test and have therefore inadvertently included patients with CPPS, rather than true CBP, in their studies.

In adult men with recurrent UTIs caused by the same organism (usually, the organism demonstrates the same antibiotic sensitivities during relapses) and in whom urinary tract imaging (by ultrasound or urography) does not demonstrate a structural basis for recurrent UTI, the most likely diagnosis is CBP. This is a rare condition, whose precise incidence is unknown. However, anecdotally, CBP has become less common in recent years, possibly because of widespread use of quinolone antibiotics.

The pathogenesis of CBP includes abnormalities of the prostatic parenchyma that are associated with chronic bacterial infection, notably disrupted architecture with scarring and microabscess formation. In addition, calcifications (including prostatic calculi) may form the basis for bacterial persistence. Chronic infection may follow an initial UTI, and CBP can arise following surgery or instrumentation of the prostate.

The value of the four-glass test in confirming the diagnosis of CBP is unknown. In the authors' experience, the four-glass test often fails to identify the organism that is repeatedly cultured during symptomatic episodes.

In the treatment of CBP, co-trimoxazole (trimethoprim-sulfamethoxazole) was used traditionally, with poor results (anecdotally, 40% cure rates). Penetration of the sulfamethoxazole component of co-trimoxazole into the prostatic parenchyma was known to be poor. The advent of quinolone antibiotics (such as ciprofloxacin) made a great impact on therapy of CBP—a number of small controlled trials reported cure rates of 70% or so after 1 month of quinolone treatment. Nonresponders are a challenge because of lack of evidence from controlled trials. Such patients should generally be managed by urologists with an interest in prostatic infection; options include more prolonged therapy (using an antibiotic guided by antibiotic sensitivity results and with good tissue penetration) and continuous low-dose antibiotic treatment. Structural factors that may require a combined surgical/medical approach to therapy should be excluded. Treatment regimens of 6 weeks to 3 months are not uncommon. Urologic consultation should be obtained in recurrent disease.

CHRONIC PELVIC PAIN SYNDROME

Among the prostatitis syndromes, CPPS is by far the commonest category, which regularly presents to primary care physicians, urologists, and STI clinics. It encompasses the conditions formally called chronic nonbacterial (or abacterial) prostatitis and prostatodynia. In general, published case series from prostatitis clinics indicate that CPPS form more than 95% of attenders. The National Ambulatory Medical Care (NAMC) survey in the United States reported that chronic prostatitis (i.e., what we would now call CPPS) was the commonest urological diagnosis among men aged younger than 55 years in the 1990s. More recently, a number of population surveys have suggested that CPPS is a common condition affecting 2–10% of otherwise healthy males.

Clinical Features

CPPS typically presents with perineal or penile tip pain, lasting more than 3 months. The pain may be more widely distributed and may affect the scrotum, upper inner thighs, and retropubic regions. Associated features include urinary symptoms, typically mild or moderate in severity, for instance, frequency and reduced or variable urine flow. Sexual dysfunction, including ejaculatory pain, erectile dysfunction, and occasionally hematospermia, may also be associated features. There is a wide spectrum of pain severity; some men are very disabled by severe chronic or relapsing symptoms.

Etiology/Pathogenesis

CPPS remains an enigmatic condition for which the etiology remains unknown, and information on pathogenesis is limited. The research literature presents a somewhat confusing picture on the role of infections in the causation of CPPS, and some investigators have reported a role for chlamydia or ureaplasma. Recent studies using molecular methods do not support a significant role for these organisms. These studies identified DNA sequences of a number of unusual, nonculturable, organisms in the prostates of men with CPPS. However, similar findings were detected in a proportion of symptomless males, and their significance therefore remains unknown. Infections, including chlamydia, may sometimes form the triggering event that initiates CPPS (see Figure 27-1), but this has not been studied systematically.

Urodynamic studies have demonstrated mechanical disturbances (tension or spasm) of the bladder neck and pelvic floor mechanism that point to a neuromuscular basis for CPPS and form the rationale for alpha-blockers in therapy. In addition, an inflammatory response is a feature of the pathogenesis—recent studies have shown elevations of proinflammatory cytokines, such as interleukin (IL)-1beta and IL-8, in the genital tract (EPS

FIGURE 27-1 Conceptual Model for Chronic Pain Syndrome

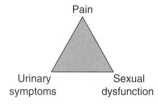

and semen) of men with CPPS. The factors driving this inflammatory process remain unknown. The possibility of an autoimmune process is being studied, and a neural mechanism for inflammation (causing neurogenic pain) has been proposed.

Investigation

CPPS is a clinical diagnosis, based on typical clinical features and the exclusion of other diagnoses. In practice, the syndrome is not difficult to identify, and an exhaustive search for alternative diagnoses is not required. The urine should be tested to exclude UTI. In sexually active males with features atypical for CPPS or urethral or testicular symptoms, testing for chlamydia (and where indicated *N. gonorrhoeae*) should be done by PCR or other nucleic acid amplification method. In the further workup of men with CPPS, the evidence does not support routine use of imaging the urinary tract or prostate, semen analysis or culture, PSA testing, or cystourethroscopy.

The Four-Glass Test

Historically, the four-glass localization study was used to investigate and categorize men presenting with chronic prostatitis symptoms. The technique involves collecting urine samples before and after prostatic massage (first-void, midstream, and postmassage urines) and expressed prostatic secretions (EPS). The samples are examined by microscopy for leucocytes and cultured using quantitative bacteriological techniques. In theory, this allows diagnostic classification into CBP, inflammatory CPPS (formerly CNBP), or noninflammatory CPPS (formerly prostatodynia). However, the four-glass test has the following problems:

1. The test has not been evaluated against an independent standard, so its sensitivity, specificity, and predictive values are unknown, both for CBP and CPPS.

2. Although historically the finding of leucocytes in the EPS was considered significant in men with relevant symptoms, more recently it has been shown that leucocytes are present in the EPS of a large proportion of healthy, symptomless adult males. Therefore, this finding may have no clinical significance.

3. The presence of bacteria or white cells in the EPS does not correlate with the presence or severity of symptoms.

4. The distinction between inflammatory and noninflammatory CPPS has no clinical relevance.

5. Cytokine elevations (for instance, IL-8 in EPS or semen) have been demonstrated in CPPS regardless of whether leucocytes are visible in the EPS.

For more than a decade, some experts have argued that the four-glass test should be confined to research contexts. Surveys in the 1990s showed that urologists in the United States did not generally employ the test. On the basis of current evidence, we recommend that the four-glass test is confined to research studies in which the test is evaluated. This principle also applies to variations of the test, such as the two-glass version in which only the pre- and postprostatic massage urine samples are examined.

Management

The range of options described in the medical literature for treating chronic prostatitis/CPPS is extensive. However, interpreting studies is hampered by the lack of a uniform definition, and study design and methodologies have often been of poor quality. A systematic review for the Cochrane database in 2000 demonstrated the lack of high-quality evidence for diagnosing and treating CPPS and concluded that no diagnostic test had been properly validated, and no therapeutic approach could be recommended on the basis of evidence from randomized trials. Over the subsequent five years, evidence from a number of well-designed, if small, randomized trials suggested that alpha-blockade may be beneficial in a proportion of men with CPPS. However, a recent large randomized trial in the United States demonstrated that long-standing CPPS is usually unresponsive to treatment with alpha-blockers.

A lack of effective treatment for this condition remains. The current clinical approach is based on general measures that may help anecdotally and specific therapy that is based on a mixture of observational evidence and limited evidence from randomized trials. Established or commonly used treatment approaches are listed in Table 27-3. The search for effective therapy for CPPS continues, and a number of investigational treatments are being studied (see Table 27-4).

The distressed patient with severe, unremitting chronic pelvic pain syndrome remains an all-too-frequent challenge for primary care physicians and genitourinary clinicians today. CPPS is similar to chronic somatoform disorders, and it is likely that a complex interaction of somatic, psychological, and social factors interact to promote persistence of the problem.

For some decades, researchers have investigated the association between chronic prostatitis (more recently CPPS) and the role of personality and psychological

TABLE 27-3   Management of Chronic Pelvic Pain Syndrome

Commonly Tried Therapies

Treatment	Comment
General	
Reassurance, explanation	Use diagrams and written information
Regular ejaculation	Anecdotal; one observational study
Anti-inflammatory	
Nonsteroidal anti-inflammatory agents	Often disappointing
Antibiotics	
Doxycycline	Observational data; avoid prolonged courses
Other antibiotics	Limited observational data; no rationale
Alpha blockers	
Tamsulosin 400 mcg nocte	Supported by small randomized trials but clinical
Alfuzosin modified release 10 mg nocte	effectiveness has not been confirmed in recent trials
Antidepressants	
Tricyclic, e.g., amitriptyline 10–50 mg nocte	No controlled trials; established in chronic pain control
Phytotherapy	
Quercetin 500 mg bd	Naturally occurring bioflavonoid; small, controlled trial

TABLE 27-4   Management of Chronic Pelvic Pain Syndrome

Investigational Therapies

Treatment	Comment
Hormonal	
Finasteride	Small, controlled studies; possible role if coexistent prostatic hyperplasia
Mepartricin	Small uncontrolled studies
Anti-inflammatory	
Pentostan polysulphate .	Used in female interstitial cystitis; one small, controlled trial in CPPS; not widely used
Corticosteroids	Anecdotal; not supported by controlled trials
Anticonvulsant	
Gabapentin	Observational data; possible role in severe intractable pain
Physical	
Transurethral microwave thermotherapy	Small, controlled trials; risk of complications; not widely used
Transurethral needle ablation (TUNA)	Small, uncontrolled studies
Repetitive prostatic massage	Anecdotal; not widely adopted
Electromagnetic pulsed therapy	Small, controlled trial; requires confirmation
Complementary therapy	
Acupuncture	Small, uncontrolled trials
Psychological	
Cognitive behavioral therapy	No trials; deserves systematic study

variables. One controlled study demonstrated that the CPPS population is a heterogeneous group of men, some of whom (perhaps 20%) have no major psychological issues and are amenable to simple reassurance. The remaining majority are made up of two broad groups: (1) men with a tendency to somatization, who may benefit from a cognitive approach to therapy, and (2) a group in whom depression or anxiety are a feature, who may benefit from psychological or psychiatric evaluation and treatment for depression or anxiety as appropriate. In men with the most severe and intractable pain, a multidisciplinary team approach, for instance, in a pain clinic may be appropriate.

In the follow-up assessment of patients with CPPS, the validated NIH Chronic Prostatitis Symptom Index (NIH-CPSI) (Litwin et al. 1999) is a useful questionnaire that scores symptoms in three domains (pain, urinary symptoms, impact on quality of life), and this instrument now forms the basis of outcome evaluation in most therapeutic trial and natural history studies conducted worldwide. The long-term natural history of CPPS is the subject of ongoing study; it seems that, regardless of therapeutic intervention, a significant proportion (roughly one-third) of patients experience resolution of symptoms within 1 year of diagnosis; patients with long-standing symptoms are less likely to experience resolution but a significant minority report improvement after a 1-year follow-up interval. This information can be helpful in discussions with patients.

■ CONCLUSION

Since the turn of the century, significant advances have been made in understanding the prevalence, natural history, and, to some extent, pathogenesis of CPPS. These insights are largely attributed to a collaboration of North American investigators, the Chronic Prostatitis Collaborative Research Network (CPCRN). In the early part of the twenty-first century, the modern concepts of prostatitis and CPPS have emerged, signaling a shift toward more precise definition of prostatitis as an infective disease of the prostate, in acute and chronic forms; and recognition of CPPS as a complex noninfective syndrome with inflammatory, neuromuscular, and psychosocial dimensions. Acute and chronic bacterial prostatitis remain uncommon entities for which the etiology is understood, and therapy relatively clear-cut. In contrast, CPPS represents a continuing and formidable challenge, both in elucidating the fundamental cause and, conditional upon this, in identifying therapeutic options for the future.

■ KEY POINTS

- Acute and chronic infections of the prostate should be distinguished from the much commoner problem of chronic genital and pelvic pain in men (chronic pelvic pain syndrome).

- Acute prostatitis is a distinctive infective syndrome causing abrupt onset of symptoms of severe UTI with systemic features.

- Chronic bacterial prostatitis is caused by a chronic focus of bacterial infection in the prostate and presents with recurrent UTI.

- Chronic pelvic pain syndrome (CPPS) has replaced the entities called chronic nonbacterial prostatitis and prostatodynia.

- CPPS is common and causes perineal or penile pain lasting more than 3 months. The pain may be more widely distributed and associated with urinary symptoms and sexual dysfunction. The etiology of CPPS remains unknown.

- There is a lack of effective treatment for CPPS. In severe cases, use of alpha-blockers is supported by a number of small, controlled trials although results in more recent trials have been disappointing and clinical effectiveness has not been confirmed.

REFERENCES

Krieger JN, Nyberg L, Nickel JC. NIH consensus definition and classification of prostatitis. *JAMA*. 1999;282:236–237.

Litwin MA, McNaughton-Collins M, Fowler FJ, et al. The National Institutes of Health chronic prostatitis symptom index: development and validation of a new outcome measure. *J Urol*. 1999;162:369–375.

Luzzi GA. Chronic prostatitis and chronic pelvic pain in men: aetiology, diagnosis and management. *J Eur Acad Dermatol Venereol*. 2002;16:253–256.

McNaughton-Collins M, MacDonald R, Wilt TJ. Diagnosis and treatment of chronic abacterial prostatitis: a systematic review. *Ann Intern Med*. 2000;133:367–381.

Nickel JC, ed. *Textbook of Prostatitis*. Oxford: Isis Medical Media Ltd; 1999.

Pontari MA, Ruggieri MR. Mechanisms in prostatitis/chronic pelvic pain syndrome. *J Urol*. 2004;172:839–845.

28

Prevention Counseling and Condom Use

Richard A. Crosby and Beth Meyerson

■ INTRODUCTION

Clinicians who treat sexually transmitted infections (STIs) recognize that many clients return with either a reinfection or a newly acquired STI. STI prevention researchers have documented that the best predictor of subsequent infection with an STI is a history of one or more STIs. Studies have generated relatively consistent findings regarding the prevalence of subsequent infection among persons attending STI clinics. Repeat infections are typically acquired from the same or from new sex partners, meaning they are typically not attributable to failed treatment. In most populations studied, about 1 of every 6 persons diagnosed with a treatable (i.e., bacterial or parasitic) STI will be reinfected within 12 months, usually within 3–4 months of the initial episode.

Our objective is to focus on skills building for clinic staff to be able to increase condom use and other protective measures among clients, resulting, it is hoped, in a reduced repeat infection rate. It is our belief that sexual health care providers and STI clinic staff have opportunities to effect tremendous change in risk behaviors associated with STIs.

■ A PARADIGM SHIFT?

Traditionally, the clinic approach to STIs has been episodic treatment, medicalized because of the ability to offer curative treatment. Behavioral approaches to reduce STIs were left to others in the public health community, primarily community-based organizations or health department programs focused on HIV. STI clinicians and staff members have an opportunity to effect tremendous change in the population of STI clinic patients by shifting from a paradigm in which the clinic solely provides episodic medical treatment to traditional clinic activity enhanced by employing comprehensive and community-linked strategies. This approach includes activities that may be new to STI clinics from a practice standpoint and from an organizational–cultural standpoint.

The success of such a shift requires clinic teams to think differently about the clinic environment. The goal here is to identify opportunities for maximum client education and reinforcement. For managers, this will mean leading the STI clinic staff in assessment and planning activities, as well as developing staff skills in counseling and condom education. For clinicians, this will mean greater use of socially ascribed authority as the communicator of information to clients. For communities engaged in prevention of STIs and HIV, this may mean forming a deeper relationship with STI clinic operations and programming. Although clinic operational efficiency may be challenged in the short run, the benefit of changing organizational behavior will be felt in reduced STI recidivism.

Effective counseling and appropriately delivered instruction regarding condom use are the mainstays of efforts to prevent repeat STI infections among persons newly diagnosed with an STI. Counseling and condom instruction are critical assets in the public health effort to avert repeat infection, thereby fostering reductions in the population prevalence and, therefore, incidence of STIs.

■ WHAT HAPPENS IF WE MAINTAIN THE STATUS QUO?

The paradigm of treating clients medically without also addressing behavioral issues ignores subsequent infections. As a rule, it should never be assumed that clients will somehow begin to practice safer sex after they have been diagnosed with an STI and received prevention education. Studies have consistently shown that although their self-reported STI history was associated with increased prevention knowledge, it was not associated with increased motivation to use condoms, and with higher levels of risk behaviors, including sex while under the influence of alcohol and multiple partners.

An STI diagnosis or attending an STI clinic may not be a sufficient source of motivation to change behavior because of the deeply complex and socially prescribed nature of sexual decision making. In the absence of adopting protective behaviors, reinfection becomes a function of the sexual network. In addition to patients returning with a repeat STI, other members in their sexual network may be drawn into this cycle of infection. This cycle may, in turn, greatly magnify the prevalence of STIs within sociosexual networks, thereby making STI acquisition more likely.

■ WHO SHOULD DELIVER CLINIC-BASED STI PREVENTION COUNSELING?

In the traditional clinical setting, STI clinics have historically relied on disease investigation specialists (DIS) in the United States and health advisers (formerly called contact tracers) in the United Kingdom to counsel clients who come to the clinic and to locate potential sex partners of these clients (see Chapter 30 on partner notification). Although DIS have been important staff assets in the public health effort to reduce STIs, their success is contingent on the support of the clinic environment. For example, DIS may not have ample time to engage patients in prevention-oriented counseling. If DIS are the only clinic staff providing counseling, then opportunity for reinforcement and appropriate/effective counseling is lost because of a busy clinic environment. Two solutions exist: (1) efficacious prevention counseling methods that are relatively brief can be identified and DIS can be trained to use them, and (2) all clinic staff can be trained in such methods so that patients are exposed to several different and mutually reinforcing counseling opportunities.

An example of a brief risk reduction program is Project RESPECT (Kamb et al. 1998). A 40-minute program (divided over two sessions) was shown to increase self-reported condom use and reduce STI recidivism in five U.S. STI clinics between 1993 and 1996. STI clinics in Baltimore, Maryland; Denver, Colorado; Long Beach, California; Newark, New Jersey; and San Francisco, California, made a training and clinic flow adjustment to accommodate this counseling protocol as a prevention strategy. The extent to which DIS would be the "frontline" providers of any clinic-based STI prevention efforts, such as the Project RESPECT protocol, is likely to become a primary question for clinics that adopt a prevention-oriented philosophy.

Another, more recent, example of an effective clinic-based intervention program is known as Focus on the Future (Crosby et al. 2009). This initial efficacy trial of this program produced an effect size much larger than that obtained from Project RESPECT. Focus on the Future is a brief (45-minute) program delivered by a lay health adviser to high-risk men newly diagnosed with an STI. Evidence suggests that lay health advisers have been instrumental in achieving intervention success among various populations and across a broad range of health behaviors. The essence of the concept is that the most effective change agents are people from the community for which the intervention program is intended. The concept goes far beyond the concept of "matching" by race, age, and gender.

The adoption of formal prevention programs is not the only option available to clinics. Recently, clinics are building on the work of the DIS by asking other personnel (e.g., nurses and physicians) to reinforce counseling messages. The success of this approach is due to the message repetition and reinforcement, and, in some cases, the authority of the clinic worker, particularly if this staff member is a physician. The potential power of a "medical authority" to reinforce prevention messaging cannot be overstated. In the words of V. Campbell, a DIS working with urban Midwest (United States) STI prevention efforts:

> I'm not sure that clinic physicians and managers are aware of the STI cluster, that is, how a STI continually re-infects member of a social circle. Too many times we treat the same STI infection in a patient who does not disclose all, or any, of the partners. I have seen many cases where one partner will continually re-infect several partners. Many times the partners are aware of one another but do not disclose the names for various reasons. They fear being ostracized from the

group, losing their drug connection and even violence. They also do not understand the long-term health effects of an STI and they don't usually believe what a DIS will tell them. They are much more likely to believe these facts if they are explained to them by the doctor or nurse.

The power of the social authority possessed by the medical profession cannot be underestimated when thinking about opportunities to reinforce behavior change. Yet STI clinicians do not always have adequate training or skills in client history or sexual health counseling, as clinics have traditionally assigned client counseling to nonmedical staff. STI clinic and organizational practice history as well as professional–cultural roles may pose barriers to the clinic adoption of more integrated staff approaches to client counseling. These can be overcome. STI clinic managers and staff are encouraged to work together so that all staff have strong counseling and condom instruction skills, and clinic physicians are prepared and available to engage in counseling and condom instruction as well.

■ WHAT ARE THE KEY OBJECTIVES OF A COUNSELING SESSION?

Issues pertaining to relationships between sex partners inevitably permeate all aspects of STI counseling and instruction about condom use. This adds complexity to the role of the person providing the counseling and instruction. To compound the situation, it must be kept in mind that any intervention will be occurring with only one person within at least one dyad (i.e., the sexual relationship dyad). Stated differently, the counselor intervenes with only one of at least several persons who contribute to the likelihood of a subsequent infection. The limitations of this reality are especially pronounced when the client is a female in inequitable relationships with men where the balance of power favors male decision making about sex and sexual protective behaviors. With this limitation firmly in mind, the counseling/teaching session can then be thought of as posing four basic objectives:

1. Clients need to *gain awareness* about the "silent" nature of STIs (i.e., their frequent ability to be asymptomatic) and their modes of transmission. This awareness should be used to build a contaminant stance of sexual caution/protection with any of their sex partners. Sexual protection measures should transcend penile–vaginal sex, as many clients are likely to engage in oral or anal sex, thinking these acts pose less, if any, risk.

2. Clients should also learn how to *recognize symptoms* of STIs given that sometimes symptoms will occur. This recognition ability will (in some situations) allow them to refrain from having sex until their timely return to the clinic for diagnosis and treatment. The primary value of avoiding treatment delay is that many clients will not refrain from sex during the symptomatic period, thereby greatly enhancing the odds of STI transmission to their partners.

3. Clients should recognize that adopting sexual protective behaviors can be challenging. Like other health behaviors, sexual behaviors may be socially and culturally proscribed and people can easily become frustrated in their efforts to change and thus stop trying. If the counseling session can *instill a commitment* within the client to long-term behavior change, then the stage is set for teaching skills needed to achieve this goal.

4. Together, the client and counselor should *identify skill deficiencies* that can best be addressed to help the client practice safer sex. The key word here is "together"—it clearly implies that the session should be interactive rather than didactic. Given that long-term abstinence from sex is not a realistic possibility for clients, many of the skill-related needs will center on condom use.

Objective 1: Gaining Awareness

Clinics have many options and avenues to increase client awareness of risk and potential risk reduction strategies even outside of the counseling session. The first step, however, is to understand the client base. Who are the people attending the clinic? What can be learned about them based on demographics such as age, race, or geography? What is their cultural background and how does that background influence their sexual risk taking? Most important, working to increase client awareness of a risk for STIs is predicated on understanding the population and their perceptions of STI risk and protection. In the United States, STI clinics are part of a national planning effort for HIV and STI prevention programs. Such planning requires population-based assessments of need for prevention services. These assessments are available through state and city departments of health and can be a first step toward understanding populations who share characteristics with local clinic populations.

Once an ample amount of understanding about the clinic population has been gained, awareness "messages" can be developed. Careful attention should be given to language and literacy issues. The next step is to determine how these messages will be disseminated. Clinic managers and staff can initiate a review of the clinic environment to identify structural opportunities for this dissemination. Table 28-1 lists examples of opportunities that exist in the STI clinic environment. These can also be adapted to other primary care settings. Clinic managers and staff may identify other opportunities by reviewing clinic flow and functioning. Opportunities for client engagement can use technology, they can be conversational, or they can be brief and advertising/marketing oriented.

The structural opportunities shown in Table 28-1 are intended to occur in conjunction with a comprehensive client counseling approach. Using multiple and culturally appropriate means of communicating with clients about STI risk can raise STI prevention awareness and simultaneously build client trust in the clinic.

Each clinic or clinic system should, ideally, initiate an assessment of the clinic space to identify structural/environmental opportunities to increase client awareness. Engaging clients in the environmental assessment would enhance this evaluation, as clients themselves would have a role in shaping the clinic environment. Clinics are also encouraged to enlist the help of clients in tailoring awareness messages. For example, pamphlets with a lot of wording will probably be ineffective. Instead, a maximum use of images and culturally appropriate media may be optimally effective. Success with increasing client awareness in clinic environments could have the additional impact of diffusing into clients' so-cial networks, thereby having a potentially substantial influence on network STI risk perceptions.

Finally, the STI clinic may be the first place for "straight talk" about STIs. Thus, awareness about STI prevention may be greatly enhanced by simply explaining basic facts to clients. Such explanations need not be elaborate and should be provided in terms consistent with the clients' vocabulary and culture.

Objective 2: Recognizing Symptoms

One of the greatest "survival advantages" that STI pathogens have is their asymptomatic presentation. For example, symptoms for STIs such as gonorrhea or chlamydia while short lived and irritating, often go unrecognized particularly in men. For example, studies have shown that about 20% of men with symptomatic gonorrhea reported having unprotected sex while symptomatic. Therefore, educating patients about the symptoms of STI is critical. This portion of the counseling session need not be elaborate and may be addressed by a visual aid. For example, a large chart could use the word STOP as a learning device (see Box 28-1).

This acronym could be printed on a small card (perhaps the size of a business card) and laminated. Clients could then obtain a laminated copy to keep in their wallet or purse. If time allows, clients might also benefit from being shown pictures of ulcerative STIs, such as syphilis, chancroid, and herpes. Unlike clinical training, the goal is not to distinguish among these STIs or to attach names to them. Instead, the goal is to let clients see what symptoms may look like.

Although teaching people about STI symptom recognition may seem challenging, the task is likely to be

TABLE 28-1   Clinic Opportunity to Increase Awareness about STI Risk

Structural Element	Opportunity to Increase Awareness of Risk
Clinic exterior (doors, walls in outside hallways); street signage	Poster images (few words) appealing to the clinic target population
Clinic waiting room	Use of walls with images appealing to the clinic target population. Messages with these images being brief and focused on awareness and risk reduction strategies
Television/video communication	Use of clinic video stream into the waiting room with appealing (and evaluated) medium for conveying STI awareness and risk. Example: Voices/Voces (Crosby et al. 2009).
Staff–client communication	Several opportunities: on way to exam room, while history taking, during blood draw and exam, in counseling (see section on counseling)

BOX 28-1 STOP Acronym

STOP sexual activity and return to the clinic if even one of these conditions occurs!

S – Severe pain in the genitals of men or vaginal/lower abdominal pain in women

T – Temporary blisters or sores found on or near the genitals

O – Obvious and abnormal discharge from the genitals

P – Pain when urinating

---

eased by something called the *teachable moment*. The teachable moment represent an opportunity to intervene with clients who otherwise may not be receptive to learning. Their enhanced receptivity is a product of the STI diagnosis. The diagnosis signals that their health and well-being may be threatened and thus corrective measures for the future may be in order. Indeed, when the teachable moment occurs, clients may be receptive to learning and to asking questions about STI symptom recognition. They may be particularly keen to talk about any symptoms they may have recently experienced. Again, talking with clients in a clear and open manner (avoiding, for example, medical jargon) may be the best approach.

Finally, it is critical that clients know that symptom recognition is "good" because it signals two actions: (1) returning to the clinic for evaluation and possibly treatment and (2) cessation of sex until treatment is complete. However, it is important for clients to know that the absence of symptoms does not equal "safety." Moreover, clients should be specifically informed that they cannot judge the potential STI risk of sex partners based on the absence of symptoms in those partners.

Objective 3: Instill a Commitment

Ultimately, awareness and recognizing symptoms are not sufficient to effect behavior change. A long-term commitment to change is necessary. The challenge then for STI clinics is to promote a commitment that will be sustained over time. Client commitment to change will involve clinic staff learning how to conduct and document risk reduction plans for each client counseled. Behavioral change to reduce the risk of reinfection with STIs may involve several different steps, including, but not limited to, the consistent and correct use of condoms. Actively involving the client in developing a risk reduction plan can help reduce recidivism. Indeed, the active involvement was one of the primary strategies employed in Project RESPECT and in the Focus on the Future program.

A crucial dimension of obtaining a sustained commitment is understanding where STI acquisition "ranks" in a client's personal hierarchy of prevention needs. STI acquisition may also be related to one of several other prevention needs in the client's hierarchy of needs. For example, clients may face several obstacles, such as domestic violence, homelessness, or drug addiction, or they may be engaging in sex trade for drugs or money. Clinicians and clinic staff will need to key into these related needs, that is, develop treatment plans, prevention/risk reduction planning, and educational approaches) based on the needs.

Some STI clinics have developed relationships with community-based organizations to form peer educator or mentor relationships with persons attending STI clinics. For example, clients diagnosed as HIV positive are paired with a friend or mentor in the community who is also HIV positive and culturally matched for maximum support. In the STI context, a matching or mentoring scenario may be tailored to clinic reality and could be based on a peer network. Peer educators or mentors could follow up with clients in the field for up to a 12-month period following diagnosis and with reference to the risk reduction plan developed in the initial counseling session. The availability of such a program could be a valuable aid in obtaining long-term commitment to change.

Objective 4: Identify Skill Deficiencies

Table 28-2 displays a list of possible identifiable skill deficiencies. For each, the counselor should gain more detail from the client before proceeding. The client can then be engaged in a more active (and interactive) form of counseling—one that teaches specific skills. For example, consider a client who claims that he or she has a strong dislike for condoms because they are difficult to use and greatly detract from pleasure. Indeed, evidence suggests that one reason clients may not like condoms is that they do not "fit well" or they do not "feel right." Imagine, that further probing yields the following dialogue.

> *Client:* Condoms really pinch me when I put them on—they hurt a little.
>
> *Counselor:* What part of you is pinched?
>
> *Client:* Ahh, mostly my pubic hairs—they get trapped by the rim on the condom.

Counselor: Okay, and what do you mean by "they hurt"?

Client: I just get the feeling that my penis is being squeezed—it is not a good feeling.

This brief exchange is informative on two levels. First, it is apparent that the male client is inadvertently pulling the rim of the condom so far down toward the scrotum that pubic hairs are being caught, causing discomfort. This problem can be corrected by teaching the client how to apply condoms. With the aid of several condoms and a realistic penile model, the client can be taught to slide the rim gently down the shaft of the penis with one hand while pulling the public hair back with the other. Second, it is likely that the client is using a condom that is too small. This problem can be easily rectified by explaining how to find the right size when selecting condoms. The client could then be shown a variety of condoms in different sizes and encouraged to take one or more of each to eventually determine which size (or brand) gives him the best feeling.

Counselors must remember a paramount principle when counseling clients about condom use or any other STI protective practice. The counselor must respect the client's sexuality. The counseling/teaching process requires that the client disclose a great deal of personal and intimate information about his or her sexual behavior. Each act of disclosure to the counselor should be viewed as an invitation to establish trust. This trust will quickly erode when even subtle hints of the counselor's judgment. Sexual behavior expresses a person's sexuality, and sexuality is an important aspect of a person's well-being. Thus, challenges to a person's sexual behavior can threaten the "self," meaning that mental defense mechanisms may be engaged to cope with the threat. Consequently, counselors must become impervious to client's disclosures, for example, about same-gender sex, sex with large numbers of partners (perhaps in group settings), sex in exchange for money or drugs, and sex that involves anal penetration, the use of dildos, or sex toys.

■ CONDOM USE INSTRUCTION

The male condom can be a highly reliable method of preventing HIV and the transmission of many STIs when used consistently and correctly. The efficacy of condom use for HIV and STI prevention has been widely established. Condom efficacy diminishes if use is incorrect or inconsistent. Indeed, incorrect use may be common, and people may experience a broad spectrum of problems when attempting to use condoms. Unfortunately, persons who experience problems with condom use may be less likely to use condoms in the future. Thus, strategies to promote the correct use of condoms are essential and must be combined with efforts to motivate consistent condom use among persons at risk of HIV and STI acquisition and transmission. Figure 28-1 displays a continuum of condom use, ranging from no use at all to consistent and correct use. Clearly, one important function of clinic-based STI counseling is to "move" clients progressively farther to the right-hand end of this continuum.

TABLE 28-2 Possible Skill Deficiencies

Deficiency	Comment
Cannot control sexual impulsivity	Clients may suggest that they "lose control" and engage in risky sex.
Dislikes condoms because they are difficult to use and they detract from pleasure	Clients will often express various reasons why they do not like using condoms. Most can be addressed by improving condom use skills.
Cannot plan ahead for the use of condoms	Clients may state that, "condoms are never available" when they are having sex.
Lacks confidence or ability to initiate condom use in a new relationship	Condom initiation requires communication skills that may not be part of the client's repertoire.
Lacks the relational power needed to negotiate if/when sex will occur and whether condoms will be used	This reality is powerful and it is not one that is amenable to change in a brief counseling session.

FIGURE 28-1 A Continuum of Condom Use

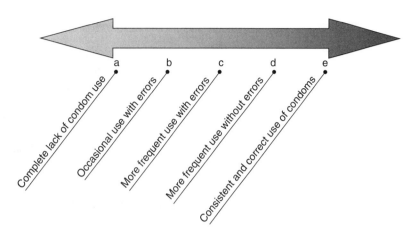

Similar to contraceptive effectiveness, condom effectiveness can be conceptualized at two distinct levels: (1) effectiveness given perfect use and (2) effectiveness given typical use. Clearly, the difference between perfect and typical condom use may be quite large. For example, the authors' study of men found that 43% reported recently putting a condom on after starting sex and 15% recently reported taking a condom off before sex was over. It is possible that this "incomplete use" of condoms is based on ejaculation. That is, the condom may be used only immediately before and during ejaculation. However, given the potential for sperm and semen (carrying pathogens) to be emitted from the male urethra well before ejaculation, the former finding alone is quite telling and supports the notion that typical use and perfect use are not one in the same. Because other studies have found that men report this type of incomplete condom use, it is conceivable that the practice is common.

Indeed, a broad spectrum of user errors may exist in relation to condom use. Table 28-3 displays a list of more than 20 potential errors and 4 common problems that may occur in conjunction with condom use. Two of the problems listed (breakage and slippage) are most likely the result of various errors. The other two problems are related to erection difficulties associated with condom use. From a behavioral perspective, intervention regarding the problems associated with erection is important to help men move toward point "e" in Figure 28-1. Much of the problem in moving to point "e" may involve "fit and feel" of condoms—a problem that can be addressed in a brief, clinic-based intervention.

Breakage and slippage of condoms are critical concerns. Given the imperative to promote consistent and correct use of condoms, clinic-based protocols designed to achieve this goal carry great potential to help prevent the acquisition and transmission of STIs. Although such protocols need to be tailored to the client population, it may be helpful for clinic managers to begin with a template. Thus, we have provided a template as part of this chapter.

■ TEMPLATE PROTOCOL FOR CONDOM USE INSTRUCTION

1. Begin by establishing an effective rapport with the client. First ask simple questions unrelated to STIs and slowly shift the conversation to condom use questions. As clients answer these questions, demonstrate a nonjudgmental response mode and let the client know you appreciate his or her honesty.

2. Begin to fill gaps in understanding as misconceptions become apparent during the exchange with the client. Be aware that clients may have little accurate information about the correct use of condoms. Common areas to address are

   - Why oil-based lubricants should not be used

   - Using condoms from start to finish of penetrative sex

   - Avoiding contact of sharp objects (including teeth) with condoms

   - Not reusing condoms when changing sexual acts

   - Withdrawing the condomized penis carefully to avoid slippage

TABLE 28-3 Potential Errors and Problems Relevant to Correct Condom Use

Technical Errors

Did not check condom for visible damage

Did not check expiration date

Put condom on after starting sex

Did not hold tip and leave space

Put condom on the wrong side up (had to flip it over)

Used condom without lubricant

Took condom off before sex was over

Condom slipped off while withdrawing penis

Started sex before condom was unrolled to base of penis

Used a condom that was stored more than 1 month in a wallet

Ejaculate dripped onto partner's mouth, genitals, or anus

Used oil-based lubricant on condom

Did not store condom in a cool and dry location

Unrolled condom and then tried to put it on the penis

Condom contacted sharp object (teeth, jewelry, fingernails)

Knowingly used expired condom

Reusing a condom

Knowingly used a damaged condom

Technical Errors Under Specific Circumstances

Switched between vaginal, oral, or anal sex

Of these, did not change to a new condom when switching

Availability Errors

Wanted condom, but did not have one

Had a problem with a condom, another not available

Wanted a water-based lubricant, but not available

Communication Error

Did not discuss condom use before sex

Problems

Condom broke

Condom slipped off during sex

Lost erection before condom was put on

Lost erection after condom was on and sex had begun

- Lubricating condoms adequately (and frequently throughout sex) to ensure minimal friction and maximum pleasure

- Knowing that erection problems may be normal and learning not to let these problems interfere with condom use

3. Ask about clients' negative condom use experiences and attempt to address issues that may be correctable. For example, if a client states that she finds men are "always unwilling to use condoms because they take the fun out of sex," the counselor could proceed to inform (and show) her that condoms come in many different sizes, shapes, colors, scents, and packages. The woman could then be invited to take several of these "novelty condoms" and offer these to sex partners as an enticement to "try something new." Some problems may not be easily correctable, and these may become a signal for referral. For example, a woman might explain that her current boyfriend would react negatively and may even become abusive if she suggested he use condoms. Clearly, the skill of negotiating condom use only extends so far and providing women with the ability to navigate this type of situation is beyond the scope of a brief, clinic-based intervention. Thus, referral to more extensive, community-based programs should always be a ready option.

4. Allow clients to practice condom application by providing a large supply of condoms and a realistic (rubber) penile model. Penile models are available in all skin tones. Although many clients will have perfected applying condoms, many may struggle through this action in a somewhat cumbersome manner. Some clients may view the mechanical act of applying condoms as antithetical to lovemaking and sex. The counselor needs to have a clear image of the potential dilemma clients face—clients engage in sex using actions that have become ritualistic and condoms may not be a welcome part of that ritual. Condom use may represent a "break in the action." Therefore, putting on a condom may need to become less of a burden and more of a fluid action, part of the sexual advance. Thus, practicing condom application may not only help clients use condoms correctly, it may also promote frequency of use.

Clients, especially heterosexual men, may initially be reticent to handle the penile model. The counselor can ease this anxiety by "going first" and proceeding to deftly show how to apply the condom without undue hassle. Next, the counselor should demonstrate the entire process again but in a carefully narrated, step-by-step sequence carefully and allow for questions.

One difficult and therefore important step in the sequence will be finding which side of the condom is "up." Most clients with experience using condoms will quickly identify with placing the condom on the head of the penis only to discover that it cannot be efficiently unrolled because it has been placed upside down. An efficacious teaching method shows clients how to use a thumb and forefinger to test the direction of unrolling. Show clients that the test should only involve unrolling a fraction of an inch. Clients should also be informed that this test should occur before placing the condom on the penis. Moreover, take care to explain that placing the condom on the penis and then turning the condom over (to get the right side up) must be avoided as this practice can inadvertently introduce pathogens to the external surface of the condom, thereby causing the transmission of an STI to the partner.

Other application steps may also be problematic for clients and therefore such actions deserve protracted time and attention in the counseling session. For example, many clients will not be able to apply condoms without the formation of excessive air bubbles. The counselor can address this problem by demonstrating the technique of squeezing the receptacle tip with the thumb and forefinger of one hand while carefully unrolling the condom to the base of the penis with the other hand. This task, like other tasks that compose condom application, will become more fluid with practice. Thus, the majority of time devoted to this session should be dedicated to client practice rather than counselor demonstration. When counselors observe clients make mistakes they should gently correct these while at the same noting that the task is not necessarily easy. Conversely, the moment counselors observe success (for any step in the process) they should be quick to provide an appropriate level of positive feedback and praise.

Four points should be made before the counselor and client terminate this practice session. With the condom being properly applied to the penile model, the counselor should note these points.

1. Holding onto the rim (point to the rim) is important during the process of removing the penis from the vagina or rectum. Either partner can do this, but it must be done. Otherwise, the condom could easily slip off, and the fluid inside could then become the source of an infection.

2. Condoms may become dry during sex (stroke the condom to show that it currently has plenty of lubrication) even though they appear to have ample lubrication after being applied. Thus, don't hesitate to briefly remove the condomized penis for the purpose of quickly adding a water-based lubricant (at this point, it may be helpful to actually supply clients with pocket-sized containers of water-based lubricant).

3. Condoms provide the best protection against STIs. Most are made of latex. Holding a new or used condom between your hands, show clients that latex material is tremendously elastic and durable and then proceed to explain that the material is not porous compared with natural skin condoms. Some persons, however, are allergic to latex, which may require use of nonlatex condoms (see Chapter 12).

4. Again, using the condomized penile model as a visual aid, explain that "men" come in all shapes and sizes and thus condoms are not a one-size-fits-all commodity. Encourage male and female clients to take an ample supply of condoms before they leave the clinic and suggest that they sample from a variety of sizes and brands. Emphasize that finding the right "fit and feel" is important. This portion of the counseling session implies that STI clinic managers will be economically savvy, and therefore, recognize that value of paying for condoms rather than pharmaceuticals. The cost of condoms is clearly a much smaller part of the clinic budget than the larger costs associated with continued transmission and repeat acquisition of STIs.

5. Conclude the counseling session by supplying clients with a "help card." This should be a laminated card (the size of a business card) that displays contact information for the counselor on one side and an acronym for condom application on the other. While the acronym is an important strategy to aid clients with condom application, the contact information is far more valuable. The phone number listed should be a direct line to the same counselor who delivered the teaching/learning session. Even though the session may have been brief (e.g., 30 minutes), the rapport developed during that time represents a significant achievement that should not be squandered. Indeed, this newly established relationship should ideally become the basis for an "easy connection" that allows the client to interface with the STI clinic using the counselor as a liaison. In many instances, the interface

will not need to extend beyond the counselor as the questions clients pose may pertain only to the correct use of condoms. However, clients may also ask (at some in the future) about potential STI symptoms they may have observed or about problems with medication they have been prescribed. The counselor then becomes a convenient form of an outreach worker.

■ A CASE STUDY IN CONDOM USE INSTRUCTION

The previously mentioned program known as Focus on the Future can be instructive at this juncture. The efficacy trial evaluated the effects of a brief counseling program delivered to young African American men immediately after their diagnosis and treatment. The lay health adviser who provided the individualized counseling was an African American male from the same community as the clients. He began each session by establishing a rapport with the client and then proceeded to show them a wall poster that displayed a bar graph depicting the racial disparity pertaining to AIDS rates among African American men compared with Hispanic and white counterparts. The ensuing discussion typically led men to realize that they can help change the grim reality of HIV/AIDS for African American men, which can begin with their own use of condoms.

Next, men were engaged in a conversation about various aspects of condom use emphasizing how condoms should be used and how they can find the brand and size that gives them an optimal sense of "fit and feel." This portion of the counseling session typically became quite interactive and naturally varied, depending on the needs of the client. Two active learning exercises are built into this portion of the session. The first involves asking men to demonstrate condom application skills using a penile model. The lay health adviser carefully observes this demonstration and proceeds to teach the men how to avoid any errors they may have made in the application process. Men then repeat the application process (with guidance) until they achieve mastery.

The second activity is designed to add some levity to the session and to illustrate the dangers of using an oil-based lubricant. Many men have been unaware that added lubricants must only be those with a water base. The lay health adviser explained the importance of adding lubricant to condoms as they become dry during sex and then informed men that only water-based lubricants should be used. He then inflated a condom with air and rubbed a few drops of baby oil on the "condom balloon."

Within seconds, the condom balloon typically shattered into small pieces, sometimes traveling several feet across the room. Men were normally quite impressed with this display, and they frequently commented that they will show others.

The counseling session also includes a "condom bar" comprising at least 12 different types of condoms. Men were told about the value of finding the right size and brand and encouraged to take a large variety of condoms so they can experiment with options that may enhance their pleasure and reduce their perceptions (as well as their partner's perceptions) that condoms ruin sex.

Discussion about specific problems regarding condoms is the basis for the final portion of the session. For example, men often reported that they experience erectile difficulty when applying or using condoms. The lay health adviser used this opportunity to point out that condom-associated erectile problems are typical and may subside (1) when he gains more confidence in his application ability, (2) when condoms are adequately lubricated during sex, and (3) when condoms fit and feel optimally comfortable. The session closes by giving men a laminated card (the size of a business card) that lists eight steps of condom application. Although men ask questions throughout the session, many ask questions after they leave the clinic. Thus, men are also provided with a cell phone number so they can easily reach the lay health adviser in the coming days and weeks with any questions that arise.

■ KEY POINTS

- STI clinics and particularly clinic physicians have opportunities to effect tremendous change in risk behaviors associated with STIs.

- The success of such a shift will require clinic teams to think differently about the clinic environment.

- Counseling and condom instruction are critical assets in the public health effort to avert repeat infection, thereby fostering reductions in the population prevalence and incidence of STIs.

- Never assume that clients will somehow begin to practice safer sex after they have been diagnosed with an STI.

- Issues pertaining to relationships between sex partners inevitably permeate all aspects of STI counseling and instruction about condom use. Naturally, this adds complexity to the role of the person providing the counseling and instruction.

- Crafting thoughtful prevention objectives and messages is critical as well as creating a clinical environment that supports awareness and fosters behavior change.

- The counseling process comprises four objectives: (1) gaining awareness, (2) recognizing symptoms, (3) instilling a commitment to change, and (4) recognizing deficiencies in skills needed to achieve change.

- A paramount principle should be kept in mind when counseling clients about condom use or any other STI protective practice: the counselor must respect the client's sexuality.

- A broad spectrum of user errors and problems may exist in relation to condom use; these can be rectified through teaching and practice.

- Practicing condom application may not only help clients use condoms correctly, it may also help promote increased frequency of use.

REFERENCES

Advocates for Youth. *Building Cultural Competence*. Washington, DC: Advocates for Youth. www.advocatesforyouth.org/publications.htm.

Crosby RA, DiClemente RJ, Charnigo R, Snow G, Troutman A. A brief, clinic-based, safer sex intervention for heterosexual African American men newly diagnosed with an STD: a randomized controlled trial. *Am J Public Health*. 2009;99:S96–S103.

Crosby RA, Graham CA, Yarber WL, Sanders SA. If the condom fits, wear it: a qualitative study of young African American men. *Sex Transm Infect*. 2004;80:306–309.

Crosby RA, Liddon N, Martich FA, Brewer T. Correlates of engaging in unprotected sex while experiencing dysuria or discharge: a study of men with confirmed gonorrhea. *Sex Transm Dis*. 2004;31:421–423.

Crosby RA, Sanders S, Yarber WL, et al. Condom use errors and problems among college men. *Sex Transm Dis*. 2002; 29:552–557.

Crosby RA, Sanders SA, Yarber WL, Graham CA. Condom use errors and problems: a neglected aspect of studies assessing condom effectiveness. *Am J Prev Med*. 2003;24: 367–370.

Crosby RA, Yarber WL, Sanders SA, Graham CA. Condom discomfort and associated problems with their use among university students. *Am J College Health*. 2005;54:143–148.

DiClemente RJ, Wingood GM, Sionean C, et al. Association of adolescents' STD history and their current high-risk behavior and STI status: a case for intensifying clinic-based prevention efforts. *Sex Transm Dis*. 2002;29:503–509.

Goode TD, Jones W, Mason J. A guide to planning and implementing cultural competence: organizational self assessment. HRSA Monograph. Winter 2002. http://gucchd.georgetown.edu/nccc/documents/ncccorgselfassess.pdf.

Holmes KK, Levine R, Weaver M. Effectiveness of condoms in preventing sexually transmitted infections. *Bull World Health Organ*. 2004;82:454–461.

Kamb ML, Fishbein M, Douglas, et al. Efficacy of risk-reduction counseling to prevent human Immunodeficiency virus and sexually transmitted diseases: a randomized controlled trial. *JAMA*. 1998;280:1161–1167.

Mehta SD, Erbelding EJ, Zenilman JM, Rompalo AM. Gonorrhea reinfection in heterosexual STD clinic attendees: Longitudinal analysis of risks for first reinfection. *Sex Transm Infect*. 2003;79:124–128.

Mertz KJ, Finelli L, Levine WC, et al. Gonorrhea in male adolescents and young adults in Newark, New Jersey: implications of risk factors and patient preferences for prevention strategies. *Sex Transm Dis*. 2000;27:201–207.

O'Donnell LN, San Doval A, Duran R, O'Donnell C. Video-based sexually transmitted disease patient education: its impact on condom acquisition. *Am J Public Health*. 1995;85(6):817–822.

Wingood GM, DiClemente RJ. Applying a theoretical framework of gender and power to understand the exposures and risk factors for HIV among women. *J Health Educ Behav*. 2000;27:539–565.

29

HIV Counseling and Testing

Louise Brown and Penny Goold

■ INTRODUCTION

Human immunodeficiency virus (HIV) testing has since the 1980s been considered a specialist skill in which structured pretest and posttest counseling of patients was required. This was previously further complicated by statutory requirements for specific informed consent, which is beyond the standard consent for medical care completed by most hospital and clinic patients. In recent years, this was termed *HIV exceptionalism*. Because of the statutory-mandated counseling, consent, and regulatory burden, as well as the time required, this gradually became appreciated as a barrier to testing. These barriers became more important as the effectiveness of HIV prevention and treatment interventions improved and as discrimination against HIV-infected persons receded. The public health consensus currently is to facilitate HIV testing widely.

Expanding HIV testing has evolved as a major public health priority. With dynamic infection rates, changing epidemiology, and major advances in treatment, early diagnosis allows public health officials to become aware of new transmission patterns and can be potentially lifesaving to newly diagnosed patients and their intimate partners. From an actuarial standpoint, it is estimated that the projected life span of persons with HIV approaches that of HIV-uninfected persons, when they have early diagnosis and treatment, with highly active antiretroviral therapy (HAART). Nevertheless, the rates of undiagnosed HIV in the United Kingdom and the United States remain unacceptably high, especially in minority and disenfranchised populations. Up to one-third of prevalent infections remain undiagnosed.

In response to these imperatives, changes in consent procedures have evolved. Traditional HIV counseling and testing requires an active consent process. In contrast, *opt-out programs* have begun to develop and have been actively promoted by organizations such as the Centers for Disease Control and Prevention (CDC) in efforts to expand and "deexceptionalize" testing. *Opt-out* (when consent is inferred, unless the patient declines after being informed the test will be done) aims to increase the uptake of HIV testing by normalizing the process, reducing the associated stigma, and helping healthcare workers (HCWs) to feel empowered to test their patients. Opt-out testing policy still requires that pretest and posttest counseling be documented in the medical records. It does remove the necessity for specific consent forms and government-mandated counseling scripts.

HIV testing requires informed consent. There is some essential information about an HIV test that needs to be provided to all patients to enable them to make an informed decision. (Depending on the context, consent can be given verbally or as written information). Oral consent is acceptable as long as documentation of counseling is made in the medical or clinic record. For example, the US has transitioned to oral consent as part of routine medical care in most clinical settings.

Assessment of an individual's risk of HIV infection will determine what additional discussion is necessary before testing, such as the implications of a positive HIV test. This chapter aims to cover all aspects of HIV testing, including risk assessment, the basics necessary to obtain informed consent, further information for patients who are high risk or have a positive result, the testing procedure, as well as other issues to consider such as testing without consent. This information should equip all HCWs to confidently and competently undertake HIV testing within their practice as part of routine care.

RAISING THE ISSUE OF HIV TESTING

Discussing HIV testing with patients will require different approaches, depending on the individual and the context of the consultation. When HIV testing is offered only to persons perceived to be "at-risk," there is increased stigma and sensitivity associated with counseling and testing. Patients are more likely to expect direct questions regarding HIV testing when they have attended a specialist sexual health service or if they raised the issue themselves. It is sometimes unexpected and therefore more difficult when an HIV test is offered as part of a general health check, as an opt-out program or when it is deemed appropriate by the HCW because of presenting symptoms that might be related to HIV. Assessing an individual's risk of HIV infection could be the first step in introducing the concept of or making the decision to offer HIV testing. Some settings have introduced HIV testing into routine care regardless of individual risk. For example, the CDC in the United States now recommends HIV testing for all patients admitted to the hospital and suggests testing at emergency department visits for persons who have not been recently tested. Implementation of these recommendations, however, is inconsistent.

ASSESSING RISK

In more general clinical settings, assessing an individual's risk for infection may help to target HIV testing. However, remember that not all people with undiagnosed infection have a clearly identifiable risk and testing should not be dismissed in these instances. In settings such as antenatal care in which HIV testing has a disproportionate benefit in diagnosis, a risk assessment is not required to target testing, a policy adopted by all opt-out programs. Assessing an individual's risk of having HIV may instead help to determine how much further information an individual needs before taking an HIV test (specifics discussed later in the chapter). In opt-out programs, a leaflet maybe given with information for the individual to assess his or her own risk, giving them the opportunity to raise the issue with the HCW for further discussion where necessary.

Risk factors for acquisition of HIV would currently include:

- Intravenous drug use in which needles or other paraphernalia are shared

- Unprotected sexual intercourse with someone in which HIV infection is more likely (owing to higher prevalence and sexual practices)
  - Men who have sex with men (MSM)
  - Multiple heterosexual partners
  - Intercourse with commercial sex workers
  - Originating from or traveling to countries where HIV prevalence is high, such as sub-Saharan Africa, eastern Europe, or South Asia, or highly impacted areas in other parts of the world

- Blood transfusions/operations in areas where screening donors is not rigorous or health and safety measures are minimal (e.g., shared equipment without adequate decontamination)

Considering the type of sex is also important. For example, receptive anal sex carries more risk than insertive vaginal sex, which, in turn, carries more risk than oral sex (BASHH Clinical Effectiveness Group).

In general settings, it may be useful to have some "lead-in lines" to raise the issue of HIV testing or assessing risk of HIV, for example:

1. "While reviewing your need for contraception we are routinely including an assessment for infections that can be passed between people. I will just need to ask you a few possibly sensitive questions."

2. "The symptoms you describe may be caused by many different things some of which are much less likely than others, and so I would like to do a number of tests to exclude them. I need to ask you a few more questions to help me with this."

3. "We now offer HIV testing as part of everybody's routine care. I would just like to ask you some potentially sensitive questions about your risk for this infection."

ESSENTIAL INFORMATION

Once you have identified that there is a need to undertake HIV testing you will need to explain to the patient what this involves. This usually occurs through discussion but can be provided as written information. It is helpful first to briefly assess what the patient already knows.

- *Distinguishing between HIV and AIDS* is sometimes necessary.

- *Explaining the nature of the test and how the results will be relayed.* This will depend on which test is used, that is, the point-of-care tests (POC) (finger prick or saliva) in which the result is often available within minutes or conventional laboratory-based tests (sample obtained by venepuncture).

- *Explaining the "window period."* The "window period" is the time taken for the HIV test to become positive following the risk exposure(s). Traditionally, it was the time at which an individual had developed detectable antibodies to the HIV (seroconversion), about 3 months. The blood tests now (fourth-generation HIV tests) routinely include an antigen test alongside the antibody test, which includes an early antigen thus making it highly sensitive, effectively reducing the real time of the window period to approximately 6–8 weeks. Three months is still used as a safety net, and a repeat test is recommended if the risk exposure falls within this period.

- *Clarifying the routes of transmission.* Assumptions may be made by patients that transmission is not possible or at least highly unlikely during oral sex, or if a condom is used but not consistently or correctly. Patients may therefore not disclose contacts of this nature. Risk in these situations is lower but still a definite possibility. Some people still think HIV only effects homosexual males.

- *Discuss concerns regarding confidentiality* as these sometimes prevent an HIV test from occurring. Common concerns include
  - *Identification*: The patients name on a sample sent to an external laboratory. Reassure patients that confidentiality applies to all HCWs. However, concerns may be valid if a patient knows another person who works within this setting, where privacy is more of an issue than confidentiality. In this instance, anonymized testing would be appropriate.
  - *Reporting*: In many areas, HIV is now a reportable communicable disease. In most states of the United States, HIV is reportable by name to the health department, similar to reports of other sexually transmitted infections. Patients should be aware of this before testing. This, however, is not the case in the United Kingdom.

- *Life insurance*: Changes in regulations in the British Association of Insurers (BAI) in 1994 advised insurance companies against asking whether an HIV test had been taken. This ruling does not necessarily apply to companies that are not a member of the BAI, and HIV testing may actually be a compulsory requirement of some policies. In the United States, HIV testing is often part of the standard examination performed by insurance companies as part of the underwriting process, and insurance may be denied to HIV-infected persons.

- However, because of advances in HIV treatment and prolonged life expectancy, some insurance companies have reevaluated the cover they provide to those persons living with HIV (PLWHIV). It is possible for PLWHIV to obtain life insurance and even critical illness cover (which offer reassurances when obtaining a mortgage). However, the rate structure for HIV-infected persons will be higher than standard rates.

■ FURTHER INFORMATION FOR PATIENT DISCUSSION

For patients identified as high risk for HIV infection, and those with symptoms highly suggesting an underlying HIV diagnosis, it would be appropriate to discuss further issues with the patient before undertaking the test. The prior knowledge and needs of the patient must always be considered.

Discussing the implications of a positive HIV test result may include many different topics that the patient wishes to discuss. Explaining to patients the benefits of them knowing their HIV status is an essential part of this discussion.

Health Benefits

The health of individuals with HIV can be maintained much more effectively through regular monitoring and appropriate medication. The estimated life expectancy for a person with HIV has improved dramatically because of new developments and increasing experience in HIV therapy over the past two decades. This is likely to extend with increasing knowledge, better-tolerated drugs, and further scientific breakthroughs. Comparing HIV with a disease such as diabetes rather than cancer helps the patient to appreciate the nature of the infection as a lifelong illness with good outcomes instead of a possible death sentence. These improvements in health care have enabled PLWHIV to continue to lead a fairly normal life.

Transmission

If a positive diagnosis is made, ensure the patient is fully aware of the risks of transmission. Reassurance is often needed regarding family and household members, especially children. It is advisable not to share toothbrushes or razors but general sharing of items such as towels, cutlery, and glasses does not pose a risk to others. The risk of transmission through sexual contact, including oral sex, must be emphasized and the recommendation of consistent condom use for sexual intercourse is vital to help prevent transmission to others, as well the acquisition of other infections.

In UK law, offenses against the Person Act (1861), and similar laws in some U.S. states, enable the prosecution of those recklessly transmitting HIV infection. Those persons who aware of their status or are aware they are at higher risk of HIV (even without having had a test) may be subject to prosecution by their partners if their (potential) status has not been disclosed. Criminal law also has been used in other parts of the world, such as Canada and Australia, although actual prosecutions are rare. Using barrier methods of contraception, that is, condoms, may be regarded as a defense, because if transmission did occur, it may not be seen as reckless. However, this has yet to be tested in the UK courts. Patients are aware of these new developments. Unprotected sexual intercourse not only contributes to the transmission of HIV to others, the transmission of resistant strains of HIV, and the acquisition of other infections; it now also exposes the PLWHIV to prosecution.

Occupation

In some jobs, an HIV diagnosis must be disclosed, which is likely to lead to redeployment. In the United Kingdom, disclosure is required for healthcare workers, such as surgeons, dentists (although, currently, this is under revision in the United Kingdom), or midwives. In the United States, there are no such requirements. In both the United States and the United Kingdom, members of the armed forces are subject to periodic routine testing and can be medically discharged or restricted from active duty if they are found to be positive.

Life Insurance Policies

Any life insurance policies would require disclosing the diagnosis. Many insurers are now more open to providing coverage for PLWHIV but practice varies greatly. Some companies still offer cover, others may refuse, and others may exclude any HIV-related problems.

Having Children

Having children may be an issue for some patients. Artificial insemination enables HIV-infected women in a serodiscordant relationship to conceive without putting their HIV-negative partners at risk of transmission. Advances in medical care have also provided an opportunity for an HIV-negative woman to conceive without being infected by her HIV-positive partner by the use of sperm-washing. Unfortunately, sperm-washing is not yet widely available or routinely provided on the National Health Service (NHS) in the United Kingdom. Coverage in the United States for this procedure varies by state and medical insurance plan, but there is wide availability of free testing at municipal health departments and other sites.

Treating an HIV-positive woman during pregnancy with antiretroviral drugs, giving the neonate antiretroviral drugs for 4–6 weeks, and abstaining from breastfeeding helps to reduce the risk of vertical transmission to less than 1%.

Dealing with a Positive HIV Test

After a test, it may be important to discuss how the patient may cope if he or she were diagnosed with HIV infection. Acknowledging the difficulties this may bring, highlighting the benefits of knowing the diagnosis, and discussing the patient's support may be sufficient. However, if the patient expresses any serious negative thoughts, such as suicide, these need to be dealt with before the test is administered. It may be possible to address negative thoughts easily during a short discussion to reassure the HCW that these were not true feelings. However, if there are concerns, it would be appropriate to delay the test and arrange further discussion and appropriate support.

Discussing the emotional and psychological support a patient believes they would have from friends and family helps them to focus their own thoughts on how they may deal with a positive diagnosis and with whom they could discuss this. It may be useful to suggest they confide in one close individual even before the test; this person may also accompany the patient to the test and to receive the result. There are often voluntary organizations and local services that provide support, counseling, and advice to those recently diagnosed and living with HIV (e.g., the Terence Higgins Trust in the UK; AVERT in the United States, Canada, and United Kingdom provides help-line information). Informing patients about these services may also help them feel less isolated. The specialist HIV medical clinic can and offer support and advice.

Once further appropriate discussion has taken place, establish whether the patient agrees to proceed with the HIV test. If the patient has decided against the test, suggest that the patient make an appointment within a week to return to discuss the situation further; highlight that you recommend the patient take the test but that the decision remains with the patient. You are there to provide further information and support as required.

However, be aware of potentially life-threatening conditions in which underlying HIV infection would help to inform the differential diagnosis. Examples include:

- Pneumocystis pneumonia
- Cerebral toxoplasmosis
- Cryptococcal meningitis
- Disseminated tuberculosis

It would be inappropriate to delay a test in these situations, so testing to enable appropriate treatment must be discussed with the individual. If the patient agrees to proceed with the test, then continue as follows.

Consent

Testing for HIV should be voluntary and undertaken only with the patient's knowledge and consent. Pretest information can be given orally or in writing. Consent may be inferred if testing is not declined as long as the patient has been adequately informed of an opt-out policy, or it may simply be obtained verbally and recorded. Obtaining the patient's written consent is not essential.

Testing Without Consent

In exceptional circumstances, testing a patient without consent may need to be considered.

When testing patients under age 16 years, the previous guidance can be used if you judge that they have sufficient maturity to understand the implications of testing (General Medical Council, CDC). In most U.S. states, adolescents who present for reproductive health care, where sexual activity was consensual, are considered emancipated and can legally consent for HIV tests and other STI clinical interventions.

Where a child cannot give or withholds consent, seek consent from a person with parental responsibility for the child. If you believe the person's judgment is distorted, for example, because he or she may be the cause of the child's infection, you must decide whether the medical interests of the child override the wishes of those with parental responsibility. Whenever possible you should discuss the issues with an experienced colleague before deciding. If you test a child without obtaining consent, you must be prepared to justify that decision (see Chapter 37 for further discussion).

Testing an unconscious adult may be justifiable for an urgent situation deemed in the patient's best interest. Test results should not be passed on to anyone not involved with the patient's care, including a partner, until the patient has either regained consciousness or dies.

If a HCW suffers a sharps injury or other occupational exposure to blood or body fluids, the index patient's consent should be obtained before the test is undertaken. If the patient is unconscious when the injury occurs, consent should be sought once the patient has regained full consciousness. If appropriate, the injured person can take prophylactic treatment until consent has been obtained and the test result is known. Healthcare clinics and hospitals have often developed policies to address these specific contingencies.

◼ TESTING PROCEDURE

Common practice for HIV testing is a venipuncture sample taken from the antecubital fossa area. Requests to laboratories may need to state the reason for the test, but simple "screening" or "risk factor" should be sufficient. Many laboratories will do same-day HIV tests. Therefore, if a rapid result is required and if the local procedure is not known, it may be worth contacting the laboratory to establish when the test result will be available. If the initial screening test is positive, further confirmatory tests will be required on the same sample, which will obviously delay the result by a day or two, depending on individual laboratories.

Other tests are available, including finger-prick blood test or oral fluid samples. These are useful in outreach settings and for patients who have difficult venous access. These tests can also allow for point-of-care (POC) testing by providing the results within a matter of minutes. It is important to confirm a positive result from a POC test, as the positive predictive value of the tests is low in situations of low prevalence. These tests will also not measure HIV antigen, and if acute (early) HIV infection is suspected, then HIV antigen, or RNA (viral load), must be requested or the test repeated after a suitable interval.

■ GIVING RESULTS

Once the test has been taken, arrange how the patient will obtain the result. POC tests give patients the opportunity to wait for their result. For all other laboratory-based tests, other arrangements need to be in place. A specific appointment may be appropriate for the patient to return, but in many high screening settings alongside other infection testing, alternative methods for sending results to patients have been implemented. These include telephone, letter, mobile telephone, text messaging, or simply "no news is good news," in which the patient is only notified of positive results. In these situations, if the result is positive, re-calling the patient for an appointment to discuss test results is much more appropriate than disclosing the diagnosis within the correspondence.

When giving results, confirm that the result is correct for the patient by checking such details as date of birth, name, and date of the test.

■ GIVING NEGATIVE RESULTS

- Need to acknowledge the window period
  - Is there a need to retest?

- Reiterate appropriate safer practices
  - Safer sex—offer condoms
  - Safer injecting drug use—consider referral to needle exchange program

■ GIVING POSITIVE RESULTS

When pretest discussion includes the possibility of a positive diagnosis, the patient is more prepared. The issues that were discussed before testing are important to reiterate in particular that HIV infection is a treatable condition. It helps to reinforce the benefits of knowing the diagnosis to maintain health and to help prevent transmitting HIV as well as acquiring other infections.

Acknowledge the patient's support at this early stage. It is often useful for the patient to identify one person they feel they could tell. Reassurance should be offered regarding your support and the support of the HIV specialist team. Signposting to other support agencies, such as voluntary charities in the area, may also be appropriate. Emphasize that a positive HIV result often comes as a shock, even in patients who are expecting a positive diagnosis. Under such conditions, the patient may not take in all the information at that visit. Arrange for an early follow-up to answer patients' questions and to check how much of the information has been absorbed. All seropositive test notifications should include either the initial HIV staging workup or expedited referral for clinical care.

Special Situation: Evaluating for HIV Acute Seroconversion Syndrome

In some situations, evaluating for acute HIV seroconversion syndrome is warranted. This is a critical public health issue because these patients will be negative by standard serological evaluation but will have extremely high HIV viral loads and therefore pose substantial transmission risk. These settings include the following:

1. Patients who are sexual contacts to known HIV-infected persons and have an acute febrile illness or other manifestations of acute HIV.

2. Homosexual or heterosexual patients who have new partners or are drug users with signs or symptoms of acute HIV. These signs and symptoms may include an acute febrile illness, lymphadenopathy, rash (usually macular), arthralgias/myalgias, odynophagia, oral thrush, mucositis, hepatitis, and even encephalitis. Clinically, these may appear as a nonspecific viral syndrome, and therefore the risk history should establish the need for testing.

In these situations, a standard HIV test should be performed. However, in addition, a *qualitative viral load determination* should be ordered. A diagnosis of acute HIV is made when the standard serological evaluation is negative, but the viral load is positive.

■ CONCLUSION

Increasing HIV testing in all appropriate settings, including using opt-out programs, will contribute to reducing the rates of new and undiagnosed infection and improve the health and well-being of PLWHIV. All healthcare professionals working in any area can be equipped to undertake HIV testing.

HIV testing should be regarded in the same manner as any other test. The patient is provided with all appropriate information, and then the patient decides whether to take the test.

■ HIV TESTING CHECKLIST

1. Risk assessment

2. Information provided
   - Benefits explained
   - Implication of positive result
   - Insurance
   - "Window" period/seroconversion
   - Result giving explained

3. Consent obtained (this may be verbal, written, or inferred, depending on system adopted)

4. HIV test taken

■ KEY POINTS

- The benefits to testing outweigh the disadvantages.

- Consent to HIV testing need not be written.

- "Counseling" is not necessary.

- Normalize the testing process.

- Assess risk factors associated with HIV acquisition.

- There are a number of testing options.

- Insurance implications may relate to a positive diagnosis.

- HIV should be considered as a lifelong illness and not necessarily a death sentence.

REFERENCES

BASHH Clinical Effectiveness Group. United Kingdom national guidelines on HIV testing. BASHH 2008. http://www.bashh.org/guidelines.

Burke RC, Sepkowitz KA, Bernstein KT, et al. Why don't physicians test for HIV? a review of the US literature. *AIDS*. 2007;21(12):1617–1624.

Centers for Disease Control and Prevention. HIV/AIDS statistics and surveillance. CDC 2007. http://www.cdc.gov/hiv/topics/surveillance/basic.htm.

Centers for Disease Control and Prevention. HIV infection reporting. CDC 2008. http://www.cdc.gov/hiv/topics/surveillance/reporting.htm.

Centers for Disease Control and Prevention. Revised recommendations for HIV testing of adults, adolescents, and pregnant women in health-care settings. *MMWR*. 2006; 55. http://www.cdc.gov/mmwr/preview/mmwrhtml/rr5514a1.htm.

Health Protection Agency. HIV in the United Kingdom. HPA 2008. http://www.hpa.org.uk/web/HPAweb&HPAwebStandard/HPAweb_C/1227515299695.

Hutchinson AB, Branson BM, Kim A, Farnham PG. A meta-analysis of the effectiveness of alternative HIV counseling and testing methods to increase knowledge of HIV status. *AIDS*. 2006;20(12):1597–1604.

Obermeyer CM, Osborn M. The utilization of testing and counseling for HIV: a review of the social and behavioral evidence. *Am J Public Health*. 2007;97(10):1762–1774.

Opt-out system for HIV testing proves successful. More are tested and referred to care. *AIDS Alert*. 2006;21(6):69–71.

Rogstad K, Palfreeman A, Rooney G, et al; Clinical Effectiveness Group, British Association of Sexual Health and HIV. UK national guidelines on HIV testing 2006. *Int J STD AIDS*. 2006;17(10):668–676.

Rotheram-Borus MJ, Leibowitz AA, Etzel MA. Routine, rapid HIV testing. *AIDS Educ Prev*. 2006;18(3):273–280.

UNAIDS. UNAIDS/WHO AIDS epidemic update. December 2007. http://data.unaids org/pub/EPISlides/2007/2007_epiupdate_en pdf.

30

Partner Notification and Management

Janette Clarke and Jonathan M. Zenilman

▦ INTRODUCTION

> I got it from Agnes
> She got it from Jim
> We all agree it must have been
> Louise who gave it to him . . .
> Now she got it from Harry
> Who got it from Marie
> And ev'rybody knows that Marie
> Got it from me . . .
>
> *Tomfoolery* and *Songs*
> *and More Songs* . . .
> Tom Lehrer, 1952

Sexually transmitted infections (STIs) need rapid and effective interventions to prevent reinfections, complications, and spreading around communities. Identifying, contacting, and treating sexual partners are essential elements in controlling these infections. Partner notification (PN) has been an integral part of STI control programs since the 1930s and was based on the premise that early identification and treatment of sexual partners would have a community-wide impact. Clinicians need to gain the trust of infected persons to disclose their sexual history and then negotiate about how the partner(s) are contacted to be screened and treated in turn. PN is applied in different ways, depending on the STI identified. The care pathway for PN varies between the United States and the United Kingdom health systems. Research into patterns of sexual behavior and sexual mixing in communities and new means of treat-

ing partners will be discussed. In many cases diagnosed in the community, PN may be possible to manage outside specialist services, given some training and support. The scope for, and limitations of, partner notification for sexually transmitted infections in primary care are discussed here.

▦ PARTNER NOTIFICATION IN PRACTICE

To succeed, partner notification strategies need to obtain from the index patient details of all sex partners from whom he or she may have acquired the infection or whom he or she might have subsequently infected. These partners are then informed of the potential risk of contracting a sexually acquired infection and offered options for testing and treatment.

Three main approaches to partner notification have been developed (Mathews et al. 2006):

Provider referral uses healthcare workers to notify partners. In the United States and the United Kingdom,

---

BOX 30-1 Why Seek Out Sexual Contacts?

- Reduce risk of spread to others
- Prevent reinfection of treated patients
- Treat asymptomatic disease before complications result

BOX 30-2 Who Seeks Out the Contacts?

- The patient
- The healthcare worker
- A combination approach

PN has been handed over to specialist personnel working in public health departments (disease intervention specialists [DIS] or sexual health advisers [HA] from genitourinary medicine clinics, respectively). Standard methods of approach are adopted, combining counseling skills, giving information, and taking the sexual history. The index patient is interviewed promptly after diagnosis. Confidentiality is assured; for example, the worker does not disclose the name of the index to any named contacts. A plan of action is agreed on with the index, and the healthcare worker may text, telephone, mail, or visit named contacts to persuade them to be screened. Contact attendance is confirmed by ensuring all persons attending clinics as contacts are also referred for PN.

This process is time consuming but gives the highest success rate. Some provider referral may be feasible in primary care, depending on the workload. Smaller clinics may combine resources to use a peripatetic worker if their caseload is small.

Patient referral refers to healthcare workers encouraging index patients to notify their partners. This may be simply telling them the benefit of having partners seen and treated—an ineffective method—or supporting the index patients by coaching them about the nature of the infection and how to approach their own partners. This approach needs some knowledge of sexual infections and sexual history taking. Follow-up, also advisable, may be done by telephone.

Contract referral (or *conditional referral*) is when healthcare workers encourage index patients to notify their partners, understanding that the healthcare worker will notify those partners who do not visit the health service by an agreed date. This process is almost as effective as provider notification and is probably more cost effective for uncomplicated cases.

■ STRATEGIES IN PARTNER NOTIFICATION

From an intervention standpoint, partner notification requires an organized effort that integrates the healthcare system, providers, and the public health authori-

ties. A number of limiting factors affect the potential effectiveness of partner notification.

Should We Trace All STIs?

This depends on which disease is diagnosed. For curable STIs, PN impact partly depends on the incubation period. For example, syphilis is the prototype disease for PN, because it has the prolonged critical period during which time a patient is infected but not infectious. Therefore, during this 3-week period, public health authorities have an opportunity to prevent further transmission of infection in a sexual network. In contrast, with gonorrhea, the time course from being infected to being infectious can be less than 48 hours. Therefore, unless sexual contacts are identified and treated within a short period, gonorrhea can be difficult to control.

Partner notification may not be beneficial for chronic viral infections. In genital herpes, human papillomavirus (HPV), and other chronic viral infections, PN is largely not used because most of these infections are latent, persistent, or recurrent, with little indication of when infection may have originally occurred. Furthermore, diagnosis can be problematic, and so it is difficult to justify any further management strategies.

HIV Infection

HIV, in contrast, is unique. Partner notification has a number of objectives.

1. *Counseling opportunity*: With partner notification for HIV infection, it may not be possible to provide preventive therapy in most situations; however, PN provides the opportunity for further testing and counseling individuals who may or may not perceive themselves as at risk.

2. *Identification of latent cases*: Partner notification of HIV-infected individuals may identify approximately 10–15% of contacts who were previously undiagnosed HIV-infected individuals. This allows providers to implement public health interventions, to offer safer-sex counseling, and to track these individuals into care, which can have profound implications for the individual and for the community.

3. *Identifying unrecognized acute HIV infection*: Aggressive intervention in patients with diagnosed HIV infection may occasionally identify a contact that

is undergoing acute HIV infection. This is critical time because estimates suggest that individuals undergoing seroconversion syndrome are particularly at higher risk for further transmission of HIV within a community. In particular, individuals undergoing HIV seroconversion syndrome may have viral loads into the millions and, therefore, are highly infectious to their sexual partners.

4. *Identifying discordant partners*: Patients may have partners yet uninfected by HIV. In such serodiscordant couples, counseling in infection prevention strategies, such as consistent condom use and post-exposure prophylaxis with antiretroviral drugs after any risky encounter like a condom accident, is an essential part of management.

5. *Liability and duty to warn*: In the UK, persons newly diagnosed with HIV are strongly encouraged to discuss active disclosure of HIV status to all traceable sexual partners to avoid possible criminal liability; all such discussions need to be carefully recorded because of serious implications. In some U.S. states, knowingly exposing a sexual partner is a criminal offense, although rarely enforced. However, clinicians may have a "duty to warn" and may even consider breaking patient confidentiality if ongoing risky behavior with a known partner persists and disclosure is not made after a reasonable time (as negotiated between patient and healthcare worker). This step may put professional registration in jeopardy and is not taken lightly.

IS HIV PARTNER NOTIFICATION FOR EXPERTS?

HIV partner notification can be complex and time consuming; all known sexual partnerships from an estimated time of infection need to be traced. This intervention is best attempted by expert DIS or health advisers and should not be seen as a primary-care-level intervention.

WHAT CAN WE DO IN PRIMARY CARE?

After testing for STIs, clinicians have remember not only what to do with the positive result but also how to approach PN and treatment (Trelle et al. 2007). Even if the clinician's aim is to refer the patient to a specialist center for full management, what is said in the initial interview can be critical to the patient's understanding and complying with a chosen care pathway.

Initiating and maintaining a frank conversation with patients about their sexual behaviors and partners requires the clinician or public health worker to have extraordinary communication skills and a high level of comfort. Inexperienced physicians or nurses may be reticent for social, moral, or personal reasons to discuss sexual experiences different from their own. Patients may notice this unease and be unwilling to disclose relevant details because of embarrassment or criticism.

Training courses and distance-learning packages on sexual history taking and managing STIs can enhance interviewers' confidence. Developing skills of health education and disease prevention in this delicate area of practice may reap rewards in other areas of patient care.

WHAT DO WE TALK ABOUT?

A clinician managing STI in primary care needs to be aware that the infected person's knowledge about the disease and his or her behavior and the behavior of the sexual partner(s) are critical to any successful intervention. Sexual infections are often asymptomatic and clear health education for patients is needed to explain the disease, routes of transmission, treatment, and prevention of further infection. The discussion of an index patients' sexual history with current and past partners as possible source(s) of the infection and the risks of infection to partner(s) because of contact with the index patient then should be followed by attempts to seek out these contacts (2006 National Guidelines). The risk of reinfection from an untreated partner and consequent complications might also be useful to address at this time. Manuals of PN and guidelines for taking sexual histories are available online (http://www.ssha.info/public/manual/index.asp).

WHO NOTIFIES PARTNERS?

Who notifies partners depends on the sexual infection. For those patients needing complex interventions or protracted follow-up, as in syphilis or HIV, provider notification by DIS/HA from an expert center is still appropriate. For most patients diagnosed in the community, however, it is likely that primary care, working in association with specialist providers, could offer a holistic care package, including PN. This is especially true for chlamydia, where evidence is building that community interventions for uncomplicated disease are at least as good as sexual health clinics in PN success.

For people with chlamydia infections diagnosed in primary care, a strategy of practice-based partner notification by trained nurses with telephone follow-up by health advisers may be more effective than specialist referral. In a randomized controlled trial of 140 adults with chlamydia infection (Low et al. 2006), it was found that 47 out of 72 participants whose partners were notified by practice nurses had at least one partner treated, compared with only 39 partners out of 68 participants referred to a genitourinary clinic, where 21 participants never turned up. The cost was the same for both strategies (http://bmj.bmjjournals.com/cgi/content/full/332/7532/0-c-FIG1#FIG1). The English National Chlamydia Screening Programme (www.chlamydiascreening.nhs.uk) has shown that tracing contacts through community-based health advisers and practice nurses outside GU medicine has achieved the standards of partner recall expected by specialist services. Another option is expedited partner therapy in which, when legally possible, patients can deliver medications directly to their partners.

■ Barriers to Partner Notification in Primary Care

Lack of knowledge and time constraints are often quoted as barriers to PN in primary care. Most of these concerns can be overcome by experience and training. Practices already devote some time to managing STIs; how they use that time may change. The time to explain the referral process to a specialist clinic could be spent taking a sexual history and carrying out PN on-site. Managing contacts not registered with a practice can be overcome with community-level networking to other services and specialist centers. In the near future, novel technological interventions such as website-mediated PN- or text-(SMS) based referral may help practices in supporting patients to contact partners.

■ Commissioning Partner Notification in Primary Care—Limitations to Effectiveness

In public health settings with limited budgets, managers need to consider the costs and benefits of interventions and their effectiveness compared with other strategies. PN is an integral part of managing STIs, but this is under challenge. In modernization strategies, commissioners may consider simple case finding and treatment could be sufficient. However, incomplete PN has been shown to be a crucial factor in reinfection of those treated for chlamydia

in community settings (LaMontagne et al. 2007), with subsequent risk of complications and further transmission events. Therefore, PN is a necessary activity, but some limitations of PN have to be recognized.

■ Anonymous Sex Means PN Is Impossible

PN will be unsuccessful in settings in which partners cannot be identified. There have been particular situations in syphilis epidemics wherein large numbers of anonymous male sex partners were involved at gay sex venues or infection was associated with heterosexual crack cocaine and "sex for drugs." In both settings, identifying large numbers of sex partners was impossible because the index patients either did not know their identity or were under the influence and could not recall.

■ Illegal Activity Means PN Is Difficult

Some STI epidemic settings have been associated with high rates of illicit activity, such as drug use, commercial sex work, and immigrants. Despite health personnel who go to great lengths to demonstrate that they are not part of the governmental structure involved in police work or immigration enforcement, suspicion can influence patient perceptions about whether to cooperate with health authorities.

■ Provider-Led PN Needs Skill and Time

Although most PN can be patient led, the need for expert intervention to achieve contact tracing in certain circumstances has to be recognized. Provider-led PN requires highly trained personnel, especially trained in nonjudgmental interviewing. This can be emotionally taxing and is expensive, as most contact tracing personnel do not engage in direct patient contact but detective work. Attracting, training, and retaining a core of expert DIS/HA workers within a sexual health clinical service area is an expensive but essential core requirement for disseminating basic PN skills into primary care.

■ Research Developments and Alternative Approaches to Traditional Partner Notification

Expedited/Accelerated Partner Management

A major role of partner notification has been to identify individuals who may be potentially infected and to bring them in for treatment. A novel and effective means of achieving this is expedited partner therapy (EPT), which has been evaluated in the United States in a number of venues. Under this scenario, index patients who are diagnosed within the healthcare setting are provided with medications to deliver to their partners, offering treatment without prior testing (Centers for Disease Control and Prevention 2006). EPT may be useful for gonorrhea and chlamydia treatment because this can be done with nontoxic, oral, single-dose medications. Variations of EPT acceptable within the English legal system have been piloted with successful outcomes (Sutcliffe et al. 2009). Clearly, EPT approaches would not work well for syphilis or other infections in which injections or courses of therapy are required. The status of EPT is changing—it is legal in about half of the U.S. states but is still not practiced in the UK.

An informal approach to EPT could be to arrange with local pharmacies where trained pharmacists could give therapy for chlamydia or gonorrhea based on the presentation of a treatment note given to the contact via the index case. This process is open to abuse by personation—wherein a noneligible person obtains treatment—and misses any opportunity for identifying other STIs in the partner. It could be practical in areas where pharmacy-based sexual health services are being developed, as in the National Health Service (NHS) in England.

Finally, partner notification characterizes traditional public health outreach efforts that have been extended to a number of areas. In particular, PN is the STI equivalent of directly observed therapy, which is seen in tuberculosis. More recently, directly observed therapy approaches have also been used on HIV infection in identifying individuals at high risk for HIV complications and nonadherence, providing outreach efforts to support medication adherence.

Social Network Approaches

Because of known and recognized outcome issues in partner notification with traditional approaches, other authorities have suggested using a social network approach to ensure treatment of partners. The social network approach consider a number of known epidemiological characteristics of STI epidemics. These include the following:

Core transmitters: Most STI epidemics are propagated by a small group of individuals with high rates of sexual partner turnover. This group is known as the "core," which is seen as the major target group in im-

plementing STI prevention interventions. Sometimes, these individuals can be clearly identified, such as commercial sex workers in syphilis epidemics or long-distance truck drivers in propagating the HIV epidemic in sub-Saharan Africa and Asia. The distribution of STIs such as gonorrhea may be concentrated into certain neighborhoods, and mapping the case distribution can allow for focused interventions in those specific areas. Nevertheless, in many situations, core members cannot be conclusively identified.

Places of social significance, or *"hot spots"*: Another well-known factor in STI epidemics is that there are usually community venues that are clearly identified as important for propagating STIs. These may be geographically identified neighborhoods with high prevalence of gonococcal or chlamydial infections or cases of syphilis and HIV. A large amount of data suggest that "places of social significance" have an important role. These venues could gay bars, bathhouses, or even truck stops or parks.

Alternative approaches—networks: Recognizing that a small group of individuals operating within a known venue or definable demographic maintain STI transmission, STI epidemiologists have suggested that, in an alternative approach to the "sexual network" or, in other words, the traditional partner notification strategy, would be identifying and treating a "social" network. A social network approach considers that individuals, friends, and acquaintances are often similar to their sexual partners, and therefore, it may be more efficient to identify sexual networks through the social networks surrogate approach. The disadvantage of this approach is that it does require a new theoretical approach to understanding partner notification and does not result in definable outcomes, which may have some evaluation problems from the standpoint of public health authorities.

In all of these new approaches, evaluation with definable outcomes can be hard to achieve; comparative trials of different approaches are rare.

▨ BARRIERS TO EFFECTIVE IMPLEMENTATION OF PARTNER SERVICES

From an intervention standpoint, partner notification really requires an organized effort, which integrates the healthcare system, providers, and the public health authorities. There are a number of important barriers to full implementation of partner notification.

Resources: PN is an extremely resource-intensive strategy. Budget considerations often preclude implementation of adequate resources to ensure good impact.

Anonymous partners: PN has been unsuccessful in settings where partners cannot be identified.

Illicit activity settings: Some patients engage in illicit activity, in particular drug use, which can influence patient perceptions to cooperate or not to cooperate with the health authorities.

Underlying disease epidemiology and practical concerns: PN effectiveness, even when fully implemented, depends on the incubation period. For example, syphilis is the prototype disease for PN, because it has the prolonged critical period during which time a patient is infected but not infectious. Therefore, during this 3-week period, public health authorities have an opportunity to prevent further transmission of infection in a sexual network.

In contrast, gonorrhea is difficult to control because the time course from being infected to being infectious can be less than 48 hours. Therefore, unless sexual contacts are "surrounded" and treated within a very short period, gonorrhea can be difficult to control. Experience bears this out. Trying to impact the spread of antibiotic-resistant gonorrhea has largely failed on multiple levels and on multiple contents, because identifying contacts is difficult.

CONCLUSION

Partner notification for sexually transmitted infections has been seen as a public health function delegated away from primary care at diagnosis. Community-based screening programs for genital chlamydia infections have now challenged that model of care. Screening site personnel can be trained and supported by specialist staff to offer holistic sexual health care, including PN to anyone found positive. This option appears to be effective in uncomplicated cases as long as follow-up is completed, is popular with patients, and may be more cost effective than the specialist services. There will remain a need to have DIS/HA support for other STIs, for vulnerable index patients in which anonymity is essential or when the index patient is unwilling to approach their partners.

Providing PN in primary care offers rare opportunities to counsel and support patients in a sensitive area of their lives at a time of crisis, protects others in the community from the risk of infection and complications,

and enhances the communication skills and knowledge base of the clinicians providing it. This new skills area can seem daunting at first but is clearly rewarding for the clinician, the patient, and the community.

KEY POINTS

- "Partner notification" describes a range of supportive interventions at the time of diagnosis and treatment of a sexually transmitted infection to help patients get their partners tested and treated.

- Partner notification of HIV and syphilis require expert intervention, involving disease intervention specialists in United States or health advisers in the UK.

- Most PN for uncomplicated STIs can be commenced in community settings by nonspecialist staff, supported by expert practitioners, coaching patients.

- Follow-up of initial interventions is essential to confirm partner treatment and assess risk of reinfection; skilled practitioners may do this by telephone interview.

REFERENCES

Annual reports of the NCSP in England. November 2004–8. Department of Health. Downloaded at www.chlamydia screening.nhs.uk.

CDC. Recommendations for partner services programs for HIV infection, syphilis, gonorrhea, and chlamydial infection. *Morb Mortal Week Rep.* 2008 Nov 7;57(RR-9):1–83; quiz CE1–4.

Centers for Disease Control and Prevention. *Expedited Partner Therapy in the Management of Sexually Transmitted Diseases*. Atlanta, GA: US Department of Health and Human Services; 2006.

French P on behalf of BASHH. 2006 national guidelines—consultations requiring sexual history-taking. *Int J STD AIDS.* 2007;18(1):17–22.

Hogben M, McNally T, McPheeters M, Hutchinson AB. The effectiveness of HIV partner counseling and referral services in increasing identification of HIV-positive individuals a systematic review. *Am J Prev Med.* 2007;33(2)(suppl):S89–100.

LaMontagne DS, Baster K, Emmett L, et al. Incidence and reinfection rates of genital chlamydial infection among women aged 16–24 years attending general practice, family planning and genitourinary medicine clinics in England:

a prospective cohort study by the Chlamydia Recall Study Advisory Group. *Sex Transm Infect.* 2007;83:292–303.

Low N, McCarthy A, Roberts TE, et al. Partner notification of chlamydia infection in primary care: randomised controlled trial and analysis of resource use. *BMJ.* 2006;7;332(7532):14–19.

The manual for sexual health advisers. http://www.ssha.info/public/manual/index.asp. Accessed October 12, 2009.

Mathews C, Coetzee N, Zwarenstein M, et al. Strategies for partner notification for sexually transmitted diseases. *Cochrane Database Syst Rev.* 2006;1.

National Institute for Health and Clinical Excellence. Public Health Intervention Guidance PH1003. Preventing sexually transmitted infections and reducing under 18 conceptions: guidance. February 27, 2007. http://www.nice.org.uk/Guidance/PH3. Accessed October 12, 2009.

NHS Quality Improvement Scotland. Scottish standards—sexual health. March 2008. http://www.nhshealthquality.org/nhsqis/files/SEXHEALTHSERV_STANF_MAR08.pdf.

Sutcliffe L, Brook MG, Chapman JL, Cassell JM, Estcourt CE. Is accelerated partner therapy a feasible and acceptable strategy for rapid partner notification in the UK? a qualitative study of genitourinary medicine clinic attenders. *Int J STD AIDS.* 2009;20:603–606.

Trelle S, Shang A, Nartey L, Cassell JA, Low N. Improved effectiveness of partner notification for patients with sexually transmitted infections: systematic review. *Br Med J.* 2007. doi: 10.1136/bmj.39079.460741.7C.

31

Counseling the Patient with Genital HSV Infection

Terri Warren

INTRODUCTION

Many clinicians think genital herpes is a minor albeit annoying medical problem, but nonmedical people do not view herpes in the same way. In a telephone survey, conducted by the American Social Health Association in 2004, 96% of randomly called respondents said they would find a diagnosis of HIV infection "very traumatic," and not far behind, 68% of patients gave the same response about receiving a diagnosis of genital herpes. In comparison, 54% found breaking up with a significant other "very traumatic," and 51% said the same about getting fired from their job (Gilbert et al. 2005). Genital herpes can have a remarkable effect on people's lives, even though its physical symptoms are often limited. At this writing, about 1 in 4 people older than age of 18 years in the United States are infected with herpes simplex virus type 2 (HSV-2) and of those infected, almost 90% don't know it. So the infection is very common and mostly unrecognized by both patients and clinicians. However, with increased availability and utilization of type-specific antibody testing (TSST) for HSV-2, more cases of herpes will be coming to the attention of clinicians.

When a diagnosis of genital herpes is made, patients need information and support. We have traditionally put these two things together under *herpes counseling*. The first, what might be called *medical counseling*, is just providing information about their infection. Topics here include the wide range of possible herpes symptoms, recurrence expectations, transmission to partners and strategies for transmission reduction, medication

options, and asymptomatic viral shedding. The second kind of counseling deals more with the emotional aspects of having herpes; its impact on sexuality, self-esteem, and social interactions with others. Both kinds of counseling are important, and one without the other leaves gaps in essential areas for patients to have a full understanding of their infection and to come to terms with what it means in their lives. Herpes is never just a medical diagnosis alone nor an emotional diagnose—it is always both.

There are some significant patient and clinician roadblocks to herpes counseling. Gilbert et al. (2005), in a study of patient's perceptions of the adequacy of counseling, identified some common barriers that patients perceived while discussing herpes with their clinician. The most common one listed by 57% of respondents was embarrassment. If you are going to talk about genital herpes, you have to talk about sex; both past and future sex acts. Discussing sex with people you know well is difficult enough, but discussing it with a clinician you may not know well or who, in the past, has only dealt with nonsexual issues like your blood pressure, is even harder. For example, people who have same-gender partners may never have raised this issue with their clinician in the past. But now, the gender of sex partners needs to come up for an accurate diagnosis and guidance about transmission reduction. A difficult topic is the specific sexual behaviors that could transmit infection in the future, such as oral and anal sex and who can do what with whom involving various body parts while minimizing transmission risk. Twenty-four percent of patients described time constraints as an obstacle to talking with their clinician. Clinicians may have time limitations. Patients may feel awkward or guilty when asking questions that take up too much time. Because herpes is a complex issue, patients often feel unprepared to deal with all issues raised by this infection, particularly if they are having a first infection. They are often too surprised or saddened to be able to formulate good questions at the time of a first diagnosis.

Clinicians also feel barriers to counseling. The physician, nurse practitioner, or physician assistant who has patients waiting to be seen in other exam rooms may feel the time constraint more acutely than the herpes patient. The 10-minute, uncomplicated UTI appointment, a patient scheduled because of painful urination evolves into a first-episode herpes infection, can throw off a schedule in no time. Though the clinician may want to take the time to address the patients' questions, they also need to respect other people, who are also waiting to be seen. Keeping abreast of all the latest information about herpes can also be challenging. When clinicians have to stay up to date on diabetes, hypertension, respiratory problems, birth control, cancer treatments, and so forth, herpes updating can fall through the cracks. No clinician likes to talk about a subject about which he or she is ill informed. While patients may be upset by this diagnosis, clinicians are distressed by the lack of a cure and find the emotionally charged response to this STI difficult to handle and may, in fact, dread the interaction in which the diagnosis must be given. Clinicians have a completely different perspective about herpes than their patient. When the clinician schedule includes a young mother with breast cancer, a teenager with uncontrolled asthma, a gentleman with a blood pressure of 190/120, the distress of the herpes patient may appear medically disproportionate. The patient receiving the herpes diagnosis does not have the benefit of the broader perspective; they have only their own life situation and their imagined bleak future with a lifelong, highly stigmatized STI about which they know nothing. Advising patients to "get a grip, there are worse things," does little to improve their situation; it only distances patients from their clinicians.

Let's assume the clinician has plenty of time, is really up to date on the latest information about herpes, has a patient eager to learn about their infection, and the clinician wants to do the counseling (rather than refer the patient to someone else, which is also a legitimate option). What messages are important to share with the patient and what do patients want to know?

■ PREVALENCE AND NATURAL HISTORY

The medical counseling (or information sharing) could start with the prevalent nature of the infection, that 1 in 4 adults (United States), or 1 in 10 (United Kingdom) has HSV-2 but most have no clue about their infection. A study by Fleming et al. (1997) found that women are 45% more likely to be infected than men, mostly because of vulnerable anatomy during intercourse. Due to the natural motion of intercourse, a virus is quite likely to penetrate the mucous membrane of the vagina. However, a penis approximating a labial lesion intermittently during intercourse is much less likely to acquire the same virus.

People in all life situations are vulnerable to acquiring genital herpes; people who are well educated, who live in both the inner city and affluent suburbs, and of all races and ethnicities can be infected with HSV-2. Having more sex partners does put someone at greater risk of infection, but a person can be infected after having only one partner, even by receiving only oral sex, or participating in "outercourse" and never having penetrative intercourse.

Patients need to know that HSV is a recurrent infection; it will most likely come back, and there is currently no cure for herpes. However, it may be better to avoid the word *incurable* and to substitute *lifelong*. Incurable has a scary meaning for most patients. HSV-2 genital infection will recur significantly more often than HSV-1 genitally, with type 2 genitally recurring about four to six times per year and HSV-1 genitally recurring less than once per year. About 20% of people with HSV-2 will have 10 or more recurrences per year. Should someone acquire HSV-2 orally, it rarely recurs nor is it shed often from the skin of the healthy adult. The good news is that recognizable outbreaks of genital HSV-2 decrease in frequency over time in most people. Recent research has show that people probably shed less virus over time, but for some people, extensive shedding continues for many years.

■ ASYMPTOMATIC SHEDDING

Patients must be told that herpes virus can be shed from the body when they have no symptoms, which is called asymptomatic viral shedding. This is probably the most difficult news for herpes patients to hear. There is no day that patients can say to their sex partner, "Today I know I will not infect you." We know more about asymptomatic viral shedding through an investigative process called *daily home swabbing*. Patients who enrolled in herpes research studies were taught to swab their genitalia at home, with a specific and standardized technique, on a daily basis, for some extended period (2, 4, or 6 months). People who are newly diagnosed will shed virus quite often, around 42% of the days sampled so they are most infectious to others during the early days of their infection. Patients with HSV-2, including those with newer and more established infections, will shed, on average, about 8–28% of the days swabbed. People with genital HSV-1, a common cause of first-episode infection, shed significantly less, one-third the rate of HSV-2 shedding.

Another approach was to study couples in which one partner was infected with HSV-2 and the other was not (a discordant couple, in herpes lingo). Seventy percent of new cases of genital herpes in this study were transmitted at a time when the infected person had no recognized symptoms. In the valacyclovir transmission trial (Corey 2004), about half the transmissions that occurred between discordant couples, happened when the infecting person had no symptoms at all. Patients need to understand, believe, and accept information about asymptomatic viral shedding as the cornerstone for understanding their herpes infection. If they do, they will have the greatest opportunity to reduce the risk of transmitting herpes to future partners. Clinicians and patients both must move beyond focusing on outbreaks to focusing on underlying infection if they are to have any impact on the frequency of new infections. A good model for understanding this concept is hypertension. We wouldn't know that patients had high blood pressure unless we monitored it (similar conceptually to herpes antibody testing), and patients wouldn't know their blood pressure was elevated, just by how they felt during the day (similar conceptually to asymptomatic shedding). For the patients who respond that they "know their body" and would know when they were shedding, I would ask, "Do you think people can tell from their body when their blood pressure is really elevated, or do you think they would simply know some situations might cause their blood pressure to rise?" The same is true for viral shedding—patients might know they were shedding during outbreaks but cannot be aware of times between, when shedding might be occurring without symptoms.

With the improved quality of herpes antibody tests and their increased availability, clinicians will identify many more patients who test positive for HSV 2 by blood test but cannot recall ever having any symptoms of genital herpes. These patients will very likely shed virus from their genital tract, with or without symptoms. This provides strong motivation for testing and identifying those who are infected but do not know it. It also tells us that herpes is not about outbreaks, it is about underlying infection. Moreover, truly asymptomatic infection is uncommon. In this same study, after careful instruction about the subtleties of herpes symptoms and their potential locations, 87% of those who were infected but "asymptomatic," learned to identify a symptom consistent with herpes by the end of 2 months of daily home swabbing.

■ TREATMENTS

Although shedding and recurrences are not good news for patients, there are effective treatments for herpes. These treatments can change the frequency of recurrences, duration of outbreaks, and reduce transmission to others. Daily antiviral therapy reduces the frequency of recurrences by about 75%. Medication taken at the start of a recurrent outbreak reduces the duration of pain, viral shedding, and lesions by 1–2 days, though most patients in one study appear to prefer daily therapy. There are many easy options for dosing herpes medication—one-day treatment is effective for treating herpes outbreaks and once daily suppressive therapy is available for the person who chooses that option, making treatment more convenient and compliance improved in both situations.

There are several ways to reduce the risk of transmitting herpes to sex partners, and patients are eager to hear about the various options and their effectiveness. In discordant couples, a large study demonstrated that transmission was reduced by 48% when the infected person took 500 mg of valacyclovir therapy once daily. Adding regular condom use can cut the risk of transmission even more significantly, by about 30–50%. Suppressive antivirals and condom use can provide a psychological benefit as well. Because transmission of this infection is a major concern among those who have herpes, an effective method to reduce transmission is important to patients: They feel proactive and have some control over their infectiousness. People with recurrent genital herpes who start on daily suppression had significantly reduced illness concern and anxiety.

Medications for genital herpes are acyclovir, valacyclovir, and famciclovir. These nucleoside analogs are demonstrated to be safe and effective when taken daily over long periods. Neither laboratory tests nor drug holidays are necessary while patients are on long-term therapy. Drug holidays, in the discordant couple, afford an opportunity for transmission. However, in patients who have a creatinine clearance of less than 50, it may be necessary to reduce the dose of antiviral medication (see package inserts for these medications).

■ PREGNANCY

Women with herpes should be counseled that they can definitely have healthy babies. Transmission rates from women who are HSV-2 antibody positive at the time of delivery, in the absence of symptoms, is less than 1%. The incidence is even lower in the United Kingdom. However, women who are antibody negative and acquire HSV-1 or HSV-2 genitally in the third trimester are at greatest risk of infecting their newborns: 30–50% of those shedding at term will do so. Susceptible women who have infected partners should be carefully counseled about abstinence and condom use to reduce transmission to the neonate. Infected men who are concerned about passing herpes to their partner while trying to impregnate them should be offered suppressive therapy to reduce the risk of transmission during the procreation process.

Testing for herpes in pregnancy is controversial, and there are strong feelings on both sides of this issue. Neonatal herpes is not reportable in most states or European countries and accurate statistics are not easily available about the frequency of infection. Until those numbers are available, it is difficult to assess the actual effect of testing and treating more pregnant women and their partners. It is often helpful to offer serologic testing to partners of patients who are infected with genital herpes. Because almost 90% of those infected with HSV-2 do not know it, couples that think they are discordant (one infected and the other not) are often not discordant. When both partners have accurately been diagnosed with the same type of virus (i.e., both have HSV-1 or both have HSV-2), they do not need to be concerned about getting each other's virus or triggering outbreaks through sex. Though there is more than one strain of each serotype, transmission of other types appears to be rare. They can feel free to enjoy sex without genital herpes as a factor in their relationship.

■ SEROLOGICAL TYPING

The Centers for Disease Control and Prevention in the STD Treatment Guidelines (2010) and recent British Association for Sexual Health and HIV (BASHH) Guidelines have all said typing herpes tests (i.e., de-

termining whether the virus is HSV-1 or HSV-2) was essential, yet some clinicians still don't ask for typing of swab tests and fail to see a benefit in knowing the serotype of a genital lesion. As discussed earlier, HSV-1 and HSV-2 have different recurrence rates in the genitals. Someone with HSV-1 is still susceptible to getting HSV-2 genitally. Couples should be made aware of their viral type so that they can better understand how they became infected. Couples who believe they have been exclusively monogamous their whole lives will be greatly upset with a diagnosis of genital herpes, questioning each other's fidelity. But in the United States and in Western Europe, HSV-1 causes more than one-third of primary genital herpes cases. Therefore, if the viral isolate is typed as HSV-1, and the couple participates in oral sex, then transmission within their own completely monogamous relationship is a plausible and parsimonious explanation and that knowledge may help to save or repair a previously good relationship. HSV-1 can be and often is shed from the mouth in the absence of symptoms, just as HSV-2 can be shed from the genitals asymptomatically. A cold sore need not be present for oral-to-genital transmission to occur.

Patients should be made aware that, usually, genital herpes infections have no long-term impact on general health. Two exceptions are increased HIV-acquisition risk and neonatal herpes infection. A person with HSV-2 genital infection has triple the risk of acquiring HIV, should they be exposed. Recent data suggest that HIV transmission is more likely in the person who is coinfected with both HSV-2 and HIV; however, modification of this particular risk is not amenable to HSV suppressive therapy.

■ PSYCHOSOCIAL ISSUES

The medical counseling issues described earlier are fairly straightforward. The psychosocial issues raised by a diagnosing genital herpes are more complicated, more difficult to discuss, more time consuming, and more problematic for herpes patients in the long run.

People newly diagnosed with genital herpes may not listen very well. Their initial emotions include shock, fear, denial, guilt, grief, blame, and confusion. It may be helpful to say, after some concise herpes messages are given, "I know there are so many questions on your mind right now. We can get together again in a few weeks for a follow-up visit, but right now, can you share with me your number one concern?" This will help them focus down a bit and allow you to help them with their most immediate need, even in a time-pressured situation.

Listed here are the most common questions that arise at the diagnostic visit and suggestions about responding.

1. *Who gave this to me and how long have I had it?* If they have had more than one partner in their lifetime, this may not be answerable. Consider the timing of their last sexual contact as it relates to the presentation of symptoms or testing. If the sexual contact occurred more than 2 weeks before symptoms developed, then the current symptoms are not likely related to that sexual contact. Genital herpes symptoms most always present within 2–14 days after infection, though certainly not everyone who is recently infected develops recognizable symptoms at that time. Suggest that your patient ask his or her current partner to get a type-specific serology test (TSST). If a partner is positive for the same type, that does not necessarily mean the infection came from that person, but if the partner is negative, then he or she is an unlikely source of the infection. For example, if your patient has a positive PCR swab test for HSV-2 and the HSV-2 TSST is negative, then the patient has an episode infection—the virus is present on the skin but not enough time has passed to make antibodies. A baseline serology combined with the swab test can help clarify how long someone has been infected. Similarly, if this is the first time the patient has recognized a herpes symptom, the swab test is positive for HSV-2 and the antibody test is strongly positive for HSV 2, then the infection is not new but a recurrence. Up to a third of patients experiencing a first-recognized outbreak have antibody already to that same serotype, indicating that this would be a recurrence, not a first infection. It is best never to make statements about a new infection or an old infection without laboratory confirmation, regardless of the clinical presentation. Such statements involve not only a medical question but also a relationship one as well and can be complicated. You cannot tell by looking whether someone has a new or an old infection nor can you tell whether it is type 1 or type 2 by looking—both types look the same.

2. *Can I ever have children or father children? Can I ever have sex again?* The answer is, of course, a resounding yes. Women should be reassured that, if their obstetric care providers know about the her-

pes, babies can be safely carried and delivered with an incredibly low risk of complications. Men with herpes can certainly father children, and if on suppression, the risk of infecting their female partner is probably low. For even less risk of transmission, especially for the fearful, artificial insemination is an option. A full and rewarding sex life is still possible. Yes, adjustments will need to be made. Potential sex partners should be told about herpes and tested if their HSV status is unknown. Risk reduction strategies will be useful if the couple is discordant—daily suppressive antiviral medicine, condom use, symptom recognition skills, and an open dialogue about the issue.

3. *Did my partner cheat on me for me to get this?* Anger is often present at the first visit. Questions about fidelity quickly come up. Patients should be reassured that they could have had herpes for a long time and not known it or that the partner could have been infected for a long time, with or without knowing it and recently infected them. Or if they give and receive oral sex as a couple, the herpes could be genital type 1 as a result of sex practices within their relationship. A third party could have been involved, but it is best not to jump to that conclusion when other reasonable explanations are possible.

4. *Can I give this to other people?* If you strongly suspect herpes, even as you wait for the lab results, transmission should be discussed right away. Patients need to know that they could be infectious with and without symptoms.

As you conclude the visit, medicines should be prescribed if new herpes is suspected before the lab results come back. Provide resources for patients to learn about herpes. You do not have to provide all of the education, just point patients in the right direction for additional help. Be ready with a list of good books, accurate Web sites, videos (if you have them), and toll-free phone numbers for herpes support groups, especially local ones, if you have them in your town. (Look them up on ashastd.org, bashh.org, ihmf.org.) Patients will be hungry for information that you may not have time to provide. Finally, at that first visit, clearly state that herpes does not change the core of who the patients are. It does not make them less worthwhile or "damaged goods."

Follow-up visits allow you to talk with patients in-depth because an appointment time has been set aside, specifically for education and discussion. Typical topics that come up during follow-up visits include transmission reduction, asymptomatic viral shedding, telling future partners about herpes, self-esteem, and sexual functioning related to transmission concerns. Medication options should be discussed at this time. Recent studies suggest benefits obtained from early use of suppressive therapy, or patients may choose to get a prescription to treat outbreaks only or opt for no medication until some time passes and they gain more experience about how herpes affects them. Some patients will experience high levels of anxiety or depression related to the diagnosis of HSV. Patients should be encouraged to tell at least one other person about their herpes—this can be a lonely secret to carry. Referrals to therapists who counsel patients with herpes will be useful. For billing for medical services, based charge on time spent, not complexity of the visit.

Patients often ask about stress and its relationship to herpes outbreaks. Studies have found mixed results on this issue.

Finally, say something good for your patients to hold on to when they leave, something to read or a video to watch at home. Remind patients that having herpes is not a judgment; it is simply a viral infection. The virus didn't do a personality inventory or check the number of past sexual partners a person had before it invaded a cell. It just invaded a cell. Making this concept clear may be one of the most effective tools to help people with this infect to accept themselves.

Clinicians can make a significant difference in how people adjust to herpes. With practice, the herpes counseling message can be concise, useful, and kind. Patients will benefit greatly when time is spent addressing these challenging issues.

■ KEY POINTS

- An accurate and type-specific diagnosis is the foundation for living with genital herpes.

- People with genital herpes can live full, sexually active lives, can bear children, and can find partners who will love them fully.

- Medicines are available that can reduce outbreak frequency, reduce risk of transmission to others, reduce viral shedding, and shorten recurrences.

- Herpes is common and largely unrecognized or misdiagnosed.

- Clinicians should ideally provide both medical information and psychological support for this diagnosis to patients.

- The only two significant medical problems associated with herpes is increased risk of HIV acquisition and neonatal herpes.

■ ACKNOWLEDGMENT

With thanks to Dr. Rajul Patel for contributions and editorial comment and to Dr. Raj Patel, FRCP, Consultant , GUM/HIV, Senior Lecturer, University of Southampton, Royal South Hants Hospital, Southampton, United Kingdom.

REFERENCES

Ashley RL. Performance and use of HSV type-specific serology test kits. *Herpes*. 2002;9(2):38–45.

Brentjens MH, Yeung-Yue KA, Lee PC, Tyring S. Recurrent genital herpes treatments and their impact on quality of life. *Pharmacoeconomics*. 2003;21(12):853–863.

CDC. STD treatment guidelines, 2010. *Morb Mort Week Rep*. 2010;59(RR-12):1–110.

Celum C, Levine R, Weaver M, Wald A. Genital herpes and human immunodeficiency virus: double trouble. *Bull World Health Organ*. 2004;82(6):447–453.

Corey L, Wald A. Maternal and neonatal herpes simplex virus infections. *N Engl J Med*. 2009;361(14):1376–1385.

Corey L, Wald A, Patel R, et al.; Valacyclovir HSV Transmission Study Group. Once-daily valacyclovir to reduce the risk of transmission of genital herpes. *N Engl J Med*. 2004;350(1):11–20.

Fleming DT, McQuillan GM, Johnson RE, et al. Herpes simplex virus type 2 in the United States, 1976 to 1994. *N Engl J Med*. 1997;337(16):1105–1111.

Gilbert L, Scanlon K, Peterson R, Ebel C. Patient and partner perceptions about preventing genital herpes transmission. *Herpes*. 2005 Dec;12(3):60–65.

Gupta R, Wald A, Krantz E,. Valacyclovir and acyclovir for suppression of shedding of herpes simplex virus in the genital tract. *J Infect Dis*. 2004;190(8):1374–1381.

Gupta R, Warren T, Wald A. Genital herpes. *Lancet*. 2007;370 (9605):2127–2137.

Herpes on-line toolkit. http://www.ashastd.org/herpes/herpes_toolkit/.

Schiffer JT, Abu-Raddad L, Mark KE, et al. Frequent release of low amounts of herpes simplex virus from neurons: results of a mathematical model. *Sci Transl Med*. 2009;1(7):7ra16.

Sen P, Barton SE. Genital herpes and its management [review]. *BMJ*. 2007;334(7602):1048–1052.

Tyring SK, Baker D, Snowden W. Valacyclovir for herpes simplex virus infection: long-term safety and sustained efficacy after 20 years' experience with acyclovir. *J Infect Dis*. 2002;186(suppl 1):S40–S46.

Wald A, Zeh J, Selke S, et al. Reactivation of genital herpes simplex virus type 2 infections in asymptomatic seropositive persons. *N Engl J Med*. 2000;342:844–850.

Warren T, Ebel C. Counseling the patient who has genital herpes or genital human papillomavirus infection. *Infect Dis Clin North Am*. 2005;19(2):459–476.

Xu F, Sternberg MR, Kottiri BJ, et al. Trends in herpes simplex virus type 1 and type 2 seroprevalence in the United States. *JAMA*. 2006;296(8):964–973.

32

Counseling the Patient with Genital HPV Infection

Allison Friedman, Charles Ebel, and Raymond Maw

▣ INTRODUCTION: GENITAL HPV INFECTION

Issues that complicate counseling for herpes patients (see Chapter 31) also have relevance for persons diagnosed with genital human papillomavirus (HPV). The sexually transmitted nature of the infection, the ongoing potential for asymptomatic transmission, the lack of curative treatment for the underlying viral infection, and the lack of a highly effective prevention strategy for future sex partners—all potential stressors to those diagnosed with genital HPV types. Clinicians often characterize psychosocial issues as the most difficult aspect of management for those who test positive for HPV. In the context of cervical cancer screening, patients' emotional reactions to an HPV diagnosis have been noted to divert attention from discussing needed follow-up care for cervical cancer prevention.

An HPV diagnosis also carries with it additional counseling and education challenges stemming from the scientific complexity of HPV and the uncertainty of the future course of infection. Until recently, the dearth of appropriate patient educational materials and the widespread lack of HPV awareness among the public and patients have only added to these challenges. While recent public health efforts, industry advertising, availability of effective vaccines, and media attention have raised general HPV awareness and changed the social landscape in which HPV is understood by the public and by patients, most women still have little knowledge about HPV. HPV knowledge remains lowest among women who may be at highest risk for cervical cancer.

An estimated 50–80% of sexually active adults are infected with genital HPV at some point in their lives. Annual incidence of genital HPV infection in the United States, including both high- and low-risk types, is estimated at 6.2 million among Americans 15–44 years of age. Prevalence nationwide, based on the most recent published data, is estimated at 26.8% among females between the ages of 14 and 59 years, with the highest prevalence in the 20- to 24-year-old age group. While only a small proportion of these infections are high risk and progress to cervical cancer, in 2005, there were approximately 12,000 cases of invasive cervical cancer in the United States. Meanwhile, external genital warts (EGW), which are usually associated with low-risk HPV types 6 and 11, remain one of the leading lesion-causing sexually transmitted infections (STIs). An estimated 1% of sexually active adults have visible genital warts at any point in time.

The availability of safe and effective HPV vaccines now offers the potential to reduce the future number of patients diagnosed with genital warts and cervical dysplasia. Declines in genital warts cases have been reported in countries that have implemented national vaccination programs. At the same time, however, there is an increased need for effective HPV education and counseling as the use of HPV DNA testing expands for cervical cancer screening and management and as new HPV vaccines become available to larger segments of the population (see Chapter 6). Providers are the primary and most trusted source of HPV information for patients and the public. They can alleviate patient concerns, offer needed psychological support, clarify confusing issues, facilitate informed decision making about treatment and partner management, and promote adherence to recommended follow-up.

■ PSYCHOSOCIAL ASPECTS OF GENITAL HPV DIAGNOSIS

The psychosocial impact of genital HPV has been examined by a number of investigators. Historically, an HPV diagnosis has been characterized in much the same way as a genital herpes diagnosis, provoking emotional patient reactions such as anger and shame, and concerns about partner rejection and social isolation because of having a potentially chronic viral infection. This is perhaps especially true of genital warts, a diagnosis that may be experienced as embarrassing and shocking and may elicit fear, guilt, and perceived stigma. The psychological distress associated with genital warts has been noted in several studies to outweigh the actual medical consequences of the condition. Patients with genital warts have reported low self- and sexual esteem, depression, concerns about rejection, and sexual anxiety. Patient self-esteem and self-image may be particularly affected when warts are recurring or disfiguring. The potential psychosexual impact becomes more severe with higher numbers of treatments, more painful techniques, and more extensive scarring.

In the context of cervical cancer screening, an overwhelming majority of studies suggests that HPV has an adverse psychosocial impact, with increased anxiety, distress, and concern about sexual relationships, at least in the short term. The sexually transmitted nature of HPV can introduce feelings of stigma, anger and shame, and partner concerns about infidelity. Some data suggest that concerns about partner infidelity may be less salient for older women with high educational status, who are confident their relationships are monogamous. The diagnosis of HPV can compound the distress and fear already associated with borderline or abnormal Pap test results, eliciting confusion and anxiety about the many unknowns of HPV. Paradoxically, confusion, anxiety, and distress about screening test results have been shown to reduce the likelihood of follow-up; yet research suggests that clear, accurate information delivered in a nonstigmatizing manner can resolve many of these patient concerns.

The counseling challenge is likely to be greater with persistent HPV. A second HPV-positive test result appears to be more distressing than the first, even after women have been informed about HPV and overcome their initial anxiety and distress. This second positive result may make the prospect of cancer more real to patients, as their hopes or expectations of HPV regression are not met.

Studies suggest that a genital warts diagnosis may create tension between partners in existing relationships and impact aspects of a patient's sexual self-concept (including sexual desirability) and levels of sexual satisfaction. Different stages of diagnosis and treatment may differentially affect the patient and his or her relationship. The diagnosis often raises questions about fidelity, causing suspicions on the part of both the diagnosed patient and his or her partner. Patients whose HPV infection strongly suggests partner infidelity, who are single, and who had some form of sexual dysfunction before HPV diagnosis may be more vulnerable to sexual impairments from HPV. Patients have also reported sexual impairments following treatment of genital warts, resulting from their physical condition, pain during intercourse, forced condom use, or fear of infecting their partner. Fear of transmission to partners is one of the more common concerns among HPV-positive patients.

It is not surprising that HPV has been found to cause patient anxiety about disclosure and fear of rejection. For many patients, it may be difficult to understand that their current partner may actually have been the source of infection, even in the absence of symptoms. Keller and colleagues (2002) found that while more than half of HPV-positive persons believed that they should disclose their diagnosis to future sex partners, only 31% of them actually reported doing so. It may be that HPV disclosure is more likely to occur in the context of current relationships, particularly long-lasting relationships. Despite patient worries about partner rejection, studies suggest that HPV disclosure rarely results in rejection or a negative impact on sexual relations, and that those in relationships who have disclosed their HPV report more positive feelings of sexual self-concept.

■ PATIENT INFORMATION NEEDS

Gilbert and colleagues (2003) analyzed the most frequently asked questions received through the American Social Health Association's National HPV and Cervical Cancer Resource Center. This list is generally consistent with other studies describing patients' immediate concerns following an HPV diagnosis and can provide guidance on what types of counseling messages are needed. The major questions included those about transmission and potential for transmission to partners, the potential for nonsexual transmission to casual contacts, availability of testing for HPV, treatment options, and risk to newborn children. It reflects patients' attempts to identify the source and duration of their infection; to find out whether their partner can be tested for HPV; to understand the likelihood of HPV transmission to new partners; and to seek recommendations regarding future prevention, disclosure, treatment, and follow-up care. The large numbers of questions about testing and treatment indicates a substantial need for providing information in these areas, recognizing that the issues are highly complex and not amenable to simple answers.

With genital warts, both patients and their partners can benefit from informative counseling, including discussion of potential psychological or sexual issues. Addressing some of the potential challenges or misunderstandings within a relationship and offering practical suggestions to overcome both the physical and emotional problems can help patients and their partners cope.

With cervical cancer screening, women may have difficulty comprehending a diagnosis of "high-risk" HPV without first knowing what HPV is and what it means for their health, how common it is, the likelihood of progression to cancer, how to control it, and the impact of HPV on future sexual activity. Finally, the information and counseling needs of women who receive repeated positive HPV test results may differ from those receiving an initial diagnosis.

■ EDUCATIONAL CHALLENGES AND FACILITATORS

HPV information may be challenging to convey to patients for a number of reasons, the most salient of which may be the scientific complexity of HPV. Many aspects of HPV have been identified by patients and members of the general public as confusing, contradictory, and seemingly counterintuitive (see Table 32-1). Patients are often left wondering how concerned they should be about HPV. For many, the information they receive does not fit within their familiar constructs about identifying and treating disease. HPV concepts may be especially challenging to explain to patients who lack any scientific

background or understanding of biomedical concepts. As Hunter points out, in some cultures and among individuals with limited education, basic medical concepts such as "cells" or "virus" may have no clear meaning.

A second challenge to providing HPV counseling is the lack of clearly defined answers to console patients about their concerns regarding acquisition, stigma, and future prevention. Particularly with cervical cancer screening, these concerns can overwhelm the clinical encounter and distract from the medically important discussion of patient management and follow-up. Studies suggest that framing HPV with other STIs and emphasizing multiple sex partners as a risk factor may provoke anxiety and stigma among women. In contrast, providing information about HPV in a neutral context that emphasizes its high prevalence, long latency period, and transient nature (spontaneous clearance) may reassure patients and reduce perceived stigma. Patients in relationships may be comforted to know that an HPV diagnosis does not necessarily imply partner infidelity, nor need it cause concern about transmission to a partner. Finally, patients can be reassured to know that, in most cases, the serious health consequences of HPV can be prevented and that there *are* ways to prevent future transmission, although the *consequences* of HPV infection (rather than the virus itself) should be the primary motivation for prevention.

This raises a third challenge to counseling in the context of cervical cancer screening. Providers need to carefully balance information about the commonness and transience of HPV infection, on the one hand, with its potentially serious sequelae on the other. HPV information can be anxiety provoking for patients, in that the virus is usually invisible and potentially harmful, has no cure or foolproof prevention strategy short of abstinence, and no approved or recommended detection tests for partners. Research suggests that women diagnosed with

TABLE 32-1   Potential Contradictions and Scientific Complexities of HPV

- Distinction between "low-risk" and "high-risk" types; how can a virus possibly be "low-risk"?
- The connection between HPV, cervical cancer, and genital warts.
- Treatability of HPV: how can HPV be both incurable and transient?
- Distinction between the Pap test and HPV test
- Lack of general HPV testing recommendation: why shouldn't men and women be tested for a virus that can cause cancer?

high-risk HPV tend to overestimate their cancer risk and that too much anxiety and fear of cancer can serve as a barrier to recommended follow-up. Thus, it falls to clinicians to portray the facts about HPV without creating complacency—and without creating undue anxiety.

Finally, effective patient counseling and education may be difficult because of patients' limited capacity to absorb new information at the time of diagnosis as a result of shock and distress. Both patients and providers have identified the need for quality, low-literacy-level materials, toll-free help-lines, and other free resources that patients can use after the diagnostic visit. Yet until recently, most print materials have suffered from several serious flaws: They have been too medically complex; too broad in content or too limited in scope; lacking in cultural diversity and appropriateness; or unresponsive to the social, emotional, and behavioral aspects of HPV. Similarly, most Internet-based information on HPV was either inaccurate or too complex for the average patient. While better and more appropriate information is constantly emerging, it may be difficult for patients to navigate through these resources and to identify which are accurate and reliable, so it is best to point patients to specific resources known to have scientific credibility, such as professional or medical associations and government agencies.

■ KEY COUNSELING MESSAGES FOR PATIENTS WITH HPV

In recent years, key researchers and leading medical and public health agencies have contributed to the body of behavioral and communication research aimed at understanding and addressing the educational and emotional needs of HPV-positive patients; offering insights on how to relay HPV information to patients in clear and meaningful ways while minimizing associated stigma, confusion, and fear; and providing accurate perceptions of cancer risk. A number of these organizations, such as the Centers for Disease Control and Prevention (CDC), the British and American Cancer Societies, the British Association for Sexual Health and HIV (BASHH), the Association for Reproductive Health Professionals, and American Social Health Association (ASHA), have published consumer education materials or developed messages that providers can use in various clinical scenarios with patients diagnosed with HPV. However, there remain only a small number of materials that adequately address the range of emotional, behavioral, and psychosocial and information needs specific to patients with genital warts.

Research suggests that patients undergoing cervical cancer screening want HPV information tailored to their specific risks, based on their type of HPV, their age, culture, and literacy level. Therefore, even the best educational materials will likely leave the individual with the specific question, "What does this mean *for me?*" The Internet allows for customization and tailoring to a user's specific information needs, and private and public health agencies are increasingly taking advantage of this (e.g., www.thehpvtest.com). But HPV-positive women prefer conversations with a trusted clinician and the opportunity to ask questions (Gilbert 2003). This is where providers can play a critical role, personalizing the information so that it is relevant and actionable to the patient. To support patients, take-away materials should be provided. Patients can retain more health information if it is conveyed both verbally and in writing, and they can refer to the information on their own, when they are better able to absorb it at their own pace.

Taken together, the literature suggests a number of key points to emphasize in HPV-related counseling. A synopsis of 10 key points are presented, adapted from CDC materials. Clinicians can draw from this list to address the questions and concerns raised by individual patients.

1. *HPV is a common virus in men and women.* There are many types of HPV passed on through genital (skin-to-skin) contact, most often during vaginal or anal sex. HPV may also be passed on by oral sex. HPV is common, and most people contract it at some time in their lives.

2. *Most people never know they have HPV because the virus usually causes no signs or health problems.* In most cases, the body's natural defenses fight off HPV within a couple years. But this is not always the case.

3. *Some types of HPV can cause genital warts. Other types can cause cervical cancer in women and other less common cancers, such as penile and anal cancers.* It is only in rare cases, when the body does not fight off HPV over many years, that HPV can cause cancer.

4. *There are treatments for the problems caused by HPV, such as genital warts, early signs of cancer, and cancer.* Treatment does not necessarily kill the virus (HPV). Therefore, you may need follow-up visits to make sure the problem does not come back.

5. *There is no sure way to know when (or from whom) you got HPV.* Most of the time, HPV is passed on

when there are no visible signs of infection. A person can have HPV for many years before it is found or starts causing problems. An HPV diagnosis does not mean that you or your partner has had sex outside of your relationship.

6. *Sex partners are likely to share HPV, especially if they have been together for a while.* Both partners may be infected with the same HPV types, even when neither or only one has signs of HPV. You and your partner may benefit from talking openly about your sexual health and HPV. Talking to partners can be challenging. But if you are well informed and able to put HPV in perspective, you are likely to feel better about discussing it. In most cases, partners are supportive.

7. *If you have HPV, there are ways to prevent or treat its potentially serious health effects.* Women can prevent cervical cancer by following up with recommended testing or treatment. Most men with healthy immune systems do not develop serious health problems from HPV; but treatments are available for HPV-related cancers in men. Individuals with genital warts need not worry about warts turning into cancer; the types of HPV that cause warts are different from the types that cause cancer.

8. *If you have HPV, there are ways to prevent getting new HPV infections.* A person can have more than one HPV type. If you are 26 years of age or younger, HPV vaccines are available to prevent the HPV types that cause the most common HPV-related health problems. If you're sexually active, using condoms every time you have sex may lower your chances of getting other types of HPV or developing HPV-related diseases. Limiting your number of sex partners can also lower your chances of exposure to a new HPV infection. But HPV is so common that the only sure way to prevent HPV is to avoid sex (skin-to-skin sexual contact).

9. *If you have HPV, there are ways to prevent passing it to new sex partners.* If you are sexually active, condoms may lower your chances of passing HPV to a new partner if they are used all the time and in the right way. But HPV can infect areas that are not covered by condoms, so condoms do not fully protect against HPV. Partners aged 26 years and younger may also choose to get an HPV vaccine.

10. *There is no test for men or women to check their "HPV status."* But HPV usually goes away on its own, without causing health problems. So an HPV infection that is found today will most likely be gone a year or two from now. There *are* ways to find the most common problems caused by HPV. A healthcare provider can inspect the genitals for warts. For women, there are tests to find early signs of cervical cancer. The HPV tests on the market are only meant to help screen for cervical cancer.

Providers should recognize that some of these points may seem confusing or contradictory to patients. Some medical terms and anatomical references, such as *virus* or *cervix*, may not be familiar to patients and may require further explanation. The best way to ensure that patients understand what has been communicated to them is to have them "teach back" what they have learned and ask questions about any points they find confusing. Providers should use their discretion in determining the amount and level of detail appropriate for each patient, recognizing that too much information can actually be overwhelming and *diminish* a patient's ability to make informed decisions. Research suggests that patients are likely to absorb even less when they are under the emotional stress of a new diagnosis.

■ SPECIAL CONSIDERATIONS FOR HPV

External Genital Warts

Although genital warts do not pose a serious health threat to patients, the psychological distress associated with warts often outweighs the medical consequences. Counseling should be nonjudgmental and sensitive to patients' psychological and emotional needs, stressing the need to maintain a balanced perspective, and that patients *can* and will still live normal, healthy lives. The messages in Table 32-2 were adapted in part from the CDC.

■ SUBCLINICAL/HIGH-RISK HPV

Experts have recommended that clinicians deliver pre-test counseling about HPV before administering HPV DNA tests, so that patients are not blind-sided by sexual transmission at the time of a diagnosis. With cervical cancer screening, distinguish HPV from most other STIs and disconnect it from notions of promiscuity and stigma. Avoiding the use of stigmatizing labels (e.g., STI, multiple sex partners), and using nonjudgmental language and tone can help reduce perceived stigma. Balance the commonness and transience of

TABLE 32-2 Counseling Messages for Genital Wart Disease

- Do not blame yourself. You are not alone. Millions of other people have HPV.

- It is still possible to have a normal, healthy life, even with HPV. Genital warts can be treated, and your feelings will improve over time.

- There are treatments for genital warts. Some treatments can be applied at home; other treatments require a visit to the doctor.

- If you don't treat genital warts, they may go away, remain unchanged, or grow in size or number. They will *not* turn into cancer—even if left untreated.

- It is common for genital warts to recur (come back after treatment), especially in the first 3 months after treatment.

- You can still pass HPV on to sex partners, even after the warts are treated. It is not known how long a person remains contagious after warts are treated. In most cases, HPV goes away in time.

- If you have genital warts, you may benefit from screening for other sexually transmitted infections (STIs). Your current partner may also benefit from seeing a health professional for counseling and being checked for genital warts and other STIs.

- Genital warts can be very infectious to partners. Avoiding sex (including genital-to-genital contact) is the only sure way to prevent passing HPV to partners. If you have sex, using condoms (all the time and the right way) can help lower your chances of passing HPV to your partner(s). Also, if your partner is 26 years old or younger, he or she may consider getting a vaccine to protect against most genital warts.

- It is not clear whether there is any health benefit to telling future partners about a past diagnosis of genital warts (once warts are treated). It is not known whether or how long you would remain contagious after treatment.

- Women with genital warts do not need to get Pap tests more often than usual, but they do need regular Pap tests (at least every 3 years).

- There is a small chance that a pregnant woman with genital warts can pass HPV to her baby. In the rare case that this happens, the baby could develop warts in the throat or voice box. Cesarean births are not generally recommended because they do not seem to prevent a mother from passing HPV to her baby.

HPV infection with its potentially serious sequelae and promote accurate portrayals of HPV risk without creating undue anxiety—or complacency. There is no consensus on appropriate partner management and prevention, particularly for women in long-term, monogamous relationships, and clinicians should tailor their recommendations to the individual circumstances of the patient. Promote recommended follow-ups to empower women to take control of their health, emphasizing their ability to prevent cervical cancer now.

Table 32-3 identifies additional counseling messages, adapted from the CDC, to deliver to patients.

■ CONCLUSION

Patients with genital HPV infection are highly likely to have questions about the impact of these infections not only on their long-term health but also on their most intimate relationships. Educational counseling therefore plays a vital role in managing patients, and clinicians do well to be familiar with patient needs and key researched and tested counseling messages. Given the lack of a curative therapy for HPV, patients may require long-term management and may need to attend to recurring symptoms. An HPV diagnosis may raise issues of persisting infectiousness along with a need for patient counseling about potential risk to partners and risk reduction strategies. While the promotion of HPV vaccines may help to create a change in perceptions of HPV, the existing literature suggests the potential for psychosocial distress among patients diagnosed with HPV. Clinicians can make a significant difference in patient adjustment and addressing these challenging issues will greatly benefit patients.

TABLE 32-3 Counseling Messages for Subclinical HPV

- You have already taken the first step to prevent cervical cancer by getting screened.

- A positive HPV test means that you have HPV on your cervix. This does not mean that you have or will get cervical cancer. But you could have a higher chance of developing cervical cancer in the future.

- HPV is so common that anyone who has ever had sex—even married adults (if they had other sex partners before marriage)—may be at risk for HPV.

- Most of the time, the body fights off HPV naturally within 2 years. But if HPV stays on a woman's cervix for many years, it can cause cell changes that lead to cervical cancer over time.

- There are ways to treat the cell changes caused by HPV so that they do not turn into cervical cancer in the future.

- Most women who have HPV do not get cervical cancer as long as they follow their doctor's advice for more testing or treatment. Be sure to come to all recommended appointments and tests.

- Having HPV or cell changes does not make it harder to get or stay pregnant. It will not affect the health of your future babies, but if you need treatment for any cell changes caused by HPV, the treatment could affect your chance of having children. Most treatments do leave the cervix intact so you can have children in the future.

- There is no HPV test for men. But a vaccine is available to protect against most genital warts, which are the most common problem caused by HPV in men. Men aged 26 years and younger can receive this vaccine.

KEY POINTS

- Growing numbers of patients today are confronted with the need to understand human papillomavirus (HPV), both because of the expanded use of HPV DNA testing as a cervical cancer screening and management tool, and because of increased HPV vaccines promotion.

- Persons diagnosed with HPV may be confused and distressed to learn it is sexually transmitted, may persist even after treatment, and carries the potential for subclinical transmission despite risk reduction measures.

- Providers are the primary and most trusted source of HPV information for patients. They can address patient questions, alleviate their concerns, reduce anxiety, and promote appropriate follow-up.

REFERENCES

Friedman A, Shepeard H. Exploring the knowledge, attitudes, beliefs, and communication preferences of the general public regarding HPV: findings from CDC focus group research and implications for practice. *Health Educ Behav.* 2007;34: 471–485.

Gilbert L, Alexander L, Grosshans JF, Jolley L. Answering frequently asked questions about HPV. *Sex Transm Dis.* 2003;30(3):193–194.

Goldsmith MR, Bankhead CR, Kehoe ST, Marsh G, Austoker J. Information and cervical screening: a qualitative study of women's awareness, understanding and information needs about HPV. *J Med Screen.* 2007;14(1):29–33.

Graziottin A, Serafini A. HPV infection in women: psychosexual impact of genital warts and intraepithelial lesions. *J Sex Med.* 2009;6(3):633–645.

Keller M, von Sadovszky V, Pankratz B, Hermsen J. Self-disclosure of HPV infection to sex partners. *West J Nurs Res.* 2000;22(3):285–302.

Maissi E, Marteau TM, Hankins M, Moss S, Legood R, Gray A. Psychological impact of human papillomavirus testing in women with borderline or mildly dyskaryotic cervical smear test results: cross-sectional questionnaire study. *BMJ.* 2004;328(7451):1293–1299.

Maw RD, Reitano M, Roy M. An international survey of patients with genital warts: perceptions regarding treatment and impact on lifestyle. *Int J STD AIDS.* 1998; 9(10):571–578.

McCaffery K, Waller J, Nazroo J, Wardle J. Social and psychological impact of HPV testing in cervical screening: a qualitative study. *Sex Transm Infect.* 2006;82(2):169–174.

Tiro JA, Meissner HI, Kobrin S, Chollette V. What do women in the U.S. know about human papillomavirus and cervical cancer? *Cancer Epidemiol Biomarkers Prev.* 2007;16(2):288–294.

Waller J, Marlow LA, Wardle J. The association between knowledge of HPV and feelings of stigma, shame and anxiety. *Sex Transm Infect.* 2007;83(2):155–159.

Waller J, McCaffery K, Nazroo J, Wardle J. Making sense of the information about HPV in cervical screening: a qualitative study. *Br J Cancer.* 2005;92:265–270.

33

Care Following Rape and Sexual Assault

Jan Welch

■ INTRODUCTION

Sexual violence is a common problem throughout the world. In the United Kingdom, about 1 in 20 women 16 years and older have been raped, and a lifetime risk of up to 20% for attempted or completed rape has been reported from some areas. Similar figures are reported from the United States. Although anyone can be sexually assaulted, adolescent and young women are especially susceptible. Other factors increasing vulnerability to sexual assault are disability, poverty, homelessness, and residing in an institution or conflict zone. Sex workers are at particular risk. Sexual assault is often associated with the consumption of alcohol and drugs; alcohol is implicated much more often than the so-called date-rape drugs Rohypnol and ketamine.

Most perpetrators of sexual assault are known to their victims; in one study, 38% of women experiencing domestic violence also suffered forced sexual activity. Perpetrators are often motivated by power and control and may specifically seek out vulnerable individuals. Most sexual assaults are not reported to the police, but survivors commonly seek medical help although they may not disclose the crime. Women often delay seeking care for months or even years. Assaults by strangers are less common but are more likely to be reported to the police, resulting in higher conviction rates.

Different jurisdictions vary in their approach to sexual offences. Gender equality is a major issue; for example, in some countries it is not recognized that a married woman can be raped by her husband. In the United Kingdom, the 2003 Sexual Offences Act reflected a comprehensive revi-

sion of the law in England and Wales and variants of this definition exist in most U.S. states: Rape is now defined as nonconsensual penetration of the vagina, anus, or mouth by a penis, which means that both females and males can be raped. Assault by penetration is the intentional insertion of an object other than the penis, into the vagina or anus, without consent. In addition, there are specific offenses that relate to children as victims.

Rape and sexual assault result in significant short- and long-term physical and psychological sequelae. These include genital and nongenital injuries, unwanted pregnancy, sexually transmitted infections, including HIV, depression, and posttraumatic stress disorder (PTSD). Management should be determined by the individual's wishes and needs, and to some extent will depend on the time since the assault. In this chapter, I will primarily focus on the immediate medical management and other aspects of aftercare, including the diagnosis and treatment of potential sexually transmitted infections.

The management of someone who has been sexually assaulted requires coordinating medical and forensic services and providing psychosocial support. The main considerations will be managing any injuries, collecting and preserving physical evidence of the assault, preventing unwanted pregnancy and sexually transmitted infections, and providing appropriate psychosocial support. Survivors of sexual assault may, understandably, find it hard to access different services and to repeat explanations of what has happened to them. Therefore, care should be provided in a coordinated and timely fashion, where feasible, in one place at one time, by sensitive and nonjudgmental clinicians (WHO 2003). Where feasible, female staff should be available to conduct examinations, as most female and many male victims prefer them. In many countries, sexual assault centers (SACs) have been established that offer a team approach, with highly trained personnel, to provide all necessary services in a safe, private, and forensically secure environment (Lovett et al. 2004). Although SACs generally receive many police referrals, their facilities may enable victims to provide anonymous intelligence and evidence to assist in identifying serial perpetrators.

■ THE ROLE OF SEXUAL HEALTH SERVICES

People who have been sexually assaulted usually will be referred by law enforcement to specialized forensic centers. However, victims may present initially to sexual health services or are referred by the police or other clinicians or agencies for aftercare. Although sexual health services' primary responsibility is to prevent and manage sexually transmitted infections, it is important that other needs are considered.

Many sexual assaults are first reported to the police. The police can, in many cases, provide officers with specialist training to provide excellent initial support, to arrange forensic examination as appropriate, and to access further services. In some situations, however, an individual may first disclose a sexual assault while obtaining care for STI management or other sexual health service. It is therefore essential that healthcare providers in such settings be aware of local legal reporting requirements.

Documentation

Many people who attend sexual health services following sexual assault will say they intend not to report to the police but good documentation is still essential. They may change their minds or a statement may be required for other purposes, such as criminal injuries compensation, even years after the event. A pro forma is useful to ensure that necessary information is captured as well as to remind the clinician of important aspects of management. When the patient is a minor, child protection issues should also be considered where necessary.

Assessment of Injuries

Minor injuries are found in at least 50% of people reporting sexual assault and should be documented, if this has not already been done at the forensic examination, and any necessary treatment provided. Nongenital injuries such as bruises and abrasions are more common than genital injuries. The absence of any injury does not mean that the victim consented. Major injury, for example, vaginal or anal bleeding following genital assault with a foreign body, such as a broken bottle, is unusual but may be life threatening and so should be assessed in an acute hospital setting.

Preserving Evidence

Preservation of evidence is important when the victim presents soon after the assault and before forensic examination, as otherwise the opportunity will be lost (Newton 2004). Careful documentation is important, and the victim should be asked whether she or he would like the assault reported to the police and arrange a forensic examination for full documentation of any injuries and collection of samples for DNA and other evidence (Rogers 2004). DNA evidence is unlikely to be found if more than 7 days have elapsed since an adult woman's assault or 3 days since a man's or a child's assault but later examination for injuries may still be worthwhile. A forensic examination should be performed in specialized centers, and this is usually beyond the scope of the sexual health service or sexually transmitted infection clinic.

Even before the forensic examination, early evidence ideally should be preserved, as even a few hours delay may reduce the chance of finding useful evidence such as DNA in a mouth sample or drugs in the urine sample. Gloves should be worn to prevent DNA contamination, consent obtained, and samples carefully labeled. Ideally, a mouth swab for the assailant's DNA is taken before the victim has anything to eat or drink, and a urine sample is taken to test for alcohol and drugs. Other samples that may yield DNA evidence are used tampons, sanitary towels and condoms, and chewing gum. All forensic specimens are subject to "chain of custody" requirements (detailed guidance on www.careandevidence.org). Because of the potential for legal proceedings, clinicians managing these individuals, even if they are not involved in forensic specimen collection, should carefully document all aspects of the history, physical examination, and assessment. Specially trained examiners using specific collection kits usually conduct subsequent full forensic examination, ideally in a forensically secure environment, such as an SAC.

■ CONTRACEPTION

Without adequate contraception, the risk of the rape of a woman of reproductive age resulting in pregnancy is about 5%. Adolescents are most at risk and may be too frightened or ashamed to admit the pregnancy until too late to be offered a termination. Emergency contraception should therefore always be considered and provided, unless effective contraception is already used. A single 1.5-mg dose of levonorgestrol (Levonelle-1500) is effective up to 5 days after intercourse but may be more effective when given earlier. Insertion of an intrauterine device is also effective and can be used up to 5 days after the earliest predicted date of ovulation in the menstrual cycle. If an IUD is considered, antibiotic prophylaxis to cover the insertion should be considered.

SEXUALLY TRANSMITTED INFECTIONS

The risk of acquiring sexually transmitted infections (STIs) from sexual assault depends on the local epidemiology of STIs and the nature of the assault. For example, risks and concerns of a woman raped by her husband will be different from those of a teenager raped by several youths. People who have been sexually assaulted are often understandably reluctant to attend follow-up services such as those for screening or treatment of STIs and may perceive an internal or speculum examination as an additional violation. It is therefore important to consider ways of minimizing intrusive medical appointments and examinations, for example, by offering prophylactic antibiotics and by offering noninvasive screening tests carried out on urine samples rather than requiring speculum examination.

PROPHYLAXIS

Epidemiological studies have shown that the actual risk of STI following sexual assault is low. Patients should be counseled and reassured. Despite the low risk, most authorities and practitioners recommend preventive therapy

TABLE 33-1 Sexually Transmitted Infections for Which Screening Should Be Offered Following Rape

- Gonorrhea
- Chlamydia
- Trichomoniasis
- Syphilis
- Hepatitis B
- HIV

effective against typical STI pathogens. Chlamydia and gonorrhea are the most potentially serious bacterial infections, as they may result in pelvic inflammatory disease and infertility in women. They are not always easy to diagnose, especially if only one set of samples is taken a suboptimal time after the assault. A single dose of antibiotics effective against local strains of gonorrhea, and chlamydia, for example, cefixime and azithromycin, is likely to minimize the chance of sequelae if the client does not return for further tests (Mein 2003; Centers for Disease Control 2010), and is acceptable to patients. Vaccination against hepatitis B infection should also be considered for persons who have not been previously vaccinated and who are susceptible. HIV is discussed later in this chapter.

CHAIN OF EVIDENCE

Chain of evidence refers to documenting the origin and history of a sample to produce an unbroken chain from its source to the court. It can refer to forensic or microbiological samples and should include records of individuals handling the samples, their signatures, and the places and conditions of storage together with details of dates and times.

Ideally, sexual health services should agree to protocols for managing samples taken from sexual assault victims with local microbiological services, advised by national guidelines where available. These could include the following:

- Identifying such samples, for example, medicolegal

- Determining when to use chain-of-evidence documentation

- Managing medicolegal samples, that is, tests, confirmatory tests, storage, and documentation

- Supervising a senior laboratory clinician or scientist

SEXUALLY TRANSMITTED INFECTIONS AS EVIDENCE

Finding a sexually transmitted infection in someone who alleges sexual assault does not necessarily mean that the information will assist his or her case in court. It is often impossible to determine whether the STI predated the assault, and in an adversarial legal system, the defense lawyer may use this finding to denigrate the victim, depending on the jurisdiction and local rules on disclosure and admissibility in court.

STIs are most likely to provide relevant evidence in

- Victims at the extremes of age, that is, children and the elderly

- Sexually inexperienced individuals

- Sexually inexperienced orifices (for example, the rectum of a heterosexual man)

CHOICE OF TESTS

In the past, chlamydia and gonorrhea culture was advocated in medicolegal cases, but, as in routine practice, it has largely been superseded by more sensitive tests such as nucleic acid amplification tests (NAATs). Cultures have therefore become less available, even in reference settings. NAATs can also be carried out on urine samples rather than on a cervical swab, thereby avoiding the use of a speculum. In medicolegal cases, however, it is essential to confirm an infection found by NAAT with an additional test to minimize false-positive results. Ensure that the laboratory processing samples has adequate quality assurance documentation and that samples are archived for potential further testing.

PREVENTING HIV INFECTION

Concern about HIV infection is common in people who have been raped. The actual risk is usually low in developed countries but much higher in some areas of the world, such as sub-Saharan Africa, especially in conflict settings. In general, the risk will depend on the local prevalence of HIV and features of the assault.

Risk of HIV transmission = Risk that source is HIV positive × risk of exposure

(Fisher 2006)

BOX 33-1 Postexposure Prophylaxis for HIV

When to consider HIV postexposure prophylaxis (PEP) following rape:

- Assailant HIV positive
- Assailant with risk factors
- Anal rape
- Trauma and bleeding
- Multiple assailants
- Assault within 72 hours

Establishing whether an individual perpetrator has HIV is usually impossible, but some degree of risk assessment is usually feasible although highly subjective. High-risk perpetrators are those known to have HIV (although prisoners not uncommonly state they have HIV when they do not) or risk activities such as men having sex with men, injecting drug use, or coming from a high prevalence area for HIV. Multiple assailants, as in group rape, increase the chance that one assailant has HIV. The risk of exposure of the actual assault is increased by factors reducing the effectiveness of host defenses, such as anal rape, defloration, trauma, and bleeding.

Postexposure prophylaxis (PEP) against HIV is estimated to reduce the risk of transmission by about 80% following occupational exposure and is known to be effective in reducing mother-to-child transmission. There is now some evidence of its effectiveness following sexual exposure. It is most likely to be beneficial when given as soon as possible after the assault, ideally within 24 hours or less and continued for 28 days but unlikely to be effective if started later than 72 hours (Fisher 2006).

A number of different drug combinations have been used, without any shown to be more effective than others. The choice is therefore generally based on safety, tolerability, and local guidelines and formularies. Since HIV prevention and treatment guidelines can change rapidly, we are not offering specific recommendations here. Typically, two to three drugs are recommended. Side effects include nausea and diarrhea and reduced efficacy of oral contraception. The drugs are expensive and so initially a starter pack of three to five days medication

BOX 33-2 HIV Prevalence Figures

Example

- Woman raped by 4 men from high-prevalence area#:
- 1 in 14 (their chance of having HIV) × 1 in 1000 (risk of receptive vaginal intercourse) = 1 in 14,000 × 4 * = 1 in 3500
- Man raped by a homosexual man
- 1 in 7 (chance of assailant having HIV) × 1 in 33 (risk of receptive anal intercourse) = 1 in 231 *

HIV prevalence figures available via www.who.int/hiv/en/.
* Risk increased by trauma and bleeding.

may be provided as many people decide not to continue with the full course. Follow-up should include general and adherence support and the offer of HIV testing at 3 months after completion of PEP. Drugs should be selected in consultation with local HIV experts.

■ Psychosocial Aspects

Rape and sexual assault commonly result in major short-term and long-term psychological sequelae. Individuals vary in their responses and may appear quiet and controlled, distressed and tearful, or in denial. Common early symptoms include anxiety, interrupted sleep, feelings of shame and guilt, and powerlessness. Many individuals will recover spontaneously over subsequent months, but others develop longer-term problems, including depression, posttraumatic stress disorder (PTSD), difficulties with social and sexual functioning, and misuse of alcohol and other substances. In fact, sexual dysfunction and depression may be presenting symptoms related to a sexual assault in the distant past.

Health advisers and counselors within sexual health services are well placed to provide useful initial support and advice and to help reduce feelings of humiliation and self-reproach. General written information should be provided, as well as details of local support agencies such as victim support and rape crisis services. General practitioners may also be able to provide invaluable support and help with symptom control, for example, the short-term use of hypnotics in improving sleep and reducing flashbacks. Antidepressants are helpful for marked depressive symptoms or to treat an established depressive illness. If PTSD supervenes treatment with cognitive behavior therapy or eye movement desensitization and reprocessing should be offered (NCP Guidelines 2005), usually via a specialist.

■ Key Points

- Rape and sexual assault are common and can affect both females and males, although young women are most at risk; the perpetrators are usually known males.

- Most sexual assaults are not reported to the police, but medical help is often sought, although this may not be until weeks, months, or years later.

- Good documentation is essential, and sexual health services should also consider evidence collection when the assault was recent, so that perpetrators can be identified and prosecuted.

- Main sexual health needs following sexual assault include the prevention and management of sexually transmitted infections and bloodborne viruses, and emergency contraception.

References

Websites

www.rcne.com:
Rape Crisis Network Europe—provides information about counseling, legal, and support services in more than 30 countries

www.rapecrisis.co.uk:
Rape Crisis—provides information to help survivors of sexual violence, friends, and family access services

www.careandevidence.org:
Provides training and other resources such as flowcharts and a free DVD, in the care of and evidence collection from people who have been sexually assaulted, for healthcare professionals

www.victimsupport.org_independent:
UK charity helping people cope with the effects of crime, providing free and confidential support and information to help survivors deal with their experience

www.uktrauma.org.uk:
UK Trauma Group—contact information for UK health professionals about specialist resources advising on the assessment or treatment of people with psychological reactions to major traumatic events

Publications

Centers for Disease Control and Prevention. *Sexually Transmitted Disease Treatment Guidelines*. Atlanta: CDC; 2010.

Fisher M, Benn P, Evans B, et al. UK guidelines for the use of post-exposure prophylaxis for HIV following sexual exposure. *Int J STD AIDS*. 2006;17:81–92.

Lovett J, Regan L, Kelly L. *Sexual Assault Referral Centres: Developing Good Practice and Maximising Potentials*. London: Home Office Research, Development and Statistics Directorate; 2004.

Mein JK, Palmer CM, Shand MC, et al. Management of acute adult sexual assault. *MJA*. 2003;178(5):226–230.

Newton M. The sexual assault medical examination kit. In: Dalton M, ed. *Forensic Gynaecology*. London: RCOG Press; 2004.

Rogers D. The general examination. In: Dalton M, ed. *Forensic Gynaecology*. London: RCOG Press; 2004.

Scott-Ham M, Burton FC. A study of blood and urine alcohol concentrations in cases of alleged drug-facilitated sexual assault in the United Kingdom over a 3-year period. *J Clin Forensic Med.* 2006;13(3):107–111.

Sugar NF, Fine DN, Eckert LO. Physical injury after sexual assault: findings of a large case series. *Am J Obstet Gynecol.* 2004;190(1):71–76.

WHO. Guidelines for medico-legal care for victims of sexual violence. World Health Organisation, Geneva. 2003. http://www.who.int/violence_injury_prevention/publications/violence/med_leg_guidelines/en/.

White C, McLean I. Adolescent complainants of sexual assault; injury patterns in virgin and non-virgin groups. *J Clin Forensic Med.* 2006;13(4):172–180.

34
Sexually Transmitted Infections in Homosexual Men

C. Wayne Sells and Gary Remafedi

▨ INTRODUCTION

The prevention and control of sexually transmitted infections (STIs) in men who have sex with men (MSM) is important to the health of all members of society. Although in-depth discussions of specific pathogens and disease syndromes are featured elsewhere, this chapter offers an overview of the unique aspects of STIs among MSM. Available information about the epidemiology, detection, treatment, and prevention of common STIs will be presented. Evaluating and managing oropharyngitis, urethritis, ulcerative lesions, hepatitis, proctitis, proctocolitis, and enteritis will be emphasized. However, current knowledge is limited by wide gaps in disease surveillance and other research relevant to MSM. Since STIs can be asymptomatic or present with nonspecific symptoms, suggestions for a comprehensive sexual history and risk assessment will be highlighted. Regardless of their sexual orientation, MSM who engage in unprotected sexual intercourse continue to face a high likelihood of exposure to a wide variety of infections, some of which are incurable and fatal. Primary prevention must couple immunizations with targeted behavioral interventions. Early identification and treatment of infected individuals and their contacts can contain the secondary spread of disease, while tertiary interventions employ pharmacotherapy to reduce morbidity and mortality. A comprehensive public health strategy that coordinates primary, secondary, and tertiary interventions is essential to reduce the devastating impact of STIs on MSM.

▨ RISK FACTORS FOR SEXUALLY TRANSMITTED INFECTIONS

Characteristics of the Host

A complex interrelationship between the host and specific sexually acquired pathogens accounts for the variable prevalence of sexually transmitted infections within different populations. The spread of STIs among MSM may be attributed to physiological factors, as well as specific sexual behaviors. For example, the penis, through deep penetration and forceful ejaculation provides an efficient mode for transmission of sexual pathogens, especially when coupled with damaged rectal or oral mucosa.

▨ STIs AMONG MEN WHO HAVE GENITAL–ANAL INTERCOURSE WITH MEN

Genital–anal intercourse is an efficient transmission route for many STIs (see Chapter 23 for a discussion of the diagnosis of anorectal syndromes). Consequently, MSM have been reported to have significantly higher rates of syphilis, scabies, HIV, human papillomavirus (HPV), cytomegalovirus (CMV), and hepatitis B (HBV) than heterosexual men and women. Urethral gonorrhea is independently associated with both insertive genital–anal sex and insertive oral intercourse. Despite overall decline in gonorrhea cases throughout the United States since 1972, the incidence of disease among MSM has been increasing, and MSM have accounted for an increased proportion of total gonorrhea cases since 1999. Fluoroquinolone-resistant gonococcal isolates are especially prevalent among MSM in the United States and in western Europe. These trends were important considerations in the Center for Disease Control and Prevention's decision in 2007 to remove quinolones as first-line therapy for gonorrhea. Similarly, the syphilis rise in the United States and western Europe since 1997 have been almost exclusively due to increases in gay men, who also have high prevalence of HIV infection.

HIV remains an important sexually transmitted infection in homosexual men, and since the late 1990s, there has been major concern about relapses in high-risk behaviors in this group. Homosexual men from racial and ethnic minorities are at particularly high risk. The strongest predictors of HIV infection among MSM are unprotected genital–anal intercourse and multiple partners.

STIs Among Men Who Have Oral–Genital/Anal Sex with Men

Unprotected oral–genital sex is widely practiced. Anilingus (oral–anal sex) is a common practice among MSM, which may explain why enteric illnesses such as *Giardia* are more prevalent among MSM than in the general population. Hepatitis A and B infections may be transmitted by fecal–oral contact, often occurring during oral-anal sex (see Chapter 25 on hepatitis). Herpes (HSV-1 and HSV-2), gonorrhea, and HPV can be easily transmitted via oral–genital sex. Thus, STI prevention efforts should emphasize the need to reduce unprotected oral–genital and oral–anal contact.

Characteristics of Pathogens

The pharyngeal and rectum environment may each harbor strains that have specifically adapted to the local environment. For example, some studies have suggested that rectal gonococcal strains have reduced antimicrobial susceptibility because of the reduced permeability to the toxic hydrophobic molecules found in feces.

Comorbidities

In particular, MSM may be exposed and infected with multiple STIs. In particular, anogenital STIs increase the risk of other STIs, including HIV (see Chapter 10).

Genital ulcers, such as those produced by herpes or syphilis, have also been shown to increase the risk of transmission of HIV (See Chapter 18 on herpes and Chapters 9 and 17 on syphilis).

Barriers to STI Prevention

Consistent condom use is highly effective for reducing STIs and HIV transmission. However, a significant proportion of MSM continue to have unprotected intercourse. In a longitudinal cohort study of HIV seroincidence in six U.S. cities (Boston, Chicago, Denver, New York, San Francisco, and Seattle), 2216 men reported receptive genital–anal intercourse in the previous 6 months (Koblin et al. 2003). Twenty percent reported that they never used condoms. More than 75% of those who had genital–anal intercourse reported condom use more than 80% of the time. Younger MSM are more likely to engage in unprotected anal intercourse than older MSM. A study of Minnesota youth who identified themselves as gay or bisexual found that those who had unprotected anal intercourse were more likely than those who had not to report more frequent intercourse, having a steady partner, substance abuse, noncommunication with partners about risk reduction, and greater perceived likelihood of acquiring HIV (Henning 1995). Thus, despite generally accurate beliefs and knowledge, some MSM and men who have sex with men and women (MSMW) remain at significant risk for HIV and STIs.

Condom failure rates vary and can occur due to breakage, slipping off, use of oil-based lubricant, or improper application at the beginning of intercourse. There has been increased interest in the developing and evaluating topical microbicides and virucides that may be used during anal intercourse to prevent the transmission of HIV and STIs. Postexposure prophylaxis for both HIV and STIs have been proposed and some pilot projects implemented. However, efficacy of these interventions will be difficult to ascertain, and these programs require a substantial amount of support.

Sexual History

The Clinical Interview

The healthcare professional should approach the patient who presents with concerns about a sexually transmitted infection in an open, caring, and nonjudgmental manner.

Both clinician and patient need to achieve a level of comfort that promotes trust and the sharing of the patient's most intimate personal concerns. The patient is likely to have questions concerning confidentiality and privacy that need to be clarified, addressed, and respected. Clinicians must talk with teenagers and their parents about how they will maintain confidentiality and when it might be violated, such as when the teen or others are in danger, in circumstances of sexual abuse, and when required for public health reporting.

■ ENHANCING COMMUNICATION: IDENTIFYING AND OVERCOMING HOMOPHOBIA

The social stigma associated with homosexuality may inhibit the patient's willingness to freely discuss his or her concerns. Healthcare professionals caring for a gay, lesbian, or bisexual patient must examine their knowledge and personal beliefs concerning homosexuality. Medical practitioners may carry societal prejudice that are present in educational, health, religious, and governmental systems.

An understanding of sexual identity development is important, while recognizing the social and emotional isolation experienced by gay, lesbian, and bisexual individuals. The first stage of homosexual identity development begins in childhood with a period of "sensitization" in which the child feels different. Development spans adolescence and adulthood through periods of "identity confusion" and "identity assumption" toward "commitment," at which time the individual achieves a level of self-acceptance that incorporates sexual identity into all aspects of life. The patient's stage of development may be reflected in sexual behaviors as well as the degree of openness during the clinical interview. As many clinicians must overcome discomfort with homosexuality, the patient often experiences some degree of conflict and internalized homophobia. Even when unspoken, nonverbal cues can communicate the practitioner's discomfort. Individuals who have "come out" and who have acknowledged their homosexuality frequently use the term *gay* and *lesbian* to describe their personal and social identities.

Patient Assessment

Clinicians should routinely assess behaviors that place an individual at risk for STIs. Questionnaires should use inclusive language that does not assume a client's heterosexuality. The patient should be prepared for a sexual history with an explanation that he or she will be asked personal questions that are discussed with all patients. This introduction will facilitate later discussions of sexual orientation and activity. For example, for adolescents, a sexual history should include a detailed review of health issues identified through a structured Adolescent Risk Profile Interview—HEEADSSS Assessment. Such an assessment includes evaluation of the **H**ome environment, **E**ducation and employment history, **E**ating issues, peer-related **A**ctivities, **D**rugs, **S**exual activity and orientation, **S**uicide or depression issues, and **S**afety from injury and violence. The HEEADSSS assessment may be adapted for adult patients.

Components of the Sexual History

Establishing an open, caring relationship is fundamental to obtaining an accurate sexual history. The patient's perception of risk, methods of protection, past history of sexually transmitted infection, previous testing for STIs/HIV, sexual experiences and relationships, communication skills, and alcohol and substance use history all are important components. Introductory statements for sexual history questions will provide additional preparation for the patient; for example, "I am going to ask you about your sexual experiences and relationships. I understand that this is personal information but it will help me understand your risk for sexually transmitted infections and HIV." Self-reported condom use could be a helpful indicator of exposure to STIs in sexual experiences with recent partners. Specific questions about recent sexual experiences are better predictors of STIs than more global impressions of high-risk behaviors. While the individual's sexual attractions and sexual orientation are not relevant for STI detection, these components of the sexual history may be helpful for risk reduction counseling and for reaching a better understanding and rapport with the patient. Open-ended as well as more specific questions are useful in analyzing STI risk factors.

The patient's concerns about STIs should be discussed in the context of his or her sexual practices, number of partners, and history of substance use. While professional terminology may sometimes enhance the comfort level during the clinical interview, terms (Table 34-1) that are more familiar to the client may also help clarify historical information and HIV/STI risk status.

TABLE 34-1   Sexual Terminology

Fellatio	Oral–penile sex, giving head, sucking
Cunnilingus	Oral–vaginal sex, licking
Genital–anal intercourse	Top (insertive partner) Bottom (receptive partner)
Anilingus	Oral–anal intercourse, rimming
Manual–anal intercourse	Fisting or fingering

PHYSICAL EXAMINATION

The general STI physical examination is covered in Chapters 3 and 4. Rectal examination is best reserved for those who report genital–anal intercourse or have lower gastrointestinal symptoms and is also described in Chapter 23. When anorectal pain or discharge is present, anoscopic examination is indicated.

CLINICAL SYMPTOMS, ASSOCIATED PATHOGENS, AND TREATMENT— SPECIFIC ISSUES AND CHALLENGES IN MSM

Oropharyngitis

Suspicion of oropharyngeal STI requires a comprehensive sexual history is obtained. *Neisseria gonorrhoeae* is the most common sexually transmitted cause of pharyngitis and may be asymptomatic or clinically indistinguishable from viral or streptococcal pharyngitis. Herpes simplex virus often presents with gingivostomatitis and

systemic symptoms. Syphilis may present with large atypical-appearing lesions, most commonly on the lips. Human papillomavirus may also present on the oral mucosa. Patients with a history of unprotected receptive oral–genital contact and oropharyngeal lesions should be evaluated for *N. gonorrhoeae*, HSV, and syphilis, the latter especially in persons who are from, or who have traveled to areas where syphilis is epidemic. Syphilis is diagnosed by presence of lesions and accompanying serological evaluation. *Chlamydia trachomatis* of the pharynx is asymptomatic and not thought to be an important pathogen, thus routine pharyngeal culturing is not recommended. Since coinfection at other sites is common, in individuals with pharyngeal *N. gonorrhoeae*, treatment for both gonorrhea and chlamydia should be considered, especially if chlamydial infection has not been ruled out (Table 34-2).

Urethritis

The presentation of urethritis is no different in MSM than in heterosexual men who have sex with women (see Chapter 14). Urethritis is defined as inflammation of the urethra, which may be asymptomatic or present with discharge or dysuria. The presence of urethritis can be confirmed by *any* of the following: mucopurulent or purulent discharge, Gram stain of urethral secretions showing ≥5 WBCs per oil immersion or intracellular gram-negative diplococci (*N. gonorrhoeae*), positive leukocyte esterase test on first-void urine, or ≥ 10 WBCs per high power field on first-void urine. The leading causes of urethritis include *N. gonorrhoeae, C. trachomatis, Ureaplasma urealyticum, Trichomonas* and *Mycoplasma genitalium, and Trichomonas.* Men who have had insertive rectal intercourse are at increased risk for

TABLE 34-2   Diagnosis and Treatment of Sexually Transmitted Oropharyngeal Pathogens in MSM

Organism	Diagnosis	Treatment
Neisseria gonorrhoeae	Culture (NAAT testing)	Ceftriaxone 250 mg IM PLUS *Treatment for chlamydia if chlamydial infection is not ruled out*
Treponema pallidum (primary syphilis)	Nontreponemal (VDRL or RPR) confirmed by treponemal test (FTA-ABS or MHA-TP)	Benzathine penicillin G 2.4 million units IM in a single dose

TABLE 34-3   Diagnosis and Treatment of Urethritis in MSM

Infectious Agent	Diagnosis	Treatment
Neisseria gonorrhoeae	Culture, nucleic acid hybridization, or nucleic acid amplification tests	Ceftriaxone 250 mg IM OR Cefixime 400 mg orally, PLUS *Treatment for chlamydia if chlamydial infection is not ruled out*
Chlamydia trachomatis	Culture, nucleic acid hybridization, or nucleic acid amplification tests	Azithromycin 1 g orally OR Doxycycline 100 mg orally twice a day for 7 days
Nongonococcal Urethritis (C. trachomatis, Mycoplasma genitalium, or Ureaplasma urealyticum)	Culture, nucleic acid hybridization, or nucleic acid amplification tests to evaluate for gonorrhea and chlamydia	Azithromycin 1 g orally OR Doxycycline 100 mg orally twice a day for 7 days
Trichomonas vaginalis (Trichomoniasis)	Wet prep or culture	Metronidazole 2 g orally OR Tinidazole 2 g orally

urethritis due to *E. coli* and other enteric gram-negative rods. Further discussion of urethritis can be found in Chapter 14.

The availability of urine-based nucleic acid amplification techniques may enable expanded screening for both *N. gonorrhoeae* and *C. trachomatis* in clinics and in community settings.

Ulcerative Genital Lesions

Most sexually active persons in the United States who present with genital ulcers will be diagnosed with herpes or syphilis. Outbreaks of lymphogranuloma venereum have occurred in the United States and western Europe, and should be suspected in cases where there is prominent lymphadenopathy, especially MSM. Chancroid and granuloma inguinale are rare (Table 34-4). The evaluation of genital ulcers is similar among men who have sex with men or women. Of importance to MSM is that painless ulcers (syphilis) may be difficult to detect in rectal crypts without a high index of suspicion and a careful examination. Although the incidence of these diseases varies throughout the United States, HSV is prevalent in most parts of the country.

Beyond the history and physical examination, a minimal workup for all genital ulcers should include a culture or PCR for HSV and a serologic test for syphilis. Dark-field examination or direct immunofluorescence test for *Treponema pallidum* may be helpful if available. Herpes cultures may be negative if the lesions have begun to crust. If LGV is suspected, serological assessment (which is provided by the public health reference laboratory) should be performed. It should also be remembered that individuals may be coinfected with multiple STIs, including HIV. Therefore, HIV counseling and testing should be offered to all individuals with genital ulcers. Further discussion of genital ulcer disease can be found in Chapter 17.

Human Papillomavirus

Many types of human papillomaviruses (HPV) can infect the genital area. Although the most HPV infections are subclinical, asymptomatic, or unrecognized, the majority of visible genital warts are causes by HPV types 6 and 11. Treatment is focused on these visible genital warts (Table 34-5). Perianal HPV may be present in men and women who do not have a history of

TABLE 34-4   Diagnosis and Treatment of Sexually Transmitted Infections Presenting with Genital Ulcers in MSM

Infectious Agent	Diagnosis	Treatment
Herpes simplex virus (first clinical episode)	Culture	Acyclovir 400 mg orally three times a day for 7–10 days OR Acyclovir 200 mg orally five times a day for 7–10 days OR Famciclovir 250 mg orally three times a day for 7–10 days OR Valacyclovir 1 g orally twice a day for 7–10 days
Herpes simplex virus (recurrent)	Culture or serum type-specific antibody in clinical context	Acyclovir 400 mg orally three times a day for 5 days OR Acyclovir 800 mg orally twice a day for 5 days OR Acyclovir 800 mg orally three times a day for 2 days OR Famciclovir 125 mg orally twice a day for 5 days OR Famciclovir 1000 mg orally twice a day for 1 day Valacyclovir 500 mg orally twice a day for 3 days OR Valacyclovir 1 g orally once a day for 5 days
Treponema pallidum (Syphilis)	Dark-field examinations and direct fluorescent antibody tests of lesion exudates or tissue, or nontreponemal (VDRL or RPR) confirmed by treponemal test (FTA-ABS or MHA-TP)	Benzathine penicillin G 2.4 million units IM in a single dose for primary syphilis
H. ducreyi (Chancroid)	Culture on special media, or by clinical criteria	Azithromycin 1 g orally, OR Ceftriaxone 250 mg IM OR Ciprofloxacin 500 mg orally twice a day for 3 days OR Erythromycin base 500 mg orally three times a day for 7 days
Chlamydia trachomatis serovars L1, L2, or L3 (Lymphogranuloma venereum)	Culture, serology, direct immunofluorescence, or nucleic acid detection and exclusion of other causes of genital ulcer or lymphadenopathy	Doxycycline 100 mg orally twice a day for 21 days
Klebsiella granulomatis (Granuloma Inguinale or Donovanosis)	Donovan bodies on tissue crush preparation or biopsy	Doxycycline 100 mg orally twice a day for at least 3 weeks or until all lesions completely healed

TABLE 34-5 Treatment of HPV in MSM

Infectious Agent	Diagnosis	Treatment
External Genital Warts *Patient applied*	Diagnosis is clinical but may be confirmed by biopsy	Podfilox .5% solution or gel twice a day for 3 days, then 4 days no therapy for up to 4 cycles OR Imiquimod 5% cream daily at night, 3 times a week for up to 16 weeks
External Genital Warts *Provider administered*	Diagnosis is clinical but may be confirmed by biopsy	Cryotherapy with liquid nitrogen weekly as needed OR Trichloroacetic acid or Bichloroacetic acid 80–90% weekly as needed, OR Podophyllin resin 10–25% weekly as needed OR Surgical removal
Urethral Meatus Warts *Provider administered*	Diagnosis is clinical	Cryotherapy with liquid nitrogen weekly as needed OR Podophyllin resin 10-25% weekly as needed
Anal Warts *Provider administered*	Diagnosis is clinical but may be confirmed by biopsy	Cryotherapy with liquid nitrogen weekly as needed, OR Trichloroacetic acid or Bichloroacetic acid 80–90% weekly as needed, OR Surgical removal

anal sex. However, intra-anal warts are seen primarily in individuals who engage in receptive anal intercourse. Among MSM, the presence of intra-anal HPV is common. Although the CDC does not suggest routine classification of HPV, types 16, 18, 31, 33, and 35 have been associated with penile and anal squamous intraepithelial neoplasia. HPV-infected MSM are at significant risk for anal cancer, especially if they are HIV positive or immunocompromised.

Anal cancer may be a preventable disease; and, in the future, screening programs similar to cervical cancer screening may be recommended. In some clinical settings, especially those with is a large HIV-infected population, routine anal Pap screening has been implemented. However, generalizing this strategy is difficult because of a lack of standardized guidelines for reading and classifying anal Pap smears, lack of specimen standardization, and most important, a paucity of skilled cytopathologists with skills specific to this test. However, this situation will probably change in the near future with dissemination of the technology, as well as development of evidence-based screening guidelines. Because the majority of anal neoplastic lesions are the same HPV

subtypes covered in the newly developed vaccines (HPV 16 and 18) primary prevention strategies for anal squamous intraepithelial neoplasia in the future will likely involve immunization.

Hepatitis A, B, and C

Although the natural histories of hepatitis A, B, and C infections differ, their presenting symptoms may be indistinguishable. Hepatitis A, B and C are more frequently diagnosed in MSM. Symptoms may include fever, malaise, jaundice, anorexia, and nausea, or mild nonspecific manifestations. Asymptomatic infections are common. When the etiology of viral hepatitis is not obvious by history, the clinician should consider testing for hepatitis A with anti-HAV IgM, hepatitis B with IgM anti-HBc, total anti-HBc and HBsAg, and hepatitis C with anti-HCV or HCV RNA. A complete discussion of the workup of viral hepatitis is in Chapter 25.

In MSM, hepatitis A (HAV) may be transmitted sexually through oral-genital contact, specifically analingus. The incubation period ranges from 15 to 50 days, with a mean of average of 30 days. Individuals who have been exposed to hepatitis A within the previous 2 weeks should be given immune globulin (.02 mL/kg) unless they have been vaccinated in the previous month. Hepatitis A vaccination is recommended for all men who have sex with men, persons with chronic liver disease, as well as those reporting illicit drug use.

Hepatitis B (HBV) is a relatively commonly transmitted STI, with sexual transmission accounting for most HBV infections in Europe and North America. Before the availability of vaccination, HBV seropositivity rates were 10 times higher than those in heterosexuals, and receptive rectal intercourse was defined as an extremely efficient mode of transmission. In the 1990s, transmission among MSM accounted for 15% of infections, while 40% were among heterosexual partners. Hepatitis B vaccination is the most effective way to avert infection, although other methods used to prevent STIs also should be effective against HBV. Immunization of all newborns, children, and adolescents is expected to drastically reduce the numbers of new infections of HBV, but it has not been universally implemented. Current recommendations for routine vaccinations to prevent the sexual transmission of HBV include sexually active MSM; sexually active heterosexual men and women in whom an STI has been diagnosed; people with more than one sexual partner in the previous 6 months; people who report sex with an injection-drug user; household members, sex partners, or drug-sharing partners of a person with chronic HBV infections; or those who report prostitution and illegal drug use. MSM and those who report injection drug use are at high risk for HBV. Therefore, screening for hepatitis B core antibody before vaccination may be cost effective in MSM and other high-risk groups. Many authorities recommend giving them the first dose of vaccine at the time of taking blood for hepatitis B core antibody (see Chapter 25). Sexual contacts of individuals with acute hepatitis B should receive hepatitis B immune globulin as soon as possible (preferably ≤24 hours) after exposure and begin the vaccination schedule.

Acute hepatitis C (HVC) is indistinguishable from HBV or HAV by signs and symptoms alone. Although the parental route is the primary mode of transmission, there is a subset where sexual transmission is likely. In the CDC's sentinel counties surveillance system, which has evaluated hepatitis transmission for >30 years, 11% of patients with acute hepatitis C report sexual exposure without other risk factors. Overall, it appears that prevalence rates of HCV among MSM and heterosexual individuals are similar. The incubation period for

HCV averages 6 to 7 weeks, with a range of 2 weeks to 6 months.

PROCTITIS, PROCTOCOLITIS, AND ENTERITIS

MSM who present with persistent gastrointestinal symptoms require a comprehensive history and physical (for a full discussion see Chapter 23). Evaluation may include microscopic examination of stool for ova and parasites, and culture for *Salmonella*, *Shigella*, or *Campylobacter*. In addition, diagnostic testing for *N. gonorrhoeae*, *C. trachomatis*, and herpes simplex virus should be obtained through anoscopy, if proctitis is suspected.

Proctitis

Proctitis is defined as inflammation of the distal 10–12 cm of the rectum and is predominantly seen in individuals who participate in receptive anal intercourse. Symptoms of proctitis commonly include rectal discharge, tenesmus, and pain. Asymptomatic infections are common. The most common causes of proctitis are *N. gonorrhoeae*, *C. trachomatis* (including LGV serovars), *T. pallidum*, and HSV. Herpes proctitis may be especially severe in individuals who are coinfected with HIV. Patients presenting with symptoms consistent with proctitis should be examined by anoscopy and tested for *N. gonorrhoeae*, *C. trachomatis*, HSV, and *T. pallidum*. Traditionally, rectal *N. gonorrhoeae* and *C. trachomatis* have been diagnosed by culture. However, recent studies have suggested that nucleic acid amplification techniques are sensitive and specific alternatives. If anorectal exudate or polymorphonuclear leukocytes are found on Gram stain, the patient should be treated empirically for *N. gonorrhoeae* and *C. trachomatis* (Table 34-6).

Proctocolitis

Proctocolitis is an inflammation of the colonic tissue extending beyond 12 cm above the anus. Presenting symptoms include symptoms of proctitis plus diarrhea and abdominal cramps. Individuals usually report a history of oral–fecal contact or receptive anal intercourse. Common pathogens associated with proctocolitis include *Campylobacter* sp., *Shigella* sp., *Entamoeba histolytica*, and LGV serovars of *C. trachomatis* (serovars L1, L2, or L3). More frequently now, in an HIV-infected person, cytomegalovirus (CMV) and opportunistic agents may be involved. There is significant overlap between organisms that cause protocolitis and enteritis.

TABLE 34-6 Diagnosis and Treatment of Sexually Transmitted Pathogens Which Can Present with Symptoms of Proctitis

Infectious Agent	Diagnostic Tests	Treatment
Neisseria gonorrhoeae	Gram stain Culture (NAAT)	Ceftriaxone 250 mg IM OR Cefixime 400 mg orally PLUS Treatment for chlamydia
Chlamydia trachomatis	Culture or NAAT	Doxycycline 100 mg orally twice a day for 7 days OR Azithromycin 1 g orally
C. trachomatis L1, L2, L3 (Lymphogranuloma venereum)	Culture, serovar-specific serologic tests not widely available	Doxycycline 100 mg orally twice a day for 21 days
Treponema. pallidum (syphilis)	Nontreponemal (VDRL or RPR) confirmed by treponemal test (FTA-ABS or MHA-TP)	Benzathine penicillin G 2.4 million units IM in a single dose for primary or secondary syphilis
Herpes simplex virus	Culture	See Table 34-4

Enteritis

Sexually transmitted enteritis usually presents with diarrhea and abdominal cramping, but without rectal discharge, tenesmus, and anorectal pain. Enteritis is often acquired by oral–fecal contact. *Giardia lamblia* is by far the most frequently reported cause of sexually transmitted enteritis in otherwise healthy individuals (Table 34-7). Asymptomatic infections are common. HIV may be the primary cause of enteritis. HIV-infected individuals frequently have enteritis that is not sexually transmitted due to CMV, *Mycobacterium-avium intracellulare, Salmonella* sp., *Cryptosporidium, Shigella* sp., *Microsporidium,* or *Isospora.* Multiple-stool examinations may be needed to detect *Giardia,* and special preparations are needed to diagnose cryptosporidiosis or microsporidiosis. Sigmoidoscopy of the distal 25 cm of the colon typically is normal. Treatment depends on identifying the offending organism.

■ PREVENTION OF SEXUALLY TRANSMITTED INFECTIONS

The prevention of STIs among MSM is critical to all members of society. Men who engaged in unprotected sex with men face a high likelihood of exposure to a wide variety of illnesses that do not regard the sociopolitical boundaries of sexual orientation. Preventive interventions can be categorized as primary, secondary, and tertiary. Primary strategies aim to avert disease in uninfected parties. Infected persons are the focus of secondary efforts to prevent the spread of disease beyond an index case. Tertiary interventions help reduce morbidity and mortality among infected person. A cohesive public health disease prevention and control strategy requires coordination at all three levels of intervention. This discussion will primarily focus on the prevention approach to homosexual men.

Primary Prevention

Primary prevention couples immunization with behavioral interventions to prevent infection. Although effective hepatitis A and B vaccines have been widely available and recommended for men who have sex with men, they have not been well utilized. Impediments include lack of awareness among providers and patients alike, poor communication about sexual matters in traditional healthcare settings, the perceived social stigma of homosexuality, and all other barriers to health care for marginalized populations.

TABLE 34-7 Diagnosis and Treatment of Sexually Transmitted Pathogens That Present with Symptoms of Proctocolitis or Enteritis

Infectious Agent	Diagnosis	Treatment
Enteritis		
Giardia lamblia	Stool for ova and parasite, ELISA or Enterotest	Metronidazole 250 mg orally three times a day for 5 days, OR Nitazoxanide 500 mg orally twice a day for 3 days Tinidazole 2 g orally
Proctocolitis		
Chlamydia trachomatis L1, L2, L3 (Lymphogranuloma venereum)	Culture, serovar-specific serologic tests not widely available	Doxycycline 100 mg orally twice a day for 21 days
Entamoeba histolytica	Stool ova and parasite	Metronidazole 750 mg orally three times a day for 7–10 days, OR Tinidazole 2 g once daily for 3–5 days
Shigella sp. (bacillary dysentery)	Stool culture	Trimethoprim-sulfamethoxazole DS orally twice a day for 5 days
Campylobacter sp.	Stool culture requiring special isolation techniques	Erythromycin 250–500 mg orally for 5–7 days OR Ciprofloxacin 500 mg orally twice a day for 3–5 days

Behavioral interventions encompass strategies to avoid risky sex or to reduce the risk associated with sex. Correct and consistent use of condoms during intercourse has been the mainstay of HIV-risk reduction guidelines. As an adjunct or alternative to condom use, some MSM favor other means to avoid exposure to HIV and other STIs, such as monogamy, selection of seronegative partners, reducing numbers of partners or frequency of sex, or avoiding intercourse altogether. Even modest reductions in risky behaviors can profoundly affect the incidence of disease in a population.

Knowledge about STI transmission and prevention is necessary but insufficient to sustain behavioral change. Beyond information, effective prevention programs use the tools of social marketing, small-group discussion, and individual counseling to build personal and community-wide awareness, self-esteem, self-efficacy, intentions to enact healthy behaviors, and social norms of safe sexual behavior. Other desirable programmatic features are a solid conceptual framework, clear behavioral objectives, developmental and cultural appropriateness, repetition and rehearsal of lessons, opportunities to learn from credible peer educators and role model, and attention to the contextual issues that place people at risk. Alcohol and other drug use in sexual situations consistently has been found to impede safer sex among MSM.

Secondary Prevention

When primary prevention fails, secondary prevention describes other strategies to prevent the spread of infection beyond an index case. These include prompt diagnosis and treatment and, where appropriate, partner notification, and treatment partners.

Tertiary Prevention

We define tertiary prevention as pharmacological approaches to reduce infectivity of chronic infection. The development of effective antivirals for HIV/AIDS, hepatitides, and herpes virus infections facilitate this prevention modality. "Treatment to prevent transmission" has been conclusively shown in herpes infections—where chronic suppressive treatment of individuals with asymptomatic infection reduces transmission to their uninfected (susceptible) partners. Similar trials are now ongoing for HIV, and there is also additional interest in postexposure prophylaxis, such as microbicides for STI and antiviral-containing microbicides for HIV Such possibilities underscore the public health imperative for a coordinated and multifaceted approach to STI prevention for MSM and their communities.

■ SUMMARY

Sexually transmitted infections continue to pose a serious threat to the lives and well-being of men who have sex with men. A comprehensive history and careful physical examination are essential to ensure that MSM receive appropriate evaluation and treatment for STIs and HIV. All men who engage in unprotected oral or anal intercourse with men should be offered periodic STI screening, even in the absence of symptoms.

The growing availability of noninvasive diagnostic tests for urethritis and HIV infection is creating opportunities for expanded access. When one STI is detected, other infections, including HIV, should be suspected. The early detection and treatment of STIs can reduce morbidity, mortality, and secondary spread of disease.

The advent of potent antiviral agents and immune system modulators represents a major breakthrough in controlling chronic viral illnesses but should not cause complacency. The apparent resurgence of gonorrhea among MSM and the significant rates of transmission of HIV among youth give reason to increase primary prevention efforts through immunization and intensive behavioral intervention, although evidence of long-term efficacy of the latter remains to be determined. Effective topical microbicides and vaccines against currently incurable viral illnesses may enhance the success of future preventive efforts.

■ KEY POINTS

- MSM who engage in unprotected sexual intercourse continue to face a high likelihood of exposure to a wide variety of infections.

- All men who engage in unprotected oral or anal intercourse with men should be offered periodic sexually transmitted infection (STI) screening, even in the absence of symptoms.

- Rarely is an oropharyngeal STI suspected unless a comprehensive sexual history is obtained.

- The availability of urine-based nucleic acid amplification techniques to screen for *Neisseria gonorrhoeae* and *Chlamydia trachomatis* have decreased barriers to testing.

- Painless ulcers (syphilis, granuloma inguinale) may be difficult to detect in rectal crypts without a high index of suspicion.

- Individuals may be coinfected with multiple STIs, including HIV.

REFERENCES

CDC. STD treatment guidelines 2010. *Morb Mort Week Rep.* 2010;59(RR-12):1–110.

Ekstrand ML, Coates TJ. Maintenance of sager sexual behaviors and predictors of risky sex: the San Francisco Men's Health Study. *Am J Public Health.* 1990;80:973.

Ekstrand ML, Coates TJ, Morin SF, et al. Longitudinal predictors of reductions in unprotected anal intercourse among gay men in San Francisco: the AIDS Behavioral Research Project. *Am J Public Health.* 1990;80:978.

Handsfield HH, Schwebke J. Trends in sexually transmitted diseases in homosexually active men in King County, Washington, 1980–1990. *Sex Transm Dis.* 1990;17:211.

Henning KJ, Bell E, Braun J, et al. A community-wide outbreak of hepatitis A: risk factors for infection among homosexual and bisexual men. *Am J Med.* 1995;99:132.

Koblin BA, Chesney MA, Husnik MJ, et al. High-risk behaviors among men who have sex with men in 6 US cities: baseline data from the EXPLORE Study. *Am J Public Health* 2003;93:926–932.

Lafferty WE, Hughes JP, Handsfield HH. Sexually transmitted diseases in men who have sex with men: acquisition of gonorrhea and nongonococcal urethritis by fellatio and implications for STD/HIV prevention. *Sex Transm Dis.* 1997;24(5):272.

Short LS, Stockman DL, Wolinsky SM, et al. Comparative rates of sexually transmitted diseases among heterosexual men, homosexual men, and heterosexual women. *Sex Transm Dis.* 1984;11(4):271.

35
Sexually Transmitted Infections in Homosexual Women

Christine A. Bowman

■ INTRODUCTION

Individuals may define themselves as lesbian, gay men, or bisexual on the basis of their preferred sexual partner, their desires, or actual sexual activity (past or present). These factors may change during a lifetime. In this chapter, I will use the term *women who have sex with women* (WSW) to facilitate discussion on the impact of this expression of sexual behavior on sexual and reproductive health. Misconceptions about the sexual behavior and healthcare needs of WSW are common and have adverse consequences for the delivery of appropriate services to these women.

To address the health needs (including sexual and reproductive health) of any particular group of individuals, we need to be able to clearly define and identify them. An inability to do this has impeded research and service development for WSW. In addition, misperceptions of needs and factors related to service provision and staff attitude may contribute to the "low visibility" of lesbian healthcare users.

Providers often assume that women attending sexual and reproductive health services are heterosexual. Sexual and reproductive healthcare services have been often justified on the basis of preventing infertility and adverse pregnancy outcomes. They therefore emphasize screening and treating bacterial sexually transmitted infections (STIs) such as chlamydia and gonorrhea, which are difficult to transmit from woman to woman. Reproductive healthcare services also focus on pregnancy prevention, ensuring prenatal services for pregnant women, and pregnancy termination services. In most settings, these services are often assumed (wrongly) to be irrelevant to lesbians. Many lesbians may feel anxious or even intimidated in health consultations and consequently elect not to confide the nature of their sexual partnerships

The detection and clinical management of HIV infection is another important component of sexual healthcare services. Recognizing the increased risk of HIV infection and STIs among men who have sex with men (MSM) and the important role of other STIs in facilitating HIV transmission led to the development of specific programs to address these issues. Furthermore, in some communities, MSM may misrepresent themselves as heterosexual men or may have also had sexual relationships (or long-term commitments, including marriage) with women. These trends have fostered an enormous body of behavioral and service-delivery research to develop appropriate means of delivering prevention services to these groups. In contrast to MSM, transmission of HIV between sexually active WSW is extremely rare. This has made lesbians invisible to HIV research and service development. However, there are hidden risks; WSW may have other high-risk activities, including sex with men (for pleasure, for financial gain, for procreation, or as a result of rape/abuse), or may have intravenous drug exposure. While sex between women may not be a high-risk activity for HIV transmission, WSW may have other HIV risk factors that need to be addressed as part of their sexual and reproductive health (see Table 35-1).

TABLE 35-1 High-Risk Factors for HIV Among WSW

Past or current sex with men:
- Casual or regular male partners
- Partners from high-risk groups (e.g., men who have sex with men)
- Commercial sex work
- Rape

Artificial insemination

Injection drug use

Defining "Lesbian"

Sexual orientation has been defined by self-identity, by sexual attraction, or by behavior. For women, as for men, these factors may not be congruent and often change over time. If sexual behavior is used as the defining factor, there are important issues in the definition. Should we consider only women currently having sexual contact with one or more women, those women who have had sex with a woman in the last year or ever in their lifetime, even if they are currently celibate or only having sex with men? Should the term *lesbian* rather than *bisexual* or *bi-curious heterosexual* be applied only to women exclusively having sex with women, and, if so, for how much of their lifetime? A critical factor is that current or past sexual contact with men (which is often unreported to providers) increases the lesbian's risk of STIs, HIV, or unwanted pregnancy. For some infections (such as human papillomavirus, or HPV) and cervical cancer, any sexual contact, homosexual or heterosexual, can increase health risks (see Table 35-2). For example, lesbian women can be at substantial HPV risk, either because of past exposure to an infected male partner, or through current exposure to an infected female partner. However, many lesbian women do not received periodic cervical cytology (Pap) or HPV screening because of the misperception that they are at low risk if they are exclusively in a WSW relationship.

How Common Is Female Homosexuality?

The sensitivity of the issue, stigma, and inaccuracies in self-reporting significantly impair accurate data collection. According to the U.K. National Survey of Sexual Attitudes and Lifestyles (2000), 5% of women in Britain in 2000 aged 16–44 years report one or more female sexual partners at some point in their lives, with higher figures of 7% of women living in Greater London. Similar results have been reported from the United States, with 4% of 18- to 59-year-old women across the United States (6% in largest cities) having had one or more female sexual partners at some point in their lives. In 2004, available U.S. estimates of lifetime WSW ranged between 8% and 20%, with current sexual female same-sex relationships in 1.4% to 4.3% of women. It is estimated that 2.3 million self-defined lesbians lived in the United States at that time.

High levels of previous or concurrent heterosexual experience in WSW are supported by a large literature.

TABLE 35-2 Malignancies and WSW

Malignancy	Predisposing Factors
Increased risks of cancer in: • Breast • Uterus • Ovary	More unopposed menstrual cycles: • Fewer pregnancies • Less breast-feeding • Less use of oral combined contraceptive Increased BMI Alcohol use Smoking
Cervical malignancy	Failure to screen for premalignant change or HPV • Poorer uptake of cervical cytology • Misconceptions about risk by patient and healthcare worker

NATSAL 1990 data indicated that 96% of women who have had a female sexual contact have also had a male sexual contact at some time in their life.

■ BARRIERS TO LESBIAN SEXUAL HEALTH

What Is Sexual Health?

In 1975, the World Health Organization defined sexual health as "the integration of the somatic, emotional, intellectual and social aspects of sexual beings, in ways that are positively enriching and that enhance personality, communication and love." An alternative view on sexual health is one that involves "the enjoyment of sexual activity of one's choice without suffering or causing physical or mental harm . . . It can be interpreted as uniting all the positive aspects of sex as a life-enhancing source of self-fulfillment and pleasure given by mutual consent, be it heterosexual, gay or lesbian sex" (Greenhouse 1994, 22–23).

Failure to recognize that a woman attending healthcare services may identify as lesbian or may have issues related to being a WSW is the first barrier to lesbian sexual health care (see Table 35-3). Women attending with sexually transmitted infections, HIV, or pregnancy-related issues are generally expected to be heterosexual women. Some WSW will have healthcare issues resulting from consensual or nonconsensual heterosexual contact. Some may have infections contracted through sex with other women, such as genital warts, herpes, or bacterial vaginosis. Others may wish to discuss dysmenorrhea, vulval skin conditions, menopausal symptoms (including dyspareunia), or assisted pregnancy.

Studies of WSW attending sexual or reproductive healthcare clinics report that women are frequently not asked the sex of their partner and that they are too embarrassed or fearful of unsympathetic responses to volunteer this information. A nonjudgmental approach in taking the medical and sexual history is therefore critical (see Chapter 2 on taking the history and Chapter 34 on MSM) Research in the United States and in the United Kingdom suggests that healthcare providers commonly hold or are perceived to hold prejudiced, condemnatory, and ignorant views about lesbian, gay, and bisexual patients. In addition to causing difficulty in seeking care for specific symptoms or advice, this may result in reluctance to engage in routine screening programs (e.g., cervical cytology and mammograms). The introduction of the Civil Partnership Registration in the UK (2005) and similar legislation in a number of U.S. states affords lesbian and gay couples most of the legal rights of married heterosexuals and has marked greater acceptability of gay and lesbian couples in society. This may improve recognition of these groups and their healthcare issues by health services and professionals.

■ SEXUAL BEHAVIOR

What Do Lesbians Do?

Details of sexual practices among WSW are often lack research and epidemiological reports. Bailey et al. (2003) published some UK data based on a sample of 803 lesbian and bisexual women attending two London lesbian sexual health clinics and 415 WSW from a community sample recruited through listings in the lesbian and gay press, conferences, focus groups, and snowballing (a recruitment technique in which participants are asked to invite other relevant members from their social networks to join the

---

TABLE 35-3   Barriers to Sexual Health for WSW

Failure to identify WSW:
Woman reluctant to disclose

- Privacy
- Embarrassment
- Shame
- Feel of stigma/mistreatment

Healthcare worker

- Ignorant of possibility
- Embarrassed to ask
- Fear of offending patient
- Issues around sexuality

Lack of perception of healthcare needs for:

- STIs/HIV
- Cervical cytology
- Other malignancies
- Pregnancy
- Menopause

Prejudice

Legal issues—varies geographically

- Sexual practice
- Civil partnership/marriage
- Assisted conception/adoption

study). In this study, 85% of the WSW had had a sexual contact with a man at some stage in their life, 12% of these within 12 months of the survey. The most commonly reported sexual practices between women were oral sex, digital vaginal penetration, mutual masturbation, and tribadism (frottage with genital-to-genital contact or rubbing of genital areas against another part of the partner's body), each of which occurred in around 85% of WSW. Less common practices (in decreasing order of reported frequency) included anal penetration with fingers, vaginal penetration with sex toys, rimming (oroanal contact), sadomasochistic sex, and anal penetration with sex toys. Use of dildos and other sex toys was by no means a universal sexual activity by WSW. Only 16% reported often having vaginal penetration with a sex toy (and 37% occasional sex toy vaginal penetration) during sex with women. This compared with 4% often and 16% occasional use of a sex toy for vaginal penetration in WSW sexual encounters with men.

Similar preferences have been reported from the Pride Survey (Creith 1996), based on a sample of 278 lesbians attending London's annual Pride festival, and the Boston Lesbian Health Project (2000), a U.S. national survey of 1633 lesbians recruited by snowball sampling.

Safer Sexual Practices

Some STIs, including *Trichomonas vaginalis*, can be spread by exchange of cervicovaginal fluid and direct mucosal contact. Penetrative sexual practice therefore might be expected to increase the risk of transmission. Proposed preventive measures proposed include handwashing, using latex gloves, cleaning sex toys, and using condoms on toys. Studies, however, often report limited and inconsistent use of these methods in WSW. There is no good evidence to show that using a dental dam (a piece of latex applied to the genitals as a protective barrier during oral sex) reduces the transmission of STIs or

HIV between WSW. Studies show these to be unpopular and rarely used. Unwillingness of WSW to adopt "safer sexual practices" may be the result of having limited knowledge about the possibilities of STI transmission or feeling less vulnerable to STIs and HIV.

Patterns of Partner Change

Numbers of sexual partners, frequency of new partners, and multiple concurrent sexual contacts increase the risk of transmitting STIs and HIV. Although there is clearly a wide range of reported numbers of partners in cohorts of WSW, partner numbers remain relatively low: Only 23% of women in a study of Bailey et al. (2003) had more than 10 lifetime partners. This is similar to figures for heterosexual women reported in NATSAL (2000).

■ SEXUALLY TRANSMITTED INFECTIONS AND OTHER GENITAL INFECTIONS

The likelihood of transmitting genital infection in any one sexual act depends on: the presence of active infection in one of the sexual contacts, the infectivity of the infecting agent, the infectious dose delivered by the sexual act performed, the receptiveness of the contact site to that particular infection and cofactors for transmission (e.g., trauma, inflammation). In population terms, spread of STIs and HIV will depend on sexual networking (see Table 35-4). As genital herpes (HSV) and infectious syphilis both produce highly infectious lesions on oral and genital mucosal surfaces, it is no surprise that they are potentially transmissible through most WSW sexual activities. *Trichomonas vaginalis* (TV) and bacterial vaginosis (BV) are easily visualized by microscopy in the vaginal secretions of most affected women; transmission through exchange of vaginal fluids gives a plausible explanation for the documented WSW transmission of these conditions. The usual mode of hepatitis A transmission

TABLE 35-4   STIs or Other Genital Infections in WSW

Common (easily transmitted by WSW contact)	**Occasional**	**Uncommon** (usually due to additional heterosexual contact)
Bacterial vaginosis	*Trichomonas vaginalis*	Gonorrhoea
Vulvovaginal candidiasis		Chlamydia
Genital papilloma, infections, and warts		Syphilis
Genital herpes		HIV

is by feco–oral spread, and WSW sexual transmission has also been reported.

In contrast, *Chlamydia trachomatis* and *Neiserria gonorrhoeae* are both organisms that in adults infect the cervix, urethra, pharynx, and rectum. They do not establish infection in the adult vulval or vaginal epithelium. It is probably necessary to "inoculate" a sufficient infectious bacterial load directly onto one of these sites during sex to transmit these infections. It may therefore be technically more difficult to spread infection of these agents from one woman to another. Woman-to-woman transmission of chlamydia and gonorrhea has not been documented but does occur in WSW who have also had heterosexual contact.

The prevalence of STIs is lower in lesbians than in heterosexuals and much lower than in MSM. This may reflect biological factors, frequency of partner change, and sexual network dynamics. The risks of STIs and HIV are increased in WSW who have previous or ongoing sexual contacts with men, are current or previous intravenous drug abusers, or have attempted artificial insemination by donor.

Unlike other genital infections, BV is reported as more common in WSW than in heterosexual women. The prevalence of BV is reported to be 27–52% in WSW compared with women attending prenatal clinics (16%) or STI clinics (24–37%). BV is a condition in which the normal bacterial flora of the vagina is disturbed, resulting in a reduction in lactobacilli and a predominance of commensal anaerobic bacteria, often associated with *Gardnerella vaginalis mobiluncus* species and *mycoplasma* species (see Chapter 7). It is one of the most common causes of abnormal vaginal discharge in women and occurs in most women at some time in their lives. BV often resolves spontaneously but may recur, sometimes frequently, despite treatment. It is often asymptomatic but may cause an unpleasant malodorous vaginal discharge. It has been associated with increased risk of preterm labor, low birth weight, postpartum and postabortal endometritis and may increase the risk of acquiring HIV. In heterosexual women, BV is not considered a sexually transmitted infection, and treating the male partner does not reduce recurrence of BV. Asymptomatic women may not need any specific treatment unless they are pregnant or about to undergo an invasive gynecological procedure.

Studies in WSW have shown significant concordance of the presence or absence of BV in monogamous lesbian couples. BV is associated with a higher lifetime number of female partners, failure to consistently clean insertive sex toys before use or between sharing, and oral–anal sex with a female partner. Recent douching and a new male partner are risk factors for BV in heterosexuals; their im-

pact on increasing the finding of BV in WSW is less clear. Future studies comparing the incidence of BV in WSW exclusively and women having sex with men exclusively using penetrative sex toys would add weight to the lesbian sexual transmission of BV-related organisms. These studies need to control for hormonal cofactors, such as the contraceptive pill and pregnancy, as there is evidence that vaginal flora changes through the menstrual cycle and can be affected by mode of contraception in heterosexual women. It has been suggested that female saliva may have an inhibitory factor on vaginal lactobacilli, but there is yet no data to support this.

A number of BV issues are worth exploring (does this represent a colonization of flora issue?) that may or may not require intimate contact. Furthermore, because most BV prevention and treatment activity are recently focused on the perinatal period, providing care to lesbian women may be affected. Finally, diagnosis of BV requires clinical suspicion and ability to screen, which is another part of service provision.

■ HIV

Can HIV Be Sexually Transmitted Between Women?

In 2003, an isolated case of female-to-female genotype-concordant HIV was reported. However, epidemiological data have failed to show HIV positivity in WSW who have no other risk factors, and transmission via WSW contact is exceedingly rare and not an issue of public health importance. In heterosexual women, HIV is thought to enter via receptors on the cervix during vaginal penetration or in the rectum during anal intercourse. A relatively large inoculum of HIV is usually required to achieve sexual transmission, which explains the marked risk reduction seen in couples using condoms. HIV-positive patients with high viral loads (e.g., during seroconversion or in late-stage HIV without antiretroviral therapy) are more infectious to sexual partners as are patients with STIs and other genital infections, which increase HIV levels in genital secretions. HIV-negative partners with STIs and genital infections are more at risk of acquiring HIV from an infected partner because of up-regulation of HIV receptors in their genital tract.

HIV transmission in WSW is biologically plausible during particularly high-risk activities involving contamination with fresh blood, for example, sharing unwashed penetrative sex toys during menstruation of an infected individual. The risks would be increased if the vulnerable partner had BV or a sexually transmitted infection.

A woman's sexual identity is not an accurate predictor of behavior. A large proportion of "lesbian women" report sex with men either consensually (for pleasure, conception, commercial gain, or even within the context of a marital relationship) or nonconsensually (rape or abuse). Female and male homosexuality are stigmatized in a number of countries and is illegal in some countries as well. Substantive HIV-transmission risks include unprotected sex with men, artificial insemination with unscreened donor semen, and injecting drug use (IDU). For example, Australian studies reported increased risk taking among WSW with more sexual contacts with MSM, riskier IDU use (sharing needles, etc.), and participation in commercial sex work. "Do-it-yourself" artificial insemination by donor or sex with a male friend (often gay) is a risk some WSW take to overcome their lack of access to legitimate fertility services.

■ Cervical Cytology and Dysplasia

HPV is the leading cause of anogenital intraepithelial neoplasia (squamous intraepithelial lesions) and genital warts (see Chapter 22). Lesbians can acquire HPV from sexual contact with either men or women. In one study, HPV DNA was detected in 19% of WSW with no history of male contacts. Intimate genital contact with or without digital penetration or penetration with toys is a likely mode of sexual transmission. Oral transmission of HPV has also been postulated. Routine cervical cytology and HPV testing where appropriate is indicated for all sexually active women, independent of sexual preference. Because of the long latency in the presentation of HPV sequelae, this would include women who are not sexually active currently but have been so in the past.

Providing preventive health and gynecological services to lesbian women can be challenging. Poorer uptake of cervical screening services by lesbians, compared to heterosexual women is well documented. This may reflect a lack of perception of risk of both HPV and cervical cancer in WSW and in their sexual healthcare providers. In addition, lesbians may find it more difficult to access services because of real or perceived prejudices and hostilities of staff.

■ Risks of Other Gynecological Cancers: Uterus and Ovary

Pregnancy (even those terminated or miscarried), breastfeeding, and using hormonal contraception reduce the risk of upper tract genital cancer. Smoking and high-body mass index are also adverse risk factors for ovarian cancer. Studies of lesbian groups have shown increased prevalence of these malignancies compared with heterosexual women associated with these risk factors.

In addition, increased risk of breast cancer in lesbians is well recognized. This malignancy shares the risks of unopposed menstrual cycles and increased body mass but is also associated with increased alcohol consumption, frequently reported in studies comparing lesbians to heterosexual women.

These increased cancer risks emphasize the importance of access for WSW to good preventive advice (about smoking, alcohol, and obesity) in addition to encouraging uptake of screening and seeking appropriate diagnostic health care when indicated.

■ Other Gynecological Problems

An increase in prevalence of polycystic ovary syndrome has been reported among lesbians. This condition may present with infertility, hirsuitism, or obesity. Because it is associated with insulin insensitivity, it may be associated with increased cardiovascular risk. Menstrual, premenstrual, and menopausal problems can affect all women, whatever their sexual orientation or behavior. Women exclusively having sex with women, however, may be more reluctant than their heterosexual counterparts to take the combined oral contraceptive pill to reduce dysmenorrhea.

The menopause may be associated with vulval atrophy and decreased natural secretions, which reduce sexually aroused natural lubrication and lead to superficial dyspareunia. Many WSW may find discussion of these problems particularly difficult or embarrassing.

■ Pregnancy

Being lesbian does not eliminate the strong biological drive that many women have to conceive, carry their own children, or raise a family.

Access to fertility and adoption services for lesbians varies widely. Social barriers can include legal constraints, societal stigma, and insurance reimbursement issues. In settings in which WSW parenthood is marginalized, WSW may resort to high-risk approaches to conceive, including unprotected heterosexual sex with or artificial insemination by an unscreened man. Studies show that these partners are often gay or bisexual men who are themselves at high risk for STI and HIV.

■ DESIGNING A SEXUAL HEALTH SERVICE FOR WOMEN WHO HAVE SEX WITH WOMEN

Sexual and reproductive healthcare staff need to demonstrate their awareness of the range of human sexuality and avoid assumptions of heterosexuality. All patients hope to be cared for by clinicians who are friendly, professional, and nonjudgmental. Improved education and training on sexual diversity may help.

Specialist clinics for lesbian and bisexual women have proved popular with some WSW. However, these types of dedicated services require catchment populations large enough to sustain them. Many other lesbians enjoy a good sense of integration into their wider community and prefer to access friendly mainstream services. In either setting, staff need to address behavioral risks or requests for services appropriately and empathetically.

What Sexual and Reproductive Health Care Do Women Who Have Sex with Women Need Access to?

- Information on alternative lifestyles and relationships, identifying and managing risks, support networks

- Information on sexual health issues for WSW

- Access to routine cervical cytology and colposcopy

- Access to hormonal contraceptives for menstrual problems or as birth control

- Information and screening for breast cancer

- Management of symptomatic genital infections and skin conditions

- Screening for STI, HIV, and viral hepatitis if at risk

- Advice on and access to fertility services, safe assisted conceptions, fostering, and adoption

- Advice on and management of menopausal symptoms, including dyspareunia

■ KEY POINTS

- Women who have sex with women may identify themselves as lesbians, bisexuals, or bi-curious heterosexuals.

- All sexually active women need access to appropriate sexual and reproductive health care.

- Determining the most appropriate advice, screening, and clinical management depends on eliciting an accurate sexual history.

- Most lesbians will have had some previous heterosexual contact that may have put them at risk of certain STIs (e.g., chlamydia and gonorrhea) and HIV, which are difficult to transmit between women.

- Some STIs, including herpes, genital wart virus, and TV, are easily passed between women.

- BV may be sexually transmitted between women and appears to be more common in lesbians than in heterosexual women.

- Screening for abnormal cervical cytology should be offered as part of the routine program.

- Lesbians are at increased risk from ovarian, uterine, and breast cancer if they have not had exposure to hormonal contraceptives or pregnancy. Smoking, alcohol, and obesity increase the risks of these (and other) malignancies, so lifestyle advice may be useful.

- Many lesbian women aspire to have children, which may result in high-risk sexual contacts or unscreened artificial insemination.

REFERENCES

Bailey JV, Farquhar C, Owen C, Whittaker D. Sexual behaviour of lesbians and bisexual women. *Sex Transm Infect.* 2003;79(2):147–150.

Creith E. *Undressing Lesbian Sex: Popular Images, Private Acts and Public Consequences.* London: Cassell; 1996.

Fenton KA, Johnson AM, McManus S, et al. Measuring sexual behaviour: methodological challenges in survey research. *Sex Transm Infect.* 2001;77:84–92.

Greenhouse P. A sexual health service under one roof. In: Pillaye J, ed. *Sexual Health Promotion in Genitourinary Medicine Clinics.* London: Health Education Authority; 1994:22–33.

Johnson AM, Mercer CH, Erens, et al. Sexual behaviour in Britain: partnerships, practises and HIV risk behaviours. *Lancet.* 2001;358:1835–1842.

Marrazzo JM. Barriers to infectious disease care among lesbians. *Emerg Infect Dis.* 2004;10:1974.

Marrazzo JM, Coffey P, Elliott MN. Sexual practices, risk perception, and knowledge of sexually transmitted disease risk among lesbian and bisexual women. *Perspect Sex Reprod Health.* 2005;37:6–12.

National Centre for Social Research et al. (2000). National Survey of Sexual Attitudes and Lifestyles II, 2000–2001. Colchester, Essex: UK Data Archive [distributor], August 2005. SN: 5223.

Roberts SJ, Sorensen L, Patsdaughter CA, et al. Sexual behaviours and sexually transmitted diseases of lesbians: results of the Boston Lesbian Health Project. *J Lesbian Stud.* 2000;4:49–70.

World Health Organization (WHO). Education and treatment in human sexuality: the training of health professionals. Geneva, Switzerland: WHO; 1975:WHO Technical Report Series No. 572.

36
Sexually Transmitted Infections in Drug Users

David C. Perlman, Holly Hagan, Benny Kottiri, Nadim Salomon, and Samuel R. Friedman

▮ INTRODUCTION

The relationship between sexually transmitted infections (STIs) and illicit drug use has been recognized for nearly a century. High rates of STIs continue to be observed in more recent cohorts of injection drug users (IDUs), with up to 60% reporting histories of STIs. High rates of STIs are seen among noninjection drug users, such as users of crack cocaine and methamphetamine. STIs have also been shown to be independent risk factors for the sexual transmission of human immunodeficiency virus (HIV).

Despite the high prevalence and incidence of STIs, and the HIV transmission implications, drug users can be a difficult-to-reach population who may be incompletely or inconsistently engaged in longitudinal or preventive health care, and for whom adherence to therapeutic interventions can be problematic. Yet, with appropriate preventative interventions and healthcare delivery models, drugs users have been shown to be capable of both significant risk-reducing behavior change and of adhering to diverse therapies.

▮ INCIDENCE AND PREVALENCE

There are approximately 5 million IDUs worldwide. In the United States alone, there are 1.1 million IDUs and 4.6 million persons who use illicit drugs by various routes. The term *drug users* is a construct applied to a heterogeneous group of individuals who use diverse

drugs by diverse routes at varying frequencies. The medical issues affecting drug users may vary, with differences in the background prevalence of conditions and with diverse drug use, environmental, behavioral, and social exposures. Sniffing or snorting drugs may be associated with the risk of infection either through mucocutaneous exposure to shared implements to administer drugs or drug-related sexual risk behavior. Further, drug users may transition between periods of drug injection, periods of noninjection illicit drug use, and periods of no drug use; yet they may acquire chronic infections such as HIV, hepatitis B virus (HBV), hepatitis C virus (HCV), syphilis, or others during periods of drug use with the potential for subsequent transmission.

Incidence rates for early syphilis in drug users are substantially higher than for the general population. Since the late 1980s, outbreaks of primary and secondary syphilis have been associated with crack cocaine and methamphetamine associated with the exchange of money or drugs for sex. Among IDUs, youth, multiple sex partners, and paid sex are associated with higher rates of syphilis. Multiple studies have suggested that the risks for STIs in drug users are not homogeneous. For example, the relationship between drug use and STI rates may be weaker for gonorrhea or chlamydia compared with syphilis, the viral hepatitides, and HIV.

Although chancroid is rare in the developed world, previous outbreaks have usually been associated with crack cocaine use and sex-for-drugs exchanges. Genital ulcer diseases (syphilis, herpes, and chancroid) are all associated with HIV transmission (see Chapter 17). Smoking crack or methamphetamine can cause blisters and sores on the lips and oral mucosa of smokers; such ulcers have been proposed to facilitate the transmission of infectious pathogens.

Syphilis is associated with HIV seroconversion among drug users; while syphilitic genital ulcer disease can directly facilitate HIV transmission; in some instances, HIV seroconversion may precede syphilis (see Chapters 9 and 10). In these circumstances, the association may be due to such behaviors as unprotected sex and exchanging sex for money or drugs, which put drug users at risk for both HIV and syphilis.

Injection drug users are at risk for acquiring HIV, HBV, and HCV, predominantly through nonsterile injection practices, and syphilis can be transmitted parenterally. Yet once acquired, these agents can be transmitted through sexual routes as well as through subsequent drug use behaviors. Studies of HCV seroconversion and seroprevalence suggest that, after onset of injection, the median time to acquisition of HCV is between 3 and 4 years. Seroconversion rates do tend to be higher in the initial period, suggesting the existence of a high-risk subgroup of injectors. However, the potential for rapid acquisition of infections among new injectors highlights the importance of developing means to both prevent injection drug use and to identify recent onset injectors for preventive vaccinations (e.g., HBV) and sociobehavioral interventions.

■ RELATIONSHIP BETWEEN SEXUAL AND DRUG USE BEHAVIORS

Although the prevalence of HIV and the prevalence of injection-related HIV risk behaviors have fallen significantly among IDUs, there is still a substantial risk. Injection practices among IDUs have changed in response to endogenous and public health initiated programs such as a greater availability of clean syringes through syringe exchanges and pharmacies, greater awareness of HIV risks among IDUs and the development of new subcultural norms about injection behaviors. In contrast, sexual transmission is increasingly an important route of HIV infection among IDUs. Injection-related risk behavior has declined, sexual HIV transmission has persisted, and an increasing proportion of new infections are attributable to sexual exposures, which has been demonstrated in a number of longitudinal cohort studies. Higher rates of HIV infection have been observed among IDUs who

also engage in male–male sex, and among female new injectors, suggesting another avenue role of sexual transmission (Friedman 1999). Another pattern observed is that age disparity (younger injectors injecting with older IDUs conferred increased HIV risk). Drug use practices may be linked to sexual practices and embedded within specific social and sexual networks. In addition to the links between drug use and exchanging sex for drugs or for money to acquire drugs, drug users may be more likely to engage in both high-risk injection drug use practices and in noninjection drug use practices, such as drug smoking, with sexual partners and within social or sexual networks.

Among drug users, consistent condom use is more frequent in relationships involving HIV seropositive IDUs and in relationships with non-IDUs. Causes of such differential condom use are likely due to behaviors prompted by uninfected or non-drug-using partners and to altruistic desires of IDUs to prevent infections in their partners. Altruism exists among IDUs and is manifested by a variety of behaviors, including their voluntary participation in HIV-prevention programs, drug users' organizations, research studies, and clinical trials.

The observation that longer-term injectors are more likely to use condoms consistently, along with other data, also question the commonly held belief that substance use or abuse may directly (perhaps by lowering inhibition or impairing judgment) facilitate unsafe sex behaviors. Newer injectors in some settings have adopted lower risk injection practices in response to HIV prevention efforts and the adoption of new drug user cultural norms, suggesting the potential for appropriately designed interventions to reduce sexual risk behaviors among new injectors as well.

Women drug injectors may be at risk for HIV and STIs through both high-risk heterosexual behaviors and through nonsterile injection practices, particularly with older male partners who may have a higher prevalence of STIs, with viral STIs such as HSV-2 having the highest prevalence (also see Chapter 18) These women may be at great, or greater, risk for STIs and HIV as other women drug users.

Ultimately, decisions regarding condom use and other risk-reduction behaviors are not made solely by individuals, but by negotiated actions between persons in social and sexual relationships. This highlights the need for STI and HIV prevention efforts to address both the specific behaviors that contribute to risk and the social contexts within which the behaviors occur.

▪ ADHERENCE OF DRUG USERS TO TREATMENT AND BEHAVIOR CHANGE

Both drug users and alcoholics have been reported to be less adherent to a variety of therapies (e.g., antiretroviral agents, antituberculous agents, and others) than non-drug- or non-alcohol-using persons. Yet adherence issues are not unique to illicit drug users, and poor adherence to therapy is a major impediment to optimal clinical outcomes for a wide range of medical conditions and populations.

Pragmatic measures to improve adherence may include patient education, reminder systems, directly observed therapy programs, incentives, health or contingency contracts, addressing pressing socioeconomic needs, and appointment scheduling that considers the exigencies of a drug users' lifestyle. Early morning clinical appointments may conflict with methadone pickup schedules or may be less realistic than later appointments for individuals who may have more nocturnal lifestyles. Contingency contracts, frequently used in psychiatric and drug abuse treatment settings and for adherence to tuberculosis therapy, may be valuable tools to enhance the adherence of drug users to STI interventions. Positively reinforcing contingency contracts, in which a reward or benefit is provided for good adherence, in general have been shown to be more effective than negatively reinforcing contingencies in which poor adherence is penalized.

Monetary incentives have been shown to be effective in improving return rates for tuberculosis skin-test interpretation among IDUs, compared with either no incentive or with educational interventions in randomized studies. Monetary incentives have also been more effective at promoting attendance at HIV/STI prevention sessions than nonmonetary incentives, such as food coupons or gift certificates. Socioeconomic impediments to adherence such as unstable housing, no health insurance, or no transportation can be addressed by coordinating social services and medical care. It may be valuable for healthcare providers and health departments to work in conjunction with drug users' organizations, in locales where such organizations exist, to identify and address potential impediments to healthcare access and adherence.

Recognizing that adherence is a potential issue in managing patients, including, but not limited to, drug users, should be coupled with an appreciation that strategies to enhance adherence are available and that, with appropriately designed interventions, drug users can be engaged and retained in therapy. Drug users are also capable of significant risk-reducing behavior change, and significant reductions in HIV risk behaviors have led to declines in HIV incidence among new injectors and have contributed to declines in HIV seroprevalence among drug users.

▪ ISSUES IN PROVIDING STI CARE TO DRUG USERS

Many illicit drug users are not engaged in longitudinal medical care, may receive their care sporadically through emergency departments, and contribute to excess healthcare costs. Further, many IDUs may avoid traditional healthcare settings or rate their care poorly because of real or perceived inequities in care. The lack of linkage to primary care induces delays in adequate obtaining health screenings, especially for HIV testing. Therefore, many clinical services and programs that target IDUs are providing rapid point-of-service HIV screening tests. Although drug use is associated with many serious acute and chronic medical conditions, healthcare utilization among drug users is low compared with persons who do not use illicit drugs. Similarly, even though drug users have multiple risk factors for STIs and a high prevalence of infections, STI control programs do not reliably reach drug users. The threshold for seeking treatment may be higher among drug users because of direct drug effects that affect their tolerance of STI symptoms, with the result that they seek treatment only when symptoms are severe. Other barriers to seeking STI screening and treatment in drug users include a tendency to seek health care only for urgent health conditions, the perception that regular health care is a low priority, and that genital examinations are embarrassing.

Provider experience and attitudes are likely to be important determinants of outcomes in caring for drug users. Many providers report negative attitudes about caring for drug users and feel uncomfortable caring for them. Healthcare provider inexperience, discomfort, or negative attitudes may result in unproductive, negatively reinforcing interactions with healthcare systems. Drug users can be challenging patients who may engage in abusive or other problematic behaviors and often have underlying mental health issues. Addressing these problems requires both appropriate provider skills in managing behaviorally challenging patients and an appreciation that despite such behaviors drug users can be capable both of behavior change and of adherence to therapy.

Addressing a patient's need for drug treatment is a critical and appropriate part of caring for drug users both to deliver drug abuse treatment and because of the effectiveness of drug abuse treatment in preventing HIV infection. However, in many settings, the numbers of those in need of drug treatment significantly exceeds the number of available treatment slots or significant waiting lists may exist. Further, as with smoking and alcohol treatment interventions, drug treatment outcomes are highly dependent on the readiness of a user to quit. Not all drug users will have reached the stage at which they may be ready to enter drug treatment at the time they present for medical care and improved strategies to promote treatment readiness are needed.

For some medical issues, it may be appropriate to triage overall clinical needs and defer some specific aspects of care until drug abuse issues are addressed. For others, such as the treatment of STIs or tuberculosis, it is clearly necessary to provide medical care despite ongoing substance abuse. It may be particularly in these circumstances that provider attitudes and experience may be important determinants of clinical outcome. The principles of harm reduction include the concept that overall harm can be reduced even with ongoing drug use. Applying these principles may be an important clinical tool in the medical management of drug users and may facilitate engaging drug users in needed treatment. Good adherence with tuberculosis directly observed therapy has been reported despite ongoing illicit drug use. Although nonjudgmental discussions of the adverse health consequences of ongoing drug use may stimulate interest in drug treatment, focus group and ethnographic data support the concept that approaching ongoing drug use in a concerned but nonjudgmental manner may allow clinical endeavors to be viewed as an extension of harm reduction practices (such as syringe exchange or condom distribution) and may facilitate acceptance and adherence where cessation of drug use is not imminent.

The provider's attitude and clinical approach is a key factor for predicting retention in therapy. For example, retention in drug abuse treatment can be markedly better in programs that adopt flexible clinic hours and positively reinforce program strategies than in programs with a confrontational and rigid attitude.

In addition to the potential effects of provider attitudes on drug users' acceptance and adherence of treatments, provider experience may have an important effect on outcome. Among HIV-infected drug users, those whose physicians were less experienced HIV providers were significantly less likely to receive opportunistic infection prophylaxis or antiretroviral therapy than those with more experienced providers. Further, receiving care from experienced providers and in experienced clinics is associated with greater survival among HIV-infected patients. Providers may receive limited training in managing chemically dependent patients and greater levels of provider training and experience in managing chemical dependency, and its medical complications may enhance the clinical outcomes for drug users.

■ SITES FOR STI CARE FOR DRUG USERS

Specific sites and systems used for healthcare delivery to drug users may play a critical role in determining the outcomes of healthcare delivery, such as the accepting therapy, keeping appointments, adhering to medication, and patient satisfaction. Integrating drug treatment and medical care, including care for HIV ("one-stop shopping") is preferred if at all possible, as it reduces the logistical issues confronted by the patient and increases retention. Drug users are frequently incarcerated for drug-related and other offenses, and consequently, correctional facilities may represent important and valuable sites to deliver STI care to this population (see Chapter 43). Progressive corrections departments have developed procedures for communication and care coordination with the medical providers for the period of incarceration, as well as providing appropriate follow-up on release.

A substantial body of data demonstrate the feasibility and value of providing medical services for drug users in drug treatment settings. Many drug treatment programs require some medical evaluation, such as tuberculosis skin testing, at entry and periodically thereafter. With the advent of noninvasive STI tests, and saliva-based HIV screening, extension of these services into the drug treatment setting is feasible. However, at any given time 80–90% of IDUs are not in drug treatment hence, additional strategies, especially outreach approaches for delivering medical services, are needed. Syringe exchanges programs, developed primarily to reduce the risk of parenteral HIV transmission, are potentially valuable sites for delivering health services to active drug injectors who may be difficult to access through other settings. These programs typically offer a range of services, including HIV testing and counseling, drug abuse treatment counseling, and some clinical services either on site or by referral.

■ DIAGNOSTIC AND TREATMENT CONSIDERATIONS

The diagnosis of STIs among IDUs differs little from the diagnosis among nondrug users. Particular issues of importance to drug users (though not unique to them) include the prevalence of false-positive syphilis nontreponemal tests among IDUs (see Chapter 20) and persons with HIV, HBV, and HCV, emphasizing the importance of performing treponemal tests as well. Among HIV-infected persons, FTA antibody tests may fluctuate between negative and positive more frequently than among HIV-uninfected persons, emphasizing the importance of both follow-up testing and making treatment decisions within a whole clinical context.

IDUs may have difficult venous access for phlebotomy. Urine- or saliva-based testing for HIV and urine-based testing for gonorrhea and chlamydia have alleviated much of this problem.

The street use of antibiotics and self-administration of previously prescribed antibiotics by drug users may complicate clinical presentations and diagnoses and lead to selecting antimicrobial resistance, especially in gonorrhea. Single-dose regimens administered on site in the healthcare setting can potentially maximize adherence and minimize treatment failure due to incomplete therapy.

Among the antimicrobial agents used to treat STIs, none are specifically contraindicated or problematic in drug users. For individuals receiving disulfiram (Antabuse) for managing alcoholism, metronidazole can precipitate an unpleasant reaction of abdominal distress, nausea, vomiting, flushing, and headache.

■ INTERVENTIONS AND CONCLUSIONS

For drug users ready to enter drug abuse treatment, drug treatment programs, such as methadone maintenance, can reduce the risk of HIV infection and by diminishing drug use may reduce the motivations to exchange high-risk sex for money or drugs and consequently reduce the risk of STIs. Among IDUs who continue to inject drugs, the consistent use of sterile syringes can reduce the risk of parenteral HIV, HBV, and HCV transmission and, by doing so, reduce the risk of their secondary sexual transmission.

Strategies to promote consistent condom use among drug users can directly reduce the risk of both HIV infection and of STIs. These strategies may need to take into account the social contexts within which high-risk drug use and sexual behaviors occur to effect long-term behavior change and risk reduction and may need to target new and young injectors.

The development and implementation of STI screening and treatment programs, which include hepatitis vaccinations and reach high-risk persons and facilitate treatment acceptance and adherence, will be needed to diminish the spread of STIs and HIV among drug users and their partners. Measures to enhance provider knowledge of and experience with the care of drug users and drug abuse treatment options may improve the outcomes of such programs.

There has been substantial interest in both community-level interventions to reduce sexual risk behaviors in certain target populations, such as homosexual men and minority women, and community-wide empiric treatment of STIs in high prevalence communities in developing countries. The goal is to reduce both STIs and the spread of HIV. Community-wide outreach and syringe exchange interventions among drug users have been effective in promoting reductions in nonsterile injection practices. A growing body of evidence shows that peer-group and community-level interventions also help reduce high-risk sexual behaviors and HIV/STI risk among drug users.

The prevention, detection, and management of STIs among drug users represent an important challenge to public health departments, to healthcare systems, and to healthcare providers (see Table 36-1). Meeting these challenges will require multifaceted and coordinated approaches, the expansion and systematic implementation of proven strategies, and the development of novel solutions with important implications for the public health.

■ KEY POINTS

- Drug users have a high prevalence of STIs.

- STIs are associated with the sexual transmission of HIV among drug users.

- The prevention, screening, and treatment of STIs among drug users requires attention to individual-, social-, and structural-level barriers and facilitators to optimize engagement in and adherence to STI services.

■ ACKNOWLEDGMENTS

We would like to acknowledge support from the National Institute on Drug Abuse grants RO1-DA06723 R01-DA020841, P30 DA 011041, R01 DA13128, and R01 DA-03574.

TABLE 36-1   STI Preventive Interventions for Drug Users

- Offer drug abuse treatment
- Interventions to promote consistent condom use among drug users and their sexual partners
- STI risk-reduction counseling
- For IDUs who continue to inject, refer to sources of sterile syringes, such as pharmacies and syringes exchanges
- Identify candidates for, and deliver, hepatitis B vaccines
- Identify candidates for, and deliver, hepatitis A vaccines (e.g., HCV-infected persons and homosexual men)
- Evaluate for postexposure prophylaxis for HBV and HIV after risky sexual or parenteral exposure

STI Screening Interventions for Drug Users
- VDRL (or other nontreponemal test)
- FTA (or other treponemal test)
- Hepatitis B testing (HBV core antibody); may give first HBV vaccine dose while awaiting result
- HIV testing and pre- and posttest counseling
- Gonorrhea/chlamydia testing (consider urine probes)
- HCV testing

Provider Issues
- Provider education about addiction as a brain disease
- Education about drug abuse treatment options
- Education about medical complications of drug abuse
- Provider training in appropriate communication skills
- Enhanced provider skills in management of challenging patients
- Provider education in harm reduction approaches

Sites for STI Interventions and Care for Drug Users
- Medical and primary care clinics
- Emergency rooms
- STI clinics
- Drug treatment facilities
- Correctional facilities
- Syringe exchange programs
- Other community-based settings (e.g., shelters, soup kitchens)
- Community- and street-based interventions

Using Adherence Promoting Strategies
- On-site rather than referral-based services
- Single-dose regimens
- Observed dosing systems
- Flexible appointment scheduling
- Reminder systems
- Address socioeconomic issues by facilitating access to social services
- Incentive strategies
- * Health (contingency) contracts

REFERENCES

Des Jarlais DC, Friedman SR, Perlis T, et al. Risk behavior and HIV infection among new drug injectors in the era of AIDS in New York City. *J Acquir Immune Defic Syndr.* 1999;20:67–72.

Edlin BR, Irwin KL, Faruque S, et al. Intersecting epidemics: crack cocaine use and HIV infection among inner-city young adults. *N Engl J Med.* 1994;331:1422–1427.

Friedman SR, Curtis R, Neaigus A, Jose B, Des Jarlais DC. *Social Networks, Drug Injectors' Lives, and HIV/AIDS.* New York: Plenum Press;1999.

Friedman SR, Friedmann P, Telles P, et al. New injectors and HIV-1 risk. In: Stimson G, Des Jarlais DC, Ball AL, eds. *Drug Injection and HIV Infection: Global Dimensions and Local Responses.* London: UCL Press;1998:76–90.

Friedman SR, Kippax SC, Phaswana-Mafuya N, Rossi D. Newman CE. Emerging future issues in HIV/AIDS social research. *AIDS.* 2006;20(7):959–965.

Longshore D, Hsieh SC, Anglin MD. Reducing HIV risk behavior among injection drug users: effect of methadone maintenance treatment on number of sex partners. *Int J Addict.* 1994;29:741–757.

Mehta SH, Galai N, Astemborski J, et al. HIV incidence among injection drug users in Baltimore, Maryland (1988–2004). *J Acquir Immune Defic Syndr.* 2006;43(3):368–372.

Nelson KE, Vlahov D, Cohn S, et al. Sexually transmitted diseases in a population of intravenous drug users: association with seropositivity to the human immunodeficiency virus (HIV). *J Infect Dis.* 1991;164:457–463.

O'Connor PG, Selwyn PA, Schottenfeld RS. Medical care for injection-drug users with human immunodeficiency virus infection. *N Engl J Med.* 1994;331:450–459.

Perlman DC, Henman AR, Kochems L, Paone D, Salomon N, Des Jarlais DC. Doing a shotgun: a drug use practice and its relationship to sexual behaviors and infection risk. *Soc Sci Med.* 1999;48:1441–1448.

Rhodes T, Quirk A. Drug users' sexual relationships and the social organization of risk: the sexual relationship as a site of risk management. *Soc Sci Med* 1998;46:157–169.

Rolfs RT, Goldberg M, Sharrar RG. Risk factors for syphilis: cocaine and prostitution. *Am J Pub Health.* 1990;80:853–857.

US Congress, Office of Technology Assessment. *The Effectiveness of Drug Abuse Treatment: Implication for Controlling AIDS/HIV Infection.* Washington, DC: US Government Printing Office; September 1990.

37
Sexually Transmitted Infections in Adolescents

Taraneh Shafii and Gale R. Burstein

■ INTRODUCTION

Adolescence is a period of transition with significant physical, cognitive, and psychosocial growth and development. Although this young stage of life is considered the peak of health and well-being, 15- to 24-year-olds have the highest sexually transmitted infection (STI) rates; in the United States, half of the almost 19 million STI cases are diagnosed annually in this age group (Weinstock et al. 2004). Poverty, health insurance status, lack of knowledge, confidentiality concerns, and transportation, communication, and self-efficacy challenges are among the many barriers adolescents face to accessing quality sexual health services. Most STIs are asymptomatic yet may result in devastating reproductive health sequelae. Therefore, healthcare providers play a critical role in STI identification and care among adolescents.

■ THE ADOLESCENT SEXUAL HEALTH VISIT

Adolescents are a challenging population to reach and engage. Yet, despite their stereotypical outward appearance of shunning and ignoring authority figures, when medical providers are able to create a safe, confidential, nonjudgmental, and empowering atmosphere, adolescents are surprisingly open and candid about themselves, their health and their behavior, including sexuality.

Addressing sexual health, screening, and counseling to prevent sequelae of risky sexual behavior is an essential component of the *primary care* adolescent preventive health visit. Discussing sexuality and taking a sexual history may cause feelings of discomfort for the provider and the adolescent patient. For the primary

care provider who has followed a now adolescent patient since birth, and has an established relationship with the patient's parents/caregivers, acknowledging the patient's sexuality and broaching sex may feel awkward. The provider may feel conflicted about shifting roles from an allegiance with the parents/caregivers, who were previously included in all healthcare decisions for their child, to an alliance with the adolescent, by promising their young patient confidentiality of reproductive healthcare services. Yet this guarantee of confidentiality is the cornerstone to building rapport and trust; good rapport is the key to engaging adolescent patients and allowing them to discuss their personal health concerns with their provider, thereby permitting us to provide optimal care.

In this chapter, we offer an approach and recommendations to facilitate dialogue with the adolescent patient, to address special considerations for the adolescent exam, to discuss some of the newly available tests for sexually transmitted infections (STIs), and to recommend management approaches of STIs in adolescents.

■ WHY IS IT IMPORTANT TO DISCUSS SEXUALITY WITH OUR ADOLESCENT PATIENTS?

Adolescence is a period, spanning approximately 10 years, of significant physical, cognitive, and psychosocial growth and development. For most, adolescence is a time of relative good health, requiring few visits to healthcare providers. The overwhelming majority of health morbidity and mortality that plague adolescent health are from consequences of high-risk behaviors and is exemplified in adolescent sexual behavior.

The adverse health consequences of adolescent high-risk sexual behaviors are demonstrated in the astronomical rates of STIs. Adolescents and young adults have the highest STI rates compared with other age groups (Weinstock et al. 2004). Among females, the highest reported gonorrhea and chlamydia rates are among 15- to 19-year-old and 20- to 24-year-olds; and among males, the highest reported rates are among young adults aged 20–24 years, with 15- to 19-year-old males a close second (Centers for Disease Control and Prevention 2008). In the United States, HIV/AIDS is now the seventh leading cause of mortality in young adults younger than 25 years and accounts for 13% of all cases diagnosed annually. Infection diagnosed in those younger than 25 years old is acquired predominantly through heterosexual contact.

■ WHY ARE ADOLESCENTS AT HIGH RISK FOR ACQUIRING STIs?

Factors that increase adolescents' risk of STIs can be categorized as (1) biological susceptibility, (2) psychosocial development, (3) healthcare utilization and compliance, and (4) concern for confidentiality and ethical and legal issues. These four factors contribute to adolescent health risk and influence high-risk behavior in the environment of evolving sexuality and sexual behavior as youth progress through puberty (see Figure 37-1).

Biological Factors

Because of developing physiologic characteristics, adolescent females are more vulnerable to STIs than adult females. The immature and incompletely estrogenized cervix is characterized by persistence of columnar epithelium extending to the ectocervix, referred to as *cervical ectopy*. Columnar epithelium is more susceptible to invasion by pathogens, such as *Neisseria gonorrhoeae* and *Chlamydia trachomatis* than squamous epithelium, which is physiologically more resistant to STIs and covers the vagina and the mature adult female cervix. Adolescent females tend to have thinner cervical mucus than adult females, thereby presenting a weaker barrier to pathogens infecting the cervix and upper reproductive tract.

Lower estrogen present in early adolescence levels also results in thinner genital tissue. In addition, the lack of sexual arousal results in inadequate vaginal lubrication before penetration. This combination places adolescent females at increased risk for trauma or irritation to the female genital tissue creating potential portals of entry for pathogens.

Psychosocial Development

To guide their approach to the patient, before initiating an interview with an adolescent, it is helpful for providers to be sensitive to adolescent psychosocial development. Adolescence spans approximately a 10-year period, which consists of three phases: (1) early adolescence, aged 11–13 years, or middle school aged; (2) middle adolescence, aged 14–16 years, or high school aged; and (3) late adolescence, aged 17–21 years, or late high school and college (see Table 37-1). However, many of the developmental issues of older adolescents are also operative in the young adult (e.g., early 20's).

FIGURE 37-1 Schematic of Adolescent Risk for Sexually Transmitted Infections

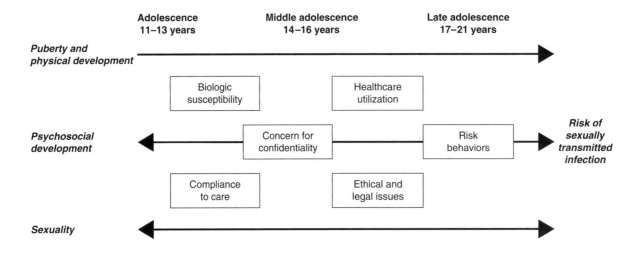

TABLE 37-1 Physical, Psychosocial, and Sexual Development in Adolescents

	Early Adolescence	Middle Adolescence	Late Adolescence
Physical growth	Onset of puberty; rapid changes at different timing and rate from peers	Full physical maturation obtained by females with menarche; more variable in males with continued growth	Full adult physical development obtained by all
Body Image	Am I normal? Concern about body and pubertal changes	Start acceptance of body changes; preoccupied with making body more attractive	Accepting and comfortable with pubertal changes and body
Cognition	Concrete, unable to think abstractedly or plan ahead; poor impulse control	Able to conceptualize and think abstractly; may revert to concrete thinking in times of stress; propensity for risk-taking behavior	Abstract thought and ability to anticipate future and plan accordingly; increased self-efficacy
Independence/Peers	Increased interest in friends with a decreased focus on family activities; Same-sex friendships predominate	Height of conformity to peer values, appearance and behavior; family conflict; Dating in couples or groups common	Establishment of personal values and goals; re-acceptance of family; conformity to and influence of peer group fades
Sexuality	Sexual myths, fantasies, masturbation; usually no sexual contact with partner	Sexual contact ranges from hand-holding to intercourse; often exploratory; serial monogamy common	Sexual intercourse achieved by most; Focus on intense relationship with one partner; serial monogamy may persist

Early Adolescence (11–13 years)

Early adolescence is marked by the onset of puberty and physical changes that are often rapid, dramatic, and may occur asynchronously and at different rates from their peers. The underlying question of this age group, "Am I normal?" is continuously being assessed in the classroom, in the locker room, and at sleepovers. During the physical exam, especially the breast and genital exam for males and females, it is important that the provider reassures the adolescent that everything looks healthy and normal for his or her stage of development.

Early adolescence marks the conscious awakening of sexual feelings and usually manifests as sexual fantasies, masturbation, and nocturnal emissions, all of which may be confusing and guilt producing to the youth. Sexual myths are common (e.g., you can get pregnant in a swimming pool; you can't get pregnant the first time you have sex) as are dirty jokes among peers (e.g., think back to the antics of middle school boys). Sexual activity at this stage is usually nonphysical and manifests as phone calls and passing notes. However, clinicians must recognize that in some populations adolescents are initiating sexual intimacy at this age, including oral, anal, and vaginal intercourse, at earlier ages. Seven percent of U.S. youth report first vaginal intercourse before 13 years of age (CDC 2008). Similar findings have been reported in the United Kingdom in the NATSAL surveys, which also show that many adolescents are unprepared for first intercourse (Mercer 2006).

Early adolescent cognitive abilities are concrete, and young adolescents are unable to think abstractly, conceptualize, or develop a plan for the future. For example, when a boy is asked whether he is sexually active, the cognitively concrete adolescent may think the provider is asking whether he is "active" during sex, or he may think the provider is asking whether he is having sex *that day* or *that week*, instead of asking whether he has *ever* had sex. The cognitive abilities at this developmental stage explain why many young adolescents do not plan or anticipate the need for condoms or contraception when they are sexually active. Using a condom presents an additional challenge for these youth, especially during heightened arousal and emotion, as their manual dexterity is limited, and they may have difficulty with complex tasks that require multiple steps, such as opening a condom package and putting the condom on the penis. These limitations are supported in the findings that younger adolescents are less likely to use condoms or other forms of contraception, and if they use contraception, they are more likely to have difficulty (Ford

and Lepkowski 2004; Kirby 2002; Shafii et al. 2004; Upchurch et al. 2004).

Middle Adolescence (14–16 years)

Most in middle adolescence attain full physical maturation with menarche for females and continued penile and testicular growth in males. Maturation rates vary more with males, and the completion of puberty may extend into late adolescence.

Sexuality is heightened during this stage, involves more physical contact, and is often exploratory and experiential rather than an expression of emotional attachment. Sexual activity at this stage progresses to dating in groups or as couples, handholding, touching, kissing, and mutual masturbation. Because the average age of sexual debut is currently 16.5 years in the United States, providers must assume (until proved otherwise) that their middle adolescent patient (1) may already be engaging in oral, anal, or vaginal intercourse; (2) therefore, is at risk for acquiring STIs; and (3) should be screened by sexual history and laboratory testing.

Adolescents in this stage develop capabilities for abstract thinking and conceptualization. However, they usually revert to concrete thinking during times of stress, which adds to their susceptibility to high-risk behaviors in intense, hormonally, or emotionally driven situations, for example, sexual activity. Traditionally, specialists have assumed that this new abstract thinking skill leads to a belief in their own "personal fable" in which they presume that "nothing bad will happen to *me* . . . those things only happen to *other people*." Although most adolescents in this age group understand that driving while intoxicated or engaging in unprotected sex can lead to deleterious consequences, their perceived *omnipotence and immortality* provides them with a false sense of security (Neinstein et al. 2008). Although these assumptions seem reckless to adults, they may point to the adolescents' level of brain and cognitive development. Rather than believing they are above harm as a driving force for high-risk behaviors, perhaps they are just not thinking about potential risks; they are instead just acting in the moment (Dahl 2004). Adolescents' seemingly cavalier attitude may, in part, reflect the paucity of life experience. Adolescents may have to validate for themselves the possibility of an adverse outcome to high-risk behavior (e.g., becoming infected with chlamydia or herpes from unprotected sex). Regardless, the concern for this middle-adolescent age group is their propensity for engaging in high-risk behaviors, which may be fueled further by peer, alcohol, or drug use influences that compromise inhibitions and result in unexpected, yet adverse, health consequences.

Late Adolescence (17–21 years)

By the end of late adolescence, adolescents have attained full adult physical maturation. Sexual orientation is established and intimacy and commitment with a single individual are the basis of sexual relationships (Neinstein et al. 2008). Abstract thought is more firmly established for most. Late adolescents are able to plan for and effectively use condoms and contraception with sexual partners. Interestingly, in older adolescents, condom use decreases as the use of hormonal contraception increases once again, providing an opportunity for STIs to be transmitted, unless both partners have been tested and are monogamous with each other.

■ SERIAL MONOGAMY: A COMMON PATTERN OF SEXUAL PARTNERING

Psychosocial and sexual development influence adolescent sexual behaviors and STI risk. However, there is also an interesting societal trend contributing to adolescent sexual behavior and associated risk. Adolescent relationships are described as *serial monogamy*: they have relationships of relatively short duration (e.g., 2 weeks or 2 months) with one partner and change partners frequently. Therefore, while they may be monogamous, which may be interpreted by both teen patients and providers as a lower-risk relationship, as they accrue an increased number of partners over time, they are in fact still at significant risk of STI exposure. To assess true STI exposure risk and obtain a more valid assessment of sexual risk behaviors, providers should inquire about the adolescent's number of partners in the past 3, 6, and 12 months instead of at just one point in time.

■ TREND FOR EARLIER PUBERTY, EARLIER SEXUAL DEBUT, AND DELAYED MARRIAGE

In the United States, the median age of menarche is approximately 12.4 years of age (12.1 years in black females); the median age of first sexual intercourse is 16.5 years (Neinstein et al. 2008); and the average age of marriage is the late 20's (an increase in approximately 5–8 years from the 1950s). Therefore, the average number of years when males and females are fertile, hormonally primed for sexual activity, and not married has increased significantly over the past 50 years, resulting in the potential for increased number of sexual partners, STI exposure, transmission, and acquisition.

■ SAME-SEX SEXUAL ACTIVITY AND HOMOSEXUALITY

Same-sex sexual activity is not uncommon in adolescence, is often exploratory, and does not necessarily predict future homosexuality. In the 2002 National Survey of Family Growth, 11% of 15- to 19-year-old females and 14% of 20- to 24-year-old females reported ever having "*any same-sex contact*" and more than 4% of 15- to 19-year-old males and 6% of 20- to 24-year-old males reported ever having "*any oral or anal intercourse with other males.*" The proportions of reported same-sex activity may vary by gender because the questions asked varies by gender, that is, "*any same-sex contact*" for female respondents versus "*any oral or anal intercourse with other males*" for male respondents. Other surveys support a higher proportion of same-sex male sexual activity, with the finding that 17% of 16- to 19-year-old males have had some male–male sexual experience (CDC 2002).

One Example of Initiating a Conversation About Sex

A 15-year-old male comes to your office for a sports physical, the provider asks, "So do you have a girlfriend?"

Adolescence is the period when sexual orientation is discovered and established. Although there have been societal trends in openness and acceptance of homosexuality in the past decade, the recognition of feeling different from one's peers, being attracted to the same sex, experiencing sexuality contrary to the messages of mainstream society, and fearing rejection and abandonment by one's family and friends, may be catastrophic for the young person. Gay, lesbian, bisexual, transgender, and questioning youth are at an increased risk for substance abuse, school failure, homelessness, sexual activity, victimization, body image and eating disorders, depression, and suicide (Strassburger et al. 2006).

If the young man in the scenario is struggling with his sexuality, asking about a girlfriend may be detrimental—the healthcare provider, as a health authority, is modeling that heterosexuality is the only acceptable orientation. The adolescent may feel embarrassed and ashamed by his doubts and the provider may have alienated the youth, when instead, the provider could have offered a safe venue for discussing sexual feelings, as well as, important sexual health information and resources of support.

Survey data suggest that from 3% to 10% of U.S. adults report being lesbian or gay. Adolescents are in the process of understanding and accepting their sexuality as evidenced in the lower proportion (1–4%) of adolescents who report being gay, lesbian, or bisexual, and the greater proportion (1–11%) who report being unsure about their sexual orientation (Neinstein et al. 2008; CDC 2002).

An Alternative Example of Initiating a Conversation About Sex

You are at the age when you start figuring out if you are interested in or attracted to guys, girls, or both. Have you thought about that yet? Have you ever had sex with a guy, girl, or both?

As healthcare providers, we are in the unique position to normalize sexuality to youth of all orientations by the words and objectivity we use to discuss the topic. By acknowledging different sexual orientations, we are sending the message that individual attractions are within the range of normal sexual behavior. This allows the struggling gay or transgender youths to begin to accept themselves and provides a medical resource for support and information to field their questions and concerns. For the heterosexual youth, providers model a position of acceptance and tolerance for sexual minorities.

■ AGE DIFFERENTIAL IN SEXUAL PARTNERS AND REPORTING LAWS

A significant number of adolescent females engage in sexual relationships with older males, increasing their likelihood of STI exposure and decreasing their power and capacity to negotiate condom and contraception use. Studies demonstrating that adolescent females with partners at least 2 years older are at increased risk for STIs and unintended pregnancy support this finding (Ford and Lepkowski 2004; Kirby 2002; Upchurch et al. 2004). Reporting laws for statutory rape and sexual misconduct vary by locality, and providers need to be aware of the laws where they practice.

■ ESTABLISHING RAPPORT

Building rapport is the most important skill a provider needs in taking care of adolescents. Most adolescent adverse health consequences result from risk-taking behaviors. To create an environment where the patient feels safe disclosing sexual behaviors and health concerns,

providers need to establish good rapport with their adolescent patients. A few simple techniques may help reassure the adolescent that their provider is trustworthy (see Table 37-2).

Acknowledge the Adolescent as Your Primary Patient

Upon entering the room, look at the adolescent first, make eye contact, address him or her, and shake his or her hand before acknowledging the accompanying caregiver. The adolescent patient is your primary patient; the parents/guardians are the secondary patients. Remember to sit down! Whether you are in the room for 5 minutes or 20 minutes, sitting down reaffirms to the adolescent (and parents/guardians) that he or she is important, you are not in a hurry, and he or she has your undivided attention.

Just as in introductions, speak directly to the adolescent when you initiate the interview, "What brings you in today?" Younger adolescents may look at the parent/guardian instead of answering the question. That is your cue to first interview the accompanying adult; yet the provider should take every opportunity to return the

TABLE 37-2 Techniques for Establishing Rapport with Adolescents

1. Introduce yourself to the adolescent first, look them in the eye, shake their hand and sit down during the interview.

2. Acknowledge the adolescent as your primary patient by directing your questions primarily to them rather than their family.

3. Use conversation ice-breakers to allow time for the adolescent to become more comfortable and get a sense of who you are.

4. Allow the adolescent to remain dressed during the interview and sit in a chair rather than on the exam table.

5. Interview the adolescent without their family present for sensitive questions.

6. Ensure confidentiality and provide a safe environment for them to be honest.

7. Practice reflective listening and take time to listen to what the adolescent is saying and not saying.

8. Facilitate a comfortable experience for the adolescent by providing adolescent-friendly and easy-to-access office and staff.

interview to the adolescent, "Do you agree?" "Is that how it feels?" "You tell me how it feels." For older adolescents, start the interview with the patient and end by asking the parents/guardians if they have anything to add and to state their specific concerns (as this may differ significantly from the adolescents). Parents/guardians are valuable in providing past medical history and family history for any age adolescent who may not know the details of their health history.

Interview the Adolescent *Without* Accompanying Adults Present

After the parents/guardians have provided necessary health information and voiced their concerns: *perform an "atraumatic parentectomy"*; in other words, *ask the parent/guardian to leave the exam room*. Separating the parents/guardians and the adolescent is imperative and serves several purposes: (1) being interviewed alone empowers the adolescent to be responsible for his or her own health; (2) the time together helps to create a therapeutic alliance between the provider and patient; (3) time alone with the patient allows providers the opportunity to obtain a confidential sexual history and screen for behavioral risks. *Never* ask an adolescent about sexual activity in front of a parent/guardian: the answer will most likely be, "no." Most adults honor the request to step out briefly, especially when you explain that they will be informed of any serious health concerns and are allowed to return to the exam room for the conclusion of the visit.

A useful technique to ensure parents/guardians will be comfortable leaving their adolescent alone with the provider is to normalize the process during the initial interview. "You are at the age where it is time to start taking on some of the responsibility for your health yourself; therefore, I would like to spend some time with you alone without your parents present." "It is my practice with all patients your age to spend some time talking to you without your parents present." "It is our clinic policy regarding adolescents to do a portion of the visit separate from the parents." Inviting parents/guardians back into the room for the end of the visit to hear the assessment and management plan (that is, with your patient's approval) prevents them from feeling alienated and allows them to continue to be engaged in their adolescent's health at some level and assists with reinforcing the care plan for the adolescent, who may have difficulty following through with medical directions.

Other simple steps providers can take to initiate the rapport and comfort-building process before they even see their patient include providing an adolescent-friendly space in the waiting room and placing age-appropriate magazines, brochures, and posters in the waiting and exam rooms. Hiring staff that like adolescents and are skilled in communicating with adolescents on the telephone and in the office helps to alleviate anxiety during the office visit. Allowing adolescents to remain dressed during the interview and covered as much as possible during the exam contributes to feelings of safety and a sense of control over their bodies and their environment.

■ THE INTERVIEW

Effective communication with adolescents requires a sensitive, flexible, and developmentally oriented approach. Since diagnosis and treatment are the emphasis of medical training, most providers have not received formal training in interviewing techniques or the opportunity to practice these skills with adolescent patients. Adolescents can be a particularly challenging to interview. Their ability to reason lies somewhere between concrete operations of childhood and formal operations of adulthood. Asking questions about sexuality can also be a particularly difficult subject to approach. Most adolescents (and adults) prefer to avoid initiating a conversation about sex. Providers must be comfortable with the subject of sexuality to be able to make the adolescent feel comfortable discussing this sensitive and private issue. It is worthwhile for providers to reflect on their own personal experiences of puberty, adolescence, and sexuality to better understand and identify with their patients. As healthcare providers, it is our responsibility to set our personal views aside and provide our patients with comprehensive reproductive health care. If providers feel uncomfortable discussing sexuality and sexual behaviors with their adolescent patients, it is the providers' obligation to refer these patients to colleagues who are able to provide appropriate care. The following are useful strategies for interviewing adolescent patients, with special emphasis on obtaining information most helpful in assessing sexual risk behaviors and risk for sexually transmitted infections.

Outline the Office Visit

Outlining what is going to take place during the office visit helps to decrease the adolescent's anxiety. "First, I am going to talk to you and your mom. Then I would like to talk to you by yourself for a bit. Then I will exam you, and if we need to do any tests, I may need to get a blood or urine sample from you." An adolescent will feel much more comfortable if he or she knows what to expect. Since genital exams are a source of great anxiety and embarrassment for youth, if a genital exam will take place, the provider should inform the adolescent patient. If a pelvic exam will be performed, a full explanation is imperative, especially if this is the patient's first exam. Showing the adolescent the speculum and even letting her handle it, usually diminishes rather than escalates anxiety. Diagrams or plastic models of genitalia and mirrors during the exam are useful to educate youth as most, especially females, are unaware of their anatomy or the proper terms, and many women—young and adult alike—have never seen their own anatomy.

Ensure Confidentiality

At the opening of the interview, the provider must define his or her confidentiality policy and under what circumstances confidentiality will be breached (e.g., suicidal/homicidal thoughts, physical/sexual abuse). "What you and I talk about is confidential from your family, which means I am not going to tell them what we talk about, unless I am worried that you are hurting yourself, hurting someone else, or someone is hurting you." An adolescent must understand that the provider is his or her healthcare provider, not the parents'. Most adolescents will not admit to engaging in any risk behaviors if they believe parents/guardians will be informed.

Ask Nonthreatening Questions First

Begin the interview with nonthreatening questions, subsequently progressing to sensitive questions. Here, small talk (e.g., ask casually about school, upcoming or past vacations, sports) can be useful because (1) it is an icebreaker and gives the patient time to feel out the provider and adjust to the surroundings; (2) it gives the provider a sense of how the rest of the interview will flow—is the patient shy or relaxed? and (3) if the parent/guardian is present, it gives the provider insight into the parent–child dynamic. Next, ask the adolescent about his or her health concerns. Convey genuine interest and concern throughout the interview— nothing is more effective in establishing rapport. An adolescent's perception of disinterest will result in loss of trust. The HEADSS (home, education, activities, drugs, sex, and suicide) (Neinstein et al. 2008) mnemonic is structured to ask progressively sensitive questions, allowing time for rapport building before personal questions are asked.

Use Written Questionnaires for Sensitive Questions

Some adolescents find it easier to admit to risk behaviors on paper rather than aloud to an adult provider. It may be useful to use paper questionnaires in a busy office practice that does not allow time for lengthy "get-to-know-you" and rapport building visits. These forms can be completed while the patient is waiting to be seen and then quickly reviewed by the provider to identify areas to focus on during the patient interview. Remember to provide a parent-free space for the adolescent to complete the questionnaire in private without fear of disclosure. Utility may be limited in patients with limited literacy skills or in populations where there are language barriers.

Interviewing Techniques

Obtaining pertinent information from an adolescent and engaging him in a comfortable conversation at the same time is an art. Several interview techniques are provided that can aid the provider in leading an informative dialogue with the adolescent patient (Neinstein et al. 2008).

Open-Ended Questions

An adolescent may be quick to answer "yes" or "no" in response to a specifically directed question. Avoid questions that yield "yes" or "no" responses. One might phrase the question, "How often do you use condoms?" rather than "Do you use condoms all the time?"

Reflection Responses

Reflection responses mirror the adolescent's feelings and can help stimulate further conversation on a topic. "So, you feel it is difficult to get your partner to use condoms? Tell me about that."

Clarification Questions

Asking the adolescent to explain anything you do not understand is not insulting but is empowering to the adolescent, because the adolescent is teaching the expert, "What do you mean when you say . . .?"

Restatement and Summation Responses

Restating and summarizing the relevant issues can clarify the question and encourage more dialogue. "It seems like you want to tell your partner that you have chlamydia, but you are afraid she will blame you and get angry. Is that right?"

Reassuring Statements and Generalization

Reassuring statements validate the adolescent's feelings, reestablish your role as an advocate, and stimulate more dialogue. "Many young women your age decide to wait to have sex until they are older, out of high school, or even married. Deciding what is right for you, does not mean there is anything wrong with you, even if it is different than what your friends are doing."

Support and Empathy

A supportive and empathetic response during the conversation acknowledging the adolescent's difficult experience can stimulate more dialogue and impart further trust. "It sounds like this has been difficult for you. I see this happen to a lot of my patients. . . ."

The Quiet Adolescent

For the noncommunicative adolescent, return to icebreakers. The goal is to get the patient to talk about anything. Ask him or her to discuss something of interest, such as school, sports, or friends to put the patient at ease.

Adolescent Sexuality and Religion

In the next decade, the ethnic makeup of adolescents will continue to diversify, bringing with it a mélange of cultural and religious traditions. Healthcare providers must be attuned to varying cultural and religious beliefs of their patient population and demonstrate cultural sensitivity to different practices. For example, some cultures engage in female circumcision, which alters the external appearance of the female genitalia and, in severe cases, affects voiding and sexual function. Knowledge of this practice can help allay the youth's fears of looking different from peers in their new culture and raises the provider's index of suspicion for the differential diagnosis when physiologic dysfunction is suspected. Youth may resist discussing sex regardless of their level of sexual experience because sexual activity before marriage is shunned by many cultures and religions. Therefore, framing information about sexuality in the context of helping their peers and friends who may be or are sexually active is a nonthreatening and effective method to provide sexual education to all patients.

How to Ask the Sex Questions; What You Need to Know About Your Patient's Sexuality; and How to Do the Exam

A comprehensive discussion of the history, physical exam, laboratory tests, and management of STIs is addressed in separate chapters of this book. However, some caveats that may assist the provider with managing STIs in the adolescent patient are offered next.

■ THE HIDDEN AGENDA

If You Ask They Will Tell You; If You Don't They Won't

The *hidden agenda* is the phenomena of adolescents seeking care for a sensitive health issue (e.g., fear of pregnancy or STI symptoms) and assuming their provider will know what is wrong with them without actually verbalizing the problem. For example, an adolescent female presents with complaints of a bellyache; the provider works up the abdominal pain but does not screen for sexual behaviors and treats the patient for presumed gastritis. The patient leaves the office reassured that she is not pregnant since she believes the provider is omniscient and would have known if she was pregnant just by virtue of her being in the office. To know whether an adolescent patient is having sex, providers must *ask* the patient; the adolescent will not always volunteer her health concerns but is surprisingly candid when asked directly.

■ WHAT KIND OF SEX?

Oral, anal, and vaginal sex and whether condoms are used and used correctly result in varying levels of STI risk: transmission, acquisition, and type of infection. As adolescents present in varying stages of cognitive development, sexual knowledge, and sexual experience, the general question, "Are you sexually active?" will be interpreted differently by individual adolescents. Providers need to ask direct and specific questions to yield the information needed to make an accurate risk assessment and extent of STI screening required. "Have you had sex with guys, girls, or both? Have you ever had oral sex? Anal sex? Vaginal or *regular* sex?" If in doubt of a youth's understanding of the definitions of oral, anal, or vaginal sex, the provider should pose the questions to ensure they are discussing the same behavior. "Tell me what 'having sex' means to you." Most likely, the adolescent will squirm, be embarrassed, and have difficulty answering the question. The provider then has the opportunity to provide the definitions for example, "I want to make sure we are talking about the same thing: so oral sex means your partner kisses or puts his/her mouth on your vagina/penis; some people call it 'going down on each other,' have you ever done that?" (see Table 37-3).

THE PHYSICAL EXAM

Foremost, the provider should always make the adolescent feel like he or she is in control. Providers should let the adolescent know what part of the exam is going to be performed next and that the physical examination will stop at any time if he or she is uncomfortable. Providers should explain that they are doing the exam to best take care of their patients' health and want to make sure that they are indeed healthy. Offer as many options as possible during the exam to empower your patient and make them feel as safe and comfortable as possible. For example, ask the adolescent if she would be more comfortable completely undressing and changing into a gown before the exam or would prefer to undress only the part of the body being examined at the time so

TABLE 37-3   Key Topics to Cover and Sample Questions for the Sexual Interview with Adolescents

Introduce the topic and establish confidentiality

"I need to ask you some personal questions that I ask all of my patients so that I can best take care of your health. What we talk about is confidential from your family unless I am worried that somebody is hurting you, you are hurting yourself, or you are hurting somebody else. You do not have to answer any question that you don't want to answer."

Sexual orientation

"You are at the age when people start to figure out who they like, are interested in or attracted to. Have you thought about that? Do you like guys, girls or both?"

Sexual activity

"Have you ever been so close to a guy/girl that you held hands or kissed? What about touching your private areas—on top of or under your clothes? Have you ever had sex? By that I mean—have you had sex where a guy puts his penis inside a girl's vagina? What about oral sex where your partner puts his/her mouth on your penis/vagina? What about anal sex – where a guy puts his penis inside your anus/bottom?"

Sexual Abuse

"Have you ever had sex when you didn't really want to? Has anyone ever touched you in your private areas in a way that made you feel uncomfortable?"

Partners and concurrency

"How many partners have you had in the past 2 months? Past year? Your whole life?

"Do you think your partner has other sex partners? Do you?"

Sexually Transmitted infections

"Has a doctor ever told you that you had a sexually transmitted infection like chlamydia? Gonorrhea? Trichomonas? Herpes? Genital warts? Syphilis? HIV/AIDS? Have any of your partners ever had one"?

Pregnancy

"Have you ever been pregnant/gotten your partner pregnant? Are you trying to get pregnant right now?"

Condoms

"What do you do to keep yourself and your partner from getting an STI? "Do you use condoms? Did you use a condom the last time you had sex? How often do you think you use condoms? Have you ever had trouble using condoms? Did they ever break or slip off during sex?

Hormonal Contraception

"What do you do to keep yourself/your partner from getting pregnant? Are you on/is your partner on any hormonal contraception like the birth control pill? The shot? The patch? The ring? How is that going? Is it hard to remember to take your pills, etc.?

that she remains partially dressed throughout the exam. Younger adolescents may prefer the latter option since they may feel insecure about their bodies. Another strategy for females, who are resistant to undressing and only require an external genital exam, is to allow them to continue wearing their underwear during the genital exam. For the exam, the provider can shift the underwear to one side allowing full visibility of the genitalia.

The stage of secondary sexual characteristic development should be documented in any adolescent exam involving the genitalia. J. M. Tanner classified the level of pubertal maturation into five levels based on breast and pubic hair development in females and genitalia and pubic hair development in males and is used as a measure of pubertal development (Tanner 1962). Figures 37-2 to 37-5 describe Tanner's classification of stages of pubertal development.

Providers need to be cognizant that some adolescents have never had a genital exam or have not been examined since the onset of puberty. All adolescents need at least one genital exam during puberty, to document normal anatomy and development, and more frequent genital exams if sexually active or clinically indicated.

With new urine-based STI testing and revised Pap smear testing guidelines (recommending first adolescent Pap smear test performed within three years after coitarche in the United States and aged 25 years in United Kingdom), many asymptomatic adolescent females do not require a pelvic exam. However, females presenting with genital symptoms and adolescents requiring their first Pap smear need to have a pelvic exam performed. A first pelvic exam can be an anxiety-provoking experience for both the adolescent patient and the provider. A reassuring and confident provider sets the tone for the exam. Providers should discuss what will occur and answer all questions before initiating the exam. Pelvic models or diagrams may be helpful to describe the procedure. Allowing a support person in the room, such as a friend, relative, or nurse, can ease the tension for the patient. As exam rooms are often cold, ensure that adolescent remains warm and as comfortable as possible with additional sheets or blankets. Visual imagery can help the adolescent relax during the exam and is easily performed by encouraging the adolescent to concentrate on imagining herself doing her favorite sport or activity in her favorite location. Visual imagery and focused breathing are helpful techniques to decrease anxiety and muscular tension thereby facilitating the successful performance of the pelvic exam and a more positive experience for the adolescent. Some providers

also place a distracting poster on the exam room ceiling for the patients to view during the exam.

Male providers may find some male patients resist an exam. Adolescent males may be in the developmental

FIGURE 37-2 Tanner Rating of Genital Changes in Boys

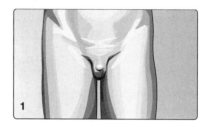
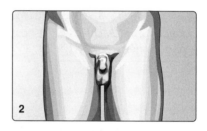
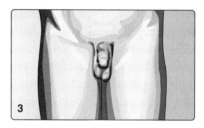
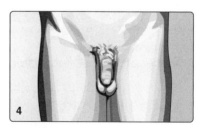
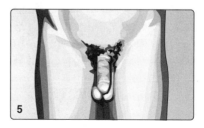

Source: Reproduced from Archives of Disease in Childhood. Variations in pattern of pubertal changes in boys, Marshal WA and Tanner JM, 45, 13–23, 1970 with permission from BMJ Publishing Group Ltd.

FIGURE 37-3 Tanner Staging of Pubic Hair in Boys

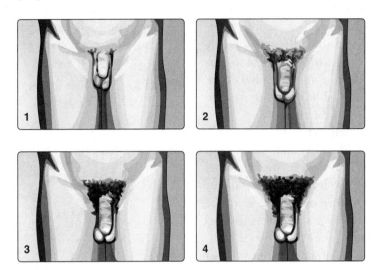

Source: Reproduced from Archives of Disease in Childhood. Variations in pattern of pubertal changes in boys, Marshal WA and Tanner JM, 45, 13–23, 1970 with permission from BMJ Publishing Group Ltd.

process of establishing sexual identity and thus may be averse to another male examining their genitalia. Similarly, adolescent females may feel embarrassed and uncomfortable with male providers. If the adolescent demonstrates discomfort, every effort should be taken, if possible, to offer a choice in the provider gender. When there is discordant gender in the provider and patient, chaperones should be used (e.g., nurse, medical assistant, or parent/guardian) as a measure of safety and comfort for the pa-

tient and to protect the provider against false impropriety claims (see Chapter 3 for a discussion of chaperones).

■ LABORATORY TESTS

Sexually active adolescents are at high risk for acquiring STIs, such as gonorrhea and chlamydia. Current guidelines for delivery of adolescent primary care services recommend yearly STI screening for all sexually

FIGURE 37-4 Tanner Staging of Pubic Hair in Girls

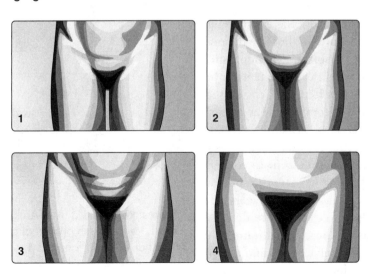

active adolescents (CDC 2010). Tests for chlamydia, gonorrhea, and trichomonas should be obtained routinely. Many experts recommend chlamydia screening every 6 months for sexually active female adolescents. Chlamydia and gonorrhea testing of self-obtained vaginal swabs and urine samples avoid invasive genital and pelvic exams as a major obstacle to many adolescents seeking care and a disincentive for providers in busy primary care practice settings to screen for STIs. Current recommendations for HIV testing are at least once for HIV and more often as indicated by sexual risk behaviors (CDC 2010).

FIGURE 37-5 Tanner Staging of Breast Development in Girls

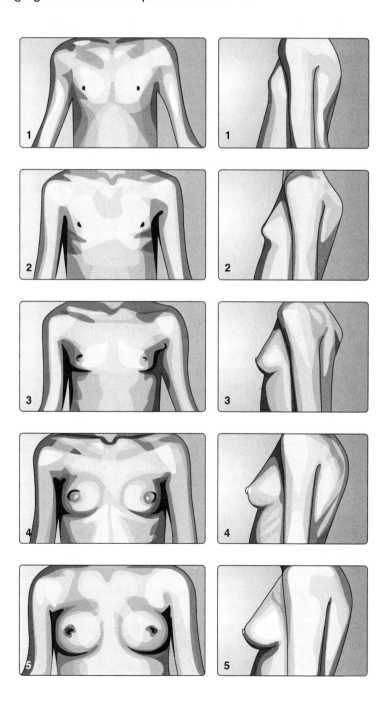

■ TREATMENT

The CDC recommended management of STIs for adolescents does not vary from that of adults, except with the caveat to ensure completed treatment. Since adolescents are notorious for poor compliance with treatment and follow-up recommendations, single-dose therapy is recommended when available.

■ CONCLUSION

Adolescence is an exciting yet arduous time of life. Their rate of physical development surpasses their rate of cognitive development. Adolescents are physically able to engage in behaviors that place them at risk for STIs, but they have not yet fully developed the capabilities to judge when and how to protect themselves. Primary care providers are in a unique position. They are a potentially valuable resource to educate adolescents about their health and their bodies in a private and safe environment where they can offer individualized information and strategies to guide adolescents and young adults toward physical and emotional health. As providers of health care for adolescents, it is our job to support our patients to remain in good sexual health, despite their developmental dichotomy between judgment and action.

■ KEY POINTS

- Establish a good rapport with all adolescent patients to create an environment where the patient feels safe disclosing sexual behaviors and health concerns.

- Interview the adolescent *without* accompanying adults present.

- When interviewing adolescents, ask open-ended questions.

- During the physical exam, the provider should always make the adolescent feel like she or he is in control.

- Providers should routinely offer noninvasive chlamydia and gonorrhea tests for all sexually active adolescent females during a preventive health visit.

WEBSITES FOR PROVIDERS

Adolescent Health Working Group:
http://ahwg.net/

American College of Obstetrics and Gynecology:
http://www.acog.org/

American Medical Association Guidelines for Adolescent Preventive Services (GAPS):
http://www.ama-assn.org/ama/pub/physician-resources/public-health/promoting-healthy-lifestyles/adolescent-health/guidelines-adolescent-preventive-services.shtml

California STD/HIV Prevention Training Center:
www.stdhivtraining.org/educ/training_module/tools.html

Centers for Disease Control and Prevention:
www.cdc.gov/std/

ETR Associates (patient brochures):
www.etr.org

Gay and Lesbian Medical Association (GLMA):
http://www.glma.org

Guttmacher Institute:
http://www.guttmacher.org/

Kaiser Family Foundation:
http://www.kff.org/

National Campaign to Prevent Teen Pregnancy:
http://www.teenpregnancy.org/

National Chlamydia Coalition:
http://www.prevent.org/index.php?option=com_content&task=view&id=242&Itemid=210

New York State Screener/Trigger questionnaire:
http://www.urmc.rochester.edu/pediatrics/training/fellowship/programs/adolescent_medicine/technicalresources.cfm#PrimaryCare

Planned Parenthood Federation of America:
http://www.plannedparenthood.org/index.htm

Society for Adolescent Medicine:
http://www.adolescenthealth.org/Clinical_Care_Resources/1529.htm

Society of Obstetricians and Gynecologists of Canada:
www.sexualityandu.ca

WEBSITES FOR ADOLESCENT PATIENTS OR PARENTS/GUARDIANS

Advocates for Youth:
http://www.advocatesforyouth.org/

American Social Health Association adolescent sexual health information:
http://www.iwannaknow.org

Campaign for Our Children:
http://www.cfoc.org/

Center for Young Women's Health (CYWH):
http://www.youngwomenshealth.org/

Children Now:
http://www.talkingwithkids.org/

Columbia University's Health Promotion Program "Go Ask Alice" website for adolescents and young adults:
http://www.goaskalice.columbia.edu/

DIPEx website (UK):
http://www.youthhealthtalk.org/

MTV collaboration with Kaiser Family Foundation:
http://www.itsyoursexlife.com/

Planned Parenthood Teens:
http://www.teenwire.com/

Rutgers, the State University of New Jersey, teen sexual health:
http://www.sexetc.org/

Society of Obstetricians and Gynecologists of Canada:
www.sexualityandu.ca

Teenage Health Websites Ltd (UK):
http://www.doctorann.org/

REFERENCES

Centers for Disease Control and Prevention (CDC). Youth Risk Behavior Surveillance—United States. *Morb Mort Wkly Rep.* 2008;57(SS-4):1–36.

Centers for Disease Control and Prevention (CDC) NCfHS. *National Survey of Family Growth.* Atlanta, GA: CDC; 2002.

Centers for Disease Control and Prevention (CDC).: Sexually transmitted diseases treatment guidelines, 2010 *Morb. Mort. Wkly Rep.* 2010; 17:59(RR-12):1–110.

Dahl R. Adolescent brain development: a period of vulnerabilities and opportunities [keynote address]. *Ann NY Acad Sci.* 2004;1021:1–22.

Ford K, Lepkowski JM. Characteristics of sexual partners and STD infection among American adolescents. *Int J STD AIDS.* 2004;15(4):260–265.

Kirby D. Antecedents of adolescent initiation of sex, contraceptive use, and pregnancy. *Am J Health Behav.* 2002; 26(6):473–485.

Mercer CH, Wellings K, Macdowall W, Copas AJ, McManus S, Erens B, Fenton KA, Johnson AM. First sexual partnerships—age differences and their significance: empirical evidence from the 2000 British National Survey of Sexual Attitudes and Lifestyles ('Natsal 2000'). *J Adolesc Health.* 2006 Jul;39(1):87–95.

Neinstein LS, Gordon CM, Katzman DK, Rosen DS, Woods ER. *Adolescent Health Care, A Practical Guide.* 5th ed. Philadelphia, PA: Wolters Kluwer; 2008.

Shafii T, Stovel K, Davis R, Holmes K. Is condom use habit forming? condom use at sexual debut and subsequent condom use. *Sex Transm Dis.* 2004;31(6):366–372.

Strassburger V, Brown RT, Braverman PK, Rogers PD, Holland-Hall C, Coupey SM. *Adolescent Medicine: A Handbook of Primary Care.* New York, NY: Lippincott Williams & Wilkins; 2006.

Tanner J. *Growth at Adolescence.* 2nd ed. Springfield, IL: Charles C Thomas; 1962.

Upchurch DM, Mason WM, Kusunoki Y, Kriechbaum MJ. Social and behavioral determinants of self-reported STD among adolescents. *Perspect Sex Reprod Health.* 2004; 36(6):276–287.

Weinstock H, Berman S, Cates W Jr. Sexually transmitted diseases among American youth: incidence and prevalence estimates, 2000. *Perspect Sex Reprod Health.* 2004; 36(1):6–10.

38

Sexually Transmitted Infections in Travelers

Karen Elizabeth Rogstad

■ INTRODUCTION

Sexually transmitted infections (STIs) are not limited by national boundaries, and outbreaks are often associated with population movements and social disruption. Travel and movement also provide opportunistic "dissociative mixing," where persons from high-prevalence STI areas interact with persons from low-prevalence areas. Much population movement occurs now as recreational travel, a by-product of increased wealth and leisure time. Travel occurs for different reasons and may be national or international. It may be voluntary for holidays, for business, or for visiting friends and relatives (VFR). Particularly in underdeveloped nations and in countries of the former Soviet Union and related states, travel may occur because of economic or political pressures, for example, refugees or forced displacement. Each of these settings provides opportunities for sexual interaction between travelers and the local population or between travelers themselves. The sexual health needs of all these groups needs to be considered. This chapter will concentrate primarily on people traveling abroad for leisure or for business, but many of the principles of management can also be applied to refugees and economic migrants, some of whom will frequently return to their country of origin to visit family (those who are traveling to VFR are less likely to access health care before travel).

■ EPIDEMIOLOGY OF TRAVEL

Worldwide, in 2004, 639 million tourists contributed US$463 billion to the world's economy, and by 2007,

the number of tourists had increased to 898 million. Residents of the United Kingdom alone made 69.5 million visits abroad in 2006, around two-thirds of these for holiday, approximately 15% for business and 15% to visit family and relatives. The number of UK residents traveling abroad for holiday increased by more than 27% between 1997 and 2007 but fell in 2009 to 60 million, possibly as a result of the of the global recession. Of holiday trips in 2006, just under half (42%) were package tours. Conversely, overseas residents made 32.7 million visits to the UK. For UK travelers, the 10 most popular travel destinations are to the developed world, with the 9 most popular to Europe and the other to the United States. Overall 80% of UK visitors traveled to Europe. In the United States, most holiday travel is within the continent. Despite the low proportion, 26 million airplane trips were made abroad (excluding Canada and Mexico), of which 44% were to VFR (2002 data), and by 2005, there were 63.5 million trips abroad.

VFR travelers are usually recent migrants or children of migrants. The countries they are likely to travel to are Latin America and Asia for U.S. residents and to Africa and the Indian subcontinent for UK residents (in 2002, 30% of new UK residents were from Africa and 24% from Indian subcontinent). Some holidays and destinations particularly attract certain demographic groups. For example, more than 250,000 young people from the UK travel annually to Ibiza, an international dance resort in Mediterranean Spain, and an even greater number of U.S. college students attend "spring break" beach vacations in Florida. There are also trips designed for specific groups, such as gay/lesbian travel junkets.

Sexual Behavior, Holidays, and Travel

There is a seasonal variation in sexual activity, with increased sexual intercourse (SI) and unsafe sex occurring around Christmas and summer vacation in the United Kingdom. Holidays provide the opportunity for increased sexual mixing at home or abroad. Travelers often feel released from the social mores of their own community and are more likely to consume alcohol and use illicit drugs while vacationing.

Increased sexual risk behaviors while on holiday has been increasingly documented, especially in studies of European travelers. Studies in the early 1990s showed significant sexual risk behavior in international travelers who attended for a "tropical check." Of UK genitourinary medicine (GUM, STI clinic) attenders who had traveled abroad in the preceding 3 months, 25% reported a new partner while away and two-thirds had not or inconsistently used condoms. Norwegian STI services, which extended the period of questioning to 5 years, found 41% had a new partner abroad. Studies on non-STI clinic attenders also show high levels of risk behavior, with 28% of Swedish family planning patients having a new partner abroad. When the travelers were studied, 48% of those traveling without a partner to Ibiza on holiday had at least one new partner while away, and 62% always used a condom. Of British vacationers in Tenerife, 35% had sexual intercourse with a nonregular partner while on holiday, with no significant difference between men and women. Most striking were results in healthcare professionals. For example, 32% of medical students who traveled reported having sexual intercourse with a new partner while on holiday. Younger people aged 16–24 years were more likely to have a new partner than older groups, which was also found in British vacationers in Tenerife, where those aged 25 years or younger were more likely to have a new sexual partner than older than 25 years (50% vs. 22%).

Travel destination has an effect on whether someone is likely to have sex. For example, people returning from Peru had lower rates than people returning from Ibiza or Tenerife. Country of residence of the traveler also affects behavior, suggesting that a larger proportion of UK residents engage in casual travel sex (27%), when compared with those of other countries (16%). Overall pooled prevalence of travel-associated casual sex is 21%, and 50% of those had unprotected intercourse.

Overseas travel should be seen as a major behavioral sexual health risk. A review by Vivancos et al. (2010) has

systematically reviewed and performed meta-analysis on sexual risk behavior in travelers and provides a valuable resource for those interested in this topic.

PARTNERING PATTERNS

Sex abroad in many cases will be with someone of the same nationality or with someone else from a westernized country. The 2000 National Survey of Sexual Attitudes and Lifestyles found that a half of the men and women from the United Kingdom had sex with another UK national, and more than a third from another European country. Less than 5% reported new partners from sub-Saharan Africa, the Caribbean, or South America. However, of "tropical check" clinic attenders who had returned from developed countries, 44% had sex with a local. This may be more frequently seen in certain groups who are likely to have an extended stay—for example, U.S. Peace Corps volunteers, expatriates, and deployed military personnel in areas where the local population is not hostile.

Traditionally it has been thought that men are more likely than women to have sex with partners from the host country, but this depends on which group of travelers are studied; for example, women in Tenerife tended to have sex with more non-UK partners than men (13/30, 43% compared with 6/32, 19%). Differences become more apparent when travel is to sub-Saharan Africa and Asia, where men are more likely to have sex with locals. The pooled rate of casual travel sex in women is 20%, while that of men was 25%.

Risk-Taking Behavior

Travelers often increase the rate of new partner acquisition. However, those who take sexual risks abroad also do so at home. For example, having any sex in Ibiza was associated with illicit drug use and more partners before the visit, and the nationwide UK studies (NATSAL) have shown that risky sex abroad is associated with having an increased number of UK partners, paying for sex (for men), intravenous drug use (women), and unsafe sex in the preceding 4 weeks. Worldwide, those most likely to have new sexual partners while abroad were young men, single, traveling alone or with friends, with a previous history of multiple sexual partners or an STI. In addition, being abroad for longer periods, and men who have sex with men, were associated with an increased risk of having new sexual partners and unprotected intercourse. There was no difference between men and women in rates of unprotected intercourse at 62.1% and 62.3%.

Alcohol plays an important contributor to sexual risk-taking behavior in nontravelers, and it is likely to be even more important in travelers, with 33% of UK residents admitting to consuming more alcohol while on holiday abroad.

An issue that is rarely addressed is that of nonconsensual sex while on holiday or traveling. Factors associated with this anecdotally appear to include alcohol use, lack of knowledge of the locality, foreign tourists as easy prey, and, increasingly, the use of the date rape drug Rohypnol. Legal recourse in countries where nonconsensual sex occurred is usually limited.

■ SEXUALLY TRANSMITTED INFECTIONS AND TRAVEL

There is marked international variation in STI prevalence, with higher rates of bacterial infections usually seen in the less developed nations. There is also wide variation in susceptibility of organisms to therapy. For example, antimicrobial resistance in *Neisseria gonorrhoeae* is highest in the Far East. In contrast, infection with antiviral-resistant HIV has been a feature of infection acquired in developed countries, although this will likely change with the increased availability of antiretrovirals in developing countries.

The risk of developing an STI is increased up to threefold in people who have casual sex abroad, and in developed countries, travelers appear to be responsible for a small but significant proportion of acute STIs. For example, in two London clinics, 12% of acute STIs diagnosed were due to sex abroad. Almost 1 in 10 (9%) of individuals with gonorrhea reported having had sex abroad in the 3 months before diagnosis. Of gonorrhea in the UK acquired abroad, men who have sex with men (MSM) mainly reported sexual contact in mainland Europe (64%) or the United States (14%), whereas heterosexual men mostly reported sex in the Caribbean (35%) and the Far East (18%). UK women with gonorrhea mainly reported sex in the Caribbean (62%). In 2008, 12% of patients in England and Wales with gonorrhea reported sex abroad, and of these, 22% were infected with a strain with high level resistance to penicillin and tetracycline. This increased to 60% in those who had traveled to India and the Far East.

Although syphilis in heterosexual men and women in the UK is increasingly acquired at home (68% by

2008), a large number of cases are still imported, with at least 18% of cases associated with travel (21% of men and 14% of women).

Other diseases rarely seen in developed nations are endemic in many parts of the world. These include chancroid, lymphogranuloma venereum (LGV), and granuloma inguinale (donovanosis). Outbreaks of chancroid in the United States have been linked to those traveling abroad. Recent outbreaks of LGV in the UK and in Holland in MSM have however occurred through transmission in those countries. Human T lymphotropic virus (HTLV I) is prevalent in the Caribbean and Japan but does not present acutely.

HIV risk is proportional to local prevalence and is therefore increased in areas such as sub-Saharan Africa, the Far East, and, more recently, India, Latin America, and the Caribbean. Between 2000 and 2002, 69% of UK-born men with heterosexually acquired HIV (235 of 342) were infected through sex while abroad, as were 25% (75 of 316) of women. Twenty-two percent of these men were probably infected in Thailand.

■ PAYING FOR SEX AND SEX TOURISM

Sex tourists are men or women who travel (often long distances) with the intention of having sex. Sex tourism is becoming a major concern by the country of origin and countries visited, not only because of its impact on the health of individuals and the public health but also because of the recognition that it often involves exploiting children. Destinations vary from different countries. It is predominantly men who are involved. Amsterdam has been a common destination in Europe, particularly for "stag parties," although more recently eastern Europe has increased in popularity. Asia has traditionally been a destination for sex tourists. Initially, Thailand, developed a sex industry to accommodate U.S. servicemen on recreational leave from the Vietnam conflict and the Philippines. German sex tourists in Thailand stated that other destinations included the Philippines, Kenya, and Brazil.

Structural interventions, such as legislation, can affect choice of destinations, and therefore, this is a dynamic process. For example, since Asia began measures to reduce sex tourism, Latin America has increased in popularity as a destination for sex tourists from the United States.

There is scant research on sex tourists. They tend to be from a slightly older group than groups traditionally at risk for STIs. In a study of German sex tourists, participants tended to be 30–40 years old, (range 20–76 years), single, and with a well-paid job. Many did not consider their Thai contacts as prostitutes but rather as "intimate friends," as a result condom use was reduced (condom use was 30–40%). Half of German sex tourists also had sexual contacts inside Germany on their return from Thailand, highlighting the risk of onward transmission when sex tourists return home. Sexual tourism also has a negative impact on the health of the prostitute or exploited child, as well as for the public health in the country visited. In some settings, the perception is that HIV is more likely to be acquired from older commercial sex workers (CSWs), leading to the increased exploitation of teenagers and children who are perceived as "clean."

There are others whose do not travel with the express purpose of paying for sex but who use sex workers while they are abroad. Groups more likely to seek commercial sex are expatriates working overseas for long periods, military personnel, and businessmen. Men who have casual travel sex are also more likely to have ever paid for sex. Military personnel deployed overseas have been found to have high rates both of casual sex with locals and paying for sex. Sex with commercial sex workers was associated with younger age and a single or divorced lifestyle; inconsistent condom users, however, were more likely to be older.

Why men pay for sex abroad has received scant attention, but one study of Japanese businessmen found that factors included a sense of freedom and anonymity, a sense of loneliness, peer influence, and low costs.

■ PRETRAVEL DISCUSSION AND PREVENTION OF STIs

More widespread prevention education is clearly necessary for holidaymakers and travelers. During a pretravel visit, besides appropriate vaccinations, malaria prophylaxis (when indicated), and counseling on reducing foodborne illness, the discussion should include information on risks of sex abroad. Studies have shown that, although there is increasing knowledge of STIs in travelers, this has little relation to their behavior, and some evidence suggests that those who do not use condoms at home also do not use them abroad. However, a single, brief, patient-centered counseling session, especially from a health provider, has been shown to reduce bacterial STI acquisition for several months. Travel advice should include information on safer sex and the

risks of sex abroad, as well as the effects of alcohol and illicit drugs on decision making. Travelers should be advised to take condoms with them, to store them correctly in hot climates, and to avoid oil-based lubricants and nonoxynol-9. Travelers should be advised that if they develop symptoms of an STI, that is, dysuria, vaginal or urethral discharge, an unexplained rash, genital lesion (e.g., ulcer), groin swelling, or genital or pelvic pain, they should seek care and refrain from sexual intercourse. They should be advised that STIs can be associated with systemic illness, particularly HIV, which may manifest as a seroconversion glandular fever-like illness. Problems may occur 6 months or more following exposure. If they have unprotected sex abroad, they should receive an STI screen on their return, whether or not they have symptoms.

The Centers for Disease Control recommends hepatitis A vaccination should be given to intravenous drug users and MSM, and hepatitis B vaccination should be offered to seronegative persons with a history of STI, multiple sexual partners, injecting drug users, or their partners and MSM. Hepatitis B vaccination should be offered to sex tourists. Women should also have a full needs assessment for contraception.

BOX 38-1 Advice and Management Before Travel

- Prevalence of STIs/HIV in area to be visited
- Safer sex, including condom use with any new partner
- Risk of sexual assault/"date rape" drugs
- Alcohol and drug consumption advice
- Information on postexposure prophylaxis for HIV (PEPSE)
- Hepatitis B vaccination for sex tourists or those taking a prolonged holiday to high risk areas, e.g., gap-year students
- Symptoms/signs that may indicate an STI
- Attendance at STI clinics if unprotected SI occurs
- Travel packs—condoms, PEPSE (starter pack) in certain situations
- Consider sexual history STI screen and contraceptive for all, particularly young people and MSM

Management of Patients Who Have Had Sex Abroad

Consider urgent referral to specialized STI services if travel was to a developing country and genital ulcer(s) or lymphadenopathy present.

Management and treatment of those acquiring or at risk of acquiring an STI from travel-related exposure requires a systematic approach that will vary according to whether they are symptomatic and the characteristics of their sexual partner(s), particularly if they are from a high-risk group or in a developing country. Tests should be undertaken on all who have had a new sexual partner abroad, and the minimum on the asymptomatic should include urine, self-taken vaginal, or endocervical swabs,

for gonorrhea and chlamydia testing; and venous blood for syphilis and HIV taken on return and 12 weeks post-sexual intercourse (the "window period") (an additional test can be done at 4 weeks if there is high risk, using a fourth-generation HIV assay. For travelers who have been at high risk, hepatitis B testing should also be done at 12 weeks. Testing for hepatitis C should also be considered for certain risk groups, for example, intravenous IVDUs or contact with them, and MSM. HIV testing should be in the context of informed consent, and this may be facilitated by using a leaflet to provide pretest discussion.

Coinfection is a particular issue if there has been sex in an area with a high STI prevalence and, for example, a

TABLE 38-1 Management of Returning Traveler Who Has Had Sex Abroad

Sample	Test
Urine, self-taken vaginal or endocervical swabs	Gonorrhea and chlamydia NAAT testing
Pharyngeal and rectal swabs	Gonorrhea culture and chlamydia/GC NAAT (MSM)
Venous blood baseline	HIV STS (all) hepatitis B and C (high risk)
4 weeks	HIV STS (high risk)
12 weeks	HIV STS (all) hepatitis B and C (high risk)
6 months	Hepatitis B and C (high risk)
Immediate	HIV test using fourth-generation assay if suspected HIV seroconversion illness
Genital ulcer swab	Herpes culture or NAAT
Sex in developing country and genital ulcers—additional tests	
Genital ulcer swab	LGV NAAT
	Hemophilis ducreyi culture
Serology	LGV
Ulcer biopsy	Microscopy for donovanosis (from South Pacific)
Management	
Hepatitis B vaccination for those at risk if they present within 6 weeks, and for sex tourists	Immediately, 7 and 21 days, 1 year
PEPSE—assess risk according to guidelines	Within 72 hours, triple HAART
Advice	Sexual abstinence/condom use until results back. Return if symptoms develop. Prevention advice for future trips
Partner Notification	If STI detected, notify partners during travel and since return

LGV, lymphogranuloma venereum; MSM, men who have sex with men; NAAT, STS; PEPSE, postexposure prophylaxis for HIV.

positive herpes result from a genital ulcer should not obviate the need to consider and test for syphilis or chancroid. If someone presents to a primary care physician/GP within 6 weeks of risk behavior with someone from an area endemic for hepatitis B, then an accelerated vaccine course may provide some protection. Postsexual exposure prophylaxis for HIV is recommended if the patient presents within 72 hours of sexual contact, according to the following criteria: (1) HIV serostatus of sexual contact if known, prevalence of HIV in that community if status unknown and (2) type of sexual act and whether there was sexual assault. Guidelines are available for the United States, the United Kingdom, and Europe from CDC, BHIVA, and Euro Surveillance, respectively. The risk of acquiring HIV needs to be balanced against drug toxicity and needs to be discussed in full with the patient. If commenced, expert opinion should be sought after initiation of therapy, and if possible before. Treatment, if given, should be with three antiretroviral drugs starting ideally within 1 hour but, at the most, within 72 hours, although some advocate it may be useful even after this period.

For patients who are symptomatic or who have had sexual intercourse in a developing country with a local resident, examination is essential. MSM also require additional investigation with a proctoscopy and rectal and pharyngeal samples for gonorrhea and chlamydia testing, as rectal and pharyngeal infections are usually asymptomatic. The presence of genital ulcers requires tests for *Herpes genitalis* (NAAT or culture) and syphilis serology, as well as tests for LGV (serology, NAAT if available), chancroid (culture for *Haemophilis ducreyi*), and granuloma inguinale (biopsy, cell culture, NAAT).

Partner notification should be attempted if an STI is diagnosed although it may be difficult and should consider sexual partners since their return. Antibiotic therapy for gonorrhea needs to take into account resistance patterns as infections from abroad often have reduced susceptibility to penicillin and ciprofloxacin.

■ TROPICAL DISEASES THAT MAY IMITATE STIs

Beware the returning traveler from the tropics with any of the symptoms or signs of fever, lymphadenopathy, malaise, myalgia, or rash. Although syphilis or primary HIV should be considered, life-threatening malaria, shistosomiosis japonicum, and dengue fever should be urgently tested for according to region of travel. In addition, some tropical infections can present with genital symptoms: *Schistosomiasis haematobium* can present with dysuria, hematuria, urinary frequency, urethritis, friable cervical, vaginal or vulval polyps; 1% of cases of dengue fever may have GU symptoms; genital ulcers, nodules, or other genital skin lesions can be caused by amoebiasis, leishmaniasis, onchoceriasis, guinea worm, cutaneous larva migrans, and myiasis.

HIV Pretest Discussion

As highly effective antiretroviral therapy has become available, there has also been a move toward normalizing testing to pick up infections earlier and thus reduce morbidity, mortality, and onward transmission either to sexual partners or vertically to infants. To ignore HIV testing in those who return from travel overseas, particularly if they have had sexual intercourse with a resident in a high prevalence area, potentially could be considered negligent (see also Chapter 29 on HIV counseling).

■ THE ROLE OF THE TRAVEL INDUSTRY, GOVERNMENTS, AND NONGOVERNMENTAL ORGANIZATIONS

Health advice in travel brochures is lacking, and only 3% were found to contain advice on safe sex. Tour operators and travel providers should address these needs, particularly for those on excursions where there is a high expectancy of sexual activity or those traveling to areas with high STI/HIV prevalence. They should advise about the risk of sexual assault abroad with advice on how to reduce such a risk.

Information provided by governments and the World Health Organization is of variable quality and quantity. The CDC in Atlanta produces the Yellow Book, which is an excellent resource for travelers. It provides advice on general travel health but also has extensive sections on HIV and other sexually transmitted infections and is available from their Web site. The UK leaflet on travel health, however, has minimal sexual health information. The UK Foreign Office's specific country information warns travelers to the Football World Cup in South Africa of the high prevalence of HIV/AIDS and recommends, "so avoid putting yourself at risk," but does not give warnings about the high prevalence of other STIs, nor advice on how to reduce risk of HIV or other STIs. The media through all its forms can inform and educate the public and play an increasingly important role in modern society. Some charitable organizations provide invaluable advice on personal protection and help-lines for those concerned about HIV and other STIs.

■ SUMMARY

Travel for whatever reason increases opportunities for new sexual encounters. Those particularly at risk are young people and sex tourists and those with risky behavior in their country of origin. Sex abroad has the potential to be a major cause of morbidity. Preventative advice should be offered to all travelers but particularly those traveling to the developing world; vaccinations should be given as required. Those who have been at risk should be encouraged to receive sexual health screens after their travel, and secondary prophylaxis for hepatitis B and HIV should be considered. Travel and sexual history taking are an essential part of a medical consultation. Clinicians should consider referral to specialized STI services where there are symptoms or signs suggesting syphilis, HIV, or tropical STIs. Healthcare professionals and the travel industry working together can improve the health of their clients with timely advice, utilizing simple tests for detecting STIs, and effective use of primary and secondary prophylaxis. Publications and organizations that provide travel advice should include information on STIs, HIV, and sexual risk behavior.

■ KEY POINTS

- There are more than 600 million tourists annually worldwide.

- Visits abroad to see friends and relatives (VFRs) by recent migrants are common.

- Those who have risky behavior in their home country are likely to have risky sexual behavior abroad.

- Destinations for sex tourists vary as local laws change.

- Travelers should be warned of the risks of sex abroad and advised on prevention of STIs, and postexposure prophylaxis for HIV.

- Hepatitis B vaccination should be considered for sex tourists and those likely to have sex abroad.

- Returning travelers should have an STI screen according to risk behavior while abroad.

- Some tropical diseases may mimic STIs.

REFERENCES

ABTA Travel trends report 2010. www.abta.com/filegrab/?ref=312&f=TravelTrendsReport2010.pdf.

Abdullah AS, et al. Sexually transmitted infections in travellers: implications for prevention and control. *Clin Infect Dis*. 2004;15(39):533–538.

Almeda J, Calsabona J, Sima B, et al. Management of HIV postexposure prophylaxis after sexual, injecting drug or other exposure in Europe. *EuroSurveillance*. 2004;9(6):35–40.

Angell SY, Behrens RH. Risk assessment and disease prevention in travellers visiting friends and relatives. *Infect Dis Clin North Am*. 2005;19:49–65.

Bellis MA, Hughes K. Sexual behaviour of young people in international tourist resorts. *Sex Transm Infect*. 2004;80:43–47.

Department of Health. Yellow book on traveller's health. www.ncid.cdc.gov/travel/yb

Fisher M, Benn P, Evans B, et al. UK guideline for the use of post-exposure prophylaxis for HIV following sexual exposure. *Int J STD AIDS*. 2006;17:81–92. *www.bashhh.org/guidelines/2006/pepse0206.pdf*.

Foreign and Commonwealth Office. Information on how to avoid sexual assault and what to do if it occurs. www.fco.gov.uk.

Hart GJ, Hawkes S. International travel and the social context of sexual risk. In: Carter S, Clift S, eds. *Tourism and Sex: Culture, Commerce and Coercion*. London: Cassell; 2000.

Health Protection Agency. Information on STI rates and Gonococcal resistance. www.hpa.org.uk.

Rogstad KE, Palfreeman A. HIV testing for patients attending general medical services. National Guidelines. Concise Guidance to Good Practice Number 3. Royal College of Physicians; 2005.

Holmes KK, Sparling PF, Stamm W, et al. (Eds). *Sexually Transmitted Diseases*. 4th ed. McGraw-Hill New York; 2008.

Hughes K, Bellis MA. Sexual behaviour among casual workers in an international nightlife resort: a case control study. *BMC Public Health*. 2006,6:39. *www.biomedcentral.com/1471-2458/6/39*.

Marrazzo JM. Sexual tourism: implications for travellers and the destination culture *Infect Dis Clin North Am*. 2005;19(1):103–120.

Mercer CH, Fenton KA, Wellings K, et al. Sex partner acquisition while overseas: results from a British national probability survey. *Sex Transm Infect*. 2007;83:517–522.

Mulhall B. Sex and travel: studies of sexual behaviour, disease and health promotion in international travellers—a global review. *Int J STD AIDS*. 1996;7:455–465.

National statistics travel trends 2006. www.statistics.gov.uk/downloads/theme_transport/TravelTrends2006.pdf.

Rogstad KE. Sex, sun, sea and STIs: sexually transmitted infections acquired on holiday. *BMJ*. 2004;329:214–217.

Travellers' Health: Yellow Book. Health information for international travel. wwwn.cdc.gov/travel/yellowBookCh1-Recommendations.aspx accessed 6 March 2008.

Vivancos R, Abubakar I, Hunter PR. Foreign travel associated with increased sexual risk-taking, alcohol and drug use among UK university students: a cohort study. *Int J STD AIDS*. 2010;21:46–51.

Vivancos R, Abubakar I, Hunter P R. Foreign travel, casual sex and STIs: systematic review and meta-analysis. *Int J Infect Dis*. 2010 Oct;14(10):e84–251

Wellings K, Macdowall W, Catchpole M, Goodrich J. Seasonal variations in sexual activity and their implications for sexual health promotion. *J Royal Soc Med* 1999;92:60–64.

Women, Health and Development Program—Pan American Health Organisation. *www.paho.org/genderandhealth*.

World Health Organization. International STI and HIV epidemiology. www.who

39

Sexually Transmitted Infections in Commercial Sex Workers

Maryam Shahmanesh

INTRODUCTION

Sex workers often have high rates of sexually transmitted infections (STIs). Rates of STIs are higher in settings where sex work is illegal or marginalized. Besides the medical and humanitarian need to treat and prevent STI, including HIV, in this population, there are substantial community benefits. Sex workers are classic epidemiological core groups, which are hypothesized to maintain HIV/STI transmission in communities. Mathematical modeling shows the effectiveness of targeting core groups (groups with high rates of sexual partner exchange) in the early and accelerated phases of an STI/HIV epidemic. A multitude of published experimental and quasi-experimental studies in sex workers have shown the effectiveness of various HIV-prevention strategies.

Besides provider-initiated and structural interventions, innovative approaches have included direct involvement of sex workers in developing and implementing prevention and treatment programs. For example, the group empowerment model implemented in Sonagachi, West Bengal, involved sex workers in designing and implementing the project through peer educators and collectives. However, structural obstacles often hamper these participatory models, such as the lack of camaraderie, high levels of mobility, invisibility, isolation, and female disempowerment among sex workers. The documented successes of Thailand, Senegal, and Sonagachi suggest a need to explicitly engage with these structural factors that either increase sex workers' vulnerability or impede implementing effective interventions in this marginalized group.

WHY DEVOTE A WHOLE CHAPTER TO MANAGEMENT OF STIs IN SEX WORKERS?

High Rates of STIs in Sex Workers

In commercial sex settings where condom use is inconsistent and access to STI treatment is limited, half to two-thirds of women typically have an STI at any given time. Up to 10% may report genital ulcer disease; one-third may have reactive syphilis serology and many have more than one infection. In many parts of the world, more than two-thirds of women have serological evidence of HSV-2. Pregnancy is also a risk, and in areas where effective contraception is not available or provided, most are terminated, often in settings that pose considerable danger to the woman.

Treating Sex Workers as Part of a Public Health Strategy

Sex Workers: A Core Group

Sex workers are the "classic" core group for STI intervention. "Core groups" are defined as a set of individuals who exhibit levels of risk behavior sufficient to maintain the net reproductive rate of an STI above 1. Their disproportionate contribution to infection transmission places them at the heart of HIV and STI prevention strategies. The equation in Box 39-1 quantifies this effect.

BOX 39-1 Equation for the Basic Reproductive Rate of an STI

$$R_0 = \beta cD$$

R_0 = basic reproductive rate

β = probability of transmission of the organism (infectivity)

c = the rate of exposure between infected and susceptible individuals

D = duration of infectivity

According to the equation, unprotected sex (constant β) with many susceptible people (increase c), and delayed treatment of infection (increase D) would lead to the propagation of an STI.

This definition of a "core" is an epidemiological concept and, with few exceptions, is not easily defined in concrete terms. Furthermore, blanket categorization of sex workers as core groups homogenizes an otherwise heterogeneous group.

Targeting Sex Workers as Part of HIV Prevention Strategies

Interventions to reduce STI prevalence in sex workers generally acknowledge the exposure risk and take a "harm-reduction" approach at three levels:

- Increasing condom use and reducing high-risk sexual acts

- Reducing the number of sex partners

- Improved STI diagnostic and treatment services

Each one of these interventions has a specific impact on the reproductive rate equation described in Box 39-1.

BOX 39-2 Rational for Targeted Interventions for Sex Workers

1. Reduce the burden of disease and STI complications (e.g., infertility, PID, and complications of syphilis in child birth) in sex workers
2. Reduce prevalence of STIs among sex workers, clients, and partners
3. Reduce the efficiency of HIV transmission within the sexual networks important in driving the HIV epidemic

For example, reducing the number of partners reduces c, the behavior term; increasing condom use reduces "β," or transmission efficiency of sexual exposure, and providing enhanced diagnostic and treatment services shortens D, the duration a person would be infectious.

■ WHAT ARE THE CHALLENGES TO IMPROVE STI MANAGEMENT IN SEX WORKERS?

Marginalization and Vulnerability

Sex workers are often hard to reach for social and legal reasons. The lack of social sanction, which can range from stigmatization to frank criminalization of sex workers, marginalizes them and pushes them underground. Migration and mobility, which is commonly observed, inhibits community building and compounds the "otherness" they are made to feel. They are often subject to physical and sexual violence. Mental health and substance abuse are often present as coexisting problems. In the absence of either formal or informal regulation requiring periodic examinations, reproductive and sexual health is often low priority. All of these combine to increase vulnerability to HIV and STIs. Young sex workers and those who have recently started work are often the most vulnerable and the least likely to have access to services.

Targeting and Spotlighting

Concepts like "core groups," although ostensibly neutral epidemiological terms, raise important ethical issues in relation to labeling, stigmatization, and discrimination. For example, epidemiological studies that identify sex work as a key driving force of the HIV epidemic can be translated in the public domain into "prostitute-bashing"—without addressing the important public health needs of these persons. In some areas, such as part of Europe, where many sex workers are migrants, this can be translated into anti-migrant sentiment. A danger of targeted interventions has been a renewed spotlight on "prostitution" as the "source of contagion," a stark reminder of similar reactions from the public following the contagious diseases acts in Europe of the 1800s.

Trafficking of Women

Trafficking of women for sex work is a major public health and human rights issue. Annually, an estimated 4 million people are trafficked, one quarter of which are younger than 18 years. Nearly a million of these are trafficked across borders. Women who are trafficked into the sex trade provide an even greater challenge for service delivery. In the source countries, they are often vulnerable for recruitment into trafficking rings because of extreme poverty, unemployment, and gender inequality. At their destination, they are often present illegally and may be coerced and trapped in unfamiliar surroundings with an equally unfamiliar language. The traffickers may seize their travel documents and confine them to brothels. Even in countries where amnesty and clinical services are available, fear of recognition, fear of authority, and unfamiliarity with the healthcare systems of the host country are barriers for trafficked women to access care and prevention services. Their lack of negotiating powers can lead to higher-risk sexual encounters, including penetrative sex without the protection of condoms.

Delivering Services to the Hard to Reach

The public health benefits of targeted interventions for sex workers depend to a large degree on coverage. The invisibility and mobility of sex workers affects both intervention delivery and evaluation of outcomes. One of the greatest challenges we face is to scale up effective interventions and reach the majority of sex workers.

Participation Is the Key to Success

Interventions implemented with the participation of sex workers improve the chances of success. Furthermore, through peer outreach, sexual health skills can diffuse through sex worker networks. The active involvement of sex workers in interventions also has an empowering effect that may become the first step to reducing vulnerability.

Participation takes many forms. At the minimum, there is strong coordination between the clinical services and the peer networks that promote safer sexual practices, such as condom distribution and use. At the other end of the spectrum, sex workers actually own and steer the intervention through strong sex worker collectives or unions. An example of this is the West Bengal program where an intervention organized and implemented through sex workers known as Sonagachi has led to levels of HIV 10-fold lower than elsewhere in India.

Looking Beyond the Reproductive Organs

When sex workers are involved in service development, they request services, which are expanded beyond the

---

BOX 39-3 Proximity of Condom to the Point of Use Increases the Likelihood of Use

A randomized controlled trial with a factoral design compared three models of condom distribution in Nicaraguan motels, with or without IEC material. Condom use was measured through retrieval of used condom from the rooms.

The two interventions were

1. The receptionist would hand condoms to the couple as they checked in.
2. An attractively packaged condom was placed on the bed in the room.

The control arm was for condoms to be made available at reception to couples only at their request.

Couples were **most** likely to use condoms if they were placed in the rooms. They were also more likely to be used if they were handed to the couples than if they had to ask for them at reception.

Paradoxically, the presence of IEC material in the rooms reduced the likelihood for condom use.

---

narrow focus of HIV and STI. Provision of broader social and health services avoids the spotlight effect and increases the credibility of the program. Examples are STI services nested within general health clinics that also cater to dependents and children of sex workers; integrated sexual and reproductive health services; one-stop centers that provide sexual, reproductive, and mental health together with substance misuse services; or integrated HIV care and prevention services. Social interventions are also effective. The growing evidence for extremely high levels of violence experienced by sex workers, and its association with higher-risk sexual behavior and mental health problems, suggests the need to integrate health services with interventions to tackle gender-based violence.

Taking Services to the Sex Workers—Outreach

In most areas, direct outreach by the healthcare system or nongovernmental organizations (NGOs) is needed to overcome the myriad of access barriers. In some areas, where sex workers live and work in a clearly demarcated red-light area, service provision can be provided in a permanent clinic, drop-in center, or community center. In settings where sex workers are mobile, outreach vans have been effective. Outreach clinics can also take services to where sex workers aggregate, such as truck stops and mines. This type of geographic proximity facilitates access, improves coverage, and can even provide services for women whose movement is restricted. For example, the Hillbrow project in South Africa tackled the social isolation of sex workers by establishing a sexual health service in the lodges where they worked. This not only provided services but also provided a social forum for the women. In Nicaragua, attractively packaged condoms placed in the hotel rooms where sex workers brought their clients were more likely to be used than if they had to be picked up at the reception.

Tackling Mobility

One of the greatest challenges to sex worker interventions is their extremely high mobility. This mobility often relates to the extent to which the trade is criminalized as well as how trafficking rings operate. Innovative interventions have attempted to address these issues. For example, in Nicaragua, an STI treatment voucher project was developed. These vouchers were redeemable at quality-approved public and private clinics. Of the 8500 vouchers distributed to more than a thousand sex workers, 40% were used. Concurrent ecologic studies through surveillance data suggested a drop in prevalent syphilis.

An alternative approach is to engage proprietors such as the pimps and brothel owners and use their access to newer women entering the area as the basis for the intervention strategy. There are dilemmas here—for example, does improving the health of women tacitly acknowledge the role of the proprietors in human rights violations?

The Trafficked Woman

Global strategies to reduce human trafficking are within the purview of the international organizations mobilized to combat this abuse. NGOs that are involved in this include the International Organization for Migra-

tion (www.iom.org) and the Protection Project (www.protectionproject.org). Assurance that trafficked women exchanging sex for money have access to appropriate reproductive and sexual health services is needed, but often difficult. A key element is to ensure that health services are kept separate from immigration and other law enforcement agencies. Interventions for trafficked women often need to be broad based, as there are often legal, social, mental health, and other health service issues involved.

■ What Is Effective?

Effectiveness studies are hampered by methodological challenges, that is, finding a representative sample in such a hard-to-reach group, and the difficulty of developing longitudinal cohorts in highly marginalized populations. Nevertheless, evidence from ecological studies, observational studies, cohorts, quasi-experimental studies, and a handful of randomized controlled trials has accumulated. which allow a number of conclusions.

Behavioral Interventions

Provision and Promotion of Condom Use

Condom promotion and behavioral interventions should be an integral part of all interventions targeting sex workers. The most effective large-scale condom promotion effort was the 100% condom campaign in Thailand, in the early 1990s. In the Thai program, brothels were required to implement a 100% condom policy, which was accompanied by a variety of clinical and structural interventions. As a result, HIV and STI rates fell by more than 90%. In Mumbai, India, for example, a careful evaluation of a peer education and condom promotion intervention lead to a threefold reduction in HIV incidence. Randomized controlled trials of different STI treatment strategies showed substantial reductions in HIV incidence in both arms of the study, which was attributed to condom availability and the behavioral component delivered to both arms. Although these observational and quasi-experimental studies have limitations, the consistency of the direction of change, the association between participation in the intervention, self- reported condom and reduced HIV or STI incidence, biological plausibility; and increase in condom consumption suggest that these observations reflect real changes. There is as yet no data to suggest that any one type of behavioral intervention is superior to another.

BOX 39-4 Delivering STI Services to Sex Workers

Sex workers should be involved in developing geographically accessible services, delivered through peer-driven networks, and responsive to their mobility and broader social and health needs.

Female Condoms

Even in the best interventions self-reported condom use falls short of 100%. One potential way to overcome dependency on male clients is female-controlled methods of prevention. In the absence of effective vaginal microbicides, female condoms have been widely promoted. Female condoms are relatively expensive and require training in their use, both of which limit acceptability.

Integrating HIV Prevention with Care

Given the high prevalence of HIV in some settings in some developing countries, and that sex workers often have regular nonpaying or romantic partners, linking HIV prevention with care makes programmatic sense. The rapid expansion of HIV care in these settings raises human rights and equity issues, and programs need to be careful not to exclude sex workers from access to treatment.

Treatment of Sexually Transmitted Infections

Treating STIs in sex workers is not straightforward. The treatment of symptomatic women on clinical, etiological, or syndromic grounds, which is the method most commonly used, is constrained because treatment relies on symptoms to identify women. Yet most women with STIs are asymptomatic and even when symptomatic the common "syndromes" of vaginal discharge and abdominal pain have poor sensitivity and specificity for diagnosing of cervical infections and STIs. Sex workers may have a higher prevalence overall of vaginal discharge. Sensitive nucleic acid amplification tests (NAATs) for diagnosing cervical infection are expensive and require good laboratory infrastructure. They are further limited by the time to diagnosis, consequent delays in treatment, and potential loss to follow-up.

Given these problems, suggested strategies for reducing STIs among sex workers are regular screening for STIs, periodic presumptive treatment (PPT), or a combination of the two. Both strategies have been associated with a reduction in the burden of STIs, but to date, neither has been shown to reduce incident HIV in randomized controlled trials.

Regular Screening for STIs

Clinical services offering regular screening for sex workers are usually part of a multifaceted approach, which includes condom promotion and prevention messages, and so the relative effect of each is hard to quantify. In

> ### BOX 39-5 Regular STI Screening Services
>
> Regular contact with clinical service reduces the burden of STIs, provides an opportunity to screen and treat syphilis, reinforces condom use, and becomes an entry point for women to access HIV treatment services.

research settings in Kinshasa, Nairobi, Abidjan, Cotounou, and La Paz, services offering regular screening were associated with increased condom use and reduced STI and HIV prevalence. The screening strategies have varied between use of highly sensitive STI screening tests, to the development of less expensive algorithms, based on evidence-based risk scores, clinical picture, and microscopy. In reality—these types of strategies can be only infrequently implemented because of resource limitations

Presumptive Treatment of Sex Workers

Because of the limitations of implementing regular screening, presumptive treatment of sex workers has been proposed as an alternative. The rationale of this approach would be to treat a population with a known increased probability of having an STI.

This strategy has been used in conjunction with behavior change to reduce the prevalence of STIs in sex workers and their clients. Quasi-experimental studies in South African mines found that this strategy led to a fourfold reduction in bacterial STIs in sex workers over time. They also found that there was gradation such that miners closer to the intervention were less likely to present to the mining clinic with an STI. However, there are substantial limitations to presumptive or mass therapy approaches. First, to be maximally effective, treatment of the community must be completed within a short period. Second, the optimum frequency of presumptive

> ### BOX 39-6 Presumptive Therapy for Sex Workers
>
> Presumptive therapy for STIs in sex workers can be an additional tool to reduce the prevalence of bacterial STIs. Presumptive treatment approaches need to be coordinated with clinical experts who understand current treatment regimens and antimicrobial resistance patterns.

treatment is not clear. Third, there are increasingly limited oral options available for bacterial infections such as gonorrhea and syphilis.

In practice, many settings use a combination of presumptive treatment and regular screening and syndromic management. This strategy has been effective at reducing the prevalence of curable STIs in sex workers working in the Avahan program districts of northern Karnataka, India. However, these strategies may have the potential to foster the development of antimicrobial resistance.

■ OTHER STRATEGIES

Treatment of Clients and Nonpaying Partners

Broadening interventions to include clients, nonpaying partners, and pimps can break the chain of transmission at various points in the network. An intervention in Bulawayo, Zimbabwe, was implemented through a peer educator program that targeted mobile men and male bar patrons. This was associated with an increase in self-reported condom use and a drop in male STI clinic attendees over time. Accessing clients, however, can be extraordinarily difficult and is often dissuaded by brothel owners.

The Future

Other strategies that are on the horizon are the development of vaginal microbicides and STI vaccines.

■ STRUCTURAL INTERVENTIONS: REDUCING VULNERABILITY

Sex work is estimated to produce an annual income equivalent to 5% of world domestic product. Four million people are estimated to be trafficked annually with the majority destined for work in the sex industry. In the context of such large global interests, notwithstanding other vulnerabilities mediated through the global economy, it is difficult to envisage a solution that does not have a global component. And yet given the complexity of the interrelationship between poverty, migration, gender relationships, and the particular cultural historical context of each locality, it is equally difficult to envisage not incorporating the uniqueness of the context. The regulatory approaches of the nineteenth century did little except drive prostitution underground. Although the improved diagnostics and advent of antibiotics may have contributed to better STI control, it is most likely to have been social changes that accompanied economic development and improvements in women's status that led to a decline in STIs.

Although effectiveness of interventions targeting sex workers has been documented for more than two decades, few interventions have been scaled up for implementation.

Many barriers to scale-up are political or legislative. Equally, it is necessary to tackle some of the broader social injustices that make women involved in sex work vulnerable to HIV and STIs. Such interventions that tackle the broader social and economic context within which sex work occurs are called *structural interventions*. Structural interventions are explicit about changing social norms, including legislative changes and economic interventions. When considering structural interventions, it is useful to divide them into

1. Those that tackle factors that increase the sex workers vulnerability to HIV.

2. Those that tackle the barriers to scaling up sex worker intervention.

The most well-described structural intervention to reduce HIV and STIs has been the Thai 100% condom project. The key feature of this strategy was that the government in liaison with sex industry led it. The main components were ensuring an adequate supply of condoms to all sex workers through the peer pressure of model brothels supported by legal sanctions, establishing STI clinics countrywide, free weekly STI tests and treatment for sex workers, and a massive media campaign aimed at clients. As this is a countrywide intervention, there are no control groups; however, various indicators suggest an impact, namely, increased condom supply through government and private manufacturers, an 80% reduction in surveillance of five major STIs in men sustained over time, and a 10-fold decrease in STI incidence in new military recruits. These declines occur in the context of worsening epidemics in neighboring

---

BOX 39-7 STI Treatment in Sex Workers

- Regular screening for STIs using risk-based algorithms, clinical examination, and microscopy
- Periodic presumptive therapy with azithromycin ± cefixime, and addition of tinidazole for cases with vaginal discharge
- A combination of screening and presumptive therapy
- Treatment of nonpaying male partners

countries. A quasi-experimental study in the Dominican Republic also suggested that brothel-based interventions were more effective where 100% condom use was enforced through regional policy in contrast with self-regulation. However, Thailand had a unique situation in that it had a vested economic interest in controlling HIV to protect a lucrative sex industry, while most other countries are either reluctant to confront the reality of a sex industry or use imported "100% condom" programs to further coerce and intimidate sex workers.

In this context, interventions like Sonagachi in India show that it may be possible to intervene at a local level to reduce vulnerability of women. Sonagachi's key feature was the participation of the sex workers, through collectivization and politicization, in confronting factors that increased their vulnerability. The result was a broad-based intervention, which in addition to HIV prevention encompassed anything from legal advice, to child immunization. Like Thailand, they engaged the structures of power, including police, brokers, and brothel owners. Without a control arm, the impact of the intervention cannot be quantified; nevertheless, HIV prevalence among sex workers of Sonagachi has remained in single figures in contrast to more than 50% elsewhere in India. More recently, the Avahan program—the massive scale-up of targeted interventions using a similar model of community mobilization of female sex workers, condom promotion, and provision of free and accessible sexual health services, throughout the high-prevalence states in the south of India—seems to have resulted in a decline in HIV incidence at a population level.

CONCLUSION

It is salutary to note that a variety of interventions with sex workers increase condom use and reduce HIV and STI incidence in participants. Therefore, the first and foremost step is to scale up these effective interventions to reach most sex workers. Most effective interventions have been part of a multifaceted approach, and it is impossible to disentangle the relative merits of condom provision and STI management. It would seem that the combination of condom promotion and improved STI treatment have a synergistic, unquantifiable effect. Syndromic management of STIs is clearly inadequate and hence some sort of regular screening with risk-based algorithms in conjunction with epidemiological treatment of STIs needs to be considered. Active treatment of the clients and nonpaying partners of sex workers can supplement these STI control methods. Nesting these

interventions among broader health care will reduce the potential negative impact of spotlighting and may increase the acceptability of the services.

Effective interventions have included components that empowered the women to collectively address the barriers to safer sex. Their participation in designing and implementing the interventions goes some way to preventing the intervention from becoming a coercive force. Any attempt to genuinely reduce the prevalence of STIs, HIV, and incurable viral STIs in sex workers will need to explicitly engage with the social, legal, economic, and human rights context that increase their vulnerability. This can only be achieved with the participation of sex workers themselves.

KEY POINTS

- Targeted intervention for core groups like sex workers reduces the burden of disease in women; reduces the prevalence of STIs in the sex workers, partners, and clients; and reduces the efficiency of HIV transmission through the sexual networks.

- Scaling up service delivery to this mobile, hidden, and hard-to-reach group is one of the largest challenges to successful HIV prevention.

- Targeted interventions run the risk of spotlighting and making sex workers the scapegoat for the HIV epidemic. Services provided as part of a broader social and health intervention are frequently more acceptable and run less risk of spotlighting.

- Provide services, which are geographically proximal to where sex work occurs.

- Consider innovative strategies, such as vouchers or franchised clinics, for mobile sex workers.

- Promote components such as peer networks and collectivization that encourage women to work collectively to address barriers to safer sex.

- Emphasize consistent condom use as the only way to effectively prevent HIV and incurable viral infections.

- Provide effective treatment for both symptomatic and asymptomatic STIs.

- Address the larger social, legal, economic, and human rights issues that increase vulnerability and risk.

- Engage sex workers in the design and implementation of the intervention.

REFERENCES

Alary M, Mukenge-Tshibaka L, Bernier F, et al. Decline in the prevalence of HIV and sexually transmitted diseases among female sex workers in Cotonou, Benin, 1993–1999. *AIDS.* 2002;16:463–470.

Anderson RMMR. *Infectious Diseases of Humans; Dynamics and Control.* Oxford: Oxford University Press; 1991.

Bhave G, Lindan CP, Hudes ES, et al. Impact of an intervention on HIV, sexually transmitted diseases, and condom use among sex workers in Bombay, India. *AIDS.* 1995;9(suppl 1):S21–S30.

Blanchard JF, O'Neil J, Ramesh BM, et al. Understanding the social and cultural contexts of female sex workers in Karnataka, India: implications for prevention of HIV infection. *J Infect Dis.* 2005;191(suppl 1):S139–S146.

Blankenship KM, West BS, Kershaw TS, Biradavolu MR. Power, community mobilization, and condom use practices among female sex workers in Andhra Pradesh, India. *AIDS.* 2008;22(suppl 5):S109–S116.

Boily MC, Lowndes C, Alary M. The impact of HIV epidemic phases on the effectiveness of core group interventions: insights from mathematical models. *Sex Transm Infect.* 2002;78(suppl 1):i78–90.

Day S, Ward H, Harris JR. Prostitute women and public health. *BMJ.* 1988;297:1585.

Egger M, Pauw J, Lopatatzidis A, et al. Promotion of condom use in a high-risk setting in Nicaragua: a randomised controlled trial. *Lancet.* 2000;355:2101–2105.

Fleming DT, Wasserheit JN. From epidemiological synergy to public health policy and practice: the contribution of other sexually transmitted diseases to sexual transmission of HIV infection. *Sex Transm Infect.* 1999;75:3–17.

Ford K, Wirawan DN, Fajans P, et al. Behavioural interventions for reduction of sexually transmitted disease/HIV transmission among female commercial sex workers and clients in Bali, Indonesia. *AIDS.* 1996;10:213–222.

Ghys PD, Diallo MO, Ettiegne-Traore V, et al. Effect of interventions to control sexually transmitted disease on the incidence of HIV infection in female sex workers. *AIDS.* 2001;15:1421–1431.

Gorter A. Improved health care for sex workers: a voucher programme for female sex workers in Nicaragua. *Res Sex Work.* 1999;2–4.

Grosskurth H, Gray R, Hayes R, et al. Control of sexually transmitted diseases for HIV-1 prevention: understanding the implications of the Mwanza and Rakai trials. *Lancet.* 2000;355:1981–1987.

Hanenberg RS, Rojanapithayakorn W, Kunasol P, et al. Impact of Thailand's HIV-control programme as indicated by the decline of sexually transmitted diseases. *Lancet.* 1994;344:243–245.

Holmes KK, Johnson DW, Kvale PA, et al. Impact of a gonorrhoea control program, including selective mass treatment, in female sex workers. *J Infect Dis.* 1996;174(suppl 2):S230–S239.

Jana S, Bandyopadhyay N, Mukherjee S, et al. STD/HIV intervention with sex workers in West Bengal, India. *AIDS.* 1998;12(suppl B):S101–S108.

Kaul R, Kimani J, Nagelkerke NJ, et al. Monthly antibiotic chemoprophylaxis and incidence of sexually transmitted infections and HIV-1 infection in Kenyan sex workers: a randomised controlled trial. *JAMA.* 2004;291(21):2555–2562.

Kerrigan D, Ellen JM, Moreno L, et al. Environmental-structural factors significantly associated with consistent condom use among female sex workers in the Dominican Republic. *AIDS.* 2003;17:415–423.

Laga M, Alary M, Nzila N, et al. Condom promotion, sexually transmitted diseases treatment, and declining incidence of HIV-1 infection in female Zairian sex workers. *Lancet.* 1994; 344:246–248.

Lowndes CM, Alary M, Gnintoungbe CA, et al. Management of sexually transmitted diseases and HIV prevention in men at high risk: targeting clients and non-paying sexual partners of female sex workers in Benin. *AIDS.* 2000;14:2523–2534.

Moses S, Ramesh BM, Nagelkerke NJ, et al. Impact of an intensive HIV prevention programme for female sex workers on HIV prevalence among antenatal clinic attendees in Karnataka state, south India: an ecological analysis. *AIDS.* 2008;22(suppl 5):S101–S108.

Ngugi EN, Plummer FA, Simonsen JN, et al. Prevention of transmission of human immunodeficiency virus in Africa: effectiveness of condom promotion and health education among prostitutes. *Lancet.* 1988;2:887–890.

Parker RG, Easton D, Klein CH. Structural barriers and facilitators in HIV prevention: a review of international research. *AIDS.* 2000;14(suppl 1):S22–S32.

Reza-Paul S, Beattie T, Syed HU, et al. Declines in risk behaviour and sexually transmitted infection prevalence following a community-led HIV preventive intervention among female sex workers in Mysore, India. *AIDS*. 2008;22(suppl 5):S91–100.

Shahmanesh M, Patel V, Mabey D, Cowan FM. Effectiveness of interventions for the prevention of HIV and other sexually transmitted infections in female sex workers in resource poor settings: a systematic review. *Trop Med Int Health*. 2008;13(5):659–679.

Steen R, Dallabetta G. Sexually transmitted infection control with sex workers: regular screening and presumptive treatment augment effort to reduce vulnerability. *Reprod Health Matters*. 2003;11(22):74–90.

Steen R, Vuylsteke B, DeCoito T, et al. Evidence of declining STD prevalence in a South African mining community following a core-group intervention. *Sex Transm Dis*. 2000;27:1–8.

Walkowitz JR. *Prostitution and Victorian Society: Women, Class and State*. Cambridge: Cambridge University Press; 1980.

Wilson D, Sibanda B, Mboyi L, et al. A pilot study for an HIV prevention programme among commercial sex workers in Bulawayo, Zimbabwe. *Soc Sci Med*. 1990;31:609–618.

40
Sexually Transmitted Infections During Pregnancy

Ahmed S. Latif and Sharon Moses

Sexually transmitted infections (STIs) in pregnancy may result in adverse pregnancy outcomes, fetal infection, neonatal infection, and a broad range of social consequences. Adverse pregnancy outcomes include ectopic pregnancy, miscarriage, and stillbirth, congenital and perinatal infections, and maternal puerperal infections. Infection before pregnancy can lead to ectopic pregnancy and infertility, and infection during pregnancy can cause miscarriage, chorioamnionitis, preterm delivery, small-for-dates infants, and congenital infection. The susceptibility to infection is increased during pregnancy, and the clinical manifestations of some STIs are altered during pregnancy. STIs present at delivery can cause maternal puerperal infection and neonatal infections.

▪ PREGNANCY-RELATED COMPLICATIONS OF STIs

Although fertility-related complications are not the specific focus of this chapter, they are the among most critical and costly complications of unprotected sexual intercourse and STI. Ectopic pregnancy and infertility are recognized complications of salpingitis; the most common causes of salpingitis are *Neisseria gonorrhoeae* and *Chlamydia trachomatis*. The risk of ectopic pregnancy increases 10-fold following an episode of salpingitis. Both chlamydial and gonococcal infection can cause salpingitis, resulting in tubal obstruction, a major cause of infertility.

Postabortal infections following surgical terminations are substantially increased in women with coexistent chlamydia, gonorrhea, or bacterial vaginosis. Screening and treating women for these infections pre-

surgery has led to a reduction in febrile morbidity rates (Qvistad et al. 1983; Crowley et al. 2001). If screening is not practical, many clinics and practitioners routinely treat all women receiving surgical abortion for chlamydia presumptively and, in high prevalence areas, would treat for gonorrhea as well.

Intrauterine infection may be the result of hematogenous or ascending infection. For example, congenital syphilis *Treponema pallidum* is hematogenously spread in the mother's blood and invades the placenta and fetal tissues. Such infection produces characteristic histologic changes in the placenta. Ascending infection from the cervix and vagina may occur through intact or compromised fetal membranes and can cause chorioamnionitis and amniotic fluid infection. HIV and hepatitis B, in contrast, are hematogenously disseminated in the mother but do not pass the placental barrier. Vertical transmission occurs in these cases at parturition, through exposure to blood and secretions.

Fetal loss, prematurity, and preterm rupture of membranes, low birth weight, and a variety of perinatal complications occur more frequently in pregnant women with reproductive tract infections, including STIs and bacterial vaginosis.

Intrauterine or perinatally transmitted STIs can have severely debilitating effects on pregnant women, their partners, and their fetuses, and are among the top causes of disability-adjusted life years lost in developing countries. All pregnant women and their sex partners should be asked about STIs, counseled about the possibility of perinatal infections, and ensured access to treatment, if needed.

SCREENING FOR STIs IN PREGNANCY

The antenatal care visit provides an opportunity for screening pregnant women for STIs and for providing critically important surveillance data to STI and perinatal program managers. The infections that are screened will depend on the prevalence of infections in the community in which the pregnant woman lives and on the individual woman's risk for acquiring infection. Screening tests are available for most STIs; however, the range of tests available in resource-constrained settings may be limited. Generally, comprehensive testing is recommended at an early prenatal visit (in the first trimester). Depending on the organism, the clinical setting, and risk profile, testing may be repeated during the third trimester as parturition approaches. Clinicians should not be deluded that once engaged in prenatal care, that patient's risk disappears!

HIV TESTING

All pregnant women should be offered voluntary HIV testing at the first antenatal visit. Repeat testing for HIV is advisable in the third trimester and at the time of delivery in women at greater risk for infection, including women that have an STI during pregnancy or have multiple sexual partners during pregnancy, those that have an HIV-infected partner, those using illicit drugs, and those that live in or come from areas where HIV prevalence is high.

HIV testing consent requirements are in transition, from the former "HIV testing exceptionalism" that requires a separate consent process, to "normalization," wherein HIV testing is routinely provided unless practitioners are specifically asked not to test. Testing should occur after the patient is notified that she will be tested for HIV as part of the routine panel of prenatal tests (Centers for Disease Control and Prevention 2010; American College of Obstetricians and Gynecologists 2003). For women who decline, providers should continue to strongly encourage testing and address concerns that pose obstacles to testing. Women who decline testing because they have had a previous negative HIV test should be informed of the importance of retesting during each pregnancy. The concept of incident infection should be reemphasized. Testing pregnant women is particularly important, because antiretroviral and obstetric interventions can reduce the risk of perinatal HIV transmission to below 2%. In settings where women present for delivery and their HIV status is undocumented, rapid testing should be performed if available.

Pregnant women identified as HIV infected should be staged with CD4 and viral load testing, as well as for opportunistic infections. As soon as possible, they should be apprised of the potential options available to them. Three options are (1) term delivery with appropriate antiretroviral prenatal and perinatal intervention, which reduces vertical transmission to <2%; (2) term delivery without antiretroviral therapy, which carries a 30% risk of vertical transmission; and (3) pregnancy termination. Women should also be apprised that current data suggest that pregnancy during HIV infection does not result in increased adverse HIV-related events or complications. Women who carry a pregnancy to term should be advised that 1–15% of seronegative infants will become infected during breast-feeding if HIV-infected women breast-feed their infants into the second year of life.

Pregnant women who are HIV infected should be counseled concerning their options (either on-site or by referral), given appropriate antenatal treatment, and advised not to breast-feed their infants if infant formula is readily available and can be safely prepared.

SCREENING FOR SYPHILIS

A serologic test for syphilis should be performed on all pregnant women at the first prenatal visit. Where prenatal care is not optimal, rapid plasma reagin (RPR)-card test screening should be performed, and if the test is reactive, treatment should be given at the prenatal visit. Women who are at high risk for syphilis, live in areas of excess syphilis morbidity, were previously untested, or have positive serology in the first trimester should be screened again early in the third trimester (28 weeks gestation) and at delivery. Ideally, women should be retested at delivery, and infants should not be discharged from the hospital unless the syphilis serologic status of the mother has been determined at least one time during pregnancy and preferably again at delivery. Any woman who delivers a stillborn infant should be tested for syphilis. Congenital syphilis is considered in most areas to be a "sentinel public health event" because it is 100% preventable through screening and treatment.

TESTING FOR HEPATITIS B VIRUS INFECTION

A serologic test for hepatitis B surface antigen (HBsAg) should be performed on all pregnant women at the first prenatal visit. HBsAg testing should be repeated late in pregnancy for women who are HBsAg negative but who are at high risk for HBV infection, including injection-drug users and women who have other STIs.

Women who are HBsAg positive should be referred for assessment and medical management and for assessment and vaccination of their sexual partners and household contacts. The hospital in which delivery is planned and the provider who will care for the newborn should be notified of the woman's HBsAg result so that the neonate may be provided with immunoprophylaxis. At time of delivery, the combined provision of hepatitis B hyperimmune globulin (passive vaccination), and initiation of the hepatitis B vaccine series is highly effective in preventing vertical transmission of hepatitis B.

In contrast to the situation with HIV, pregnant women who are HBsAg positive should be reassured that breast-feeding is not contraindicated and should receive information regarding hepatitis B modes of transmission, prevention of transmission, and the importance of postexposure prophylaxis for the neonate and hepatitis B vaccination for household contacts and sex partners.

■ SCREENING FOR CHLAMYDIAL INFECTION

Chlamydia is highly prevalent and is associated with a host of perinatal complications, including low birth weight, ophthalmia neonatorum, and neonatal pneumonia. Screening interventions have markedly reduced the incidence of these complications. Chlamydial testing should be performed at the first prenatal visit. In resource-limited areas, at-risk women should be prioritized for testing. These include women younger than 25 years old and women who have a new or more than one sex partner. These persons should also be tested again during the third trimester to prevent maternal postnatal complications and chlamydial infection in the infant. Screening during the first trimester might enable prevention of adverse effects of chlamydial infection during pregnancy, such as low birth weight (McMillan et al. 2006). Nucleic acid amplification tests (NAATs) are most convenient, as these may be performed on self-obtained lower vaginal swabs NAATs may be carried out to detect both chlamydial and gonococcal infection on the same specimen.

■ SCREENING FOR GONORRHEA

Gonorrhea during pregnancy is also associated with low birth weight but, more important, severe ophthalmia neonatorum and keratitis in infants born to infected mothers. Screening should be performed at the first prenatal visit. In resource-poor settings, screening should be reserved for women at risk or for women living in an area in which the prevalence of *N. gonorrhoeae* is high (Miller et al. 2003). A repeat test should be performed during the third trimester for those at continued risk. Testing can be performed by either culture (of endocervical secretions) or NAATs. As with chlamydia, NAATs are highly sensitive, specific, and offer the widest range of testing specimen types and may be used with self-obtained vaginal swabs, endocervical swabs, vaginal swabs, and urine. Current test formats allow a single specimen to be collected for testing for both chlamydia and gonococcal infections (Schachter et al. 2005; Bignall 2004).

■ TESTING FOR HEPATITIS C VIRUS INFECTION

A test for hepatitis C antibodies (anti-HCV) should be performed at the first prenatal visit for pregnant women at high risk for exposure, including those with a history of injection-drug use, repeated exposure to blood products, prior blood transfusion, or organ transplants.

No treatment is available for anti-HCV-positive pregnant women. However, all women found to be anti-HCV-positive should receive appropriate counseling and referral for assessment and management. Currently, no vaccine is available to prevent HCV transmission. Vertical transmission occurs, but with much reduced efficiency compared with the other bloodborne infections.

■ EVALUATION FOR BACTERIAL VAGINOSIS

Bacterial vaginosis is a clinical diagnosis that is related to alterations of the vaginal flora (see Chapter 7). BV is extremely common in some populations and is associated in particular with premature rupture of membranes (PROM), chorioamnionitis, and postpartum endometritis. Despite these clear associations, the clinical trial data conflict on whether treatment of all BV during pregnancy reduces complications. There is consensus, however, that treatment of symptomatic BV is warranted. Evaluation for bacterial vaginosis (BV) may be conducted at the first prenatal visit for asymptomatic patients who are at high risk for preterm labor (e.g., those who have a history of a previous preterm delivery), which would then warrant observation.

■ PAPANICOLAOU SMEAR

A Papanicolaou (Pap) smear can be obtained at the first prenatal visit if the patient is due for a Pap smear according to national guidelines (see Table 40-1).

TABLE 40-1   Summary of Recommendations for Screening for STIs During Pregnancy

HIV infection

All women should be screened for HIV infection at the first prenatal visit. If negative, repeat testing should be performed in the third trimester and again at delivery in women at high risk for infection.*

Syphilis

All women should have syphilis serology performed at the first prenatal visit. Women at high risk # for syphilis should be retested in the third trimester and again at delivery.

Chlamydial infection

All women should have a chlamydia screening test offered at the first prenatal visit, and those women considered to be at high risk for infection should have repeat testing in the third trimester and again at delivery. ¶

Gonorrhea

All women should have a gonorrhea screening test offered at the first prenatal visit, and those women considered to be at high risk for infection should have repeat testing in the third trimester and again at delivery. ¶

Hepatitis B

All pregnant women should be screened for the hepatitis B surface antigen at the first prenatal visit. The test should be repeated in the third trimester if it was negative initially in women at high risk for infection. §

Hepatitis C

Screening for hepatitis C should be carried out in women at risk for infection, including those with a history of injection-drug use, repeated exposure to blood products, prior blood transfusion, or organ transplants.

Bacterial vaginosis

Women with a history of previous preterm labor should have an assessment for bacterial vaginosis at the first prenatal visit.

Pap smear

A Pap smear can be carried out at the first prenatal visit in women who have are due to have the test according to national guidelines and recommendations.

* Women at high risk for HIV infection include women that have an STI during pregnancy or have multiple sexual partners during pregnancy, those that have an HIV-infected partner, those engaged in using illicit drugs, and in those that live in or come from areas where HIV prevalence is high.

Women at high risk for syphilis include those living in areas with excess syphilis morbidity, are previously untested, and those that have positive serology in the first trimester.

¶ Women at greater risk for chlamydial or gonococcal infection include those aged younger than 25 years, and those who have a new or more than one sex partner.

§ Women at greater risk for hepatitis B infection include women who are injecting-drug users and those that have an STI during pregnancy.

There is insufficient evidence of benefits of routine screening for trichomoniasis, human papilloma virus, and herpes simplex virus in asymptomatic pregnant women.

■ MANAGEMENT OF SEXUALLY TRANSMITTED INFECTIONS IN PREGNANCY

The following section briefly describes the management of STIs during pregnancy (CDC 2010). For all STIs, contact tracing and treatment and partner notification should be carried out together with appropriate screening, and all persons with STIs and their partners should be offered education and counseling for risk reduction.

■ SYPHILIS

Syphilis in pregnancy is treated the same way as in non-pregnant persons. Infection is managed according to the stage of infection. Parenteral penicillin is the treatment of choice and is most conveniently given in the long-acting form intramuscularly. For pregnant women with primary, secondary or early latent syphilis, a single intramuscular dose of 2.4 million units of benzathine penicillin is given. Please note that early latent syphilis is defined differently in the United States (<1 year) and in the United Kingdom (< 2 years duration). In pregnant women with late latent syphilis (1 year in the United States) duration or of unknown duration, 2.4 million units of benzathine penicillin is given each week for 3 weeks (total dose 7.2 million units).

Pregnant women with neurosyphilis, that is, those with neurologic signs such as cognitive dysfunction, motor or sensory deficits, ophthalmic or auditory symptoms, cranial nerve palsies, and symptoms or signs of meningitis; those with syphilitic eye disease such as uveitis, neuroretinitis, and optic neuritis; and those with abnormal cerebrospinal fluid should be given aqueous crystalline penicillin 18 to 24 million units daily administered as 3 to 4 million units intravenously every 4 hours or by continuous infusion, for 10 to 14 days, followed by 3 doses of 2.4 million units of benzathine penicillin given intramuscularly each week for 3 weeks.

Penicillin is the only antibiotic recommended in treating syphilis in pregnancy, and pregnant women who are allergic to penicillin should be admitted for desensitization and then given full treatment. Though erythromycin and, more recently, azithromycin has been suggested for treating syphilis in pregnancy, treatment failures to prevent congenital syphilis are well documented, and therefore macrolides are not recommended. Tetracyclines, which are often used to treat syphilis in penicillin-allergic patients, are absolutely contraindicated in pregnancy.

Following completion of full treatment, patients should be monitored regularly and RPR or VDRL titers should be measured at 3, 6, and 12 months.

◼ CHLAMYDIAL INFECTION

For the treatment of chlamydial infection in pregnancy, the following treatment regimens are recommended:

Azithromycin 1 g in a single oral dose. This is the preferable regimen since compliance can be assured.

Alternative regimens include

Amoxicillin 500 mg orally 8 hourly for 7 days

Alternatively, the following may be used:

Erythromycin base 500 mg orally 6 hourly for 7 days, or

Erythromycin base 250 mg orally 6 hourly for 14 days, or

Erythromycin ethyl succinate 800 mg orally 6 hourly for 7 days, or

Erythromycin ethyl succinate 400 mg orally 6 hourly for 14 days

The lower-dose 14-day regimens may be used if gastrointestinal tolerance is a problem

Erythromycin estolate is contraindicated in pregnancy because of drug-related hepatotoxicity

Considering the sequelae that might occur in the mother and neonate if chlamydial infection persists, it is recommended that tests for cure are performed using NAATs 3 weeks after completion of therapy to ensure therapeutic cure.

◼ GONOCOCCAL INFECTION

The options for treatment of gonococcal infection in pregnancy are limited. Quinolone class drugs are contraindicated in pregnancy. Therefore, only the following treatment regimens are recommended:

Ceftriaxone 250 mg in a single intramuscular dose, or

Cefixime 400 mg in a single oral dose

Pregnant women who are allergic to penicillins or beta-lactam drugs need to be referred to a referral center for consideration of alternative regimens.

As coinfection with *C. trachomatis* commonly occurs in persons with gonorrhea, it is advisable to also treat all pregnant women with gonorrhea for presumptive chlamydial infection with azithromycin or amoxicillin.

◼ GENITAL HERPES

The management of genital herpes in pregnancy is complex, and the major concern is preventing rare, but devastating neonatal herpes syndrome, which occurs through vertical transmission and exposure to maternal secretions. The following "ground rules" are useful:

1. In settings where genital HSV is common, most persons are infected before pregnancy. Women who are HSV-2 positive (seroprevalent) do not pose an increased risk to the infant, unless there are active lesions apparent at time of delivery.

2. The highest risk of vertical transmission is when a pregnant woman acquires *primary* (incident) HSV disease during the last trimester of pregnancy.

Routine screening for herpes simplex virus infection in asymptomatic pregnant women is not indicated. Cultures for herpes simplex virus may be performed in the presence of clinically suspicious genital lesions during pregnancy in women to confirm the diagnosis of genital herpes. Culture is not necessary in women who have been previously diagnosed with HSV.

Genital herpes is a chronic, lifelong viral infection. Two types of HSV have been identified, HSV-1 and HSV-2. The diagnosis of genital herpes infection may be made by virologic and type-specific serologic tests. Isolation of HSV in cell culture is the preferred virologic test for patients who seek medical treatment for genital ulcers or other mucocutaneous lesions. However, the sensitivity of culture is low, especially for recurrent lesions, and declines rapidly as lesions begin to heal. PCR assays for HSV DNA are more sensitive and have been used instead of viral culture but are not yet widely available. Type-specific antibodies to HSV develop 4–6 weeks after infection and persist indefinitely. Type-specific serology tests are now available commercially and may be performed to determine whether a pregnant woman whose partner has a history of genital herpes is susceptible to primary infection. However, these tests are costly, and routine screening is not recommended.

Because acquisition of primary herpes during late pregnancy carries the greatest risk, women without known genital herpes should be counseled to avoid intercourse during the third trimester with partners known or suspected of having genital herpes. Type-specific serologic tests may be useful to identify pregnant women at risk for HSV infection and to guide counseling regarding the risk for acquiring genital herpes during pregnancy.

All pregnant women should be asked whether they have a history of genital herpes. At the onset of labor, all women should be examined carefully for herpetic lesions. Women without symptoms or signs of genital herpes or its prodrome can deliver vaginally. In women with recurrent genital herpetic lesions at the onset of labor, delivery by cesarean section may be considered to prevent neonatal herpes, which can reduce, but not eliminate HSV transmission to the infant. Infants exposed in these settings can be treated presumptively with acyclovir for the first 2 weeks of life.

Management of Women with the First Episode of Genital Herpes in Pregnancy

All women with a first episode of genital herpes in pregnancy should be given aciclovir orally as follows (Royal College of Obstetricians and Gynaecologist 2002):

- Acyclovir 400 mg orally 8 hourly for 5 days.

- Delivery by cesarean section is *recommended* if the first episode of genital herpes lesions occurs at the

time of delivery and delivery by cesarean section may be *considered* if the first episode occurs within 6 weeks of the expected date of delivery or onset of preterm labor.

■ MANAGEMENT OF WOMEN WITH A RECURRENT EPISODE OF GENITAL HERPES IN PREGNANCY

Women with a recurrent episode of genital herpes in pregnancy may be managed as follows:

- Daily suppressive acyclovir in the last 4 weeks of pregnancy may be *considered*; in this situation, aciclovir is given in a dose of 400 mg orally 12 hourly.

- Delivery by caesarean section may be *considered* for women presenting with recurrent genital herpes at the onset of labor. However, it is generally considered that this intervention is controversial and not cost effective.

In managing pregnant women with genital herpes, it is good clinical practice that the patient is managed jointly by a genitourinary or infectious diseases specialist and obstetrician.

■ BACTERIAL VAGINOSIS

Bacterial vaginosis (BV) is a polymicrobial clinical syndrome resulting from replacement of the normal hydrogen peroxide–producing lactobacilli species in the vagina with high concentrations of *Gardnerella vaginalis*, *Mycoplasma hominis*, and anaerobic bacteria such as *Prevotella* sp. and *Mobiluncus* sp. The cause of the microbial alteration is not fully understood. However, BV is associated with having multiple sex partners, a new sex partner, douching, and lack of vaginal lactobacilli.

BV during pregnancy is associated with adverse pregnancy outcomes, including premature rupture of the membranes, preterm labor, preterm birth, intra-amniotic infection, and postpartum endometritis. Managing asymptomatic BV in pregnancy is controversial. Symptomatic women with BV and all women with BV with a history of preterm delivery should be treated as follows:

Metronidazole 400 to 500 mg twice daily for 7 days, or a single 2 g dose.

Alternatively, clindamycin is given in a dose of 300 mg orally twice daily for 7 days, OR

Intravaginal clindamycin cream (2%) is applied once daily for 7 days.

In women with a history of previous preterm delivery and BV, tests of cure should be carried out 4 weeks after completion of treatment.

Whether treatment of asymptomatic pregnant women with BV who are at low risk for preterm delivery reduces adverse outcomes of pregnancy is unclear.

■ TRICHOMONIASIS

Women with trichomoniasis may be completely asymptomatic or may have symptoms of vaginal discharge characterized by a diffuse, malodorous, yellow green vaginal discharge with vulval irritation. Trichomoniasis is usually visually diagnosed when motile trichomonads in wet mounts of vaginal fluid are examined microscopically. The organism may be cultured in special media, such as the *InPouch*. Vaginal trichomoniasis has been associated with adverse pregnancy outcomes, particularly premature rupture of membranes, preterm delivery, and low birth weight. However, metronidazole treatment has not found that there is a decrease in perinatal morbidity. Women should be treated as follows:

> Women may be treated with 2 g of metronidazole in a single oral dose.

> Alternatively, metronidazole may be given in a dose of 400 to 500 mg orally twice daily for 7 days.

■ VULVOVAGINAL CANDIDIASIS

Vulvovaginal candidiasis (VVC) occurs commonly during pregnancy is caused by *Candida albicans* but occasionally is caused by other *Candida* species or yeasts. Typical symptoms of VVC include pruritus, vaginal soreness, dyspareunia, dysuria, and abnormal vaginal discharge. None of these symptoms were specific for VVC. VVC is extremely common, and it is estimated that 75% of women will have at least one episode of VVC and up to 45% will have two or more episodes. VVC frequently occurs during pregnancy (Young and Jewell 2000).

> Only topical azole therapies, applied for 7 days, are recommended for use in pregnant women.

> Miconazole 100 mg vaginal suppository, one suppository for 7 days or

> Terconazole 0.4% cream 5 g intravaginally for 7 days

■ CHANCROID

In pregnant women with chancroid, the following treatment regimens may be used:

Azithromycin 1 g orally in a single dose, OR

Ceftriaxone 250 mg intramuscularly in a single dose, OR

Erythromycin base 500 mg orally three times a day for 7 days

Patients should be reexamined 3 to 7 days after initiation of therapy. If treatment is successful, ulcers usually improve symptomatically within 3 days and objectively within 7 days after therapy. The time required for complete healing depends on the size of the ulcer; large ulcers might require more than 2 weeks for complete healing. If no clinical improvement is evident, the clinician must consider whether the diagnosis is correct, the patient is coinfected with another STI or HIV, treatment was not used as instructed, or the strain of *Haemophilus ducreyi* causing the infection is resistant to the prescribed antimicrobial.

Clinical resolution of fluctuant lymphadenopathy is slower than resolution for ulcers and might require needle aspiration.

■ DONOVANOSIS

Pregnant women with Donovanosis (granuloma inguinale) may be treated as follows:

> Azithromycin 1 g orally once per week for at least 3 weeks and until all lesions have completely healed

> Alternatively patients may be treated with

> Erythromycin base 500 mg orally four times a day for at least 3 weeks and until all lesions have completely healed

Treatment halts progression of lesions, although prolonged therapy is usually required to permit granulation and reepithelialization of the ulcers. Relapse can occur 6 to 18 months after apparently effective therapy. Patients should be followed clinically until signs and symptoms have resolved.

■ LYMPHOGRANULOMA VENEREUM

Lymphogranuloma venereum (LGV) is caused by *C. trachomatis* serovars L1, L2, or L3. The most common clinical manifestation of LGV among heterosexuals is tender inguinal or femoral lymphadenopathy that is typically unilateral. A self-limited genital ulcer or papule sometimes occurs at the site of inoculation. However, by the time patients seek care, the lesions might have disappeared. Rectal exposure might result in proctocolitis (including mucoid or hemorrhagic rectal discharge, anal pain, constipation, fever, or tenesmus). Genital ulcer swab (or bubo aspirate) may be tested for *C. trachomatis* by culture, direct immunofluorescence, or nucleic acid detection. Genotyping is required for differentiating LGV from non-LGV *C. trachomatis* but are not widely available.

Pregnant women with LGV should be treated with:

Erythromycin base 500 mg orally four times a day for 21 days

There is expert opinion that azithromycin 1.0 g orally once weekly for 3 weeks is probably effective. Buboes might require aspiration through intact skin or incision and drainage to prevent the formation of inguinal/femoral ulcerations.

■ GENITAL WARTS

More than 30 types of human papilloma virus (HPV) can infect the genital area (see Chapters 6 and 22). The majority of HPV infections are asymptomatic, unrecognized, or subclinical. Genital HPV infection is common and usually self-limited. Genital HPV infection occurs more frequently than visible genital warts among both men and women and cervical cell changes among women. Genital HPV infection can cause genital warts, usually associated with HPV types 6 or 11. Other HPV types that infect the anogenital region (e.g., high-risk HPV types 16, 18, 31, 33, and 35) are strongly associated with cervical neoplasia. Persistent infection with high-risk types of HPV is the most important risk factor for cervical neoplasia.

In the absence of genital warts or cervical squamous epithelial lesions (SIL), treatment is not recommended for subclinical genital HPV infection, whether it is diagnosed by colposcopy, biopsy, acetic acid application, or through the detection of HPV by laboratory tests. Genital HPV infection frequently goes away on its own, and no therapy has been identified that can eradicate infection. In the presence of coexistent SIL, management should be based on histopathologic findings.

The diagnosis of genital warts is made on finding flat, papular, or pedunculated growths on the genital mucosa. The use of HPV testing for genital wart diagnosis is not recommended. The diagnosis is made by visual inspection and may be confirmed by biopsy, which is only needed if the diagnosis is uncertain.

Treatment

The primary goal of treating visible genital warts is removing the warts. Treatment of genital warts does not

eliminate HPV infection. Conventional treatments for genital warts, such as imiquimod, podophyllin, and podofilox, should not be used during pregnancy. However, cryotherapy and 80% trichloroacetic acid can be used safely. Genital warts can enlarge and become friable during pregnancy; therefore, specialists may advocate treatment during pregnancy. In addition, HPV types 6 and 11 can cause respiratory papillomatosis in infants and children. However, small warts are likely to resolve spontaneously after delivery. The presence of genital warts is not indicated for delivery by cesarean section. Cesarean delivery might be indicated for women with genital warts if the pelvic outlet is obstructed or if vaginal delivery would result in excessive bleeding. Pregnant women with genital warts should be counseled concerning the low risk for warts on the larynx (recurrent respiratory papillomatosis) in their infants or children (Silverberg et al. 2003).

■ HEPATITIS B VIRUS INFECTION

All pregnant women should be tested for hepatitis B surface antigen (HBsAg), regardless of whether they have been previously tested or vaccinated. HBsAg-negative pregnant women seeking care for STIs who have not been previously vaccinated should receive a hepatitis B vaccination. All HBsAg-positive pregnant women should be referred for assessment and further evaluation. Persistence of HBsAg and absence of anti-HBc IgM antibody for 6 months indicate chronic hepatitis B virus infection. Such patients may develop chronic liver disease and hepatocellular carcinoma and may benefit from antiviral therapy. Household, sexual, and needle-sharing contacts of persons with chronic infection should be investigated for susceptibility HBV infection and commenced on hepatitis B vaccination immediately.

■ HEPATITIS C VIRUS INFECTION

Routine testing for HCV infection is not recommended for all pregnant women. Pregnant women with a known risk factor for HCV infection should be offered counseling and testing. Patients should be advised that approximately 5 of every 100 infants born to HCV-infected woman become infected. This infection occurs predominantly during or near delivery, and no treatment or delivery method is known to decrease this risk. The risk is increased by the presence of maternal HCV viremia at delivery and is two to three times greater if the woman is coinfected with HIV. Breast-feeding does not appear to transmit HCV, although HCV-positive mothers should consider abstaining from breast-feeding if their nipples are cracked or bleeding. Infants born to HCV-positive mothers should be tested for HCV infection and, if positive, evaluated for the presence of CLD.

▌ PEDICULOSIS PUBIS

Patients who have pediculosis pubis (i.e., pubic lice) usually seek medical attention because of pruritus or because they notice lice or nits on their pubic hair. Pediculosis pubis is usually transmitted by sexual contact.

Pregnant and lactating women should be treated with either permethrin or pyrethrins with piperonyl butoxide; gammabenzene hexachloride (lindane) is contraindicated in pregnancy. Recommended treatment is as follows:

> Permethrin 1% cream rinse applied to affected areas and washed off after 10 minutes, OR

> Pyrethrins with piperonyl butoxide applied to the affected area and washed off after 10 minutes.

▌ SCABIES

The predominant symptom of scabies is pruritus. Sensitization to *Sarcoptes scabiei* occurs before pruritus begins. The first time a person is infested with *S. scabiei*, sensitization takes up to several weeks to develop. However, pruritus might occur within 24 hours after a subsequent reinfestation. Scabies in adults frequently is sexually acquired, although scabies in children usually is not.

Treatment of pregnant women with scabies is as follows:

> Permethrin cream (5%) applied to all areas of the body from the neck down and washed off after 8 hours.

▌ KEY POINTS

- Sexually transmitted infections (STIs) pose a threat to the pregnant woman and her fetus and newborn infant.

- Screening tests are available for a large number of STIs, and all pregnant women should be screened for infections during pregnancy.

- Tests that will be carried out will depend on the prevalence of infection in the community that the woman lives in and on availability of laboratory services. Any pregnant woman diagnosed with an STI should be

managed by a multiprofessional team, including obstetrician, genitourinary physician, and pediatrician.

- To prevent adverse pregnancy outcomes and morbidity and mortality, pregnant women found to have infection should be treated promptly.

- Treatment regimes for use in pregnancy need to be safe for the mother and the developing fetus.

REFERENCES

American College of Obstetricians and Gynecologists. Primary and preventive care: periodic assessment. ACOG Committee Opinion No. 292. *Obstet Gynecol.* 2003;102: 1117–1124.

Bignall CJ. BASHH guideline for gonorrhoea. *Sex Transm Infect.* 2004;80(5):330–331.

Brown ZA, Benedetti J, Asley R, et al. Neonatal herpes simplex virus infection in relation to asymptomatic maternal infection at the time of labor. *N Engl J Med.* 1991;324:1247–1252.

Centers for Disease Control and Prevention. Sexually transmitted diseases treatment guidelines 2010. *Morb Mort Wkly Rep.* 2010 Dec 17;59(RR-12):1–110.

Crowley T, Low N, Turner A, Harvey I, Bidgood K, Horner P. Antibiotic prophylaxis to prevent post-abortal upper genital tract infection in women with bacterial vaginosis: randomised controlled trial. *BJOG.* 2001;108:396–402.

Kigozi GG, Brahmbhatt H, Wabwire-Mangen F, et al. Treatment of trichomonas in pregnancy and adverse outcomes of pregnancy: a subanalysis of a randomized trial in Rakai, Uganda. *Am J Obstet Gynecol.* 2003;189:1398–1400.

Klebanoff MA, Carey JC, Hauth JC, et al. Failure of metronidazole to prevent preterm delivery among pregnant women with asymptomatic *Trichomonas vaginalis* infection. *N Engl J Med.* 2001;345:487–493.

McMillan HM, O'Carroll H, Lambert JS, et al. Screening for *Chlamydia trachomatis* in asymptomatic women attending outpatient clinics in a large maternity hospital in Dublin, Ireland. *Sex Transm Infect.* 2006;82(6):503–505.

Miller JM Jr, Maupin RT, Mestad RE, Nsuami M. Initial and repeated screening for gonorrhea during pregnancy. *Sex Transm Dis.* 2003;30(9):728–730.

Prober CG, Sullender WM, Yasukawa LL, Au DS, Yeager AS, Arvin AM. Low risk of herpes simplex virus infections in neonates exposed to the virus at the time of vaginal delivery to mothers with recurrent genital herpes simplex virus infections. *N Engl J Med.* 1987;316:240–244.

Qvigstad E, Skaug K, Jerve F, Fylling P, Ullstrop JC. Pelvic inflammatory disease associated with Chlamydia trachomatis infection after therapeutic abortion. *Br J Venereal Dis.* 1983;59:189–92.

Royal College of Obstetricians and Gynaecologist. Management of genital herpes in pregnancy. Clinical Guideline No. 30. March 2002. London, UK. http://www.rcog.org.uk/resources/Public/pdf/Genital_Herpes_No30.pdf.

Schachter J, Chernesky MA, Willis DE, et al. Vaginal swabs are the specimens of choice when screening for *Chlamydia trachomatis* and *Neisseria gonorrhoeae*: results from a multicenter evaluation of the APTIMA Assays for both infections. *Sex Transm Dis.* 2005;32:725–728.

Silverberg MJ, Thorsen P, Lindeberg H, Grant LA, Shah KV. Condyloma in pregnancy is strongly predictive of juvenile-onset recurrent respiratory papillomatosis. *Obstet Gynecol.* 2003;101:645–652.

Young GL, Jewell D. Topical treatment for vaginal candidiasis in pregnancy. *Cochrane Database Syst Rev.* 2000;(2): CD000225.

41

Sexually Transmitted Infections in a Psychiatric Setting

Andrew F. Angelino and Glenn J. Treisman

▓ INTRODUCTION

Sexually transmitted infections (STIs) have occurred at epidemic rates in a variety of historical contexts. The impact on STI prevalence of diagnosis, treatment, the role of gender issues, culture, geography, sexual mores, condom use and availability, and sexual education has been extensively analyzed. Although STIs are a direct result of behavior, little research effort has focused on psychiatric risk factors that may cause patients' increased behavioral risk. We propose that STIs will be associated with psychiatric disorders because they increase the likelihood of sexual behaviors associated with transmission. Our main objective is to provide a simple system for understanding psychiatric disorders as they pertain to STIs. Much of the recent literature on the role of psychiatric disorders in STIs is focused on HIV, with relatively less data on other STIs.

Abstinence from all sexual contact is the only absolute protection form the sexual transmission of these diseases but is neither desirable or manageable for most people. Reducing the number of sexual partners and proper use of condoms are the most widely recommended behavioral interventions to reduce STI spread; however, more focused interventions attempt to change the type of partner, to change the circumstances of sexual behavior, and to treat psychiatric disorders that lead to risky sexual behavior.

The decision to have sex falls under the province of autonomy. To make any autonomous decision, the active party is responsible for acquiring information about the benefits and risks associated with the choices and pos-sible outcomes. Further, the results of this deliberation must be communicated to be effective. Several papers have been written on the "chronically and variably impaired autonomy" in patients with psychiatric disorders and on ways that this impairment has led to pregnancy and the transmission of STIs in women. Psychiatric disorders can lead to an impairment of autonomy, but each in specific and demonstrable ways.

In *The Perspectives of Psychiatry*, McHugh and Slavney (1998) classify psychiatric disorders into four domains, or "perspectives." First, there are those illnesses that can be described as *diseases*, insofar as a particular realm of brain function is damaged. These diseases follow the laws of any medical disease, with identifiable and reproducible syndromes, pathologies, etiological factors, treatments, and prognoses. Second, there are *dimensions*, or traits of a person, such as cognitive ability and temperament, that are measurable endowments falling somewhere on a spectrum. In this category, every person has some endowment of temperament, for example, that may be a liability in a particular set of circumstances, and thus come to psychiatric attention. Third, are *motivated behaviors*, such as addictions, in which a person's behavior has developed a cycle of positive reinforcement such that the drive for the behavior has become overwhelming and out of control. Fourth are issues of *life story*, in which a person's unique life experience has created a circumstance in which he or she is vulnerable to a particular problem. We will use this method of classification to demonstrate the psychiatric nature of the transmission of STIs and outline interventions that may lead preventing spread.

■ PSYCHIATRIC DISORDERS IN THE DISEASE PERSPECTIVE

Dementia

Disorders in which a particular brain function is injured or pathologically changed play an active role in patient behavior. An obvious example is dementia. Dementia has been defined as primary impairment in at least two distinct domains of cognitive function. Typical dementias such as Alzheimer's disease and Parkinson's disease have little impact on the epidemiology of sexually transmitted infections, although in anecdotal cases they may make it difficult for a patient to control risk behaviors. Dementias in young people, such as those associated with traumatic brain and closed head injury, anoxic injury, and Huntington's disease, may significantly impair a patient's ability to understand the risk of certain behaviors and regulate his or her own behavior to take precautions. Thus, impaired autonomy takes the form of both the cognitive lack of appreciation of the risks involved in a particular sexual behavior, as well as the disinhibition associated with brain injury that makes it difficult for people to control impulses. Although studies are lacking on the impact of cognitive impairment on the risk for STIs, increased risk due to cognitive impairment would not be surprising. More subtle dementia occurs in HIV in the form of minor cognitive-motor disorder, which may make partner choice and impulsivity a factor in transmission. Similarly, neurosyphilis can also cause dementia leading to further spread.

Major Depression

Although studies have not shown a direct relationship between major depression and most STIs, depression has been linked to high-risk sexual behavior related to HIV transmission. Major depression has also been shown to be a risk factor for a variety of behavioral disturbances that may lead to HIV infection, such as substance abuse. One study has shown that HIV-negative persons with higher general psychopathology scores had some increased risk behaviors for contracting HIV. Moreover, patients without substance use disorders presenting for HIV testing were found to have a sevenfold increase in lifetime prevalence of mood disorders. Our work in the HIV clinic at the Johns Hopkins Hospital has revealed extremely high rates of major depression. Depression may incite patients to substance abuse and decrease their concern about their own well-being and safety, thereby promoting HIV risk. Prevalence of major depression in

HIV-infected populations has been variously reported at 15–40% Prevalence rates of depression in general STI clinics have been reported ranging from 10% to 25%. The latter studies are limited, however, as they relied on medical personnel to refer patients for evaluation and therefore mild cases of depression may have been missed.

Major depression usually presents with a constellation of signs and symptoms, which includes a low mood, in which patients complain of persistent sadness or flatness of emotional tone and a generalized sense of hopelessness or despair, and anhedonia, in which patients are unable to experience pleasure, satisfaction, or joy in things or activities that ordinarily would produce such response. Often present is a decreased vital sense, in which patients complain of a generalized sense of feeling ill, chest pressure, decreased energy, poor concentration, easy distractibility, and poor health and doom. Patients also complain of a decrease in self-attitude, in which they describe feeling guilty, feeling like they have failed their loved ones, feeling like they are lacking what is most important to them, in the sense of self-blame and loss of faith. Traditionally, there may be neurovegetative features of poor sleep with early morning awakening, diurnal variation of mood with mornings and late nights being particularly bad and afternoons being somewhat better, motor slowing, quiet voice, difficulty with producing thoughts, and generalized sense of being "slowed down." Major depression, with its attendant change in mood, self-attitude, and vital sense, as well as neurovegetative features, probably represents a form of brain dysfunction in the domain of affect.

Demoralization, however, is the normal psychological reaction to life stresses and may be a disorder without implying a brain pathology. In contrast to major depression, demoralization generally presents with sadness and grief, specifically related to a particular event. Patients, when distracted, often feel normal, but, when reminded of the source of their sadness or distress, have an experience of a "welling up" of sadness and overwhelming grief. Demoralized patients may experience the same type of sadness that depressed patients experience, and it may be difficult to distinguish from those suffering with major depression.

In a series in the HIV clinic with an eye to this distinction, roughly one-half of the patients suffered from major depression, while the other half suffered from demoralization, that is, DSM-IV (Diagnostic and Statistical Manual of Mental Disorders) adjustment disorder.

Major depression has led to poor compliance with medical treatment in a variety of patients. Patients who are depressed tend not to make clinic visits and tend to ignore symptoms and other medical problems. Although there is little data on the direct impact of major depression on STI transmission, depression has been shown to profoundly affect HIV treatment compliance. Patients with major depression risk noncompliance with antiretroviral treatment, and it is reasonable to extrapolate they are also less likely to comply with other forms of STI treatment.

Patients suspected of having major depression should be carefully evaluated and aggressively treated. Providers working in STI and HIV clinics should become familiar and comfortable with screening for depression and referring patients for more detailed evaluations and specialty treatment when depression is found.

■ CHRONIC MENTAL ILLNESSES: SCHIZOPHRENIA AND BIPOLAR DISORDER

Sexual High-Risk Behavior

Chronically mentally ill patients have high rates of high-risk sexual behavior. Several studies of patients with schizophrenia and chronic mental illness have been done to assess risk factors for HIV, finding high rates of multiple partners, alcohol and drug use during sex, trading sex for money, drugs or a place to stay, sex with high-risk or known infected partners, and unprotected sex. It is therefore not surprising that the prevalence of HIV in chronic mental patients has been reported between 4% and 20%.

Many reasons for the increased high-risk behaviors in this group have been proposed, including less knowledge about the disease and sexual transmission, or issues with perceptions of cognitive control and high sexual drive. However, evidence to support these hypotheses is not strong, although it is suggestive. We agree that, if definite psychosis-related reasons for risk behaviors are found, treatment of the psychosis is paramount to success in reducing high-risk behaviors.

In addition to deficits in STI knowledge and increases in sexual behavior in general, several authors have described issues related to high-risk behavior. These studies have variably shown sociocultural issues to play a role in condom use. While such issues may affect condom use in any population, the chronic mentally ill appear to have higher rates of risk behaviors, such as trading sex for money or other goods. In addition, chronic mentally ill patients appear to have more risk for contracting HIV if they meet sex partners at psychiatric clinics. This ties in well with the commonly accepted notion that chronic mentally ill patients have severe disruptions in their social functioning and may select sex partners from the pool of psychiatric patients because of availability and acceptance of their symptoms.

Interventions directed at teaching patients about safer sex practices and improved sexual hygiene have been described. Some studies have shown that such interventions result in increased knowledge or decreased risk behaviors for chronic mentally ill patients, with no detriment to the patients due to the emotionally charged nature of the sessions. All authors agree that programs to educate chronic mentally ill patients should be tailored to their specific needs. This means that the specific behaviors reported, such as coerced sex, multiple partners, partner choice, trading sex, drug use during sex, and so forth, need be addressed in the sessions. Also, providers must be prepared for impediments to learning in the patients, such as thought disorders and delusional concepts, which need to be optimally treated by appropriate medical interventions. Condoms should be distributed, and their proper application demonstrated and practiced on anatomical models.

Comorbid Intravenous Drug Use

Numerous studies have shown that patients with schizophrenia and other chronic mental illnesses have high rates of substance abuse. Various explanations have been proposed. First is the idea that mentally ill patients "self-medicate" with substances, attempting to alleviate symptoms or medicine side effects. Next, most popular is the notion that chronically ill patients have disruptions of social functioning and use substances to connect with others. These explanations help clinicians to treat dually diagnosed patients; however, patients with Axis I major mental illnesses use substances frequently and therefore may be at higher risk for STIs. Substance abuse as an independent STI risk is variable and is addressed in Chapter 36. However, substance abuse, by worsening another psychiatric disorder, may cause more symptoms or poorer coping ability and lead to increased high-risk behavior.

Health Care and the Chronic Mentally Ill

Chronic mentally ill patients may have a poor appreciation of healthcare issues, and facilities providing treatment for psychiatric disorders are generally inadequate in screening for STIs. In addition, such patients receive limited medical attention in general, and therefore are at risk for sequelae of undiagnosed disorders, such as neurosyphilis and chronic pelvic inflammatory disease. Medical providers should spend extra care in examining the chronic mentally ill when they present, as often their illnesses, or the stigma attached to them, prevent open lines of communication.

■ DISORDERS IN THE DIMENSIONAL PERSPECTIVE

Dimension refers to those human characteristics endowed from birth and distributed normally throughout the human population. A simple example of such a characteristic is height—humans have an average height, with individuals falling on a Gaussian curve to the right and left of that mean. Dimensional characteristics may be the source of problems when an individual is at an extreme on the curve for a particular trait and thus finds it hard to adapt to situations due to this endowment. An oversimplified example of such a problem arising from the height dimension would be the difficulties a four-and-a-half-foot-tall person would find if he were required to play basketball. Even if his other characteristics such as speed and manual dexterity were somewhat compensatory, the basket's distance from the floor favors taller players. Thus, the interaction of extremes of dimensional characteristics with certain tasks can lead to disorder.

Mental Retardation

Patients may have many reasons for impairment in their autonomy, and cognitive factors may play a large role. In contrast to acquired diseases that reduce a patient's attained level of cognition, mental retardation is a dimension of humanity that reflects the normal distribution of intelligence throughout the population. This is not to say that mental retardation in general is without specific causes—there is a long list of chromosomal abnormalities and birth defects from genetic or in utero malfunctions. Aside from these, however, there is a population of mentally subnormal individuals, falling more than 2 standard deviations from the mean. The cognitive ability of these individuals is limited but likely will not progress to be limited further over time.

Patients with mental retardation face specific challenges to their autonomy because of their reduced ability to acquire and process the information necessary to weigh options and outcomes and to communicate their decisions effectively. Thus, persons with mental retardation are at risk for STI transmission through such risk factors as improper understanding of STI transmission,

improper use of condoms, vulnerability to coerced unprotected sex, and failure to recognize early signs and symptoms of the illness to request treatment. Of course, this list of risk factors is incomplete, but we mention it simply to introduce that patients without an acquired disease may have impairments in autonomy due to lack of cognitive power, as a result of a normal distribution of the dimension of intelligence.

Personality Disorder

Personality is that feature of human beings that describes what they are likely to do in a given set of circumstances. Temperament can best be described in a dimensional rather than categorical way, using the model to describe cognitive ability. Each individual is endowed with cognitive abilities that can be enhanced or diminished by circumstance. These endowments can be described and even quantified using IQ tests that measure the ability to abstract. Issues of temperament and personality have a profound effect on behavior. Rather than splitting the various personality disorders into categories based on behavioral expressions of temperamental and characterologic traits, we prefer to broadly describe the temperament and show how this description can be used to generate a treatment plan.

Temperament can be divided into a basic dimension from extroversion to introversion. Persons with more extroverted temperament are reward sensitive, focused on the present more than the future or past and find their feelings to be intense and important. Persons with more introverted temperaments are punishment or consequence avoidant, focused more on the future and past than the present and find function and thought more salient than feelings. Extroverted personalities are associated with increased substance abuse risk and increased risk for impulsive, risk-taking behaviors. Introverted personality types tend to be relatively protected in these ways but are more vulnerable to obsessional features, phobias, and anxieties. Many of the patients seen in STI clinics have extroverted features. These patients are often described as antisocial, borderline, and hysterical in terms of their behaviors. At the extreme of the temperament curve, patients become vulnerable to impulsive behaviors and risk taking that make them likely to contract sexually transmitted infections. More important, however, these patients are often difficult to engage in treatment. While they are often enthusiastic and demanding at the beginning of treatment, seeming to be genuinely committed to changing their behavior and resolving their disorder, they are extremely vulnerable to distraction, noncompliance with treatment plans, and rapid changes of heart about treatment. In severe conditions that require inpatient hospitalizations, extroverts may be likely to sign out against medical advice, despite what seems like an overwhelming risk, because their judgment is so clouded by a focus on their feelings. An understanding of this pattern of behavior is paramount to success in treating extroverted persons, as treatment plans must be devised around reward systems, rather than punishments. Extroverts find future or past negative consequences to be of little salience. This explains why previous diagnosis of an STI has no effect on reducing high-risk behavior. Likewise, the immediate gratification of "more pleasurable sex" from not using a condom could be seen as a motivating factor for an extrovert, and thus it is understandable that men not using condoms are more likely to have multiple sex partners, trade sex for money or drugs, and not disclose HIV status.

These patients often present with sexually transmitted infections associated with multiple problems. They may have legal difficulties, they frequently have substance abuse disorders, and they are often embroiled in chaotic social situation. Physicians are often overwhelmed by vigorous attachments and demands coupled with an uncooperative nature in regards to changing behavior. Simple principles of treatment are important for these patients.

Clarify Treatment Goals

These patients often present with the following goals: comfort and avoiding consequences for previous behaviors. Discuss treatment goals with each patient, outlining that treatment is designed to improve longevity, function, and quality of life as primary goals, with comfort and removal of consequences secondary. Thus, the patient learns to recognize that the doctor will often prescribe treatments and behaviors that are good for him or her in the end but may require a discomfort in their application. An obvious example: insisting that the patient abstain from drugs, which requires the patient to give up a pleasurable feeling to prevent longer-term sequelae of substance dependence, such as medical morbidity, alienation from support systems, poverty, and homelessness.

Set a Clear Treatment Contract

Building on clear treatment goals, patients are required to describe what changes they will make to get the assis-

tance they wish from the physician. This often involves a clear contract, or written treatment plan. Patients with extroverted temperaments often create chaos in clinics by splitting the staff and pitting one staff member against another to get rapid accession to their wishes. A written treatment plan can allow all staff members access to what is taking place with the patient and what efforts are being made on the patient's behalf. Intervention that spares a patient from the consequences for his or her behaviors must be directly exchanged for improvement in behavior in the present time. An example would be to require that the patient submit to toxicology screens before talking to a parole officer or court appearance. Another example is requiring participation in drug or alcohol treatment for a patient requesting the completion of social security disability paperwork by the physician. Benzodiazepine and narcotic abuse in particular can be effectively dealt with using this method.

Anticipate Misunderstandings Driven by Feelings

This group of patients tends to create chronic chaos in relationships. It is an anticipated circumstance in their care that they will love the physician one day and hate him or her the next. Planning for this allows for more successful treatment. When a patient has difficulty, the physicians agrees to help rather than rescue the patient, provided the patient is willing to do more than he or she accomplished during the last encounter. For example, a patient who has failed outpatient substance abuse management may now be required to participate in a 30-day detoxification program to receive the requested aid. By raising the requirements of the patient's behavior, the physician allows the treatment to move forward instead of rejecting the patient and allows for patients to decide when they are "ready" for treatment.

The initial relationship between the patient and the provider is one in which the provider makes the treatment goals and assigns the treatment tasks. In this initial role, the physician assumes an excess responsibility regarding the treatment plan. As the patient begins to engage in the treatment plan, the physician can then allow the patient more control. Although, at first, the physician makes and sets an ultimatum requiring a certain behavior, as patients progress, the physician attempts to sway the patient to further improve his or her other behavior. Ultimately, the continued relationship with the physician results in the traditional physician/patient relationship in which the physician acts as a guide, an information source for patients so that decisions can be made in the patients' best interest but are clearly related to the patient's goals.

■ DISORDERS IN THE MOTIVATED BEHAVIOR PERSPECTIVE

In *The Perspectives of Psychiatry*, McHugh and Slavney (1998) discuss problems of motivated behaviors as arising from disturbances in the cycle of drive–behavior–satiety (see Figure 41-1). Either the drive or the behavior may be disordered in this set of illnesses. Some drives are normal and essential to maintenance of life, such as hunger, thirst, sleep, and sex, while other drives are created and modified over time by individuals with the disorder, such as drives to drink alcohol, to use drugs, or to gamble. In some cases, the drive is normal, but the behavioral response to the drive becomes misdirected by some other source, as in the case of anorexia nervosa resulting from the overvalued idea of "you can't be too rich or too thin." In any case, McHugh and Slavney teach that the behavioral disorder may spill over to affect all aspects of life and mental functioning and that the treatment for disorders of behavior begins with stopping the offending behavior. Our focus here will be on the ways that behavioral disorders increase patients' risk for acquiring or transmitting STIs.

Alcohol and Substance Abuse

Significant risks of STI transmission are associated with nonintravenous drugs, including alcohol, crack, and intranasal cocaine, and marijuana. STI spread associated with substance use disorders can be divided into either direct transmission through the behaviors of using drugs and indirect transmission through factors associated with the cycle of motivated behavior and its consequences.

Direct transmission of bloodborne STIs is accomplished by sharing infected needles, a fact known to most intravenous users in the United States and the United Kingdom. This is relevant for syphilis, HIV, and hepatitis transmission.

Data are available concerning the indirect factors of transmission, specifically concerning nonintravenous drugs of abuse. For example, cocaine and methamphetamine are reported to increase sexual desire, and use is associated with increased numbers of sexual partners. Heavy alcohol use can also lead to increased numbers of sexual partners and is associated with higher rates of risky behavior, such as receptive anal intercourse or sex with anonymous partners. People who reported having sex while intoxicated on crack cocaine or alcohol also reported a history of more STI infections.

Most interesting among these indirect risk factors is the phenomenon of trading sex for drugs or money. One might surmise that the cycle of addiction had led the user to such an impoverished state as to be forced to prostitute himself or herself, but this may be only part of the explanation. Cocaine has been reported to increase sexual desire, unlike heroin, and this may explain the finding that crack users more often exchange sex directly for cocaine, while heroin users more often exchange sex for money with which to buy drugs. For some crack users, sex may be part of the behavioral cycle of addiction.

Finally, psychiatric symptoms are frequently associated with chronic substance use. Most common is the presence of depressive symptoms, either as a direct effect, such as in cases of DSM-IV Substance-Induced Mood Disorder or, indirectly, adjustment disorders arising out of poverty or homelessness. Psychotic symptoms may also present because of substance use, either acutely or chronically, or as a result of withdrawal. All of these problems may lead to increases in risky behaviors, but

FIGURE 41-1 The Cycle of Motivated Behavior

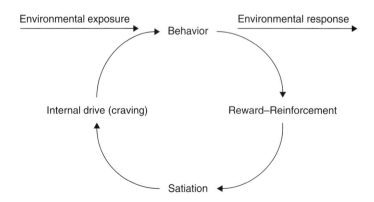

once again, we believe that depressive symptoms and hopelessness are major factors in this population.

Paraphilias and "Sexual Addiction"

The DSM-IV lists the essential features of paraphilia as "recurrent, intense sexually arousing fantasies, sexual urges, or behaviors generally involving (1) nonhuman objects, (2) the suffering or humiliation of oneself or one's partner, or (3) children or other nonconsenting persons" (DSM-IV). Given our description of a motivated behavior disorder, we would broaden the description to include any sexual behavior that has become essential to the arousal of an individual, thus limiting sexual expression. In other words, the sexual release becomes, over the course of time and practice, dependent on a scripted set of behaviors. For example, we have seen a patient who could only achieve arousal and orgasm after anally inserting a series of medical objects while fantasizing about a maternal figure performing the insertions. The patient attached no sexual interpretation to the objects but rather to the feeling of being cared for that he received from the fantasy of the maternal figure. This behavior falls slightly outside of the DSM-IV description, as he was not aroused by the objects, nor was he aroused by humiliation, yet he was unable, after a period of some months of practicing this behavior, to become aroused in any other setting.

Little has been written about paraphilias and STIs. Low rates of HIV have been found in this population, despite some high-risk behaviors. Hypersexuality outside a medical disorder, such as a testosterone-producing tumor, or psychiatric disease, such as mania or schizophrenia, may be viewed as a motivated behavior disorder in which sexual behavior leads to increases, rather than decreases, in sex drive. Every individual needs sleep but in varying amounts; therefore, everyone may have varying amounts of libido as a natural endowment. However, in some people, the pleasure achieved by the act of sex may reinforce the behavior such that the cycle of drive–behavior–satiety gets out of control, short-circuited, so to speak, out of the satiety step. Recent popular attention to this problem has labeled it "sexual addiction." In these patients, sex takes on qualities of a dependence, that is, most of the individual's time and efforts are spent thinking about sex, maneuvering to acquire it or actively engaging in it. It is not an illogical consequence that persons who spend so much time seeking sex might be at increased risk for STIs because of the sheer number of sexual contacts, even if condoms are used. However, it

is also easily imagined that such patients are at risk for practicing unprotected sex if their partners are unwilling to use condoms or a condom is not available because of the patient's feeling of urgency for sex. Anecdotal reports of such patients and their treatment exist under various nomenclatures, such as "obsessive" or "compulsive" sex. Medical castration, with agents such as medroxyprogesterone, has been used to decrease sexual drive in some of these patients.

Some individuals develop dangerous paraphilias, in which dangerous sex is the only turn-on, and thus, they cannot be aroused by sex unless there is a chance that they can contract a STI, especially HIV. Therefore, these individuals practice highly unsafe sex, such as intercourse without condoms with HIV-positive partners. The risk in these patients is obvious. To date, no data or reference can be found in the literature about the epidemiology of this problem.

In marked contrast to individuals who may be seeking higher-risk behaviors, Giannini et al. (1998) have published an interesting paper examining a trend toward lower-risk paraphilic behavior in STI epidemics. Citing historical references to the increased popularity of foot fetishism during the gonorrhea epidemic of the thirteenth century and the syphilis epidemics of the sixteenth and nineteenth centuries, these authors studied the prevalence of eroticized female feet in pornography and fashion before and after the introduction of HIV to the United States. They found an exponential increase in the number of bare feet in photographs in popular pornographic magazines (not specializing in fetishes) and in fashion magazines and shows. They also cite the increasing number of subscribers to foot-fetish sites on the World Wide Web as evidence of the increase in this behavior. The authors of editorials in foot-fetish magazines are referenced as advertising foot-fetish behavior as a safer sex alternative to intercourse.

■ THE LIFE STORY PERSPECTIVE

Last, we turn to those psychiatric problems that are not diseases, dimensions of human characteristics, or motivated behaviors but rather reflect an individual's particular past and present circumstances in such a way as to leave them vulnerable to consequences. For example, a woman whose spouse dies in an accident, leaving her with three small children to care for, may report symptoms of anxiety when alone at night, waking several times and not being reassured despite checking on her children every half-hour. Before her husband's death, she was not vulnerable to such behavior due to an extreme temperament, nor is this a sudden onset of obsessive–compulsive disease. There is no evidence of a motivated behavior disorder. Nonetheless, if lack of sleep keeps her from performing at work, the woman may be at risk of losing her job because of a perfectly understandable reaction to being the sole provider for three helpless dependents. This illness is a simple illustration of a life story disorder, and the treatment is psychotherapy, which is directed at resolving grief and at bolstering the woman's confidence in her ability to care for her children.

Life Story Problems as Vulnerabilities to STIs

There may be so many life story problems that may lead any given individual to be at risk for contracting a STI that generalizations may be impossible. This is true to a large extent, and the number of studies reporting life story issues as risk factors for STIs is small. However, some general issues can be discussed. In particular, one may examine the role of past sexual abuse on present behavior. Some reports have found that patients with past sexual abuse histories are likely to feel out of control in regards to sexual behavior and view their roles only as sex objects.

Demoralization is a the major syndrome in the life story category and arises as a result of a person's feeling that his or her current roles in life do not match his or her desired roles, with no readily apparent means of rectifying the issues. Demoralized patients are often hopeless about their future and their success.

One of the principal factors in modeling behavioral health is self-efficacy. Self-efficacy is a patient's fundamental conviction that he or she can perform the tasks required for a healthy outcome. Patients who are convinced that they can take medication have better compliance than patients who are unconvinced of their ability to comply. Improvement in a patient's conviction that he or she can do the behavior results in improved compliance. Because of this, efforts to change behavior at STI clinics require a supportive kind of psychotherapy for demoralized patients, to give them the conviction that there is value to their lives and it is worth the effort to save them. In addition, patients must have a sense of mastery over the task required, or the task further demoralizes them. A patient's conviction that he or she can persuade a partner to use a condom and that he or she is able to master the effective use of condoms allows the patient the confidence to persuade the partner to use a condom and the confidence to believe that it can be used effectively. Such attainment of mastery is the treatment for demoralization

and leads the patient to master even more tasks, allowing him or her a sense of hope for the future.

Life Story Problems Arising from STIs

There are significant psychological consequences of being diagnosed with a sexually transmitted infection. Patients may be mortified to have been infected in this particular manner. Historically, STIs are associated with uncleanliness and a staining of one's person. Discovery of sexually transmitted infection can provoke patients into suicidal feelings, self-abnegation, and self-destructive behaviors. Chronic STIs, such as condyloma, HIV, and herpes, have psychological consequences for many patients as well. These patients must learn to live with a chronic medical problem affecting the most intimate elements of life. They often are demoralized. Besides the personal problem associated with these disorders, martial and family stresses may result from infertility or chronic sexual difficulty. Sexual dysfunction in patients with chronic STIs has had relatively little attention to the literature but may play a large role in martial discord. Infertility due to complications of STIs may contribute to feelings of grief and personal loss.

■ CONCLUSION

In this chapter, we have presented a simple conceptual system for analyzing psychiatric illnesses that lead to STIs based on McHugh and Slavney's *Perspectives of Psychiatry* (1998). *Psychiatric diseases*, such as dementia, major depression, and schizophrenia; *dimensions*, such as mental retardation and personality disorders, *motivated behaviors*, such as substance use disorders and paraphilias, and *life story* disorders, such as demoralization, all overlap with STIs as causative or resultant factors. Given this outline and some of the treatment ideas we have proposed, it is our sincerest hope that practitioners will be able to identify psychiatric illnesses more clearly and improve the outcomes of patients with STIs. Such an understanding of psychiatric overlap with STIs can also lead to improvements in preventive strategies tailored to address these specific populations at risk.

■ KEY POINTS

- Psychiatric illnesses render individuals vulnerable to behaviors that may have adverse outcomes, like STIs.

- There is a high prevalence of various types of psychiatric disorders found among individuals with STIs.

- Recognition and treatment of psychiatric illnesses improves adherence to medical treatments.

- An integrated team approach is the highest standard of treatment for patients with comorbid STIs and psychiatric illness.

REFERENCES

American Psychiatric Association. *Diagnostic and statistical manual IV-TR*. Arlington VA: Author; 2002.

Brooner RK, Greenfield L, Schmidt CW, Bigelow GE. Antisocial personality disorder and HIV infection among intravenous drug abusers. *Am J Psychiatry*. 1993;150:53–58.

Giannini AJ, Colapietro G, Slaby AE, Melemis SM. Sexualization of the female foot as a response to sexually transmitted epidemics: a preliminary study. *Psychol Rep*. 1998;83:491–498.

Kalichman SC, Sikkema KJ, Kelly JA, Bulto M. Use of a brief behavioral skills intervention to prevent HIV infection among chronic mentally ill adults. *Psychiatr Serv*. 1995;46:275–280.

Lyketsos CG, Hanson A, Fishman M, McHugh PR, Treisman GJ. Screening for psychiatric morbidity in a medical outpatient clinic for HIV infection: the need for a psychiatric presence. *Int J Psychiatry Med*. 1994;24:103–113.

McDermott BE, Sautter FJ, Winstead DK, Quirk T. Diagnosis, health beliefs, and risk of HIV infection in psychiatric patients. *Hospital Community Psychiatry*. 1994;45:580–585.

McHugh PR, Slavney PR. *The Perspectives of Psychiatry*. 2nd ed. Baltimore, MD: Johns Hopkins University Press; 1998.

Perkins DO, Davidson EJ, Leserman J, Liao D, Evans DL. Personality disorder in patients infected with HIV: a controlled study with implications for clinical care. *Am J Psychiatry*. 1993;150:309–315.

Treisman GJ, Angelino AF. *The Psychiatry of AIDS: A Guide to Diagnosis and Treatment*. Baltimore, MD: Johns Hopkins University Press; 2004.

42

Syndromic Management of Sexually Transmitted Infections

Ahmed S. Latif

■ INTRODUCTION

The syndromic approach for managing sexually transmitted infections (STIs) was developed to provide high-quality care for persons with STIs at the first point of contact with a health facility without having to wait for laboratory results. Initiated in the early 1980s in southern Africa, this approach to managing STIs has become the standard of care for managing symptomatic persons in many parts of the world and has been widely promoted by the World Health Organization (WHO) as an effective method for the rapid treatment of infected persons to limit complications and to reduce transmission to others (World Health Organization 2001; Latif 1990; Lush et al. 2003). The syndromic management of STIs facilitates timely, consistent management of common clinical presentations. Local and regional epidemiology and patterns of antimicrobial susceptibility of organisms guide antimicrobial therapy that causes the infections. Syndromic management is also used in developing countries, in acute care settings, such as emergency departments, where the results of laboratory investigations are not immediately known.

In syndromic management, patients are treated for all the common infectious causes of their symptoms and signs without waiting for laboratory test results. Even when laboratory diagnostic services are available, there will be delays in reporting results, and patients may not return and risk developing complications and transmitting the infection further. The approach leads to a degree of overtreatment, but the benefits of immediate treatment outweigh this disadvantage (Dallabetta et al. 1998).

■ MAKING A SYNDROMIC DIAGNOSIS

The syndromic approach to diagnosing STIs is based on a number of sexually transmissible pathogens that produce a common pattern of easily recognizable symptoms and signs. This approach in diagnosing STI is only applicable to those persons with STI who present with symptoms and signs. Sexually transmissible pathogens produce a small number of syndromes. The syndromic management of STI is based on identifying the STI-related syndrome and providing treatment that will deal with most organisms responsible for producing the syndrome. The syndromes and their common causes are shown in Table 42-1.

Unless asymptomatically infected, infection results in the development of a pattern of symptoms and signs (a syndrome). Though a large number of different pathogens cause STIs, a number of these different pathogens produce a common set of symptoms and signs. Hence it is important to take a complete history and carry out a full physical examination in subjects presenting with genital tract symptoms. Specific etiologic diagnoses may only be made after conducting tests that may include radiologic tests or laboratory tests. An understanding of the epidemiology of STIs locally is important in informing management guidelines, and therefore, periodic surveys, etiologic studies, and antimicrobial susceptibility studies should be performed.

A syndromic diagnosis is made after taking a patient's history and an examination. A physical examination confirms the diagnosis, such as the presence of a urethral or vaginal discharge (urethral or vaginal

TABLE 42-1   STI-Related Syndromes and Their Causes

STI Syndrome	Common Causes of the Syndrome
Urethral discharge syndrome	*Neisseria gonorrhoeae, Chlamydia trachomatis, Mycoplasma genitalium*
Genital ulcer syndrome	*Treponema pallidum, Haemophilus ducreyi,* herpes simplex virus, *Klebsiella granulomatis, Chlamydia trachomatis* (LGV serovars L1, L2, and L3)
Vaginal discharge syndrome	*N. gonorrhoeae, C. trachomatis, Trichomonas vaginalis, Candida albicans,* and nonalbicans yeasts, bacterial vaginosis
Syndrome of lower abdominal pain/tenderness in women	Pelvic inflammatory disease, caused by *N. gonorrhoeae, C. trachomatis,* and other aerobic and anaerobic bacteria
Syndrome of acute scrotal swelling	*N. gonorrhoeae, C. trachomatis,* and other bacteria and viruses, such as *Escherichia coli* and mumps virus
Suppurative inguinal lymphadenitis syndrome (Bubo)	*H. ducreyi, C. trachomatis*
Syndrome of neonatal purulent conjunctivitis (ophthalmia neonatorum)	*N. gonorrhoeae, C. trachomatis,* and other bacteria

discharge syndrome) or the presence of one or more ulcers (genital ulcer syndrome). Lower abdominal pain/tenderness syndrome is diagnosed in a woman when, on examination, it is noted that the woman has lower abdominal pain and tenderness. Making a syndromic diagnosis depends entirely on taking a good medical history (including sexual history) and conducting a physical examination. Once a syndromic diagnosis has been made, it is important to exclude serious conditions that require immediate specialist attention. For this reason, clinical management protocols, or algorithms, include important steps that allow the clinician to recognize possible complications of STIs as well as to exclude conditions that require immediate specialist referral.

MANAGING STI SYNDROMES

Examples of clinical management algorithms for two common STI-related syndromes, urethral discharge in men and genital ulcers in men and in women, are shown in Figures 42-1 and 42-2.

Similar clinical management algorithms have been developed for most STI-related syndromes; however, one common syndrome, vaginal discharge in women, is quite complex and needs to be adapted locally to respond to local prevalence of infections that cause vaginal discharge. Vaginal discharge may be physiologic or pathologic (see Chapter 7). Physiologic vaginal discharge is a normal state and does not require treatment. It appears at various times during the menstrual cycle, before, during and after sexual intercourse, and during pregnancy and lactation. Therefore, all women should be carefully evaluated if they present with a vaginal discharge. An abnormal or pathologic vaginal discharge may be caused by vaginitis, cervicitis, and infection of the genital tract above the cervix, that is, pelvic inflammatory disease (PID) (see Chapter 8). In women with symptomatic vaginal discharge, attempt to distinguish whether the patient has vaginitis or cervicitis. From the clinical examination alone, it may always not be possible to differentiate between these. Vaginitis is generally caused by trichomoniasis, candidiasis, and bacterial vaginosis; though other, less common, causes of vaginitis should be kept in mind. Cervicitis is caused by gonococcal or chlamydial infection and other sexually transmitted infections, such as genital herpes and other cervical lesions. Developing syndromic protocols for managing vaginal discharge that are sensitive and specific for STIs in a range of settings has proven difficult (Pettifor et al. 2000).

The World Health Organization advises that in women with vaginal discharge a rapid behavioral and

FIGURE 42-1 Algorithm for the Diagnosis and Management of Urethral Discharge Syndrome in Men

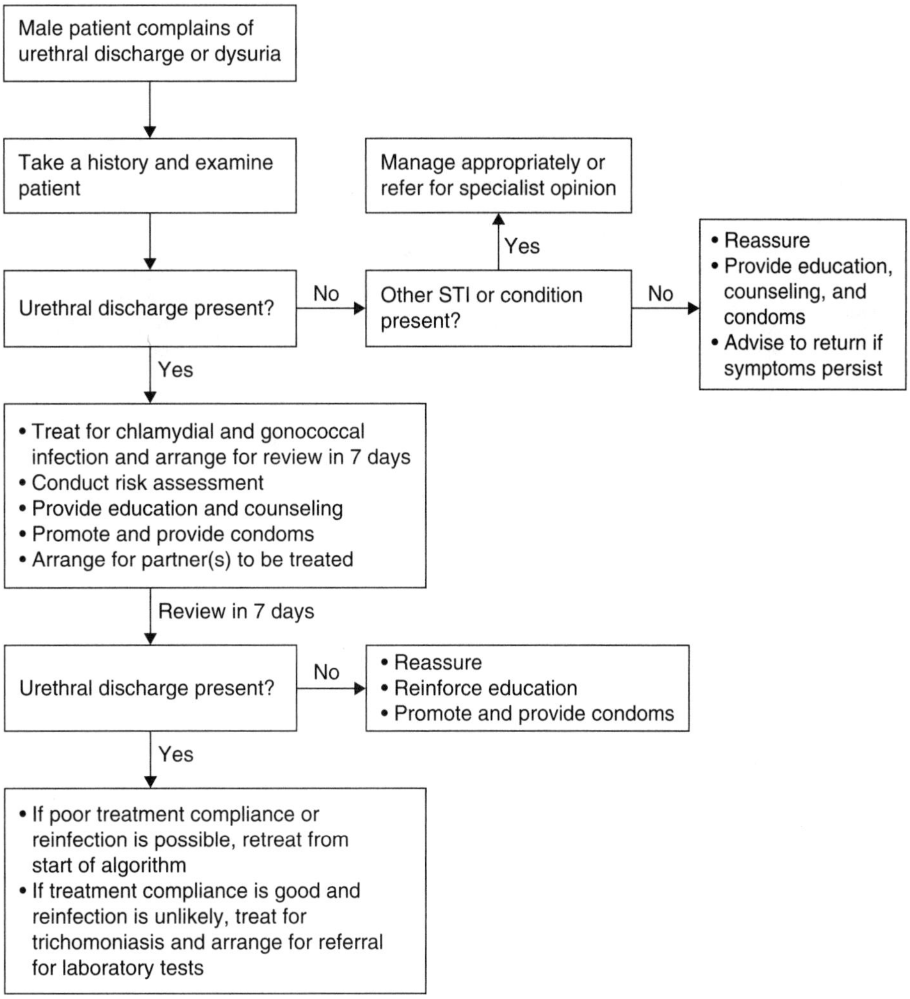

demographic screen should be carried out and has identified certain factors that predict cervicitis (World Health Organization 2001). These risk factors are as follows:

1. The patient states that her partner has an STI.

2. The patient is aged less than 20 years.

3. The patient is unmarried.

4. The patient has had sex with a new partner in the last 3 months.

5. The patient has had sex with more than one partner in the last 3 months.

WHO advises that a woman with vaginal discharge have a positive risk assessment for cervicitis if she states that her partner is symptomatic or if she has any two of

the other risks listed. An algorithm for diagnosing and managing vaginal discharge based on risk assessment is shown in Figure 42-3.

Syndromic management algorithms for managing vaginal discharge when it is possible to carry out simple laboratory tests have been developed (World Health Organization 2001). WHO has also developed algorithms to use when a speculum examination is possible. A clinical management algorithm to manage lower abdominal pain and tenderness is shown in Figure 42-4. Lower abdominal pain in women may indicate a serious, life-threatening illness, and in recommending the management of women with such symptoms and signs, causes such as acute appendicitis, ectopic pregnancy, and complications of pregnancy should be addressed (see the discussion on differential diagnosis of pelvic pain in Chapter 16).

FIGURE 42-2 Algorithm for the Diagnosis and Management of Genital Ulcer Syndrome in Men and Women

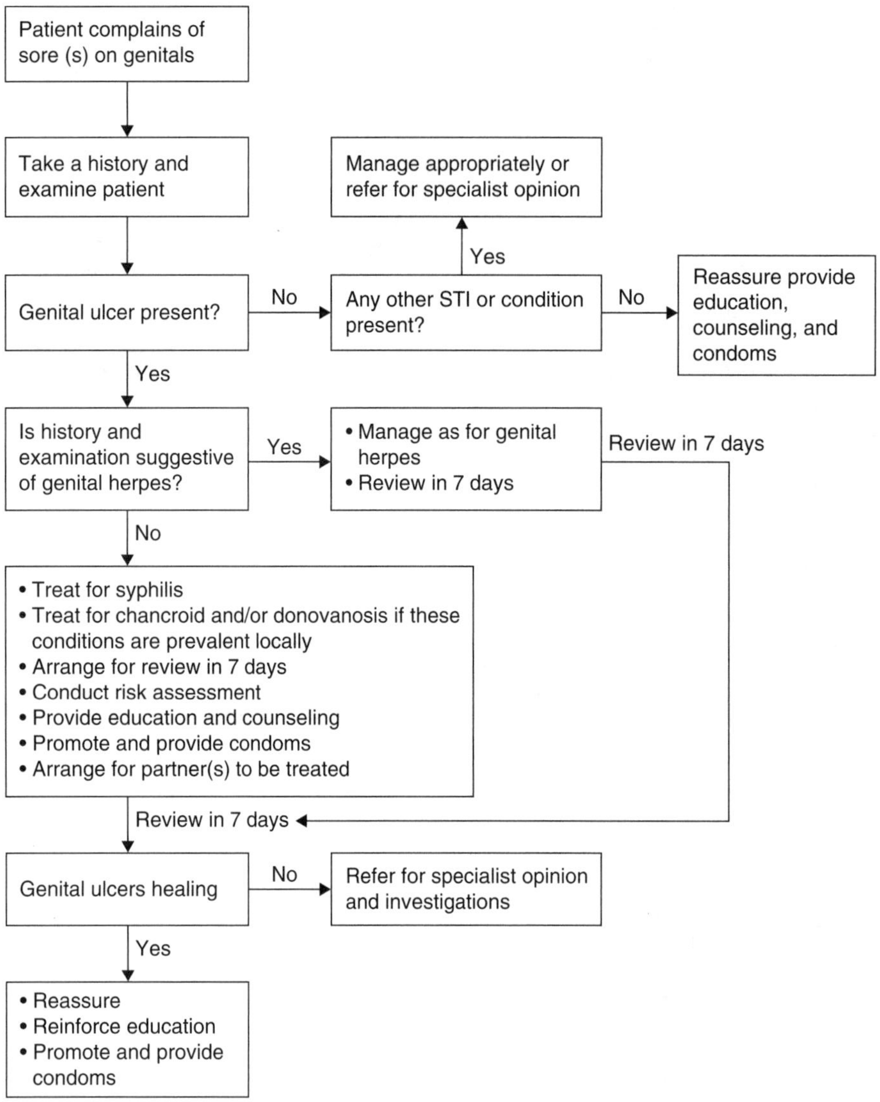

In men and women, presenting with discharge dual treatment for gonorrhea and chlamydia is now widely recommended as affordable single-dose therapy with minimal side effects is available to treat both infections adequately and because the two infections often coexist. Syndromic management protocols will vary according to local patterns of infection and antibiotic susceptibility of microorganisms responsible for the symptoms and signs.

Management of Urethral Discharge in Men

In the syndromic management of urethral discharge in men, the patient is treated for both gonococcal and chlamydial infection. In areas where gonorrhea is rare, treat-ment for gonorrhea may be omitted. The advantages of such an approach are that infections that commonly cause the syndrome are treated at the first visit, reducing the likelihood of developing complications and further transmitting infection. The disadvantages are that the patient will receive treatment for two infections when he only has one infection that causes his symptoms.

Common causes of urethral discharge in men include *Neisseria gonorrhoeae*, *Chlamydia trachomatis*, and *Mycoplasma genitalium*. In the syndromic management of men with urethral discharge, treatment should adequately cover the first two organisms, unless gonorrhea is known not be endemic in the local area. A history should be taken and the patient should be examined to determine whether urethral discharge is present or

FIGURE 42-3 Algorithm for the Diagnosis and Management of Vaginal Discharge in Women

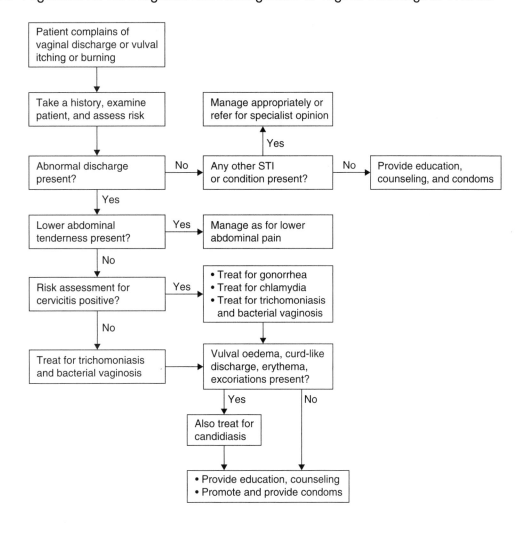

whether there is any other STI. If urethral discharge is found, then the patient should be treated for gonorrhea and chlamydia. If any other STI is found, the patient should be treated appropriately.

Treatment of Gonorrhoea

The choice of antimicrobial regimen will depend on the pattern of antimicrobial susceptibility of *N. gonorrhoeae* locally or within the region. Recommendations from the CDC 2010 STD Treatment Guidelines include:

> Ceftriaxone 250 mg as a single dose given by intramuscular injection
>
> OR
>
> Cefixime 400 mg in a single oral dose

A major, evolving issue is quinolone resistance (see Chapter 5 on gonorrhea), which has limited the utility of that class of oral, single-dose drugs. Therefore, in many parts of the world, the only oral, single-dose regimen for gonorrhea that can be recommended is cefixime.

In the few areas where quinolone resistance is known not to be prevalent, then the following regimens may be considered:

> Ciprofloxacin 500 mg in a single oral dose
>
> OR
>
> Ofloxacin 400 mg in a single oral dose
>
> OR
>
> Levofloxacin 250 mg in a single oral dose

All patients treated syndromically for gonorrhea should be also treated for chlamydial infection:

> Any one of the following regimens may be used:
>
> Azithromycin 1 g in a single oral dose
>
> OR
>
> Doxycycline 100 mg orally twice daily for 7 days

FIGURE 42-4 Algorithm for the Diagnosis and Management of Lower Abdominal Pain and Tenderness in Women

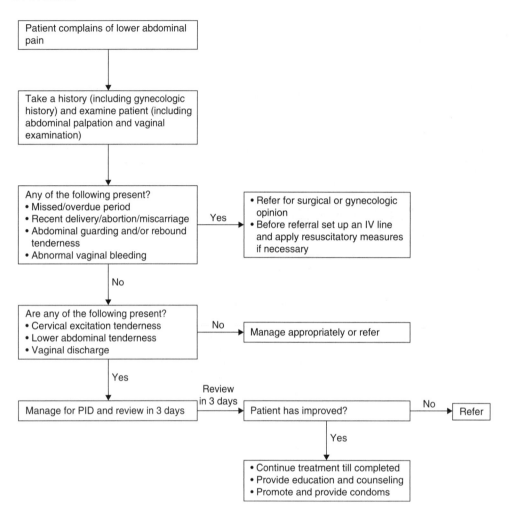

Management of Persistent or Recurrent Urethral Discharge in Men

In the syndromic management of persistent urethral discharge (also see Chapter 14), men who have received adequate treatment for urethral discharge should be treated for trichomoniasis if symptoms and signs persist after initial treatment, provided that reinfection can be excluded from the history and that treatment compliance has been satisfactory. The advantages of the approach are that unnecessary overtreatment can be reduced in the first instance and that only men who are more likely to have trichomoniasis are treated if symptoms persist. The disadvantage of the approach is a delay in treating an infection. Trichomoniasis is common in women, particularly among some ethnic groups, and there is a risk of reinfection of women may occur because the partners treatment has been delayed.

Urethral discharge in men may persist or recur. If a person has been treated adequately for urethral discharge and presents with a recurrence or persistent discharge, he may have become reinfected, may not have taken his treatment as prescribed, may have a resistant infection, or the cause of the infection may not have been gonococcal or chlamydial infection. Men with recurrent or persistent symptoms should be examined. If a urethral discharge is present, the patient should be retreated if it is likely that reinfection or poor treatment compliance has occurred. Or he should be given treatment for trichomoniasis if reinfection is unlikely and treatment compliance has been adequate. Azithromycin 500 mg stat followed by 250 mg daily for 4 days may also be added to cover for *M. genitalium.*

Treatment of Trichomoniasis

Any one of the following regimens may be used to treat trichomoniasis (also see Chapter 7):

> Metronidazole 2 g in a single oral dose (may be given in a dose of 400 mg or 500 mg orally twice daily for 7 days)
>
> OR
>
> Tinidazole 2 g in a single oral dose (may be given in a dose of 500 mg orally twice daily for 7 days)

Management of Vaginal Discharge in Women

In the syndromic approach to managing vaginal discharge in women (also see Chapter 7), all symptomatic women are treated for bacterial vaginosis and trichomoniasis, and if the discharge characterizes candidiasis, they are treated for candidiasis as well. In addition, those women with vaginal discharge who have a positive risk assessment for cervicitis are also treated for chlamydial and gonococcal infection. The advantage of this approach is that most women will be treated for common causes of vaginal discharge, that is, bacterial vaginosis and trichomoniasis. However, if the risk assessment for cervicitis (see Chapter 16) has not been properly conducted, and if, in some areas, risk factors are different from those suggested, it is possible that chlamydial and gonococcal infection will not be treated. Delaying treatment of chlamydia or gonococcal infection may result in complications. Overtreatment is another disadvantage of using the syndromic approach. In general, the syndromic approach to women with vaginal discharge is more likely to result in under- or overtreatment than the syndromic management of male urethral discharge.

Women presenting with a history of vaginal discharge should have a history taken, a risk assessment for cervicitis carried out, and an examination. If possible, a speculum examination should be performed. A spontaneous complaint of abnormal vaginal discharge, that is, abnormal in terms of quantity, color, or odor, is most commonly due to a vaginal infection. Rarely, it may be the result of mucopurulent STI-related cervicitis. *Trichomonas vaginalis*, *Candida albicans*, and bacterial vaginosis are the most common causes of vaginal infection, while *N. gonorrhoeae* and *C. trachomatis* cause cervical infection. The clinical detection of cervical infection is difficult because of the asymptomatic nature of most cases of gonococcal or chlamydial cervical infection. The symptom of abnormal vaginal discharge is highly indicative of vaginal infection but poorly predictive for cervical infection (World Health Organization 2001).

The World Health Organization recommends that all women presenting with vaginal discharge should receive treatment for trichomoniasis and bacterial vaginosis. Women with vaginal discharge who have a positive risk assessment for cervicitis should be treated for gonorrhea, chlamydial infection, trichomoniasis, and bacterial vaginosis, while women with vaginal discharge who do not have a positive risk assessment for cervicitis should be treated for trichomoniasis and bacterial vaginosis. All women with vaginal discharge should receive, in addition, treatment for candidiasis if they have vulval edema, a curdlike discharge, vulval excoriations, or erythema.

Treatment of Gonorrhoea

Any one of the following regimens may be used to treat gonococcal cervicitis:

> Ceftriaxone 250 mg as a single dose given by intramuscular injection
>
> OR
>
> Cefixime 400 mg in a single oral dose

Treatment of Chlamydial Infection

Any one of the following regimens may be used to treat chlamydial infection (also see Chapter 5):

> Azithromycin 1 g in a single oral dose
>
> OR
>
> Doxycycline* 100 mg orally twice daily for 7 days

Treatment of Trichomoniasis

Any one of the following regimens may be used to treat trichomoniasis:

> Metronidazole 2 g in a single oral dose (may be given in a dose of 400 mg or 500 mg orally twice daily for 7 days)
>
> OR
>
> Tinidazole 2 g in a single oral dose (may be given in a dose of 500 mg orally twice daily for 7 days)

---

* Doxycycline should not be used in pregnancy

Treatment of Bacterial Vaginosis

Any one of the following regimens may be used to treat bacterial vaginosis (also see Chapter 7):

> Metronidazole in a dose of 400 mg or 500 mg orally twice daily for 7 days

Alternatively, any one of the following may be used

> Metronidazole, 2 g orally, as a single dose
>
> OR
>
> Clindamycin vaginal cream 2%, 5 g at bedtime intravaginally for 7 days
>
> OR
>
> Metronidazole gel 0.75%, 5 g twice daily intravaginally for 5 days
>
> OR
>
> Clindamycin, 300 mg orally twice daily for 7 days

Treatment of Candidiasis

Any one of the following regimens may be used to treat candidiasis:

> Miconazole 200 mg intravaginally daily for 3 days
>
> OR
>
> Clotrimazole 200 mg intravaginally daily for 3 days
>
> OR
>
> Fluconazole 150 mg orally in a single dose

Alternatively, the following may be used:

> Nystatin 100,000 IU intravaginally, daily for 14 days

Management of Genital Ulcers in Men and Women

In the syndromic management approach, persons with genital ulcers (also see Chapter 17) are treated for early syphilis and for any common cause of genital ulcers in the locality the patient comes from. However, it is known that genital herpes simplex virus has become the leading cause of genital lesions globally. Treatment is not offered for herpes simplex virus in the syndromic approach. It may be possible to have separate approaches for the management of vesicular and nonvesicular lesions.

The prevalence of pathogens responsible for genital ulcer disease varies considerably according to geographic region. The clinical differentiation of cause of genital ulcers is inaccurate, hence management of genital ulcers is based on an understanding of the epidemiology and etiology of genital ulcers locally. Recommendations should

be based on local patterns of disease prevalence. In areas where both syphilis and chancroid are prevalent, it is advisable to treat all patients with genital ulcers for both conditions initially. In areas where granuloma inguinale is also prevalent, treatment for this condition should be included. In many parts of the world, genital herpes is the most common cause of genital ulcers, and in areas where HIV infection is prevalent, an increasing portion of cases of genital ulcer disease is caused by herpes simplex virus.

It is therefore recommended that in the syndromic management of genital ulcer disease patients are treated for syphilis and either treatment for chancroid if chancroid is prevalent, for granuloma inguinale if granuloma inguinale is prevalent, or for lymphogranuloma venereum if lymphogranuloma venereum is prevalent.

Treatment of Syphilis

Any one of the following regimens may be used to treat early syphilis (also see Chapters 9 and 17):

> Benzathine penicillin 2.4 million units intramuscularly (because of the volume involved this dose is usually given in two intramuscular injections in two separate sites during a single session)

Alternatively the following may be used:

> Doxycycline* 100 mg orally twice daily for 15 days

Treatment of Chancroid

Any one of the following regimens may be used to treat early chancroid (also see Chapter 17):

> Azithromycin 1 g in a single oral dose
>
> OR
>
> Ceftriaxone 250 mg intramuscularly in a single dose
>
> OR
>
> Ciprofloxacin 500 mg orally twice a day for 3 days
>
> OR
>
> Erythromycin base 500 mg orally three times a day for 7 days

---

* Doxycycline should not be used in pregnancy. In pregnancy, penicillin desensitization should be considered or the patient could be treated with erythromycin base 500 mg orally four times a day for 15 days. When using erythromycin, the newborn should be treated with penicillin, as erythromycin does not cross the placental barrier.

Treatment of Granuloma Inguinale

Any one of the following regimens may be used to treat granuloma inguinale (donovanosis):

> Azithromycin 1 g orally weekly for 3 weeks
>
> OR
>
> Doxycycline 100 mg orally twice daily for 3 weeks
>
> OR
>
> Ciprofloxacin 750 mg orally twice daily for 3 weeks

Alternatively, the following may be used:

> Erythromycin base 500 mg orally three times a day for 3 weeks

Treatment of Lymphogranuloma Venereum

The following regimen may be used to treat lymphogranuloma venereum:

> Doxycycline* 100 mg orally twice daily for 3 weeks

Alternatively, the following may be used:

> Erythromycin base 500 mg orally three times a day for 3 weeks

Treatment of Genital Herpes

There is no known cure for genital herpes; however, the course of the illness and the symptoms may be modified with antiviral treatment (also see Chapter 18). In patients with symptoms and signs that suggest genital herpes, establish whether the episode is the first clinical episode.

Management of the First Clinical Episode of Genital Herpes

Any one of the following regimens may be used to treat the first clinical episode of genital herpes:

> Aciclovir 800 mg orally twice a day for 3 days
>
> OR
>
> Aciclovir 200 mg orally five times a day for 5 days
>
> OR
>
> Famciclovir 250 mg orally three times a day for 5 days
>
> OR
>
> Valacyclovir 1 g orally twice a day for 5 days

Treatment might be extended if healing is incomplete after 5 days of therapy

---

* Doxycycline should not be used in pregnancy

Management of the Recurrent Episodes of Genital Herpes

Most patients with a first-episode of genital herpes simplex virus type 2 infection will have recurrent episodes of genital lesions. Episodic or suppressive antiviral therapy will shorten the duration of genital lesions. This needs to be discussed with patients who should be advised to start treatment as soon as symptoms of recurrence begin.

Management of Pelvic Inflammatory Disease (PID)

In the syndromic approach to managing lower abdominal pain and tenderness, women are treated for PID if surgical and obstetric and gynecologic emergencies are excluded (also see Chapter 8). Ambulatory women with PID are treated for chlamydial, gonococcal, and anaerobic bacterial infection. The advantage of this approach is that women who have PID are treated adequately. The disadvantages include overtreatment of a common symptom in women and occasionally missing a serious condition. It is advisable that a thorough history is taken and the patient examined and assessed by an experienced clinician.

Women with lower abdominal pain or tenderness should be examined carefully to exclude surgical or gynecologic conditions requiring immediate referral for specialist care. If the patient needs to be resuscitated, then resuscitatory measures should be applied before transfer and an intravenous line should be set up. The following women with lower abdominal pain or tenderness should be referred for specialist opinion if one or more categories apply:

1. The diagnosis is uncertain.

2. Surgical emergencies, such as appendicitis and ectopic pregnancy, cannot be excluded.

3. A pelvic abscess is suspected.

4. Severe illness precludes management on an outpatient basis.

5. The patient is pregnant.

6. The patient is unable to follow or tolerate an outpatient regimen.

7. The patient has failed to respond to outpatient therapy.

Women who have acute PID and are not in any of the above categories should receive treatment for gonococcal, chlamydial, and anaerobic bacterial infection as follows.

Treatment of Gonorrhea

The following regimen may be used to treat gonococcal infection:

Ceftriaxone 250 mg as a single dose given by intramuscular injection

Treatment of Chlamydial Infection

Any of the following regimens may be used to treat chlamydial infection:

Doxycycline* 100 mg orally twice daily for 14 days

OR

Ofloxacin 400 mg orally twice daily for 14 days

OR

Moxifloxacin 400 mg once daily for 14 days

Treatment of Anaerobic Bacterial Infection

The following regimen may be used to treat anaerobic bacterial infection:

Metronidazole 400 mg or 500 mg orally twice daily for 14 days

Management of Acute Scrotal Swelling

In the syndromic approach to managing acute scrotal swelling with pain, care providers should treat patients for chlamydial and gonococcal infection after excluding surgical conditions such as torsion and trauma to the testis and after ruling out irreducible or strangulated inguinal herniae. The advantage of this approach is that men with chlamydial or gonococcal epididymo-orchitis will be adequately treated quickly. The main disadvantage of the approach is that surgical causes could easily be mistaken for infection with serious consequences.

Acute epididymo-orchitis should be suspected in all men presenting with acute scrotal swelling and pain. However, other causes, including surgical emergencies such as testicular torsion, traumatic hematocele, and irreducible or strangulated inguinal herniae, should be excluded through careful history taking and examination. In men with acute epididymo-orchitis, treatment

for gonorrhea and chlamydial infection should be given as follows:

Ceftriaxone 250 mg intramuscularly

PLUS

Doxycycline 100 mg orally twice daily for 14 days

Management of Suppurative Inguinal Lymphadenitis (*Bubo*)

In the syndromic management approach, persons presenting with acute suppurative inguinal lymphadenitis (also see Chapter 17) are treated for chancroid and lymphogranuloma venereum. However, acute inguinal lymphadenitis may occur as a result of infected skin lesions on the lower limbs, buttocks, and perineum, and hence, there may be a degree of misdiagnosis and mistreatment.

Inguinal and femoral buboes are enlargements of the lymph nodes in the inguinal regions and the femoral triangles of the body. They are caused by inflammation of lymph nodes and may lead to the formation of unilocular or multilocular abscesses. Buboes are frequently associated with lymphogranuloma venereum and chancroid. However, buboes may occur in nonsexually transmitted infections as well, including infected lesions on the lower extremities and in some systemic infections as well. Patients with buboes should be managed as follows:

Ciprofloxacin 500 mg orally twice daily for 3 days

PLUS

Doxycycline 100 mg orally twice daily for 14 days, or erythromycin 500 mg orally four times a day for 14 days

Some cases may require longer treatment than the 14 days recommended. Patients in whom buboes have become fluctuant require needle aspiration of the pus.

■ PROVISION OF COMPREHENSIVE STI CARE

The simple provision of antibiotics for a sexually transmitted infection is not sufficient. The STI consultation provides an ideal opportunity to institute interventions to prevent the future acquisition of infection and to prevent further transmission. The patient–clinician encounter should be used as an opportunity to provide

---

* Doxycycline and quinolones should not be used in pregnancy. Patients with PID in pregnancy are best managed as inpatient so that an appropriate antibiotic regimen can be used.

---

* Doxycycline should not be used in pregnancy

education on the nature of infection, its mode of transmission, and possible complications. In addition, during the encounter, the patient's perception of risk and reasons for engaging in unsafe activity should be assessed and then the patient should be counseled on risk reduction. The patient should also be educated on the correct use of condoms and the association between STIs and HIV infection (see Chapter 10). Finally, the patient should be educated on how to prevent future infection through modifying sexual behavior, that is, sexual abstinence, having sex only with a mutually faithful long-term partner, or using condoms. Patients with STI have put themselves at risk of HIV infection as well. The time of the consultation is a most appropriate time to offer health education. The components of comprehensive STI care are summarized in the panel.

BOX 42-1 Comprehensive STI Care

Comprehensive STI care includes:

- Making a syndromic diagnosis after taking a history and carrying out a physical examination
- Providing antibiotics for the STI syndrome and educating the patient on the importance of treatment compliance
- Providing education on the nature of infection, possible complications, modes of transmission and prevention, and association between STIs and HIV infection
- Education on the correct use of condoms and providing the patient with condoms
- Assessing the reasons for risk-taking behavior and providing counseling on risk reduction, including not resuming unprotected sexual intercourse until the sexual partner has been treated and cured
- Education on the importance of abstaining from sexual activity until cured
- Education on the importance of attending for a follow-up examination and providing the patient with a date for follow-up attendance
- Educating on the importance of having all contacts examined and treated and initiating partner notification and contact tracing activities

---

PROVISION OF EDUCATION

As part of syndromic case management, all patients with STIs and those in whom the diagnosis of STI is considered should receive education on the prevention of STIs. The following education messages should be delivered during the consultation.

Modes of Transmission of STIs and the Nature of Infection

Patients with STI should understand that infection is acquired through unprotected sexual intercourse and that there are ways to prevent future infection. These include abstaining from sex, engaging in sex with a faithful partner, or using condoms when having sex.

The nature of the infection and the possible complications should also be explained. Patients should understand the seriousness of STIs. It has been established that HIV infection, the causal agent of AIDS, is an STI and is most commonly acquired the way other STIs are acquired. Hence, persons who engage in unprotected sex can easily become infected with HIV. Patients should also be informed that all STIs facilitate the transmission of HIV. Patients should be made aware that some STIs can cause permanent and irreversible complications, such as infertility in men and women, ectopic pregnancy, and serious intra-abdominal infection in women, fetal infections, and even blindness in neonates.

Adherence to Treatment and Follow-Up Examination

The importance of adhering to treatment and completing the full course of treatment should be emphasized. Patients should be made to understand that failure to comply with treatment may lead to complications and a reduced response to retreatment as drug resistance may develop. Patients should refrain from sexual activity altogether while taking treatment and until they are cured and their sexual partners are treated to prevent reinfection. All patients should be encouraged to attend for a follow-up examination.

Condom Promotion and Provision

Patients, males and females, should be educated on the correct use of condoms (also see Chapter 28). A demonstration of the correct use of a condom should be carried out using a penis model. All patients should then be given a sufficient supply of condoms. Patients should also be told of how to hygienically dispose of used condoms. Female condoms are now available for women to use, and these allow the woman to protect herself, especially when her male partner is reluctant to use a male condom. Patients should be provided with a supply of condoms at the time of the consultation and should be advised where condoms can be obtained in future.

Partner Notification and Treatment

Educate about the importance of partner notification and treatment (also see Chapter 30). The patient should understand that, to break the vicious cycle of STI transmission and to prevent reinfection, it is important to treat not only the index presenting with infection but also the source contact and any secondary contacts the patient may have infected. Patients should understand that many STIs remain in the body without producing any symptoms and that infected persons often do not know they have been infected until a contact informs them. To reach contacts, the full cooperation of the index patient is necessary. Different methods of partner treatment have been developed. Partner notification may be index patient facilitated or provider facilitated. Patient-facilitated partner notification is an exercise in which the patient informs her or her partner(s) to seek care. In this method, the patient is provided with contact tracing cards that he or she passes on to the partners. In the provider-facilitated method, details of contacts are obtained from the index, and then, the health services seeks out the contacts. This latter method is resource intensive and is often used for a limited number of serious infections. Currently, patient-delivered partner treatment is being evaluated. In this method, the index is provided with treatment for the partner and is left to his or her own resources to give the partner the treatment. One of the issues in syndromic management is that, because the diagnosis is not confirmed, partner notification needs to be performed with care and discretion.

The success of partner notification and treatment programs depends on the patient's trust and confidence in the health service. It cannot be overemphasized that persons with STIs are treated with respect and that healthcare provider attitudes are nonmoralizing and nonjudgmental and that confidentiality and privacy are assured at all times. The system of partner referral and treatment depends on the setting, the available resources, available, and the level of prevalence of infection in a specific community.

Assessing the Patient's Perception of Risk

To modify sexual behavior, it is necessary to assess the factors that led the patient to engage in risk-taking activity. Factors commonly associated with risky sexual behavior include, separation from the marital or long-term partner, travel away from home, economic needs, alcohol and drug use, and peer pressure. Once the possible reasons for unsafe behavior have been determined, then the patient may be counseled on ways of coping with such situations. To modify sexual behavior it is important to find out whether the patient perceives himself or herself at risk of infection. Patients who engage in casual unprotected sex should be encouraged to attend for care if any of the factors listed earlier apply to them. The asymptomatic nature of STIs should also be explained to patients.

Provision of Accessible and Acceptable Care

High-quality, effective, and acceptable STI care should be available at all health facilities in the private and public sectors and healthcare facilities providing STI care should be accessible to care seekers. The provision of STI care through designated STI clinics is at times considered unacceptable as STI care seekers feel stigmatized and fear being identified by the public. This results in the patient seeking care elsewhere. An advantage of having designated STI clinics is that specially trained personnel and laboratory-testing facilities can be made available at the center and hence all the needs of the care seeker can be met. To avoid stigmatization, persons with STIs prefer to attend facilities where they feel that privacy and confidentiality will be maintained and where they will be treated like any other healthcare seeker.

STI care is considered acceptable if the care provided is effective in relieving symptoms, preventing complications from occurring, and the care is provided in a nonjudgmental and nonmoralizing manner without any form of discrimination. It is ideal, therefore, to ensure that all health centers are capable of providing high-quality, acceptable care for persons with STIs. Healthcare providers often feel that they are unable to provide adequate care for persons with STIs as they do not have the expertise or the laboratory facilities to diagnose an STI. This is essentially true, as diagnosing based on finding the etiologic agent causing the infection requires sophisticated laboratory tests, and these will not be available at most health centers. Fortunately, however, it is not necessary, in most cases, to make a laboratory-based etiologic diagnosis before providing effective care. The syndromic case management approach permits high-quality, effective STI care to be provided at all health facilities without the need to make a laboratory diagnosis.

Persons with STIs often do not seek care, as they feel that they may be stigmatized and discriminated against at health facilities. All health facilities should provide care for persons with STIs that is both accessible (i.e., affordable, within easy reach from home or workplace and available at times convenient for the patient) and acceptable (i.e., effective, nonstigmatizing, and nondiscriminating).

EVALUATION OF SYNDROMIC MANAGEMENT PROTOCOLS

The advantage of syndromic management is that the procedures can be easily protocolized and implemented in a wide variety of settings. They can be used by a variety of reproductive health professionals and paraprofessionals, and there are numerous training curricula available. They are especially useful in areas with a high prevalence of bacterial STIs that are amenable to treatment.

However, the major limitations of syndromic management are twofold. First, these procedures offer no option for managing asymptomatic infections, which are increasingly prevalent, especially in women. As a result, a number of authorities have proposed alternative approaches, such as limited mass treatment of specific communities, but these approaches have substantial logistic, ethical, and community acceptance issues. The second limitation of syndromic management is the poor specificity of the algorithms, especially those for vaginal discharge and abdominal pain in women. Estimates are the specificity of the vaginal discharge algorithm for sexually transmitted infections may be as low as 10–30%. Furthermore, in some areas, such as sub-Saharan Africa, there are high prevalence of infections such as bacterial vaginosis (BV), but without detailed clinical examination, these women would be repeatedly treated for all STI pathogens, even when they are simply having a recurrence of their BV.

Therefore, it is important to design locally based evaluations of specific strategies. For example, if surveillance and assessment data show that gonorrhea is rare, it may be prudent to limit gonorrhea treatment to those who have had high-risk exposures or who have traveled to endemic areas. Similarly, for chlamydia treatment, it may be prudent to treat only persons in high-risk groups, such as young adults and teenagers, because the incidence of chlamydia decreases sharply after age 25 years. Syndromic management needs to be seen as a useful tool, but there are clear needs for adjunctive evaluation and developing inexpensive and accurate tests that can properly guide diagnosis and treatment.

■ KEY POINTS

- In the syndromic management approach, patients with symptoms and signs of sexually transmitted infection are examined and provided with antibiotics for all the locally common infections that cause the symptoms and signs.

- All patients should have a history taken, an examination carried out, and the pattern of symptoms and signs identified.

- All persons are offered the comprehensive case management that includes making a syndromic diagnosis, providing appropriate antimicrobials, providing education on the nature of the illness, including possible complications, its mode of acquisition and transmission, methods of preventing infection, an assessment of risk perception and reasons for risk taking, providing counseling for risk reduction, education on correct condom use and disposal, and partner notification and contact treatment.

- All patients should be encouraged to attend for follow-up examination when education and counseling are reinforced.

REFERENCES

Bogaerts J, Vuylsteke B, Martinez TW, et al. Simple algorithms for the management of genital ulcers: evaluation in a primary health care centre in Kigali, Rwanda. *Bull World Health Organ.* 1995;73:761–767.

Centers for Disease Control. 2010 Sexually transmitted disease treatment guidelines. *Morb Mort Week Rep.* 2010 Dec 17;59(RR-12):1–110.

Dallabetta GA, Gerbase AC, Holmes KK. Problems, solutions, and challenges in syndromic management of sexually transmitted diseases. *Sex Transm Infect.* 1998;74 (suppl 1):S1–S11.

Dangor Y, Ballard RC, da L. Exposto, Fehler G, Miller SD, Koornhof HJ. Accuracy of clinical diagnosis of genital ulcer disease. *Sex Transm Dis.* 1990;17:184–189.

Djajakusumah T, Sudigdoadi S, Keersmaekers K, Meheus A. Evaluation of syndromic patient management algorithm for urethral discharge. *Sex Transm Infect.* 1998;74(suppl 1): S29–S33.

Kreiss J, Willerford DM, Hensel M, , et al. Association between cervical inflammation and cervical shedding of human immunodeficiency virus DNA. *J Infect Dis.* 1994; 170(6):1597–1601.

Latif AS. Sexually transmitted diseases in Africa. *Genitourin Med.* 1990;66(4):235–237.

Latif AS, Katzenstein DA, Bassett MT, Houston S, Emmanuel JC, Marowa E. Genital ulcers and transmission of HIV among couples in Zimbabwe. *AIDS.* 1989;3:519–523.

Lush L, Walt G, Ogden J. Transferring policies for treating sexually transmitted infections: what's wrong with global guidelines? *Health Policy Plann.* 2003;18:18–30.

Moherdaui F, Vuylsteke B, Siqueira LF, et al. Validation of national algorithms for the diagnosis of sexually transmitted diseases in Brazil: results from a multicentre study. *Sex Transm Infect.* 1998;74(suppl 1):S38–S43.

Pettifor A, Walsh J, Wilkins V, Raghunathan P. How effective is syndromic management of STDs? a review of current studies. *Sex Transm Dis.* 2000;27:371–385.

World Health Organization. *Guidelines for the Management of Sexually Transmitted Infections.* Geneva: WHO; 2001.

43
Sexually Transmitted Infections in Correctional Settings

Farah M. Parvez, Alan L. F. Tang, and Susan Blank

◼ INTRODUCTION

Worldwide, an estimated 10 million persons are incarcerated, and this number appears to be increasing (Walmsley 2003). Incarcerated populations have a disproportionately high prevalence of sexually transmitted infections (STI), compared with general populations (Hammett et al. 2002); if left untreated, STIs can result in infertility, increased susceptibility to HIV, and potentially fatal cancers. Current or former inmates often engage in high-risk behaviors, such as unprotected sex, having multiple sex partners, and intravenous drug use, and are less likely to access routine health care in the community. Numerous STI outbreaks have occurred in correctional settings and transmission of STIs within and outside of such facilities has been documented (Devasia 2006). There are additional challenges as ex-offenders are released into the community. Correctional facilities are critical venues for identifying and treating STIs both to prevent acute illness and costly long-term sequelae in the individual and to prevent transmission in the communities to which inmates invariably return.

This chapter provides an overview of the (1) correctional systems of the United States (defined as 50 states, the District of Columbia, Puerto Rico, and various U.S. territories) and the United Kingdom (defined as England, Wales, Scotland, and northern Ireland); (2) demography of incarcerated populations; and (3) epidemiology of STIs in incarcerated populations. It also describes the inherent challenges to public health work in correctional settings and provides a framework for developing interventions for STI prevention and control in correctional populations.

◼ BACKGROUND

Criminal Justice and Correctional Systems in the United States and United Kingdom

The mission of the criminal justice system in both the United States and the United Kingdom is to protect public safety through legislative, law enforcement, judicial, correctional, and community correctional (e.g., probation, parole) measures. It is founded on the premise that crimes against an individual are crimes against the state. In the United States, each jurisdiction, or sphere of authority (e.g., local, state, or federal), has its own correctional procedures which are based on the stipulations of the United States and, when applicable, individual states. The overall criminal justice process is similar in the United States and the United Kingdom.

The basic chronology of events within the criminal justice system includes: (1) arrest and filing of charges; (2) judicial review at hearings; (3) arraignment with entry of a plea by the accused; and (4) trial and sentencing (Figure 43-1). Sentencing may include dismissal, fines, probation, incarceration, or parole, or alternative sentencing such as court-ordered participation in a rehabilitation program, counseling, community service, or vocational training. Arrested individuals may exit the system at any point in the process once charges are dismissed, bail is granted, or acquittal is reached. Appeals can be made to overturn conviction or change the duration of the sentence.

FIGURE 43-1 U.S. Criminal Justice System Caseflow

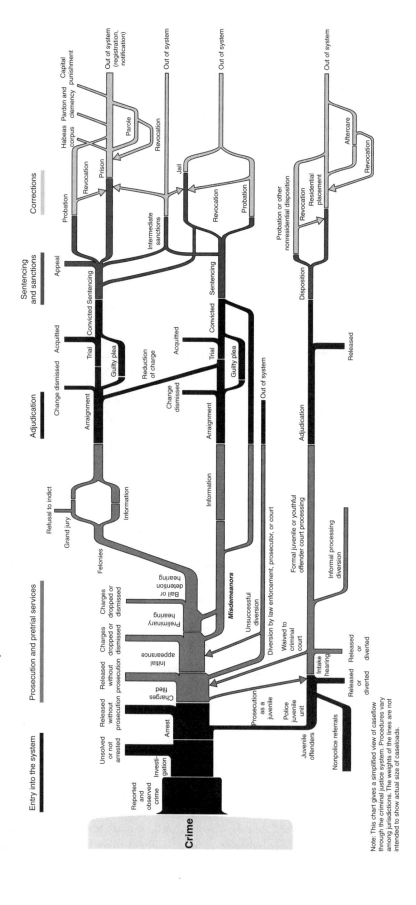

Note: This chart gives a simplified view of caseflow through the criminal justice system. Procedures vary among jurisdictions. The weights of the lines are not intended to show actual size of caseloads.

Source: U.S. Department of Justice, Office of Justice Programs. The Challenge of Crime in a Free Society: Looking Back, Looking Forward. Washington, D.C.: U.S. Department of Justice, 1997. Available from http://www.ncjrs.gov/pdffiles1/nij/170029.pdf

The correctional system is an integral component of the criminal justice system. At any point before trial and sentencing, an individual may be detained in a correctional facility, whether to ensure appearance at hearings, protect the community from an individual's potential criminal behavior, or to secure an individual's own safety. If sentenced to incarceration, an individual may serve time in a jail, prison, juvenile detention facility, or other detention centers (e.g., military, or immigration and customs enforcement), depending on the individual's age at the time of the offense, arrest, or referral to court, nature of the crime, and the duration of the sentence.

Jails

Jails (in the United States, remand centers in the United Kingdom) are detention facilities operated by municipal and county governments. They house individuals who are awaiting trial, denied bail, sentenced to one year or less of incarceration, or are awaiting transfer to other correctional facilities after conviction. In the United States, jails are generally independent and physically separate from prisons, whereas in the United Kingdom, remand facilities are often integrated with prisons.

In the United States, in 2005, there were 2,972 jail facilities, including 42 privately owned and 65 multijurisdictional sites, and 12 facilities operated by the Federal Bureau of Prisons. In midyear 2006, there were 766,010 inmates held in local jails, (Table 43-1); by midyear 2007, the number increased to 780,581. In midyear 2007, the U.S. jail incarceration rate was 259 jail inmates per 100,000 U.S. residents, an increase from 226 per 100,000 in midyear 2000. In England and Wales, at the end of March 2008, there were 139 remand centers, colocated with prisons, holding 13,073 detainees awaiting trial, up 6% from the prior year.

Most jail inmates are detainees, held in pretrial detention. The lengths of stay are often short, making public health interventions difficult to implement. Jails have a "revolving door" to the community; detainees are a part of the surrounding community, not separate from it. When charges are dropped or bail is posted, inmates are often abruptly released from jail without sufficient time for discharge planning. As such, intervening (e.g.,

TABLE 43-1 Number of Inmates in Custody, United States, 2005–2006

Facility	2005	2006	Percent Change from 2005–2006
Federal and State Prisons*	1,448,344	1,492,973	3.1
Territorial Prisons	15,735	15,205	–3.4
Local Jails+	747,529	766,010	2.5
Immigration and Customs Enforcement Facilities	10,104	14,482	43.3
Military Facilities	2,322	1,944	–16.3
Jails in Native American Country±	1,745	1,745	0.0
Juvenile Facilities†	94,875	92,854	–2.1
Total	2,320,654	2,385,213	2.8

Modified from Bureau of Justice Statistics. *Prisoners in 2006.* Washington, DC: US Department of Justice, Office of Justice Programs; 2007. Data are based on custody counts.

* Excludes federal and state prisoners housed in local jails.

+ As of June 30 of each year,

± As of June 30, 2004.

† Counts are from the *Census of Juveniles in Residential Placement,* conducted by Office of Juvenile Justice and Delinquency Prevention. The 2005 count is for October 22, 2003; for 2006, the count is as of March 29, 2006.

STI screening, treatment, and education) with inmates while they are incarcerated is critical to improving their health and preventing disease transmission in the community postrelease.

Prisons

Prisons are detention centers operated by state or federal/national governments. They often serve individuals sentenced to longer than 1 year. By definition, the turnover rate in prisons is much lower than in jails or detention facilities. In the United States, there are more 1668 prison facilities, and in 2007, the U.S. prison incarceration rate reached 509 prison inmates per 100,000 U.S. residents, an increase from 411 per 100,000 at year-end 1995.

In the United Kingdom, there were 139 prisons (including secure facilities for young offenders and juveniles) in 2008, of which at least 11 were privately owned. Unlike the U.S. system, U.K. prisons hold both sentenced prisoners and individuals on remand, as well as noncriminal persons held under the Immigration Act 1971 or for civil offenses. In the U.K., the prison population, including pretrial detainees, has grown by more than 25,000 in the past decade, reaching 91,676 in May 2008, and exceeding an operational capacity of 81,253 (Figure 43-2). Until the recent recession, such growth in prison populations is occurring worldwide (Walmsley 2003).

Inmates in prison settings have sentences of 1 year or longer and can be thought of as a community per se. In addition, inmate release dates are usually known as

enabling discharge planning. Therefore, in addition to inmate STI screening, treatment, and education, public health interventions in these settings should also facilitate notification and management of sex and needle-/syringe-sharing partners both in the correctional setting and in the community.

Juvenile Detention Facilities

Juvenile detention facilities serve youth, usually defined as persons who were younger than 18 years at the time of the offense, arrest, or referral to court. In England and Wales and some U.S. states, youth younger than 21 years of age are considered juveniles. A combination of age, offense, and prior criminal history is used to determine whether a youth will be tried as a juvenile or adult. Juvenile detention facilities include public or private detention centers, training schools, group homes/halfway houses, residential treatment centers, shelters, or boot/wilderness camps. Facilities may be nonsecure and community based or secure and confined. Like jails, juvenile detention facilities are for youth in preadjudicatory detention, awaiting sentencing, or for those serving sentences. In the United States there are 2,296 residential facilities for juveniles, which include group homes,

Group homes are the largest subset of detention centers and training schools. In midyear 2006, 92,854 youth were held in U.S. juvenile detention facilities. In England, there are 37 facilities for youth offenders including secure

FIGURE 43-2 Average Annual Prison Population, United Kingdom, 1900–2005

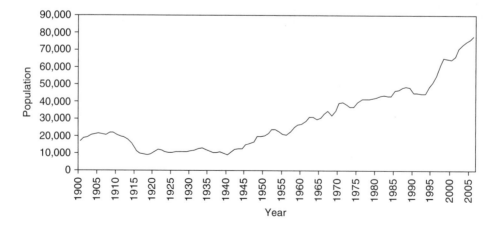

Source: Average annual prison population, United Kingdom 1900–2005. *Source:* A Five Year Strategy for Protecting the Public and Reducing Re-offending. Redrawn from data, with permission, from the U.K. Ministry of Justice.

children's homes (n = 15), secure training centers (n = 4), and young offender institutions (n = 18). In May 2008, 3006 juveniles were held in such facilities.

As with adults, detained youth may be released at any point as they proceed through the criminal justice system. Incarcerated youth have high STI rates and often engage in high-risk behaviors (e.g., unprotected sex, multiple sex partners). Thus, juvenile detention represents a unique opportunity for STI counseling and education, as well as screening and treatment, to prevent STI sequelae and transmission to sex and needle-/syringe-sharing partners.

Correctional Populations

In recent years, throughout Europe, Asia, the Americas, Africa, and Oceania, incarcerated populations have increased by 10% to 89% (Walmsley 2003). In the United States alone, the number of incarcerated persons has quadrupled over the past two decades to a census of more than 2.3 million (Table 43-1). Currently, the United States has the highest incarceration rate in the world, followed by the Russian Federation and Cuba with incarceration rates of 624 and 531 per 100,000 residents, respectively (Figure 43-3). In Europe, Ukraine, Poland, and England, and Wales have the highest incarceration rates at 314, 225, and 153 per 100,000 residents, respectively. India, Nigeria, and Nepal have the lowest incarceration rates.

Males make up the majority of incarcerated populations, accounting for 80–90% of those behind bars worldwide. The U.S. male incarceration rate is more than 10 times greater than the female rate of 134 per 100,000 female residents (Bureau of Justice Statistics 2007). However, in the United States, the female incarceration rate is growing and, in recent years, outpacing male incarceration rates.

Incarcerated populations are often young. In the United States, persons aged 18–44 years compose more than three-quarters of those who are incarcerated. In midyear 2007, more than 30% of the male incarcerated population in the United States was 20–29 years of age; more than 35% of the female incarcerated population was 30–39 years of age. In 2006, the average age among U.S. federal prisoners was 38 years; in England, in 2005, the average age of prisoners was 30 years.

In addition to being young, incarcerated populations are disproportionately composed of minority populations. In the United States, African Americans are more than six times as likely to be incarcerated as whites and Latinos are more than twice as likely (BJS 2008). At midyear 2007, in the United States, there were 4618 black male inmates per 100,000 black male residents, compared with 1747 Hispanic male inmates per 100,000 Hispanic male residents and 773 white male inmates per 100,000 white male residents. Similar racial and ethnic distributions were seen among female inmates. In England, 25% of the prison population was from minority ethnic groups at year-end 2005 compared with 9% in the general population. In the United States and the United Kingdom, foreign-born populations (citizens and noncitizens) are increasingly represented among incarcerated populations.

■ STI RISK AMONG CORRECTIONAL POPULATIONS

Incarcerated populations often come from economically disadvantaged neighborhoods and experience poverty, homelessness, substance abuse issues, mental illness, exposure to violence, and real or perceived inadequate access to health care. In addition, incarcerated populations are often sicker than general populations and have a higher prevalence of communicable conditions, including HIV, hepatitis, and STIs (Hammett et al. 2002).

Former and current inmates often report engaging in high-risk behaviors that predispose them to acquiring STIs, such as having unprotected sex, multiple sex partners, sex with illicit substance abusers, sex under the influence of drugs or alcohol, and using intravenous drug use. Incarcerated populations have a high lifetime prevalence of experiencing intimate partner violence, which is associated with risk factors for STIs (CDC 2008).

Young offenders are at particularly high risk for acquiring STIs and have higher STI rates than general adolescent populations (David and Tang 2003), and higher rates of risky sexual behavior Survival sex, including both homosexual and heterosexual commercial sex work, is common.

During incarceration, inmates may continue high-risk behavior, such as unprotected sexual activity or intravenous drug use, placing themselves at risk for both acquiring and transmitting STIs. Intracorrectional facility STI transmission has been well documented (Table 43-2). Table 43-2 references selected published reports of STI seroconversion or transmission within correctional settings in which persons were incarcerated for at least 6 months before seroconversion or there was strong evidence (e.g., epidemiology, genotyping) of intracorrectional facility STI transmission. Previous incarcerations and longer duration of imprisonment have been associated with acquiring HIV infection. A major problem in interpreting HIV incidence data within prisons is the possibility that the infection could have occurred prior to incarceration, therefore these need to be evaluated with caution unless the persons are known to be HIV-negative at entry into the correctional system.

FIGURE 43-3 Prison Incarceration Rates of Selected Countries

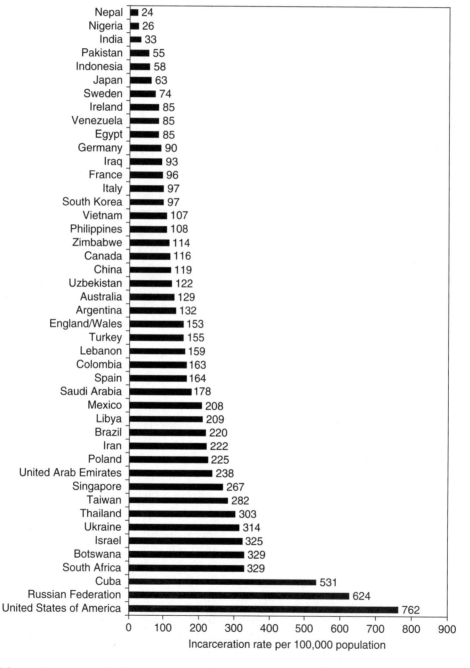

Source: Adapted from: Hartney, C. (2006). US Rates of Incarceration: A Global Perspective. Available at http://www.nccd-crc.org/nccd/pubs/2006nov_factsheet_incarceration.pdf. Source: International Centre for Prison Studies: World Prison Brief Online. Available at: http://www.kcl.ac.uk/depsta/law/research/icps/worldbrief/. Accessed and data recorded on October 4, 2009.

TABLE 43-2 Selected Published Reports of Sexually Transmitted Infections (STI) Seroconversion or Transmission During Prison Incarceration*

STI	Reference±	Study Year	Location	# Inmates	Transmission Route
HIV	CDC, 2006	1992-2005	Georgia, United States	88	Male-Male Sex, Tattoo
HIV	Krebs, AJPH 2002	1978-2000	Florida, United States	33	Male-Male Sex, Intravenous Drug Use
HIV	Mutter, Arch Int Med 1994	1978-1991	Florida, United States	18	No Unequivocal Evidence for Transmission
HIV	Dolan, 1999	1993-1994	Australia	4	Intravenous Drug Use
HIV	Taylor, BMJ 1995	1993	Scotland	8	Intravenous Drug Use
HIV	Yirrell, BMJ 1997	1993	Scotland	13	Intravenous Drug Use
HIV	Diaz, AIDS 1999	1998	Brazil	5	No Unequivocal Evidence for Transmission
HIV	Osti, Mem Inst Oswaldo Cruz 1999	1995	Brazil	3	No Unequivocal Evidence for Transmission
HBV	CDC, 2004	2001-2002	Georgia, United States	41	Male-Male Sex, Tattoo
HBV	Khan, AJPH 2005	2000-2001	Georgia, United States	18	Tattoo, Intravenous Drug Use, Male-Male Sex
HBV	Hutchinson, Epidemiol Infect 1998	1993	Scotland	7	Intravenous Drug Use
HBV	Macalino, AJPH 2004	1998-2000	Rhode Island, United States	7	Intravenous Drug Use
HBV	CDC, 2001	2000	Georgia, United States	6	Male-Male Sex, Injury, Exposure to Blood
HBV	Decker, JID 1985	1984	Tennessee, United States	4	No Unequivocal Evidence for Transmission
HBV	Hull, AJPH 1985	1982	New Mexico, United States	1	No Unequivocal Evidence for Transmission
HBV & HCV	Keppler, Sucht 1996	1992-1994	Germany	20	Intravenous Drug Use
HCV	Butler, Eur J Epidemiol 2004	1996	Australia	16	Intravenous Drug Use, Tattoo
HCV	Champion, Am J Epidemiol 2004	1999-2000	Scotland	5	Intravenous Drug Use
HCV	Haber, Med J Aust 1999	1994-1997	Australia	4	Intravenous Drug Use, Barber Shears, Fight with Exposure to Blood
HCV	O'Sullivan, MJA 2003	2000-2001	Australia	4	Intravenous Drug Use
HCV	Vlahov, JAMA 1993	1985-1987	Maryland, United States	2	No Unequivocal Evidence for Transmission
HCV	Post, MJA 2001	1999	Australia	1	Tattoo, Possible Intravenous Drug Use
Gonorrhea	Van Hoeven, AJPH 1990	1986	New York, United States	27	Male-Male Sex
Syphilis	Wolfe, AJPH 2001	1998-1999	Alabama, United States	39	Male-Male Sex

HIV= Human Immunodeficiency Virus; HBV= Hepatitis B Virus; HCV= Hepatitis C Virus

± Refer to website for full references

*Reports include persons incarcerated for at least six months prior to seroconversion or have strong evidence (e.g., epidemiology, genotyping) of intra-correctional facility transmission.

In most correctional systems, any sexual activity among inmates or involving staff is prohibited. However, consensual and forced sexual activity between inmates and between inmates and correctional staff in jails and prisons has been well documented (BJS 2007), and same-sex activity is common. Estimates of inmates who are sexually assaulted inside prison range from 3% to 28% (Krebs 2002). Recently, the U.S. Congress passed the Prison Rape Elimination Act of 2003 (PREA) to prevent, detect, respond to, and monitor sexual abuse in U.S. correctional facilities. PREA surveillance data from 2007 shows that, overall, 3.3% of jail inmates and 4.5% of state and federal prisoners reported experiencing one or more incidents of sexual victimization during incarceration (BJS 2007, 2008). In both jails and prisons, more than 50% of the alleged incidents involved correctional staff and was nonconsensual over half of the time. Incidents involving other inmates were coercive more than 40% of the time in jails and 60% of the time in prisons. In facilities where condoms are not routinely available, inmates often use makeshift devices for safer sex (e.g., latex or rubber gloves, plastic bags, or plastic wrap), placing them at risk for STI infection (Mahon 1996). Conjugal visits provide another opportunity for STI acquisition and transmission, if preventive measures, such as condoms, are not available to inmates. In the United States, six state prisons (California, Connecticut, Mississippi, New Mexico, New York, and Washington) allow conjugal visits; none are allowed in federal prisons. Conjugal visits are allowed in many countries, including Brazil, Mexico, France, and Canada; they are prohibited in Australia and, until recently, were prohibited in the United Kingdom.

Intravenous drug use during incarceration is also common. Because of the lack of available clean needles and syringes or disinfection equipment, inmates using intravenous drugs during incarceration are likely to share equipment, or "works" (e.g., needles, syringes, cookers [spoons, bottle caps], cotton, rinse water), with other inmates and are less likely to effectively clean the shared equipment between uses. Reusing dirty needles, and creating makeshift injection devices from insulin needles, basketball pump needles, and pieces of light bulbs or pens may occur (Mahon 1996). Inmates may sniff or snort drugs in an attempt to avoid acquiring hepatitis or HIV infection through injection. However, drug sniffing or snorting, particularly cocaine and heroin, can cause nasal irritation, trauma, and bleeding. The blood from the nose can remain on the surface of sniffing and snorting equipment, such as straws or rolled money, and can be passed on to the next person. Regardless of the method used, inmates who share drug paraphernalia place themselves and others at risk of acquiring HIV or hepatitis infection.

Tattooing is widespread in jails and prisons and usually is performed without fresh or sterile equipment. It involves multiple skin punctures with altered tools, such as staples, paper clips, and the inner ink tube from ballpoint pens. Body piercing is also common in correctional facilities and clean instruments for this practice similarly are unavailable. Cuts, fights, use of barber shears, and shared toothbrushes or razors also have the potential to spread HIV or hepatitis.

High-risk behavior often continues postrelease from jail or prison., and STI transmission from inmates to members of the community has been reported (Devasia 2006).

PREVALENCE OF STIs AMONG INCARCERATED POPULATIONS

Incarcerated populations have a high prevalence of STIs. Table 43-3 presents data from published reports of STI prevalences among incarcerated populations; such data are primarily reported from individual correctional facilities and are derived from heterogeneous methodologies, not from universal screening. In the United States, the CDC Corrections STI Prevalence Monitoring Project conducts surveillance on *Chlamydia trachomatis*, *Neisseria gonorrhoeae*, and syphilis in participating juvenile detention and adult correctional settings in approximately 34 states. STI surveillance in correctional institutions is not routinely conducted in the United Kingdom and many other countries. Current correctional STI surveillance systems are incomplete in coverage and should be enhanced to better estimate STI morbidity.

CHLAMYDIA TRACHOMATIS AND *NEISSERIA GONORRHOEAE*

The reported prevalence of chlamydia and gonorrhea infection among correctional populations varies by age, gender, geographic region, and correctional setting type. Among incarcerated adults, the prevalence of chlamydia infection ranges from 0.9% to 26.7% for males and 1.3% to 22.3% for females (CDC 2008). Prevalence of gonorrhea infection ranges from 1.1% to 18.3% among adult incarcerated males and 0.6% to

TABLE 43-3 Published Reports of Prevalence of Selected Sexually Transmitted Infections Among Incarcerated Populations

Sexually Transmitted Disease	Prevalence (Percent Range)			
	Adults		Adolescents	
	Males	Females	Males	Females
Chlamydia	0.9–26.7%	1.3–22.3%	0.5–46.7%	2.8–29.4%
Gonorrhea	1.1–18.3%	0.6–18.3%	0.6–6.7%	0.5–18.3%
Syphilis	0.0–7.8%	0.0–25.0%	0.0–3.5%	0.4–2.5%
Hepatitis B	8.5–47.0%	3.0–47.9%	0.0–8.0%	0.0–8.0%
Hepatitis C	7.1–39.4%	11.0–53.5%	0.32–1.8%	1.6–2.5%
Human Immunodeficiency Virus	2.1–18.1%	1.8–25.0%	0.0–3.0%	0.0–5.0%

18.3% among adult incarcerated females (CDC 2006). Among juvenile detainees, prevalence of chlamydia infection ranges from 0.5% to 46.7% among males and 2.8% to 29.4% among females (CDC 2008). The highest rates are seen in juvenile detention populations. Intra-correctional facility transmission of gonorrhea infection among male inmates, believed to be due to in-jail sexual activity with other male inmates occurs occasionally via homosexual exposure.

◼ SYPHILIS

Among incarcerated adults, the prevalence of reactive serologic tests for syphilis ranges from 0.0% to 7.8% for males and from 0.0% to 25% for females (Blank et al. 1999; CDC 2006). From 1991 to 1997, 25% of newly incarcerated females admitted to New York City jails had serologic evidence of syphilis infection, as compared with 0% to 16% reported for women in other correctional facilities nationwide (Blank et al. 1999).

◼ HIV

The prevalence of HIV among incarcerated populations is 4 to 10 times higher than in general populations. Blinded HIV serosurveys from 1989 to 2006 among newly incarcerated detainees in New York City (NYC) jails reveal HIV rates consistently higher for females than for males. In addition, although seropositivity declined during that time period, in 2006, the prevalence of HIV was nearly 10% among females and 5% among males, significantly higher than the 2005 NYC population prevalence of 0.7% for females and 1.8% for males (Figure 43-4). Similar results have been observed in other states. HIV transmission among inmates within correctional facilities has been well documented (CDC 2006a; Krebs 2002).

◼ HEPATITIS A AND B

Inmates are at high risk for having previous exposure to hepatitis A and hepatitis B infections because of close personal contacts, sexual behaviors, and illicit drug use. Surveillance data suggest that over a third have had hepatitis A, and nearly half of unvaccinated U.S. inmates have hepatitis B seromarkers. Rates of chronic hepatitis B infection may be as high as 3%, presenting both clinical care issues as well as challenges to prevent transmission, which has occurred in outbreak situations.

◼ HEPATITIS C

Incarcerated populations have significantly higher rates of hepatitis C infection than nonincarcerated populations, in part due to higher rates of intravenous drug use among inmates. HCV seroprevalence studies have estimated that hepatitis C infection rates in the United States and United Kingdom range from 7.1% to 39.4% for males and from 11.0% to 53.5% for females; 12–35% of inmates have chronic infection (Weild 2000; Weinbaum 2005). Intracorrectional facility transmission of hepatitis C has been documented (Table 43-2).

FIGURE 43-4   Findings of Blinded HIV Seroprevalence Surveys Among Newly Incarcerated Populations in New York City Jails, 1989–2006

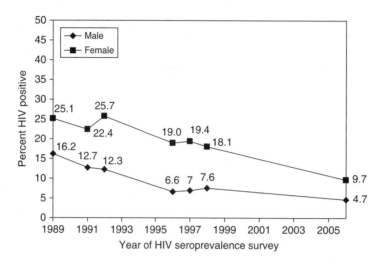

Source: http://www.nyc.gov/html/doh/downloads/pdf/dires/dires-2008-report-semi1.pdf.

■ STI STANDARDS AND PRACTICES IN CORRECTIONAL HEALTH CARE

Inmates are the only group in the United States with constitutionally mandated access to care. The Eighth Amendment of the U.S. Constitution prohibits "cruel and unusual punishment." Over time, this amendment has been interpreted by the courts not only to prohibit the infliction of pain and suffering but also to require the relief of pain and the restoration of function. This interpretation reflects the court's recognition that inmates are not at liberty to seek care elsewhere. Likewise, in England and Wales, all prisons are subject to the principle of "broad equivalence" in provision of inmate health care. The Human Rights Act of 1998 and the 2002 prison policy document, *Health Promoting Prisons,* emphasize that medical services to prisoners are seen as essential, so as not to endanger the prisoner's right to life and right not to be treated in an inhumane or degrading manner.

There are no universally accepted standards or single regulatory organization overseeing inmate health care. Adherence to any set of standards is largely voluntary. The most widely recognized policy-making group for U.S. prisons, jails, and youth detention facilities is the National Commission for Correctional Health Care (NCCHC), a nonprofit organization comprising members from law, correction, and health services. The NCCHC *Standards for Health Services* define minimum

levels of healthcare provision for voluntary adherence by U.S. correctional institutions (NCCHC 2008). Correctional health services in any jurisdiction may choose to follow NCCHC standards and may even pursue accreditation by NCCHC or by other relevant policy-making bodies, such as the American Correctional Association or Joint Commission. However, there is no mandatory accreditation process for all correctional facilities. Consequently, healthcare service delivery may vary considerably among facilities.

NCCHC recommends a complete inmate health assessment within 14 days of admission for jail inmates and within 7 days of arrival for prison inmates and juvenile detainees. Concerning STI care, NCCHC recommends that "selective early detection and treatment services be initiated for STIs" during the initial health assessment in adult facilities, where STI is defined as chlamydia, gonorrhea, HIV, and syphilis. This recommendation is for all inmates "unless the responsible physician and local health authority determine this is not necessary" (NCCHC 2008). For youth in detention, the NCCHC considers "considers education, counseling, diagnosis and treatment of STI essential." The NCCHC also recommends that "a comprehensive HIV/STI education program" and "appropriate protective devices" to reduce risk of HIV/STI be provided These guidelines are also recommended by other organizations such as the World Health Organization, the

Joint United Nations Programme on HIV/AIDS, and the British Medical Association.

In England and Wales, the 2005 publication, *Choosing Health: Making Healthy Choices Easier*, gave priority to sexual health services and health improvement initiatives in prisons (Department of Health 2005). The national recommendations for sexual health are for "targeted health promotion and prevention resources" to be earmarked in Prison Health Improvement Plans. All prisons adhere to a Local Prison Health Delivery Plan developed with their local healthcare commissioners. In the United Kingdom, STI treatment should follow British Association for Sexual Health and HIV (BASHH) guidelines, which are similar to the CDC STD Treatment Guidelines.

Despite such STI screening recommendations, most correctional facilities in the United States and the United Kingdom do not routinely screen for STIs or offer HIV testing at entry. Furthermore, in jails with policies for routine STI screening, most inmates are released before results are available In the United Kingdom, a survey of prison healthcare managers found that less than 50% had any form of STI screening policy, a third did not have an HIV screening policy, and a fifth did not have a hepatitis C screening policy (Prison Reform Trust 2007). A 1999 survey of Young Offender Institutions housing 18- to 20-year-olds found that only a minority reported providing STI testing to their inmates and, of those that did, most did not routinely provide such services (Tang 2003).

Correctional facilities also vary greatly in their harm reduction policies and practices (Table 43-4). Condoms are not widely available and in many settings, are legally disallowed. No correctional facility in the United States offers needle-exchange programs, and few provide drug harm-reduction supplies or counseling Prison-based needle- and syringe-exchange programs have been introduced in several countries and are distributed by various means, including prison healthcare staff, community-based organizations, dispensing machines, trained peer outreach workers, correctional staff, or a combination of these methods (Lines et al. 2004). Evaluation of such programs has shown reduction in needle and syringe sharing and, to date, there is no published evidence of adverse effects such as increased drug consumption or use of needles as weapons within prisons (Lines et al. 2004).

■ CHALLENGES TO STI PREVENTION AND CONTROL

Correctional settings present many challenges to STI prevention and control. Despite statutorily protected access to health care for inmates, healthcare delivery and provider-patient confidentiality in correctional facilities are often subordinated to the exigencies of maintaining security. Security is critical to prevent escapes, introduction of contraband, such as drugs and weapons, and injury to staff and inmates. Thus, healthcare providers working in correctional facilities must balance the primacy of the clinician–inmate relationship with imperatives of security, institutional policies, and state, federal/national, or local laws related to providing care to incarcerated populations. However, correctional policies that hinder STI screening or prevent provision of harm reduction resources (e.g., condoms) to inmates can severely limit STI prevention and control efforts. Without proper education and resources, inmates may continue to engage in risky sex and needle-/syringe-sharing behaviors during incarceration, placing themselves and others at risk for acquiring or transmitting STIs.

TABLE 43-4 Countries with Harm Reduction Programs in Prisons

Opioid Substitution	Condoms	Bleach	Syringe Exchange	Heroin Prescription
Albania	Australia	Australia	Armenia	Germany
Australia	Austria	Belgium	Belarus	Netherlands
Austria	Belgium	Canada	Germany	Spain
Belgium	Brazil	Denmark	Iran	Switzerland
Canada	Canada	Finland	Kyrgyzstan	United Kingdom
Czech Republic	Costa Rica	France	Luxembourg	

Adapted from Harding and Schaller (2002).

The correctional environment can pose barriers to STI control efforts. For security reasons, it is often challenging to maintain auditory or visual privacy in correctional settings. In addition, inmate concerns about the confidentiality of their medical information may hinder history-taking, physical examination, and STI screening efforts, including HIV counseling and testing. Inmates often mistrust correctional security and even healthcare staff and may provide aliases, incomplete medical histories, and erroneous postrelease contact information. Measures should be taken in policy and practice to assure inmates of their rights to healthcare privacy and confidentiality. Any breaches in confidentiality should be promptly addressed and rectified by correctional staff.

Another major challenge to STI prevention and control in correctional settings is the frequent movement of inmates into, out of, and within the correctional system (e.g., to court, other correctional facilities, or new housing areas within a facility). Such movement is rapid, unannounced, and often driven by concerns for security. Short inmate lengths of stay can also pose challenges. In jails and youth detention facilities, which account for the largest proportion of correctional facilities in the United States, inmate lengths of stay are relatively short. Thus, even if STI screening is done during incarceration, test results may not be available before the inmate's release from the facility or the inmate may be released before treatment can be initiated or completed. Discharge planning therefore needs to start at the time of STI screening and procedures for accessing test results and treatment both during incarceration and postrelease should be explained.

Finally, correctional facilities often lack the necessary financial, personnel, or space resources to implement STI screening and treatment programs, which can be labor intensive or costly. Mandatory requirements for STI reporting to public health agencies and partner notification activities can further tax already busy and overburdened correctional systems. Collaboration with public health and community partners can assist in addressing these resource needs and is invaluable to STI prevention and control efforts.

■ FRAMEWORK FOR DEVELOPING INTERVENTIONS

Despite the potential challenges, implementation of STI prevention, screening, management (e.g., treatment, reporting to public health agencies, discharge planning),

education, and surveillance programs in correctional settings is essential and can have significant impact on STI morbidity within and outside of correctional facilities. The basic framework for developing STI interventions within correctional settings involves (1) collaboration with public health and community partners, (2) defining local STI epidemiology and practices, (3) understanding the correctional environment, (4) developing feasible and effective interventions, and (5) conducting program evaluations to assess whether desired clinical and public health outcomes are being achieved.

■ COLLABORATING WITH PUBLIC HEALTH AND COMMUNITY PARTNERS

Effective STI prevention, screening, management, and education within correctional settings require collaboration between correction, public health, and community partners. Such collaboration maximizes the effectiveness of STI prevention and control efforts begun in correctional facilities. STI diagnostic and treatment procedures initiated during incarceration can be completed postrelease by public health (e.g., local or state health departments) or community partners (e.g., healthcare clinics, community-based organizations), thus ensuring continuity of care and limiting the possibility of STI transmission in the community.

Collaboration with public health or community partners can also help correctional facilities overcome some of the challenges in implementing STI programs. Public health departments or community-based agencies may be able to provide correctional facilities with financial, personnel, equipment, or educational resources needed to implement correctional STI interventions. They may be able to facilitate STI screening or assist in staff and inmate education. Public health partners can provide STI expertise and knowledge of local STI epidemiology to assist with reviewing or developing jail and prison STI policies, programs, or surveillance systems. Furthermore, public health departments can facilitate the treatment and case management of inmates diagnosed with STIs (e.g., provide timely access to the local Syphilis and Reactor Registry, assist with treatment options and compliance, establish corrections-based surveillance, assist with partner notification and STI reporting requirements). Community-based partners can facilitate continuity of care postrelease by addressing the health- and non-health-related needs of recently released inmates and supporting compliance with STI management initiated during incarceration. In addition, they can provide valuable insight about their strategies for working with correctional populations, the obstacles they encountered, and how these obstacles were overcome.

Effective collaboration requires engaging all key correction, public health, and community stakeholders and having routine and frequent communication. Correction stakeholders include security and health staff, administrators, wardens, and other correction officers. Additional stakeholders may emerge who are not apparently relevant to a public health intervention, but who may be critical in making an intervention operational. Correctional facilities should contact their local or state public health departments to identify their designated STI control staff. Likewise, STI or public health practitioners should initiate linkages with local correctional facilities. Correction and public health should identify and partner with community agencies that are both interested and experienced in working with previously incarcerated populations.

◼ DEFINING LOCAL STI EPIDEMIOLOGY AND PRACTICES

Defining the local (e.g., regional and correctional system or facility) STI epidemiology and practices is essential before developing correctional STI interventions. Knowledge of the local STI prevalence, demography, and drug susceptibility data will enable identification of program needs, development of targeted interventions, and efficient allocation of resources. If resources are limited, correctional facilities can use the STI prevalence and demography to establish disease priorities among the various STIs. For example, if infectious syphilis is less prevalent among young adults than chlamydia, then a chlamydia screening intervention may be prioritized for a juvenile detention facility over a syphilis intervention. If correctional facility or system-specific STI epidemiology data do not exist, public health or community partners can assist in conducting STI prevalence surveys and establishing surveillance systems. Surveillance data from the local or state public health departments or other comparable jurisdictions could also be used.

Understanding the local STI screening and management practices is important and forms the basis for future program planning and interventions. Assessment of correctional system STI practices should include existing (1) screening, treatment, reporting, and partner notification policies and protocols; (2) staff and inmate STI education activities; (3) STI prevention programs (e.g., harm reduction education, provision of

condoms); (4) surveillance methods; and (5) STI-related health outcomes (e.g., inmates tested, inmates with STIs treated before release from facility). In addition, policies and procedures related to inmate sexual assault prevention and management should be reviewed. Existing quality improvement or performance indicator data should be evaluated to identify potential STI interventions. For example, assessing the time between STI specimen collection and results and diagnosis and treatment may reveal process inefficiencies that could be improved. For each STI policy or practice, the correctional, public health, or community agency staff person(s) responsible for those tasks should be clearly identified.

◼ UNDERSTANDING THE CORRECTIONAL ENVIRONMENT

Designing an STI intervention must be done with a thorough understanding of the correctional setting. An intervention that potentially compromises security is unlikely to be successful or sustainable. Every correctional system is unique. Even within one system, correctional facilities may have different physical plant, staffing, and protocol issues that preclude a "one-size-fits-all" approach to implementing STI interventions and makes customizing interventions essential. In addition, state and national laws differ with respect to confidentiality (e.g., to whom disclosure of inmate's HIV test results are required) and the need for parental consent for STI testing and treatment for minors.

Early engagement of key stakeholders facilitates familiarization with the correctional environment. Stakeholders can inform the development of STI interventions by detailing relevant state-specific laws; how the correctional system is organized; how inmates enter and flow through the system; the daily inmate census and lengths of stay; and at what points in the system are opportunities for STI interventions to occur. They can also explain any security concerns or precautions that should be addressed when developing interventions.

An important step in bridging the gap between public safety and public health is to educate key stakeholders. STI or public health professionals should educate correctional agencies about STIs, their sequelae, and their public health significance, particularly in incarcerated populations. Corrections should educate public health and community partners about the correctional environment and the importance of public safety precautions. A thorough understanding by all key stakeholders of the correctional environment and the rationale for implementing STI interventions within the correctional setting will ensure the greatest chance of program success and sustainability.

■ DEVELOPING FEASIBLE AND EFFECTIVE INTERVENTIONS

Correctional facilities should employ policies and procedures for STI prevention and control, including screening, treatment, providing harm reduction education and resources, reporting to public health agencies, partner notification, discharge planning, and surveillance (NCCHC 2008; CDC 2006). In addition, policies should be instituted to prevent inmate sexual assault and facilitate increased reporting of such incidents should they occur. The ideal STI prevention and control interventions for correctional settings are those that can do so inexpensively and effectively:

1. Introduce routine STI screening

2. Employ noninvasive tests (e.g., rapid, point-of-care)

3. Integrate services (e.g., STI, HIV, hepatitis, tuberculosis)

4. Shorten the interval between diagnosis to treatment

5. Use simple treatment regimens (e.g., single-dose, directly observed therapy)

6. Conduct discharge planning to promote continuity of care postrelease

7. Facilitate mandatory STI reporting to public health agencies

8. Elicit, notify, and manage sex or needle-/syringe-sharing correctional and community partners

9. Include inmate STI and harm reduction education, counseling and resources (e.g., condoms)

10. Improve public health surveillance capabilities

Detailed STI-specific screening and treatment recommendations are presented in other chapters. In general, prompt diagnosis and treatment of STIs is imperative for correctional populations. Routine STI screening, particularly for female offenders younger than 26 years and male offenders younger than 30 years, should be prioritized, as they have the highest STI rates. Per CDC recommendations, HIV testing should be offered routinely to all inmates, regardless of risk behaviors (CDC 2006). Whenever possible, facilities should employ non-

invasive (e.g., urine-based tests versus urethral swabs for male chlamydia testing) and rapid tests (e.g., rapid HIV tests providing results within 20 minutes) to increase the likelihood of inmate test acceptance and receipt of results prior to release. STI services should be integrated with those of HIV, hepatitis, and tuberculosis (e.g., all inmates testing positive for tuberculosis or an STI should be offered an HIV test). In addition, the CDC recommends providing hepatitis testing and vaccination to high-risk inmates. Facilities should identify ways to shorten the time between STI screening and diagnosis, and diagnosis and treatment. Treatment regimens should be simplified to facilitate completion (e.g., using single-dose, directly observed treatment for chlamydia or gonorrhea in short-stay facilities such as jails or juvenile detention facilities).

Frequent inmate movement within and outside of correctional systems (e.g., to new housing facility, release to community) can complicate STI management. Tracking systems, such as electronic health records, databases, and logbooks, and discharge planning programs are necessary to facilitate continuity of care during and postincarceration. Inmate mistrust of correctional staff may lead inmates to provide false or incomplete postrelease contact information. Efforts should be made in policy and practice to inform inmates of their rights to privacy and confidentiality. In the United States, certain STIs are mandatorily reportable conditions and must be reported to local, state, or national public health agencies (e.g., health departments). Correctional facilities should promptly report STIs diagnosed among inmates, regardless of treatment or release status. In addition, public health authorities can facilitate the elicitation of names of any correctional or community sex and needle-/syringe-sharing partners and should work with public health partners to appropriately manage them. Facilities should also partner with public health and community organizations to provide inmates with STI and harm reduction education and prevention counseling, preferably through peer educators. Public health and community partners can also assist correctional facilities in improving STI surveillance efforts so that better STI morbidity estimates can be made.

Despite prohibitions, illicit sexual activities and intravenous drug use occur during incarceration. As such, facilities should consider providing preventive measures such as condoms, sterile needles/syringes, bleach, and opioid substitution therapy. Both the World Health Organization and Joint United Nations Program on HIV/AIDS strongly recommend that condoms be made available to prisoners without putting them at risk of further prosecution, stigma, embarrassment, or violence. Likewise, the feasibility of providing harm reduction measures for drug injecting inmates should be considered. By working together with key stakeholders, correctional systems can employ policies that satisfy both safety and public health goals, even if seemingly discordant. For example, though inmate sexual activity is prohibited in NYC jails, the NYC Department of Correction permits healthcare staff to provide condoms to male inmates under negotiated circumstances (e.g., distribute no more than three condoms at a time, must be distributed by health clinic staff). Security concerns are usually cited as reasons to not implement condom distribution programs in correctional settings even though program evaluations of such programs have not shown increases in security infractions or sexual assault (Stöver 2003). Because of the high prevalence of sexual assault, correctional facilities must have strong policies and sanctions against such activities. Facilities should conduct routine surveillance to identify allegations of sexual assault and should encourage and facilitate inmates' reporting of such cases without adverse consequences (e.g., prosecuting victim for participating in illegal activities, placing inmate in solitary confinement, leaving inmate in same housing unit with alleged perpetrators during investigation).

STI interventions should address identified programmatic needs, be compatible with correctional safety concerns, and be compliant with local, state, and federal/national laws or regulations. For maximal effectiveness, an intervention should be operationally feasible in the correctional setting, as well as epidemiologically sound. For example, shortening the interval from diagnosis to treatment and simplifying treatment regimens are likely to have the greatest public health impact on inmate populations in shorter-stay facilities (jails and juvenile detention facilities), whereas improving inmate counseling and prevention practices (e.g., peer counseling, condom access, hepatitis B vaccination programs) and discharge planning for inmates and their sex or needle-/syringe-sharing partners may be more feasible in longer-stay facilities. A useful approach for implementing STI interventions in correctional settings is to conduct a pilot program and evaluate its effectiveness and feasibility; successful pilot programs can be expanded into jail or prison policy. Examples of effective STI interventions are shown in Boxes 43-1 and 43-2.

Interventions that provide or enhance a sustainable public health infrastructure are of tremendous value to correctional facilities. Often public health interventions,

while creating societal savings (e.g., pelvic inflammatory disease cases averted), result in direct costs for the correctional agencies, without any apparent benefit to those agencies. Correctional facilities with limited resources may be unable to implement STI interventions without support from public health or community partners. Providing correctional systems with resources (e.g., funding, technology, staffing, education) needed to implement STI interventions can garner further buy-in and facilitate program sustainability.

CONDUCTING PROGRAM EVALUATIONS

Evaluation of STI programs and interventions in correctional settings is essential in determining whether desired clinical and public health objectives are being met, whether resources are allocated effectively, and whether program improvements are needed. The evaluation should include a systematic assessment of STI program goals, activities, and outcomes. Local STI epidemiology (e.g., STI case rates, demographics of STI cases, local drug susceptibility data) should be used to inform the program evaluation. STI program evaluation steps include (1) engaging key stakeholders, (2) describing the existing STI program, (3) focusing the scope of the evaluation, (4) gathering credible evidence, (5) identifying and justifying the conclusions of the evaluation, (6) ensuring use by formulating program recommendations, and (7) routinely providing feedback to key stakeholders and sharing lessons learned.

DISCHARGE PLANNING

Discharge planning for inmates diagnosed with STIs should begin as soon as possible after diagnosis. Every effort should be made to complete diagnostic, treatment, and partner notification activities during incarceration. In situations when follow-up may be problematic, syndromic management may be used, although diagnoses based on syndromes are more specific in males than in females. In prison, release dates are known and plans for postrelease care can be made before inmates are discharged from the facility. In jails, release dates are often unknown, and inmates can be released from jail without adequate notice of the correctional healthcare staff.

Discharge planning is essential for continuity of STI care, particularly for inmates who did not complete diagnostic workup or were discharged before initiation or completion of treatment. Inmates who do not complete diagnostic workup during incarceration risk

BOX 43-1 Male Chlamydia and Gonorrhea Screening in New York City Jails

The New York City (NYC) jail system is one of the largest in the United States with more than 100,000 admissions annually and a daily census of up to 14,000 inmates. The population comprises 90% detainees awaiting trial or sentencing and 10% who are sentenced to 1 year or less. The median length of stay is 7 days; more than 25% of inmates are released within the first 3 days after admission.

Healthcare standards for NYC correctional facilities require that all inmates undergo a medical evaluation within 24 hours of admission. The evaluation includes a comprehensive history and physical examination, testing for tuberculosis and syphilis, and routine urinalysis. All inmates are offered a voluntary rapid HIV test. Historically, incarcerated males with STI symptoms at the time of admission were tested using urethral swabs and, if clinically indicated, provided with empiric antimicrobial therapy.

Before 2003, the prevalence of male chlamydia and gonorrhea infection in NYC jail populations was unknown. In December 2003, the NYC Department of Health and Mental Hygiene Office of Correctional Public Health conducted a 2-week-period prevalence survey to assess chlamydia and gonorrhea prevalence among newly incarcerated males using a urine-based nucleic acid amplification test (NAAT). Nearly 7% of males had infections with chlamydia, gonorrhea, or both. Pilot data were shared with key stakeholders, including NYC jail correction and healthcare staff, resulting in buy-in for the screening program.

In 2005, NYC jail policy was revised to include routine chlamydia and gonorrhea screening of all newly incarcerated males 35 years and younger using the urine-based NAAT. Test results are available with 24–72 hours. Routine screening showed that 10% of males were infected with chlamydia, gonorrhea, or both. Treatment protocols included use of single-dose, directly observed antimicrobials unless there were contraindications; more than 70% of infected inmates were treated before release from jail. HIV testing is re-offered to all inmates diagnosed with STI. Inmates are educated about the need for partner notification and treatment and are provided with a brochure listing city STI clinics for postrelease follow-up. A jail-based male STI surveillance system was developed.

The NYC jail-screening program has had citywide impact on reported case rates (Figure 43-5). By the end of 2005, the number of male chlamydia cases reported from NYC jails increased from 222 in 2004 to 3854 in 2005, an increase of 1636% (Pathela et al. 2009). Thus, the citywide chlamydia case rate increased 59% from 203 cases per 100,000 (in 2004) to 322.7 per 100,000 (in 2005). Male gonorrhea cases reported from NYC jails increased 885% from 68 cases in 2004 to 670 cases in 2005, resulting in a 4% increase in the citywide gonorrhea case rate. The prompt STI diagnosis and treatment of males within jails decreases the likelihood of STI transmission upon their release into the community and may impact community female STI rates.

FIGURE 43-5 Male Chlamydia and Gonorrhea Case Rates, New York City, 1995–2007

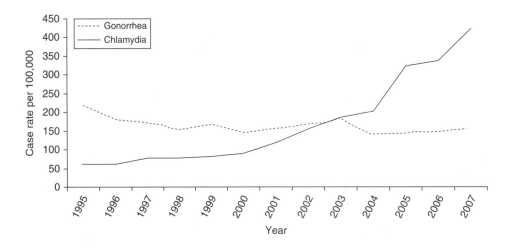

Source: http://www.nyc.gov/html/doh/downloads/pdf/std/std-quarterlyreport2008-4.pdf.

BOX 43-2 National Chlamydia Screening Program, United Kingdom

The national chlamydia screening program (NCSP) for male and female residents younger than 25 years is administered by the U.K. Health Protection Agency. Its objective is to control chlamydia infection in young adults through early detection and treatment of asymptomatic individuals, prevent adverse sequelae, and reduce transmission. NCSP surveillance data also enable determination of national chlamydia morbidity estimates.

The NCSP was established in 2002, in part, after pilots of chlamydia screening programs were shown to be feasible and well accepted in local healthcare settings (Fenton and Ward 2004). Free chlamydia screening and treatment was implemented nationwide, in phases, in both healthcare and non-healthcare settings, including general primary care clinics, pharmacies, universities, youth clubs, and military bases. Surveil-

lance data show that more than 90% of index cases are treated.

In April 2005, 49 English prisons also participated in the NCSP, representing more than 30% of prisons in England and Wales. From April 2005–March 2006, more than 1100 STI screening tests were conducted; overall, 12% were positive for chlamydia, compared with community estimates of 10% among 15- to 24-year-olds. Recent 2006–2007 data from 71 participating prisons / youth offender institutions reveal that 1942 screens were conducted and, overall, the chlamydia prevalence was 13.4%, with a male prevalence of 14.2% and female prevalence of 10.8% (NCSP 2007).

Since implementation of the NCSP, STI screening, case reports, and treatment among young adults has dramatically increased in the United Kingdom.

not only their own health but that of sex or needle-/syringe-sharing partners. Incompletely treated individuals risk treatment failure, antimicrobial resistance, and transmission to sex partners. Inmates released before receiving antimicrobial treatment are unlikely to receive any in the community; those who began multidose regimens while incarcerated are unlikely to complete their regimens postrelease. Once released, former inmates often do not access health care and fail to complete diagnostic workups or continue treatments, including HIV therapies that have been initiated during incarceration. Often they must prioritize immediate needs such as food, shelter, and employment. Efforts to locate inmates for treatment after release have had disappointing outcomes; inmates often provide incorrect postrelease contact information because of mistrust of correctional or healthcare staff.

Correctional facilities use several strategies to assist in continuity-of-care efforts. Some facilities encourage community providers to provide direct clinical services in the jail or prison, establish a therapeutic alliance with the inmates, and provide postrelease health care in the community. Other strategies include (1) community providers working with inmates for only a few months prerelease; (2) inmates not meeting the community provider during incarceration but receiving a set appointment postrelease; and (3) inmates receiving a list of community clinical providers to contact after release.

Some facilities also provide inmate education and counseling, discharge packets with male and female condoms, and aftercare letters advising recently released inmates about abnormal test results and the need to seek medical attention. Whenever possible, soon-to-be-released inmates should receive a written health summary specifying their major diagnoses, diagnostic workup, and treatment received during incarceration, along with the follow-up management required.

Public health and community partners are invaluable in the discharge planning effort. Public health departments often conduct case management for persons with certain communicable infections (e.g., syphilis). Many community partners engage former inmates as soon as possible postrelease and assist them in complying with medical care (e.g., provide transportation to medical appointments, assist with insurance applications). Discharge planning and community linkages can reduce recidivism rates and are essential in STI control efforts.

■ CONCLUSION

Incarcerated populations have a disproportionately higher prevalence of STIs than general populations. Left unrecognized and untreated, STIs can result in infertility, facilitation of HIV, and potentially fatal cancers. Feasible and effective STI interventions for both incarcerated males and females are needed within correctional systems. The prevention, screening, diagnosis, treatment, public health reporting, partner elicitation and notification, and surveillance of STIs among correctional populations must be prioritized. Continuity of care should be provided throughout incarceration and postrelease through STI discharge planning. Collaboration between correctional settings, public health agencies, and community partners is essential, if the goal of STI prevention and control both within and outside of correctional settings is to be achieved.

■ KEY POINTS

- To manage incarcerated patients, include routine STI screening and employ noninvasive tests.

- Integrated services (e.g., STIs, including human immunodeficiency virus [HIV], hepatitis, and tuberculosis) can be quite effective.

- Focus must be on shortening the intervals between examination and diagnosis and diagnosis and treatment.

- Use simple treatment regimens (e.g., single-dose, directly observed therapy).

- Conduct discharge planning to promote continuity of care and facilitate mandatory STI reporting to public health agencies.

- Elicit, notify, and manage sex or needle-/syringe-sharing correctional and community partners

- Incarcerated patients must also have access to STI and harm reduction education, counseling, and resources.

REFERENCES

Blank S, Sternberg M, Neylans LL, Rubin SR, Weisfuse IB, and St. Louis ME. Incident syphilis among women with multiple admissions to jail in New York City. *J Infect Dis.* 1999;180:1159–1163.

British Association for Sexual Health and HIV. www.bashh.org.

Bureau of Justice Statistics. www.ojp.usdoj.gov/bjs/.

Bureau of Justice Statistics (BJS). Prisoners in 2006. Washington, DC: US Department of Justice, Office of Justice Programs; 2007a.

Bureau of Justice Statistics (BJS). Prison and Jail Inmates at Midyear 2006. Washington, DC: US Department of Justice, Office of Justice Programs; 2007b.

Centers for Disease Control and Prevention. Adverse health conditions and health risk behaviors associated with inti-

mate partner violence, United States, 2005. *Morb Mortal Week Rep.* 2008;57(05):113–117.

Centers for Disease Control and Prevention (2006). 2006 National Report. Special Focus Profiles- Persons Entering Correctional Facilities. http://www.cdc.gov/STI/STATS/corrections.htm.

David N, Tang A. Sexually transmitted infections in a young offenders institution in the U.K. *Int J STI AIDS.* 2003;14:511–513.

Department of Health. (2005). Choosing Health: Making Healthy Choices Easier. http://www.dh.gov.uk/en/Publicationsandstatistics/Publications/PublicationsPolicyAndGuidance/Browsable/DH_4097491.

Devasia RA, Jones TF, Kainer MA, Halford S, Sheeler LL, Swift J, Schaffner W. Two community hepatitis B outbreaks: an argument for vaccinating incarcerated persons. *Vaccine.* 2006;24(9):1354–1358.

Dolan K, Rutter S, Wodak D. Prison-based syringe exchange programmes: a review if international research and development. *Addiction.* 2003;98:153–158.

Fenton KA, Ward H. National chlamydia screening programme: making progress. *Sex Transm Infect.* 2004;80:331–333.

Hammett TM. HIV/AIDS and other infectious diseases among correctional inmates: transmission, burden, and an appropriate response. *Am J Public Health.* 2006;96(6):974–978.

Hammett TM, Harmon MP, Rhodes W. The burden of infectious disease among inmates of and releases from US correctional facilities, 1997. *Am J Public Health.* 2002;92:1789–1794.

Harding, T.W. & Schaller, G. (1992). HIV/AIDS policy for prisons or for prisoners? In: Mann, J. et al., ed. AIDS in the world. A global report. Cambridge, Harvard University Press; 1992: 761–769.

International Centre for Prison Studies: World Prison Brief Online. www.kcl.ac.uk/depsta/rel/icps/worldbrief/world_brief.html.

Krebs CP, Simmons M. Intraprison HIV Transmission: An Assessment of Whether It Occurs, How It Occurs, and Who Is at Risk. *Aids Education and Prevention.* 2002;14:53–64.

Lines R, Jürgens R, Betteridge G, Stöver H, Latishevschi D, Nelles J. *Prison Needle Exchange: A Review of International Evidence and Experience.* Montreal: Canadian HIV/AIDS Legal Network; 2004.

National Chlamydia Screening Programme. (2007). Maintaining Momentum: Annual report of the National Chlamydia

Screening Programme in England 2006/07. http://www.hpa. org.uk/web/HPAwebFile/HPAweb_C/1204013012687.

National Commission on Correctional Health Care. Standards for Health Care in Jail (2008). www.ncchc.org.

Pathela P, Hennessy RR, Blank S, Parvez F, Woodman F, Schillinger JA. The contribution of a urine-based jail screening program to citywide male chlamydia and gonorrhea rates in New York City. *Sex Trans Dis.* 2009;36 (2 Supl):S58–S61.

Prison Reform Trust. www.prisonreformtrust.org.uk.

Stöver H, Nelles J. 10 years of experience with needle and syringe exchange programmes in European prisons: a review of different evaluation studies. *Int J Drug Policy.* 2003;14:437–444.

Tang A. Exclusively young offenders: providing dedicated adolescent sexual health clinics in English young offender instructions. *Int J STI AIDS.* 2003;14:293–297.

Walmsley R. Global incarceration and prison trends. *Focus Crime Soc.* 2003;3:65–78.

Weinbaum CM, Sabin KM, Santibanez S. Hepatitis B, hepatitis C, and HIV in correctional populations: a review of epidemiology and prevention. *AIDS.* 2005;19(suppl 3):S41–S46.

Weild AR, Gill ON, Bennett D, et al. Prevalence of HIV, hepatitis B, and hepatitis C antibodies in prisoners in England and Wales: a national survey. *Comm Dis and Public Health.* 2000;3(2):121–126.

44
Sexually Transmitted Infections in the Military

Kelly T. McKee Jr., Steven K. Tobler, Nikki N. Jordan, and Joel C. Gaydos

■ INTRODUCTION

Sexually transmitted infections (STIs) have been associated with military populations and campaigns from antiquity. Accounts of morbidity and reduced fighting effectiveness attributable to syphilis, gonorrhea, "soft chancre" (chancroid), lymphogranuloma venereum, and nonspecific urethritis abound in the annals of land and sea campaigns from at least the Middle Ages, through the American Civil War, and into the modern medical history of World War II and Vietnam. Before effective and readily accessible antibiotic therapy, the scope and impact of these conditions were substantial. During World War I, STIs ranked second only to influenza as a cause of lost productivity for U.S. forces, and the U.S. Army listed venereal disease as its most common diagnosis reported from 1965 to the end of the Vietnam War. That the problem continues is clearly evidenced in the acquisition of the "ultimate" STI agent—human immunodeficiency virus (HIV)—by nondeployed soldiers as well as soldiers engaged in international training, peacekeeping, or humanitarian assistance missions in Africa, Latin America, and Southeast Asia.

The root causes for the problem of STIs in military populations are multifactorial. Historically, civilian women were considered the source of venereal diseases, and control activities focused on ridding military settlements of prostitutes and "camp followers." More recently, it has been recognized that demographic, geographic, behavioral, and situational factors that exist in military settings combine to provide fertile ground for contracting, maintaining, and transmitting these infections.

Past interventions dealing with STIs in military populations received substantial and controversial attention. In addition to removing or restricting civilian women from installations and encampments, military leaders attempted a wide variety of control measures that included shame tactics and management of female sex workers. During the American Revolution, financial penalties were imposed on soldiers with STIs. At the end of World War I, soldiers with STIs were detained and not permitted to return home with their units. The advent of effective antibiotic treatment brought forth an enlightened attitude with abandonment of "scare" and "fear of punishment" tactics, which did not seem to work anyway. However, problems with infected prostitutes continued to be a concern into the late twentieth century. Some military leaders attempted to regulate prostitution, but this tactic was never viewed as being ethically acceptable. Current STI prevention and control efforts in the military are similar to those in the civilian sector. These consist of measures to ensure appropriate diagnosis and treatment for those seeking care, contact tracing, education, screening, and treatment in high-risk groups.

The views of the authors are their own and do not purport to reflect the views or policies of the Department of the Army or the Department of Defense.

■ Features of Military Populations

For the most part, military personnel fall into two major categories: "officers" and "enlisted." Officers and senior enlisted personnel tend to be older and hold leadership positions. While STIs certainly occur in these older leaders, young enlisted people form the bulk of the military force and are the population in which significant STI problems occur.

Military forces have an ongoing requirement for physically active, adventuresome, and, to varying degrees, risk-taking young people. The demographic features of the military population change over time and vary with the popularity of the services as employers and the availability of desirable civilian jobs. In fiscal year 2007, for example, 1.14 million, or 81%, of the active duty force were enlisted personnel as opposed to officers. During this time period, approximately 300,000 applications for admission into the active component enlisted ranks of the armed forces were processed. From these, approximately 160,000 applicants (54%) entered as new accessions into the U.S. Army, Navy, Marines, or Air Force. Accessions were predominantly male (84%), single (90%), and young; 82% were younger than 25 years of age, an age group demonstrated to be at higher risk for STI acquisition. Most (76%) were white, and 14% were black. The education level was higher than the national average; 86% had received a high school diploma, while 13% had a General Educational Development (GED) or similar credential, indicating equivalency with a high school diploma. They came to the military from all parts of the United States and its territories and brought with them the attitudes, practices, and infectious diseases that they had acquired in the societies from which they originated. More than 40% of accessions came from the southern United States, a region with higher STI rates than other parts of the United States.

As the demographics of military populations evolve, so too does the potential impact of STIs on operational integrity. For example, with rising total numbers of females in uniform, there has been a progressive integration of women into formerly all-male units and job categories. Because the physical and healthcare burden of STIs tends to be much higher in females than in males, the impact of these diseases on mission effectiveness, as well as the increase in healthcare costs associated with management of STI sequelae, are emerging as significant considerations.

After initial entry or basic training, and generally some degree of more advanced training, new enlisted personnel become members of highly mobile military units and routinely participate in training, combat, and humanitarian assistance missions throughout the world. This situation offers exposure to disease agents in multiple diverse settings, and the opportunity to import them quickly to domestic or other populations. For example, service members infected with HIV historically were more likely than the general U.S. population to be infected with exotic strains (i.e., nonclade B) of HIV, which are typically acquired overseas.

Levels of activity and anxiety in the military tend to polarize between high intensity and boredom. When engaged in demanding training or hostile action, members of the military focus on their work with commitment. However, the relief from anxiety and the boredom that fill the gaps between periods of high intensity may be accompanied by increased sexual activity with associated increases in STI rates. That military personnel frequently engage in high-risk sexual behavior, particularly during deployments, has been demonstrated. The occurrence of STIs in military populations must now be assessed with regard to interactions between members of the military, between the military and civilians in the United States, and between the military and foreign civilians.

■ STI Screening and Testing

Medical screening of volunteers who desire membership in the U.S. Armed Forces occurs at Military Entry Processing Stations (MEPS) located throughout the country. Department of Defense Instruction 6130.03 (last updated April 28, 2010) entitled "Medical Standards for Appointment, Enlistment, or Induction in the Military Services" identifies disqualifying diseases and conditions for military service. STIs and related conditions that currently are causes for rejection by the military are listed in Table 44-1. Many of these conditions are identified during a mandatory induction physical evaluation. In the case of infection due to *Treponema pallidum* or HIV, diagnosis is made by serology. In the past, evidence of active infection due to either of these pathogens immediately disqualified applicants; with syphilis, documentation of treatment or cure was sufficient to warrant reconsideration. However, declines in the rates of syphilis infection among applicants led to elimination of *Treponema* testing in 1998. Testing for HIV infection among applicants continues.

Recent studies of chlamydia and gonorrhea among army and navy recruits have demonstrated a substantial prevalence of both pathogens. Among inbound trainees at the Army's largest basic training facility, Fort Jackson, South Carolina, overall prevalence of chlamydia during 1996–1999 was 9.5% for non-healthcare-seeking

TABLE 44-1 Causes for Rejection for Military Service for Sexually Transmitted Infections and Related Conditions

- Current condyloma accuminatum or a history of condyloma accuminatum of sufficient severity to require frequent intervention or to interfere with normal function.
- Current herpes genitalis or a history of herpes of sufficient severity to require frequent intervention or to interfere with normal function.
- Current genital infection, ulceration, or condyloma, or a history of genital infection, ulceration, or condyloma of sufficient severity to require frequent intervention or to interfere with normal function.
- Current urethritis, epididymitis, orchitis, prostatitis, and chronic or recurrent urethritis or prostatitis.
- Current untreated syphilis.
- Current or history of neurosyphilis within 1 year of examination, or if residual defects present.
- Current or history of abnormal gynecologic cytology except HPV or low-grade squamous intraepithelial lesion (LGSIL).
- Pelvic inflammatory disease (PID)—acute or recurrent.
- Chronic pelvic pain.
- Presence of human immunodeficiency virus or serological evidence.
- Current or history of psychosexual conditions.

Source: Department of Defense Directive No. 6130.03, April 28, 2010. Medical standards for appointment, enlistment, or induction in the Military Services. Washington, DC.

Note: In general, the finding of acute, uncomplicated venereal disease that can be expected to respond to treatment is not a cause for medical rejection for military service. The military does require treatment of any acute communicable disease before entry.

females and 5.3% for males using urine screening by ligase chain reaction (LCR). Using the same technology, the rate for gonorrhea was 0.6% for males. At Great Lakes Naval Training Center during 1997, approximately 7% of female and 4% of male urine specimens screened by DNA probe test were found to be positive for *Chlamydia trachomatis*. About 1% of females were found to be positive for gonorrhea by DNA probe as well. On the basis of these findings, the Defense Health Board (DHB), formerly known as Armed Forces Epidemiology Board (AFEB), a civilian advisory panel to the Assistant Secretary of Defense (Health Affairs) and the Service Surgeons' General, in 1999 recommended that all new female recruits younger than 25 years throughout the Department of Defense undergo chlamydia screening using molecular-based diagnostics.

The recommendation advocated that the initial screening take place at recruit reception stations at basic training centers. These "points of entry" as well as the regimented basic training environment offer an excellent and economically sound opportunity to provide STI education, screen for STIs, and treat those infected. The Navy and Air Force each have one recruit training center, the Marine Corps has two centers (one of which trains female recruits), and the Army has five (three of

which train female recruits). STI classes that encourage recruits to seek care if they think they may have a problem are common during basic training for all services (even mandatory at some sites), but procedures vary by location. To date, the U.S. Navy, Marine Corps and Air Force have fully enacted the AFEB/DHB screening recommendations. The Army does not screen female basic trainees for chlamydia infections. Diagnosing and treating STIs in new army recruits is limited to clinical encounters when recruits seek health care or undergo physical examinations. Army policy is for women to be screened annually for chlamydia infections, beginning sometime in their first year of military service, in conjunction with annual Papanicolaou testing. Differences in chlamydia screening practices in female recruits prompted a study comparing pelvic inflammatory disease (PID) rates in the Navy and Army; higher PID rates were observed in army women during their first years of active service.

■ STI STATUS IN ACTIVE FORCES

The attention once given to STIs in the active military force has faded in recent years, especially given the ongoing Overseas Contingency Operations (OCO), formerly known as the Global War on Terrorism (GWOT). As in other segments of society, the mandate for maintaining visibility of so-called traditional (i.e., non-HIV) STIs has waned in the face of other problems perceived as more urgent in an increasingly constrained resource environment. Casualties of this evolution include not only programs to directly address specific diseases or conditions (e.g., vaccine development) but also the quality of surveillance systems that allow for accurate definition of problems. Most STI diagnoses among members of the active forces probably derive from patient-initiated healthcare encounters, contact tracing activities, or periodic physical examinations. Therefore, the current scope and nature of STIs in the military are poorly defined and must be extrapolated from available passively reported statistics and from snapshots of data obtained in focused efforts at relatively few military facilities and in limited settings.

The status of STIs in the active military during the late 1970s and 1980s is difficult to characterize. Few statistics were compiled during this period by which overall prevalence or trends in incidence could be determined. Beginning in the early 1990s, systematic surveillance systems were established that allowed for tracking of multiple communicable diseases, including STIs, for all four services. Eventually, the military developed a reportable disease list similar to the list promulgated by the Centers for Disease Control and Prevention (CDC), in Atlanta, Georgia. Each military service except the Marine Corps, which is serviced by the navy healthcare system, presently has a reportable disease reporting system. All of the systems feed data into the Defense Medical Surveillance System, which is maintained by the Armed Forces Health Surveillance Center, Silver Spring, Maryland. Military medical laboratories must comply with civilian requirements to report infectious disease diagnoses to civilian health departments in the areas in which they are located. Typically, laboratories report through military preventive medicine offices although occasionally, military labs will interact directly with the local public health laboratories. Paradoxically, however, there are no mandates for military laboratories to report laboratory data directly into Department of Defense reportable events tracking systems. Thus, available incidence and prevalence data for STIs in military populations are developed from passively reported submissions from military medical treatment facilities to central data management sites. Because submissions into the reportable medical events systems are inconsistent and frequently not validated with laboratory data, there is a systemic problem with underreporting. Nevertheless, a review

of these published statistics and extrapolation from focused surveys of specific populations yields a sense for the scope and magnitude of STIs military-wide.

Gonorrhea, chlamydia, nongonococcal urethritis, and syphilis rates reported by each branch of the U.S. military during 2003–2007 for both active duty military females and males are summarized in Tables 44-2 and 44-3, respectively. Total rates are provided as are rates for the high risk, younger than 25 years age group. As can be seen, rates vary widely among the services, and rates are consistently higher among women and individuals younger than 25 years of age. The observed intraservice variability probably reflects at least in part the passive nature of reporting alluded to previously. Reportable events data suggest that STIs are much more prevalent among army and air force personnel, as compared with the Navy and Marine Corps. However, given relatively high historical rates of STIs in studies of navy and marine corps personnel, it is possible that this difference is due to underreporting by the navy medical system. A large portion of the Navy is deployed on ships throughout the year with limited reporting capabilities, which supports this theory. That the navy/marine corps report rates are lower than the national rates provided by the CDC also suggests that at least part of the difference is methodologic.

Relative to overall U.S. rates for gonorrhea, chlamydia, and primary and secondary syphilis, STIs among military populations appear superficially to be much greater than in the general population. For example, a 1976 study of navy and marine corps personnel found that gonorrhea rates were 3–14 times greater than totals reported for comparable civilian populations. However, these differences may be influenced by screening practices. Female military members are more likely to be screened for chlamydia than their civilian counterparts; close to 70% of active duty females younger than 25 years of age are estimated to be screened annually as compared with roughly 42% nationally. Gonococcal screening may be provided in conjunction with chlamydia screening. Population denominators represented by military personnel are much more heavily weighted in favor of at-risk age, and, to a lesser degree, race/ethnicity categories. The population of the military is also quite different by gender composition when compared with the U.S. population. Legitimate comparison therefore must include appropriate statistical adjustment for these disparities before drawing conclusions. Mostly, such standardizations of rates have not been performed. A study of gonorrhea and chlamydia rates at Fort Bragg, North

TABLE 44-2 Rates of Reported Sexually Transmitted Infections: Female U.S. Armed Forces (Active Duty), 2003–2007*

		Army		Navy		Air Force		Marine Corps	
		< 25 yrs	Total	< 25 yrs	Total	< 25 yrs	Total	< 25 yrs	Total
Gonorrhea	2003	852	479	167	99	379	196	172	123
	2004	785	431	147	97	258	141	158	113
	2005	1115	589	57	39	277	137	126	92
	2006	978	537	135	76	282	142	69	54
	2007	1102	565	200	115	288	140	227	175
	2007 U.S. rates: (631/100,000 and 218 per 100,000)**								
Chlamydia	2003	5910	3402	1773	1024	5507	2861	2539	1814
	2004	6436	3611	1470	850	4679	2440	2407	1708
	2005	6790	3784	1155	675	3220	1637	2722	1951
	2006	7845	4338	1555	919	3148	1577	2834	2043
	2007	8147	4420	1679	965	5381	2544	3525	2594
	2007 U.S. rates: (2977/100,000 and 1034 per 100,000)**								
Non-gonococcal Urethritis	2003	3	1	4	2	0	1	14	9
	2004	0	0	0	0	0	0	0	0
	2005	0	0	0	0	0	0	0	0
	2006	3	1	0	0	0	0	0	0
	2007	0	0	0	0	4	2	0	0
	2007 U.S. rate not available**								
Syphilis	2003	9	5	4	4	6	3	0	0
	2004	12	7	4	4	9	7	0	0
	2005	10	4	0	0	0	1	1	0
	2006	13	7	0	4	11	6	0	0
	2007	3	4	0	0	0	3	0	9
	2007 U.S. rates: (2.9/100,000 and 1.9 per 100,000)**								

* Rates expressed as reported cases/100,000 person-years

** Rates obtained from CDC 2007 STD Surveillance report; includes comparable age groups (i.e. 15-24 and 15-54 years, respectively).

Data Source: Armed Forces Health Surveillance Center, Defense Medical Epidemiology Database

TABLE 44-3 Rates of Reported Sexually Transmitted Infections: Male U.S. Armed Forces (Active Duty), 2003–2007*

		Army		Navy		Air Force		Marine Corps	
		< 25 yrs	Total	< 25 yrs	Total	< 25 yrs	Total	< 25 yrs	Total
Gonorrhea	2003	354	214	60	40	189	99	58	57
	2004	354	225	51	31	146	75	85	63
	2005	366	232	44	27	125	66	59	44
	2006	376	230	72	42	144	71	84	63
	2007	316	201	59	41	143	72	47	37
	2007 U.S. rates: (368/100,000 and 192 per 100,000)**								
Chlamydia	2003	1115	658	233	132	1757	793	254	199
	2004	1149	690	179	107	1470	690	273	200
	2005	1250	746	137	85	1177	543	198	161
	2006	1256	787	205	126	1118	533	297	227
	2007	1278	774	243	152	1429	686	275	218
	2007 U.S. rates: (774/100,000 and 277 per 100,000)**								
Non-gonococcal Urethritis	2003	164	105	10	6	6	3	17	11
	2004	185	121	12	7	5	3	86	60
	2005	152	96	7	3	1	1	9	7
	2006	90	61	3	2	1	0.4	0	0
	2007	74	47	0	0	6	2	0	0
	2007 U.S. rates not available**								
Syphilis	2003	4	3	3	2	7	3	1	0.6
	2004	7	8	4	3	3	3	1	0.6
	2005	8	7	2	3	4	3	1	1
	2006	4	5	4	4	2	4	0	1
	2007	6	6	4	2	6	5	3	4
	2007 U.S. rates: (8.6/100,000 and 10.9 per 100,000)**								

* Rates expressed as reported cases/100,000 person-years

** Rates obtained from CDC 2007 STD Surveillance report; includes comparable age groups (i.e. 15-24 and 15-54 years, respectively).

Data Source: Armed Forces Health Surveillance Center, Defense Medical Epidemiology Database

Carolina, found that, while disparities with comparable statewide disease rates existed, the true differential was actually much smaller after standardization for age, gender, and race/ethnicity. Adjusted incidence of gonorrhea was found to decline over a 10-year period to levels lower than those observed for comparably adjusted statewide rates, while adjusted chlamydia rates remained three- to sixfold higher than state and national levels. An earlier population-adjusted study from this same installation of primary and secondary syphilis immediately preceding, during, and following the most recent nationwide syphilis epidemic found genuinely higher disease rates among soldiers in comparison to the surrounding civilian community as well.

Published reports in defined segments of military populations yield additional insights regarding STI prevalence and incidence. A shipboard study of asymptomatic navy personnel using noninvasive molecular diagnostic tests demonstrated an overall prevalence of *C. trachomatis* and *Neisseria gonorrhoeae* of 4.2% and 0%, respectively. Among predominantly asymptomatic active duty army women presenting for routine Pap testing at Fort Bragg, a 7.3% prevalence of *C. trachomatis* infection was observed (11% in women (≤25 years of age). Among women presenting for care at the Fort Bragg consolidated STI clinic because of symptoms or contact with an infected partner, the prevalence of gonorrhea, chlamydia, and trichomoniasis was 3%, 11.6%, and 6.8%, respectively. In yet another study at Fort Bragg, prevalence of *Trichomonas vaginalis* among women attending the STI clinic during 1997 was found to be 9.4% using PCR-targeting beta-tubulin genes of the organism. Although the degree to which such studies represent conditions throughout the U.S. Armed Forces is unknown, it is reasonable to conclude that STIs continue to be problematic among active military forces. Improvements in morbidity surveillance are clearly needed to better define and track STI prevalence and incidence, and efforts to reduce the burden of these diseases among military populations can be readily justified.

ISSUES PECULIAR TO MILITARY POPULATIONS

Demographic, behavioral, situational, and other external factors that contribute to STI acquisition among members of the armed forces have begun to be explored only recently. Young, nonwhite, and unmarried individuals are among those in the general population at highest risk for acquiring STIs; these demographics reflect a high proportion of the military. The recognized association of STI acquisition with alcohol consumption is particularly

problematic in the military setting. The 2002 Department of Defense Survey of Health Related Behaviors found that military personnel were significantly more likely to drink heavily as compared with civilians. Even more concerning is that military personnel between 18 and 25 years of age were almost twice as likely to drink heavily as their civilian counterparts.

Historically, high-risk behaviors occurring during overseas deployments have been recognized as significant contributors to the military STI problem. Indeed, antibiotic-resistant *N. gonorrhoeae* strains were introduced into the mainland United States during the 1960s by servicemen deployed in the Pacific basin. Reported risk factors during deployments included excessive alcohol use, inconsistent condom use, and multiple contacts with prostitutes. Where examined, the receipt by service members of standard HIV/STI education has not correlated with reduction in self-reported risk behaviors. Improved strategies for STI education and prevention have been initiated; initial attempts using such approaches as interactive video and audio, situational role-playing, and health risk appraisal have yielded promising, but as of yet inconclusive, results. Further development and future integration of such programs into routine training activities must become a major component of an overall military risk-reduction strategy.

Treatment regimens for STIs in members of the military generally follow national consensus guidelines. Travel history is particularly important in managing STIs in military personnel, because antibiotic resistance patterns vary geographically. National guidelines consider antibiotic resistance patterns found among organisms isolated from the U.S. population. Among service members that have traveled overseas, resistance among isolates may differ significantly from U.S. patterns.

Medical treatment facilities at fixed military installations in the United States and overseas have laboratory diagnostic capabilities consistent with those found in other U.S. hospitals. In contrast, military units deployed to remote geographic areas may have limited, if any, laboratory-based testing capability. Practicing medicine in remote areas is even more problematic when treating women because pelvic examinations often must be performed under suboptimal conditions or simply cannot be done at all. These shortcomings have stimulated interest in developing diagnostic kits and tests, and even self-treatment kits, which may be feasible for use in "field" settings.

Funding for HIV research in the Department of Defense is a distinct budget item. Support for other STI research in the military is much more limited, however, and generally has been directed to specific research projects of limited scope, such as "problems of women in the military." STIs research, other than HIV, is not funded as part of the Military Infectious Diseases Research Program because the morbidity from these diseases is not considered to be severe enough to have a major effect on the outcome of a military conflict. This fact notwithstanding, STIs are expensive to the military because of the cost of medical care and time away from the job for diagnosis and treatment of the sequelae of infection, such as pelvic inflammatory disease and chronic pelvic pain in women.

Variations in the incidence and prevalence of STIs observed in the civilian sector have been noted in military populations as well. Within the various military communities, networks exist that may be based on ethnic origin, social interests, job classification, or unit structure. The occurrence and importance of "core" groups of high-frequency STI transmitters, and the networks with which they have contact in maintaining and transmitting STIs in the military, have not been well studied. Recent application of Geographic Information Systems (GIS) technology to the study of STI patterns at one army installation has begun to shed light on this problem. To develop effective interventions, "core" groups and networks must be defined, the relationships between military and surrounding civilian communities in the existence and maintenance of such groups must be established, and appropriate targeted interventions must be developed for the specific network involved.

STI problems in military populations are seldom confined to the military. Sexual interactions between members of the military and civilians will occur except in the most unusual circumstances. This interaction extends beyond populations at a military installation and in nearby towns. U.S. forces are highly mobile and intensely active in training and humanitarian missions throughout the world. Military units are frequently transported great distances over short time periods. People in these units may serve as links between their usual social and sexual networks and foreign populations. In addition, with manpower reductions in the active military force and large numbers of deployments due to support OCO, Reserve and National Guard units are deploying in numbers not seen in many years. Within the Department of Defense in 2007, 26% of new enlisted and officer accession service members entered the reserve component. Members of the Reserve and National Guard maintain their civilian jobs and lifestyles but don their uniforms for military training on weekends or for short periods, typically 2 weeks to 6 months. These reservists and guard members are not restricted to their hometown or home state areas but frequently travel to remote foreign locations for short-term training or long-term operational deployments. The exotic nature of areas geographically distant from home may contribute to a relaxation of controls on risk-taking behaviors. These part-time service members are likely to appear for medical care in their civilian healthcare systems. In treating full and part-time military people, a travel history is always recommended. The high degree of interaction between the military and civilian communities requires that surveillance for, and control of, STIs be a joint effort with free exchange of data and information and coordination of intervention efforts.

■ FUTURE DIRECTIONS

STIs have gained the attention of senior military leaders in the context of a global effort to enhance Department of Defense preventive health care. The Secretary of Defense created a Prevention, Safety, and Health Promotion Council, chaired by one of the military Surgeons' General, which was charged with advancing health and safety promotion and injury/illness prevention policy initiatives consistent with Department of Defense readiness requirements. One of the task forces created by the Council was a Sexually Transmitted Diseases Prevention Committee. This committee was tasked with establishing policy and coordinating implementation of initiatives to assess the scope of STIs and providing oversight for programs targeting STI prevention and treatment. Unfortunately, the Council and Committee have been inactive.

Reporting of STIs in military populations must be improved to include the timely acquisition of laboratory diagnoses and antibiotic sensitivities, and the analysis of data on a global basis to identify adverse occurrences and trends in time to develop and execute interventions. Global, electronic, laboratory-based surveillance systems for infectious disease agents and antibiotic susceptibilities have been identified as high priorities by the Department of Defense as part of a plan to improve capabilities to detect and to respond to emerging infectious diseases. STI diagnostics have been included in these initiatives, and efforts to coordinate with appropriate civilian health authorities (e.g., participation in the CDC-sponsored Gonococcal Isolate Surveillance Project [GISP]) are ongoing. Programs are under development to enhance the quality of data collected by improving existing, or developing new, reporting systems to more accurately identify incident infections. Efforts are also under way to integrate sexual risk assessment into existing clinical prevention activities, to enhance and more effectively institutionalize STI/HIV prevention and education programs, and to expand provider educational opportunities in the areas of STI counseling, contact referral, treatment, and prevention.

Systematic screening of all active service members should be explored in an attempt to reduce the impact of STIs on the military. With the introduction of molecular-based diagnostic assays, rapid and noninvasive testing for chlamydia, gonorrhea, and potentially other genitourinary pathogens can be readily accomplished. Despite the absence of accurate statistical data to quantify the burden of STIs in military populations, that these diseases probably occur at frequencies comparable to those observed in the civilian sector provides clear impetus for establishing periodic screening programs. In conjunction with its recommendations pertaining to chlamydia screening in recruits, the DHB has also advised that all female military service members younger than 26 years of age be annually screened for chlamydia at the time of each recommended Pap smear.

The advent of emerging technologies holds promise for development of novel diagnostic modalities to support requirements peculiar to military populations. For example, a vaginal swab-based diagnostic system for STIs in females which can be self-administered and mailed to a central processing laboratory recently was shown to be at least as sensitive and specific for diagnosis of *N. gonorrhoeae*, *C. trachomatis*, and *T. vaginalis* as routine clinic-based tests. This assay system, which also incorporates detection of human papillomavirus, offers potential advantages to military women who may be deployed in remote settings for prolonged periods, and for whom access to adequate STI diagnostics or routine Pap screening may be unavailable, impractical, or awkward. Application of this or similar diagnostic systems in conjunction with algorithms for follow-up or referral to clinic-based health care, as well as development of self-treatment kits to use in conditions where access to such specialty care will be difficult, offer major advances to genitourinary health of women in the military.

The various military basic training centers must be evaluated as potential sites for STI education, screening, and treatment. The large numbers of high-risk people that pass through these locations in short periods afford opportunities for efficient and effective intervention. Studies in army trainees have shown this strategy to be cost effective for females, even when approximately half

of new recruits returned to civilian life in a matter of days, weeks, or months. In addition, anecdotal information obtained from surveying sailors has indicated that STI educational experiences provided to navy basic trainees had a lasting, positive impact. Military leaders may be reluctant to fund these programs when a high percentage of the long-term benefit will be reaped by the civilian healthcare sector, because so many service members and recruits will return to civilian life after only a brief military career. In these situations, military and civilian cost sharing should be considered.

During fiscal year 2007, approximately 2.2 million people were serving in the U.S. Armed Forces of which around 1.4 million were on active duty. Control of STIs in this population has been, and will continue to be, challenging. However, the military does not exist in isolation. Ample evidence exists to validate the interaction between civilian and military populations, and relationships between these two communities will likely increase with the passage of time. The success of future STI control efforts depends on cooperation among federal, state, and local civilian agencies, including U.S. Department of Veterans Affairs medical facilities, with their military counterparts in the design and execution of education, prevention, and intervention strategies.

■ ACKNOWLEDGMENTS

We wish to thank Capt. Megan Ryan, MD, U.S. Navy, formerly of the Great Lakes Naval Training Center, Illinois, and the Naval Health Research Center, San Diego, California, for providing data pertaining to U.S. Navy recruit screening at the Great Lakes Naval Training Center.

REFERENCES

Artenstein AW, Coppola J, Brown AE, et al. Multiple introductions of HIV-1 subtype E into the Western Hemisphere. *Lancet.* 1995;346:1197–1198.

Bauer HM, Mark KE, Samuel M, et al. Prevalence of and associated risk factors for fluoroquinolone-resistant *Neisseria gonorrhoeae* in California, 2000–2003. *Clin Infect Dis.* 2005;41:795–803.

Bloom MS, Hu Z, Gaydos JC, et al. Incidence rates of pelvic inflammatory disease diagnoses among army and navy recruits—potential impacts of chlamydia screening policies. *Am J Prev Med.* 2008;34(6):471–477.

Brodine SK, Mascola JR, Weiss PJ, et al. Detection of diverse HIV-1 genetic subtypes in the USA. *Lancet.* 1995; 346:1198–1199.

Brodine SK, Shafer MA, Shaffer RA, et al. Asymptomatic sexually transmitted disease prevalence in four military populations: application of DNA amplification assays for chlamydia and gonorrhea screening. *J Infect Dis*. 1998;178:1202–1204.

Centers for Disease Control and Prevention. Sexually transmitted diseases surveillance, 2007. http://www.cdc.gov/std/stats07/main.htm.

Clark KL, Kelley PW, Mahmoud RA, et al. Cost-effective syphilis screening in military recruit applicants. *Milit. Med.* 1999;164:580–584.

Emerson LA. Sexually transmitted disease control in the armed forces, past and present. *Milit Med*. 1997;162:87–91.

Gaydos CA, Crotchfelt KA, Shah N, et al. Evaluation of dry and wet transported intravaginal swabs in detection of *Chlamydia trachomatis* and *Neisseria gonorrhoeae* infections in female soldiers by PCR. *J Clin Microbiol*. 2002;40:758–761.

Gaydos CA, Gaydos JC. Chlamydia in the United States military: can we win this war? *Sex Transm Dis*. 2008;35:260–262.

Gaydos CA, Howell MR, Pare B, et al. *Chlamydia trachomatis* infections in female military recruits. *N Engl J Med*. 1998;339:739–744.

Gaydos CA, Howell MR, Quinn TC, et al. Use of ligase chain reaction with urine versus cervical culture for detection of *Chlamydia trachomatis* in an asymptomatic military population of pregnant and nonpregnant females attending Papanicolaou smear clinics. *J Clin Microbiol*. 1998;36:1300–1304.

Greenberg, JH. Venereal disease in the armed forces. *Med Clin North Am*. 1972;56:1087–1100.

Jenkins PR, Jenkins RA, Nannis ED, et al. Reducing risk of sexually transmitted disease (STD) and human immunodeficiency virus infection in a military STD clinic: evaluation of a randomized preventive intervention trial. *Clin Infect Dis*. 2000;30:730–735.

Lee S-e, Nauschuetz W, Jordan N, et al. Survey of sexually transmitted disease laboratory methods in US Army laboratories. *Sex Transm Dis*. 2010;37:44–48.

Madico G, Quinn TC, Rompalo A, et al. Diagnosis of *Trichomonas vaginalis* infection by PCR using vaginal swab samples. *J Clin Microbiol*. 1998;36:3205–3210.

Malone JD, Hyams KC, Hawkins RE, et al. Risk factors for sexually transmitted diseases among deployed US military personnel. *Sex Trans Dis*. 1993;20:294–298.

McKee KT, Burns WE, Russell LK, et al. Early syphilis in an active duty military population and the surrounding civilian community, 1985–1993. *Milit Med* 1998;163:368–376.

Melton, LJ. Comparative incidence of gonorrhea and nongonococcal urethritis in the United States Navy. *Am J Epidemiol*. 1976;104:535–542.

Nannis ED, Schneider S, Jenkins PR, et al. Human immunodeficiency virus (HIV) education and HIV risk behavior: a survey of rapid deployment troops. *Milit Med*. 1998;163:672–676.

Niebuhr DW, Tobler SK, Jordan N, et al. Sexually transmitted infections among military recruits. In: DeKoning BL, ed. *Recruit Medicine*. Falls Church, VA: Office of the Surgeon General, United States Army; Washington, DC: The Borden Institute, Walter Reed Army Medical Center; 2006:255–275.

Office of the Under Secretary of Defense, Personnel and Readiness. Population representation in the Military Services, 2007. http://prhome.defense.gov/PopRep2007/index.html.

Rompalo AM, Gaydos CA, Shah N, et al. Evaluation of use of a single intravaginal swab to detect multiple sexually transmitted infections in active-duty military women. *Clin Infect Dis*. 2001;33:1455–1461.

Sena AC, Miller WC, Hoffman IF, et al. Trends of gonorrhea and chlamydial infection during 1985–96 among active-duty soldiers at a United States Army installation. *Clin Infect Dis*. 2000;30:742–748.

Soeprapto W, Ertono S, Hydoyo H, et al. HIV and peacekeeping operations in Cambodia. *Lancet*. 1995;346:1304–1305.

Yoo J, Yoo C, Cho Y, et al. Antimicrobial resistance patterns (1999–2002) and characterization of Ciprofloxacin-resistant *Neisseria gonorrhoeae* in Korea. *Sex Transm Dis*. 2004;31:305–309.

Zenilman JM, Glass G, Shields T, et al. Geographic epidemiology of gonorrhea and chlamydia on a large military installation: application of a GIS system. *Sex Transm Infect*. 2002;78:40–44.

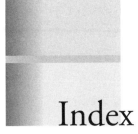

Index

Figures and tables are indicated by f and t following page numbers.